Non-Neoplastic Disorders of the Gastrointestinal Tract

AFIP Atlases of Tumor and Non-Tumor Pathology

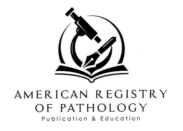

AMERICAN REGISTRY
OF PATHOLOGY
Publication & Education

ARP PRESS

Arlington, Virginia

Incoming Director of Publications: Amy Goldenberg, PhD
Production Editor: Dian S. Thomas
Technical Editor: Elizabeth Tomlinson
Copyeditor: Audrey Kahn

ARP Press gratefully acknowledges the work put into this volume by Mirlinda Q. Caton and Magdalena C. Silva.

Available from the American Registry of Pathology
Arlington, Virginia 22209
www.arppress.org
ISBN 1-933477-93-8
978-1-933477-93-0

Printed in Korea

AFIP ATLASES OF TUMOR AND NON-TUMOR PATHOLOGY

Fifth Series
Fascicle 4

NON-NEOPLASTIC DISORDERS OF THE GASTROINTESTIONAL TRACT

by

Rhonda K. Yantiss, MD
Professor of Pathology and Laboratory Medicine
Department of Pathology and Laboratory Medicine
Weill Cornell Medicine
New York, New York

Nicole C. Panarelli, MD
Associate Professor of Pathology
Albert Einstein College of Medicine
Attending Pathologist
Montefiore Medical Center
Bronx, New York

Laura W. Lamps, MD
Godfrey D. Stobbe Professor and Director of GI Pathology
University of Michigan Health System
Ann Arbor, Michigan

Published by the
American Registry of Pathology
Arlington, Virginia
2021

AFIP ATLASES OF TUMOR AND NON-TUMOR PATHOLOGY

EDITOR
Jason L. Hornick, MD, PhD
Professor of Pathology, Harvard Medical School
Director of Surgical Pathology and Immunohistochemistry
Brigham and Women's Hospital
Boston, Massachusetts

EDITORIAL ADVISORY BOARD

Manuscript reviewed by:
Elizabeth A. Montgomery, MD

EDITOR'S NOTE

The Atlases of Tumor Pathology have a long and distinguished history. They were first conceived at a cancer research meeting held in St. Louis in September 1947, as an attempt to standardize the nomenclature of neoplastic diseases. The first series was sponsored by the National Academy of Sciences-National Research Council. The organization of this formidable effort was entrusted to the Subcommittee on Oncology of the Committee on Pathology, and Dr. Arthur Purdy Stout was the first editor-in-chief. Many of the illustrations were provided by the Medical Illustration Service of the Armed Forces Institute of Pathology (AFIP), the type was set by the Government Printing Office, and the final printing was done at the Armed Forces Institute of Pathology. The American Registry of Pathology (ARP) purchased the Fascicles from the Government Printing Office and sold them virtually at cost. Over a period of 20 years, approximately 15,000 copies each of nearly 40 Fascicles were produced. The worldwide impact of these publications over the years has largely surpassed the original goal. They quickly became some of the most influential publications on tumor pathology, primarily because of their overall high quality, but also because their low cost made them easily accessible the world over to pathologists and other students of oncology.

Upon completion of the first series, the National Academy of Sciences-National Research Council handed further pursuit of the project over to the newly created Universities Associated for Research and Education in Pathology (UAREP). The Second Series was started, generously supported by grants from the AFIP, the National Cancer Institute, and the American Cancer Society. Dr. Harlan I. Firminger became the editor-in-chief and was succeeded by Dr. William H. Hartmann. The Second Series Fascicles were produced as bound volumes instead of loose leaflets. They featured a more comprehensive coverage of the subjects, to the extent that the Fascicles could no longer be regarded as "atlases" but rather as monographs describing and illustrating in detail the tumors and tumor-like conditions of the various organs and systems.

Dr. Juan Rosai was appointed as editor-in-chief of the Third Series, and Dr. Leslie Sobin became associate editor. A distinguished Editorial Advisory Board was also convened, and these outstanding pathologists and educators played a major role in the success of this series, the first publication of which appeared in 1991 and the last (number 32) in 2003.

The same organizational framework applied to the Fourth Series, meticulously edited by Dr. Steven Silverberg with Dr. Ronald DeLellis as the associate editor. With UAREP and AFIP no longer functioning, ARP remained the responsible organization. The Fourth Series volumes were hardbound with illustrations almost exclusively in color. There was also an increased emphasis on the cytopathologic (intraoperative, exfoliative, or fine needle aspiration) and molecular features that are important in diagnosis and prognosis. At the time of the Fourth Series, ARP also produced

Atlases of Non-Tumor Pathology; these volumes were numbered separately from the tumor volumes.

As in the prior series, the goal of the Fifth Series includes a continuous attempt to correlate, whenever possible, the nomenclature used in the Fascicles with that proposed by the World Health Organization Classification of Tumors, as well as to ensure a consistency of style. Including molecular diagnostics is more important than ever, as is the availability of an online component, a more nimble website (www.arppress.org), and even a social media presence linked to the website. Now in this series, the tumor and non-tumor volumes are combined and consecutively numbered as the Atlases of Tumor and Non-Tumor Pathology. Close cooperation between the various authors and their respective liaisons from the Editorial Board will continue to be emphasized in order to minimize unnecessary repetition and discrepancies in the text and illustrations.

Particular thanks are due to the members of the Editorial Advisory Board, our reviewers, the editorial and production staff, and the individual Fascicle authors for their ongoing efforts to ensure that this series is a worthy successor to the previous four.

Jason L. Hornick, MD, PhD

PREFACE AND ACKNOWLEDGMENTS

Gastrointestinal pathology emerged as a subspecialty in the 1980s when endoscopy and mucosal biopsy assumed increased importance in the diagnosis and management of patients with gastrointestinal disorders. Pathologists are now expected to generate comprehensive and accurate differential diagnoses for a variety of inflammatory conditions that occur throughout the gastrointestinal tract. They play a particularly important role in the care of patients with persistent gastrointestinal symptoms, especially those who are immunosuppressed, suffer from immune-mediated conditions, or undergo treatment for malignancies. Most of these individuals require medications that can affect the gastrointestinal tract, and emerging targeted therapies seem to cause substantial mucosal injury that may necessitate cessation of the drug. Pathologists must be able to focus on key features present in biopsy material in order to narrow the differential diagnosis and facilitate patient management.

This atlas is intended to address these needs in a succinct and pragmatic fashion. It describes practical approaches to the diagnosis of inflammatory gastrointestinal disorders, including sections that discuss biopsies in the bone marrow transplant setting and newly described medication-related injuries. The reader is provided with helpful criteria to facilitate distinction between newly recognized causes of esophagitis and gastritis. Various immune-mediated conditions that cause a malabsorptive pattern in biopsy samples from the proximal small bowel, as well as those that manifest with features of chronic colitis, are extensively discussed. We have also included sections describing important inflammatory conditions of the appendix and anus that may simulate neoplasia. I sincerely thank my coauthors for their exceptional efforts; all of the chapters are beautifully illustrated and include helpful tables that provide easy references to the reader.

Rhonda K. Yantiss, MD
Nicole C. Panarelli, MD
Laura W. Lamps, MD

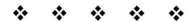

DEDICATIONS

In memory of Harvey Goldman, a pioneer in GI pathology who never stopped questioning.

Rhonda K. Yantiss, MD

To my children, Joseph Frances and Nora Scarlett, for keeping us young at heart.

Nicole C. Panarelli, MD

In memory of David L. Page.

Laura W. Lamps, MD

CONTENTS

1 NORMAL GROSS AND HISTOLOGIC FEATURES OF THE GASTROINTESTINAL TRACT

THE NORMAL ESOPHAGUS

Anatomy

Gross Anatomy. The adult esophagus is a muscular tube measuring approximately 25 cm and extending from the lower border of the cricoid cartilage to the gastroesophageal junction. It lies posterior to the trachea and left atrium in the mediastinum but deviates slightly to the left before descending to the diaphragm, where it traverses the hiatus and enters the abdomen. The subdiaphragmatic esophagus lies against the posterior surface of the left hepatic lobe (1).

The International Classification of Diseases and the American Joint Commission on Cancer divide the esophagus into upper, middle, and lower thirds, whereas endoscopists measure distance to points in the esophagus relative to the incisors (2). The esophagus begins 15 cm from the incisors and extends 40 cm from the incisors in the average adult (3).

The upper and lower esophageal sphincters represent areas of increased resting tone but lack anatomic landmarks; they are located 15 to 18 cm from the incisors and slightly proximal to the gastroesophageal junction, respectively. The gastroesophageal junction is defined as the distal extent of the tubular esophagus and, in the normal state, roughly corresponds to the mucosal squamocolumnar junction, or Z-line (fig. 1-1). There are four areas of luminal narrowing: the upper esophageal sphincter, the areas where the esophagus crosses the aortic arch and left main bronchus, and the gastroesophageal junction. Left atrial enlargement can also impinge on the esophagus.

Vascular Anatomy. The upper esophagus is vascularized by branches of the inferior thyroidal artery. Branches of the bronchial arteries, aorta, and intercostal arteries penetrate the mid esophagus, and the distal esophagus is supplied by the left gastric, left phrenic, and left hepatic accessory arteries. Veins in the proximal and mid esophagus drain into the systemic circulation, whereas the short gastric and left gastric veins of the portal system drain the distal esophagus. Linear arrays of large caliber veins are unique to the distal esophagus and can be a helpful clue to the site of a biopsy when extensive cardiac-type mucosa is present near the gastroesophageal junction (4).

Lymphatic vessels are present in all layers of the esophagus. They drain to paratracheal and deep cervical lymph nodes in the cervical esophagus, bronchial and posterior mediastinal lymph nodes in the thoracic esophagus, and left gastric lymph nodes in the abdominal esophagus.

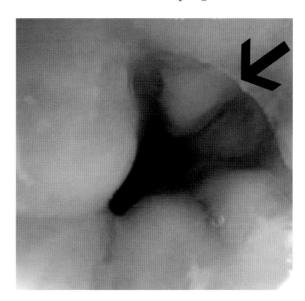

Figure 1-1

ENDOSCOPIC APPEARANCE OF THE GASTROESOPHAGEAL JUNCTION

The gastroesophageal junction normally corresponds to the squamocolumnar junction (arrow), which appears as an abrupt transition between the velvety mucosa of the rugal folds and the pink, pearly white squamous mucosa of the tubular esophagus.

Histology

The esophagus consists of mucosa, submucosa, and muscularis propria invested with adventitia, which is a nonperitonealized surface and important margin in cancer resection specimens. The left anterior aspect of the distal-most esophagus lies within the peritoneal cavity and is surfaced by mesothelium (i.e., serosa).

The pale pink, glistening esophageal mucosa is composed of multilayered, stratified nonkeratinizing squamous epithelium supported by lamina propria and muscularis mucosae (fig. 1-2A). The squamous epithelium contains a proliferative zone consisting of 2 to 3 cell layers at its base; epithelial cells in this area are ovoid with high nuclear to cytoplasmic ratios and scattered mitotic figures. Superficial squamous cells contain faintly eosinophilic cytoplasm and small nuclei with condensed chromatin arranged with their long axes parallel to the luminal surface (fig. 1-2B). Scattered CD8-positive T-lymphocytes are normally present in the peripapillary epithelium, particularly near the gastroesophageal junction, where they can number 40 to 60 per high-power field in asymptomatic patients (5).

The squamous mucosa contains occasional Langerhans cells and melanocytes (6–9). Rare eosinophils can be detected in otherwise normal biopsy samples from the gastroesophageal junction; their presence should be disregarded if unaccompanied by evidence of mucosal injury.

The lamina propria consists of loose connective tissue that supports thin-walled blood vessels, nerves, and inflammatory cells. Papillae penetrate approximately one-third of the squamous mucosal thickness. Bundles of longitudinally oriented smooth muscle cells comprise the muscularis mucosae and support the lamina propria. The muscularis mucosae is more pronounced in the distal esophagus and can be thickened or duplicated in chronic inflammatory conditions.

The submucosa contains blood vessels, lymphatic vessels, lymphoid follicles, superficial and deep nerve plexuses, and mucous glands supported by loose connective tissue. The Meissner plexus is located in the superficial submucosa and Henle plexus is present in the deep submucosa; each is composed of ganglion cells and associated nerve trunks. Smaller nerve fibers stem from the plexuses, penetrating the submucosa and lamina propria.

Acid mucin-containing glands are distributed along the length of the esophagus and are most numerous in the proximal and distal regions; lobules of glands drain into ducts that empty onto the mucosal surface (fig. 1-2C). Esophageal ducts are lined by two layers of cuboidal cells in the deep submucosa and a single layer of squamous cells near the surface.

The muscularis propria consists of thick bundles of smooth muscle cells arranged in outer longitudinal and inner circular layers. The proximal muscularis propria contains skeletal muscle fibers derived from the cricopharyngeal and inferior pharyngeal constrictor muscles. The myenteric (i.e., Auerbach) plexus lies between the muscle layers and is intimately associated with the interstitial cells of Cajal, which emanate outward through the muscle layers (fig. 1-2D).

The esophagus is ensheathed by adventitia. This layer of loose connective tissue contains nerves, lymphoid tissue, and lymphatic and blood vessels, and merges with other support structures of the thoracic viscera.

THE NORMAL STOMACH

Anatomy

Gross Anatomy. The stomach is a saccular J-shaped organ located in the left upper quadrant of the abdomen that can hold up to 2 L in the average adult. It begins at the gastroesophageal junction and extends inferiorly to the pyloric sphincter just to the right of the midline. The superomedial and inferolateral aspects are termed the lesser curvature and greater curvature, respectively.

There are four anatomic subdivisions to the stomach. The cardia is an ill-defined region that extends 1 to 3 cm from the gastroesophageal junction. The fundus is a dome-shaped bulge that lies to the left and above the gastroesophageal junction. The gastric body (i.e., corpus) is the region between the fundus and the antrum. The antrum comprises the distal third of the stomach, above the pylorus (10). The incisura angularis is a notch in the lesser curvature that roughly coincides with the transition between the corpus and antrum.

The stomach is composed of four layers. The mucosal folds, or rugae, extend longitudinally

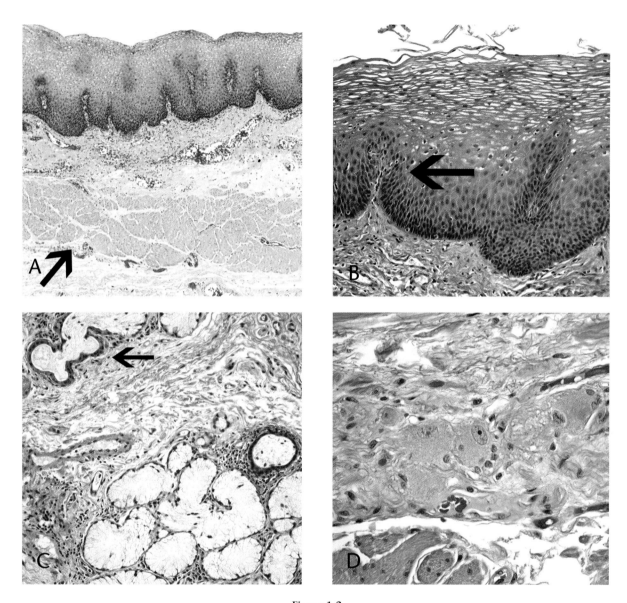

Figure 1-2

NORMAL HISTOLOGIC FEATURES OF THE ESOPHAGUS

The esophagus is lined by nonkeratinizing squamous epithelium supported by lamina propria connective tissue. The muscularis mucosae (arrow) is thickest in the distal esophagus and represents the deepest extent of the mucosa (A). Intraepithelial lymphocytes have convoluted nuclei and are most prominent around papillae (arrow). The cells in the deep mucosa comprise the proliferative zone and have higher nuclear to cytoplasmic ratios than the surface epithelial cells (B). Submucosal glands contain slightly basophilic mucin and are arranged in lobules. Their contents drain to the surface via ducts (arrow) lined by a combination of squamous and cuboidal epithelial cells (C). The myenteric plexus consists of nerve trunks and ganglion cells. The latter contain abundant amphophilic cytoplasm and large, eccentric nuclei with prominent nucleoli (D).

from the gastroesophageal junction to the pylorus and flatten with distension (fig. 1-3). The areae gastricae are shallow, horizontal grooves across the rugae. The submucosa is a loose layer of fat, collagen, and other supporting structures. The muscularis propria contains three muscle layers: the inner oblique, middle circular, and outer longitudinal layers. The middle layer thickens distally to form the pyloric sphincter.

The stomach is almost entirely invested by the serosa, except where it attached to the omentum, mesocolon, and ligaments. It has no adventitia.

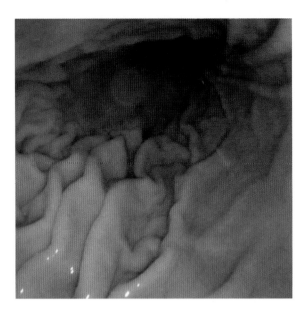

Figure 1-3

**NORMAL ENDOSCOPIC
APPEARANCE OF THE STOMACH**

The rugae are longitudinal mucosal folds that run from the gastroesophageal junction to the pylorus.

Vascular Anatomy. The gastric cardia is supplied by branches of the left gastric artery which arises directly from the celiac plexus. The greater curvature receives blood from branches of the splenic (left gastroepiploic and short gastric) and hepatic (right gastric and right gastroepiploic) arteries. The right gastric artery also supplies the lesser curvature. Anastomoses between branches of these vessels provide rich collateral circulation to the entire stomach, making ischemic gastric injury a rare event (11).

The left and right gastric veins run along the greater and lesser curvatures, respectively, and drain into the portal vein. The left and right gastro-omental and short gastric veins drain into the splenic vein, the largest tributary of the portal vein (10).

Most of the lymphatic drainage from the stomach reaches the celiac lymph nodes after passing through intermediaries. Lymphatics along the proximal greater curvature first drain to lymph nodes in the splenic hilum, whereas the distal greater curvature drains to the right gastroepiploic lymph nodes in the omentum and pyloric lymph nodes at the head of the pancreas. Lymphatics near the cardia and along the lesser curvature pass though left gastric lymph nodes to the celiac trunk before reaching the para-aortic lymph nodes below the left renal vein. The pylorus drains through the right gastric and hepatoduodenal ligament lymph nodes en route to the celiac axis (12).

Histology

The stomach functions as a food reservoir, sterilizes luminal contents, and participates in early digestion. Not surprisingly, it is home to morphologically distinct areas and several epithelial cell types. Neutral mucin-containing glands predominate in the cardia and antrum, whereas oxyntic glands containing chief and parietal cells are located in the fundus and corpus. The entire mucosa is surfaced by a monolayer of columnar foveolar cells with small, basal nuclei and tall apical vacuoles of pale pink mucin (fig. 1-4A).

Foveolar cells secrete bicarbonate and mucin. They show strong immunohistochemical staining for mucin core protein-5AC (MUC5AC) and MUC1, as well as positivity for periodic acid–Schiff (PAS) stains. The gastric pits (i.e., foveolae) represent invaginations of the superficial mucosa and are lined by similar epithelial cells. The pits occupy approximately 50 percent of the mucosal thickness in the cardia and antrum compared with only 25 percent of the mucosal thickness in the body and fundus. Intraepithelial CD8-positive T-lymphocytes are normally present in the surface epithelium but number fewer than 20 per 100 epithelial cells (13).

Mucous neck cells are located between the pits and deeper glands, and represent the proliferative zone of the epithelium. They tend to have slightly larger nuclei than other mucinous epithelia in the stomach and contain both neutral mucin and acidic sialomucins. Thus, mucous neck cells stain with both PAS and Alcian blue (pH 2.5), and show MUC5AC and MUC6 immunopositivity.

Oxyntic mucosa contains tightly packed, tubular oxyntic glands that occupy approximately 75 percent of the mucosal thickness (fig. 1-4B) (10). Sectioned tangentially, oxyntic glands may appear as "cords" or stacks of individual glands. Chief (i.e., zygomatic) cells are present in higher numbers in the deep mucosa. These cells produce pepsinogen and contain blue-gray cytoplasm, basal nuclei, and small nucleoli. Parietal cells are more numerous in the mid-region of

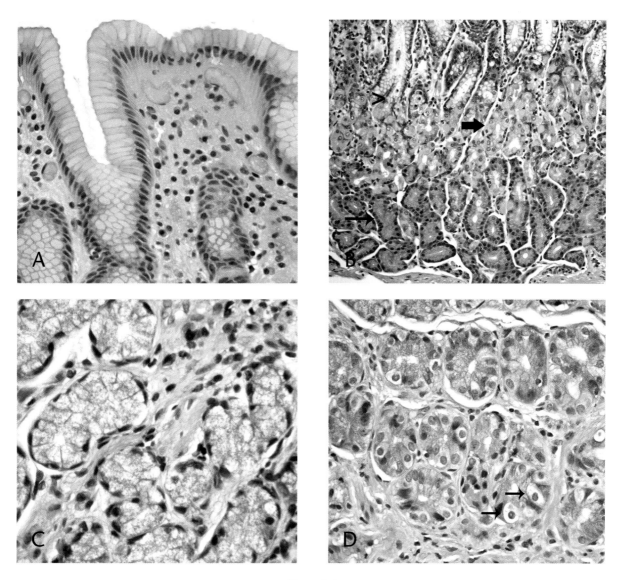

Figure 1-4

NORMAL HISTOLOGIC FEATURES OF THE STOMACH

The stomach is surfaced by a single layer of foveolar epithelial cells. These cells contain basally oriented uniform nuclei and a tall, apical mucin vacuole. The foveolar cells descend into the mucosa to form evenly spaced gastric pits (foveolae). The intervening lamina propria contains scattered inflammatory cells and capillaries (A). Oxyntic mucosa contains tubular glands that occupy 50 to 75 percent of the mucosal thickness. Chief cells are located deep in the glands and contain basophilic cytoplasm (arrow). Parietal cells have abundant eosinophilic cytoplasm and are most numerous in the mid-region (block arrow). The mucous neck cells (arrowhead) are found at the junction between the gastric pits and the oxyntic glands (B). Pyloric glands are found in the antrum and cardia. They contain pale, faintly eosinophilic, bubbly cytoplasm (C). Endocrine cells (arrows) are present throughout the stomach and are admixed with other types of epithelia in the gastric glands. They contain central nuclei and clear cytoplasm, resembling fried eggs (D).

the mucosa. They are pyramidal in shape and contain centrally located nuclei as well as abundant, granular, eosinophilic cytoplasm. Parietal cells maintain the acidity of gastric contents by releasing hydrochloric acid in response to stimulation by gastrin and histamine. They also produce intrinsic factor, a glycoprotein that aids absorption of vitamin B_{12}. Chief, parietal, and mucous neck cells are frequently commingled in glands of the superficial mucosa.

The deep compartment of the antral mucosa is populated by loosely packed lobules of pyloric-type glands with abundant intervening lamina propria (fig. 1-4C) (9). Epithelial cells in these glands contain faintly eosinophilic, slightly bubbly mucin and show strong immunostaining for MUC6. Pyloric-type glands secrete mucus that, in combination with secretions from foveolar cells, form a protective layer that prevents acid-related injury to the gastric mucosa. Scattered parietal cells are commonly identified in the antrum, particularly at the transition point with the corpus, but chief cells are rarely present. The cardia also contains pyloric-type glands that are intimately associated with oxyntic glands in almost 50 percent of adults (14).

The stomach contains three main populations of endocrine cells: gastrin-producing G cells, enterochromaffin-like (ECL) cells that secrete histamine, and D cells that produce somatostatin (15). Endocrine cells of the stomach are ovoid with pale gray to clear cytoplasm and centrally located nuclei that impart a "fried egg" appearance with hematoxylin and eosin (H&E) stains (fig. 1-4D).

The G cells are most numerous, accounting for more than 50 percent of all endocrine cells in the stomach. They reside mostly in the antrum but may be scattered in small numbers in the oxyntic mucosa. ECL cells are located in oxyntic mucosae and tend to be most numerous in glands of the deep mucosa. Scattered D cells are dispersed throughout the stomach. They secrete somatostatin in response to low gastric pH, which, in turn, inhibits release of gastrin and histamine (16). Endocrine cells are most numerous in the gastric antrum, where they number between 20 and 50 in an entire gland; oxyntic glands contain fewer than 20 endocrine cells per gland.

The lamina propria contains a supportive network of collagen, reticulin, and elastic fibers, as well as blood vessels, fibroblasts, and scattered inflammatory cells, including macrophages, plasma cells, lymphocytes, and eosinophils. It is better visualized in the superficial mucosa. Basal lymphoid aggregates are normally present the oxyntic mucosa; they often have a pyramidal configuration based on the muscularis mucosae. The muscularis mucosae is a thin bilayer of smooth muscle that forms the lower limit of the mucosa.

The submucosa contains loose connective tissue, blood vessels, and Meissner plexus. Each ganglion of the Meissner plexus consists of ganglion cells and parasympathetic nerves. Thick smooth muscle layers form the muscularis propria. Auerbach plexus lies between the middle circular and outer longitudinal layers and consists of sympathetic and parasympathetic nerves. Interstitial cells of Cajal are concentrated around the myenteric plexus and emanate through the muscle layers. A small amount of delicate collagen and adipose tissue lies between the muscularis propria and the single layer of mesothelial cells comprising the serosa.

THE NORMAL SMALL BOWEL

Anatomy

Gross Anatomy. The small intestine measures roughly 6 m in length and consists of the duodenum, jejunum, and ileum. The duodenum spans approximately 25 cm and is divided into four parts. The first part begins at the gastroduodenal junction and includes the duodenal bulb. The second part extends from the bulb to the level of the fourth lumbar vertebra on the right side of the spine where it descends a few centimeters. The ampulla of Vater is located on the medial aspect in the descending portion of the second part of the duodenum. Nearly 70 percent of healthy individuals have a minor ampulla that drains the accessory pancreatic duct of Santorini approximately 2 cm proximal to the ampulla of Vater. The third portion of the duodenum sweeps to the left across the spine to complete the C-shape that surrounds the pancreatic head and body. The fourth part rises slightly and terminates at the ligament of Treitz.

With the exception of its first portion, the duodenum lies in the retroperitoneum. The jejunum and ileum are entirely within the peritoneal cavity and supported by a mesentery. Most of the jejunum is located in the left upper quadrant; it transitions to the ileum in the mid-abdomen, and the latter passes obliquely into the right lower quadrant where it terminates at the ileocecal valve.

The small bowel consists of four layers: mucosa and muscularis mucosae, submucosa, muscularis propria, and serosa or adventitia. Mesenteric fat is normally confined to approximately 30 percent

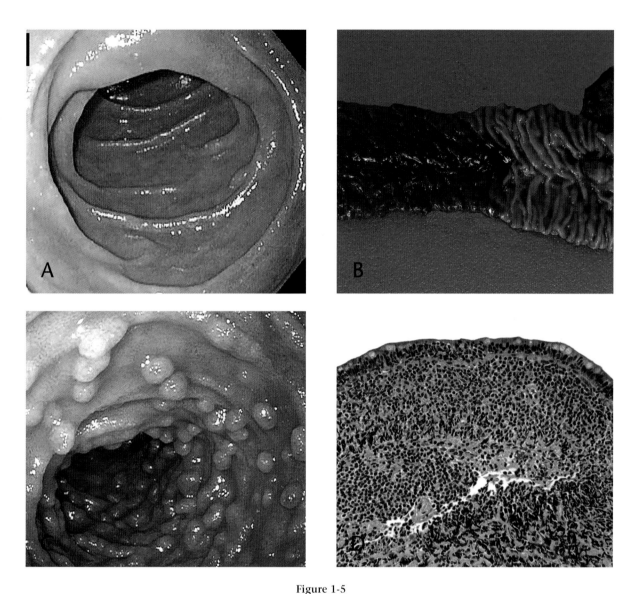

Figure 1-5

NORMAL ENDOSCOPIC APPEARANCE OF THE SMALL BOWEL

Circumferential mucosal folds are most prominent in the proximal small bowel (A). The proximal duodenum is surfaced by brown, velvety mucosa up to the region of the ampulla (right) but may have a dusky erythematous appearance more distally (B). Lymphoid aggregates impart a nodular appearance to the small intestine and are most numerous in the distal ileum (C). Lymphoid nodules extend into the lamina propria where they are surfaced by epithelium infiltrated by lymphocytes (D).

of the circumference of the jejunum and ileum. The luminal surface of the entire small intestine is arranged in transverse folds composed of mucosa and submucosa (i.e., valvulae conniventes, plicae circularis, folds of Kerckring); they are most prominent in the duodenum, which may normally show dusky discoloration compared with the proximal duodenum (fig. 1-5).

Lymphoid nodules are present throughout the small intestine and are most numerous in the distal ileum where they coalesce to form Peyer patches. These appear as small nodules, often with central umbilication that simulate aphthous ulcers (fig. 1-5C,D). Lymphoid nodules are largest in children and adolescents but gradually involute in adulthood.

Vascular Anatomy. The proximal duodenum is supplied by branches of the superior pancreaticoduodenal arteries that create a complex network of feeder vessels. The small intestine distal to the ampulla is vascularized by the superior mesenteric artery: the distal duodenum is supplied by the inferior pancreaticoduodenal arteries, and jejunal and ileal branches from the superior mesenteric artery supply the rest of the small bowel. The superior mesenteric artery courses through the mesentery and gives rise to branches from its convex aspect, forming rich, overlapping arcades (i.e., vasa recta). Short, straight branches from these arcades ramify in the serosa and penetrate the muscularis propria, ultimately terminating in arterioles that supply the villi (17). The small intestinal veins are paired with arteries in the small bowel and drain into the superior mesenteric vein of the portal venous system.

Lymphatic vessels of the duodenum drain to lymph nodes around the duodenum, pancreas, and distal stomach. Those of the jejunum and most of the ileum drain to lymph nodes in the mesentery, particularly around the superior mesenteric vessels, whereas the ileocolic lymph nodes receive lymph from the terminal ileum.

Histology

The small intestinal mucosa consists of epithelium and lamina propria arranged in villous projections into the lumen. Villi range from 0.3 to 1.0 mm in height; they are shortest in the proximal duodenum, particularly when associated with Brunner glands, reach their maximal height in the distal duodenum and jejunum, and become progressively shorter in the distal ileum (fig. 1-6). Each villus contains an arteriole, venule, central lymphatic vessel, capillaries, scattered nerve fibers, and rare, longitudinally oriented smooth muscle cells. Crypts of Lieberkühn are present in the deep mucosa near the muscularis mucosae. They are approximately 170 μm in length and contain the proliferative compartment of epithelial stem cells (18,19). The latter give rise to daughter cells that differentiate into absorptive enterocytes, M cells, goblet cells, Paneth cells, and endocrine cells, as described below.

Enterocytes are tall columnar cells arranged in a monolayer along the villous surface and upper crypt region. They contain abundant eosinophilic cytoplasm and basally located nuclei, as well as a microvillous brush border that increases the cell surface area and enhances absorption. Microvilli are supported by internal actin filaments that are cross-linked by villin and fimbrin, and tethered to the cytoplasmic membrane by myosin 1 and calmodulin. The microvillous brush border is immunopositive for CD10, EPCAM, and villin (20). Enterocytes produce glycoproteins that form a protective glycocalyx at the cell surface, as well as a variety of enzymes to break down carbohydrates and proteins. They also elaborate a secretory component, which facilitates translocation of IgA across epithelial cells.

The M cells are specialized epithelial cells overlying B-cell–rich regions of lymphoid nodules and Peyer patches. These cells play an important role in gut immunity by regulating presentation of luminal antigens to the mucosal immune system (21). Although they lack a well-developed brush border, M cells have a luminal membrane with a convoluted surface. They likely represent highly differentiated enterocytes but cannot be distinguished from other enterocytes by histochemical means (22).

Goblet cells are present throughout the small intestine, although their numbers and distribution vary in a site-specific fashion. They are more numerous in the crypt region than villous tips of the duodenum and jejunum, and increase in number toward the distal ileum. Goblet cells are distended by a large, luminally oriented vacuole of cytoplasmic mucin. The mucin tends to be colorless or faintly basophilic, reflecting the presence of sialylated glycoproteins. Goblet cells are positive with Alcian blue and PAS histochemical stains, and they express MUC2.

Paneth cells and endocrine cells are confined to the deep crypt region. Paneth cells have a columnar shape, with basally oriented nuclei, and contain large, brightly eosinophilic cytoplasmic granules rich in growth factors and antimicrobial proteins (fig. 1-6D). Endocrine cells are pyramidal in shape and also contain eosinophilic serotonin-containing granules. However, the granules of endocrine cells tend to be finer and more purple than those of Paneth cells. They are also oriented such that nuclei are located at the cell apices and granules are near the basement membrane.

Similar to the lamina propria of the colon, that of the small bowel normally contains a mixed population of inflammatory cells with

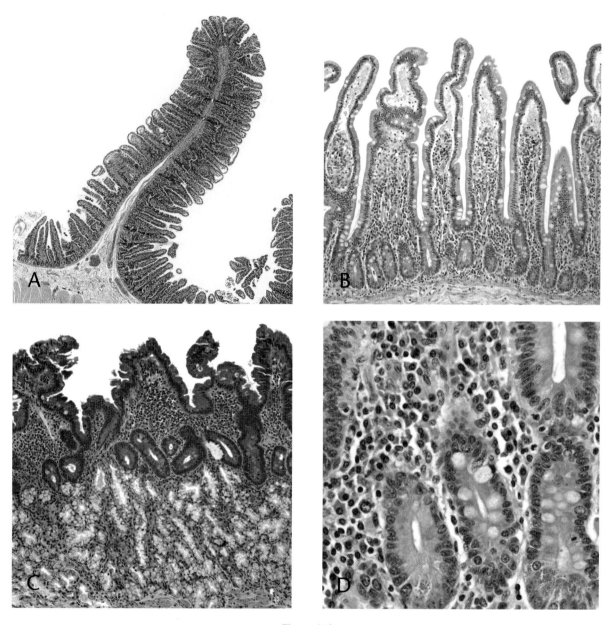

Figure 1-6

NORMAL HISTOLOGIC FEATURES OF THE SMALL BOWEL

The small bowel folds consist of submucosal projections surfaced by mucosa with a villous architecture (A). Long slender villi of the jejunum contain cellular lamina propria with small, scattered vessels and plasma cells; they are surfaced by absorptive enterocytes and interspersed goblet cells (B). Villi in the proximal duodenum are often shortened overlying Brunner glands (C). The crypts contain goblet cells and Paneth cells supported by plasma cell-rich lamina propria (D).

mononuclear cells, plasma cells, and occasional eosinophils. Neutrophils may be present, but are generally scattered and inconspicuous. Intraepithelial lymphocytes may be seen in villi of healthy patients; they number fewer than 25 per 100 enterocytes and tend to be most numerous at the bases of the villi or along their lateral aspects.

The muscularis mucosae lies just below the crypt bases. It is composed of a slender, discontinuous band of smooth muscle cells arranged in inner circular and outer longitudinal layers.

The submucosa contains linear arrays of lymphoid aggregates that may transgress the muscularis mucosae and extend into the lamina propria. They are more prominent in the distal ileum where they may be circumferential, especially in children. Lobules of neutral mucin-containing glands (i.e., Brunner glands) are numerous in the duodenal bulb and periampullary duodenum. These lobules are mostly present in the submucosa, although they can extend into the lamina propria, especially in the duodenal bulb. Medium-sized arteries are accompanied by veins and are supported by loose connective tissue, fat, and collagen fibers. Submucosal nerve plexuses are also present.

The muscularis propria is composed of two thick layers of smooth muscle cells arranged in inner circular and outer longitudinal layers. The myenteric plexus lies between these layers and contains parasympathetic ganglion cells intimately associated with the interstitial cells of Cajal. A thin layer of loose connective tissue separates the muscularis propria from the mesothelium-lined serosal surface.

THE NORMAL COLORECTUM

Anatomy

Gross Anatomy. The large intestine measures up to 1.5 m in length and has a larger diameter proximally. It is composed of four anatomic regions: the right colon consisting of the cecum and ascending colon, the transverse colon, the distal colon (i.e., descending and sigmoid colon), and the rectum. The cecum is completely surfaced by peritoneum and contains the appendiceal orifice, which is located on its medial aspect slightly below the ileocecal valve. The ascending colon is approximately 20 cm long; it is surfaced by peritoneum anteriorly but lies on the posterior abdominal wall.

The colon acquires a mesentery at the hepatic flexure. This region marks the beginning of the transverse colon, which ranges from 30 to 60 cm in length and extends to the splenic flexure. At this point, the colon is adherent to the posterior abdominal wall, where it remains throughout the length of the descending colon. The sigmoid colon is again suspended on a mesentery as it crosses the pelvic brim.

The rectosigmoid junction is located at the level of the sacral promontory. The rectum measures approximately 15 cm and extends to the dentate line. The upper third is surfaced by peritoneum on its anterolateral aspects but the remainder of the rectum is surrounded by perirectal fat and connective tissue. These soft tissues below the peritoneal reflection comprise the mesorectum, which is surfaced by adventitia, and represent the radial margin on rectal resection specimens.

Three evenly spaced longitudinal bands of smooth muscle are visible on the external surface of the entire colon. These teniae coli represent condensations of the outer layer of the muscularis propria. One of them lies adjacent to the insertion of the mesentery and the other two are located on the antimesenteric aspect of the colon. The longitudinal arrangement of teniae coli contributes to the formation of a series of saccular haustra between them, imparting a segmented appearance to the outer aspect of the colon, and producing the semilunar folds of the colonic mucosa (fig. 1-7A). The teniae coli coalesce at the base of the appendix and become progressively broader and thicker in the distal colorectum. Appendices epiploica are fatty protuberances arranged in two rows in the ascending and descending colon, and in a single row on the undersurface of the transverse colon.

Vascular Anatomy. The colon proximal to the splenic flexure is vascularized by the ileocolic, right colic, and middle colic branches of the superior mesenteric artery. The distal colon is supplied by the left colic and sigmoid branches of the inferior mesenteric artery. Anastomosing arcades link the superior and inferior mesenteric arteries through the marginal artery of Drummond, which courses parallel to the mesenteric surface of the colon. This vessel can be attenuated near the splenic flexure thereby predisposing it to ischemic injury. The vascular supply of the rectum consists of the superior rectal branch of the inferior mesenteric artery, the middle rectal arteries from the internal iliac vessels, and the inferior rectal arteries from the internal pudendal vessels. The colonic veins are paired with arteries; all of the colonic veins and those of the superior and middle rectum drain into the portal circulation, whereas veins from the distal rectum drain into the systemic circulation.

The lymphatic drainage of the colorectum is to paracolic and pararectal lymph nodes adjacent to

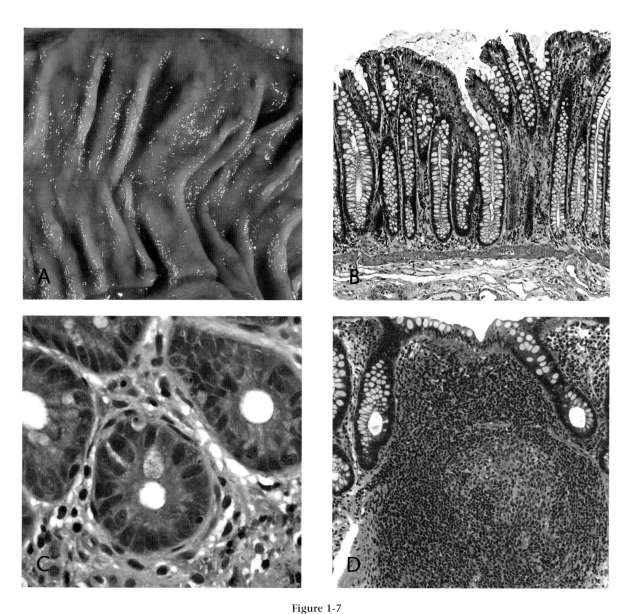

Figure 1-7

NORMAL GROSS AND HISTOLOGIC FEATURES OF THE COLON

The colonic mucosa is arranged in mucosal folds that incompletely surface the luminal circumference (A). The mucosa lacks villi, but shows an undulating surface and straight tubular crypts that extend to the muscularis mucosae (B). Deep crypts contain Paneth cells with luminally oriented granules, as well as pyramidal endocrine cells with finer, more purple granules near the basement membrane (C). Lymphoid aggregates are centered in the submucosa and frequently extend into the lamina propria; the muscularis mucosae is often interrupted in these areas (D).

the bowel wall. Lymph nodes draining the colon and proximal rectum are also dispersed along mesenteric vessels, whereas the lower rectum drains to lymph nodes along the superior rectal artery and middle rectal vessels. Lower rectal lymph nodes ultimately drain to the internal iliac lymph nodes, or even to inguinal lymph nodes through presacral lymphatic vessels.

Histology

The colorectum consists of several layers: the mucosa and muscularis mucosae, submucosa, muscularis propria, and serosa or adventitia depending on whether it is surfaced by perito-neum. The colonic mucosa primarily functions to absorb water and electrolytes, reducing approximately 1 L of liquid contents to 100 mL of feces each day. Thus, its mucosal architecture is different than that of the small intestine. The surface is flat with smooth undulations, and the epithelium is arranged in straight, regularly spaced crypts that extend to the muscularis mucosae (fig. 1-7B). Both the surface and crypts are lined by a predominance of goblet cells with interspersed absorptive cells. Colonic goblet cells are rich in sulfated or O-acetylated mucins that impart a slightly blue hue to their cytoplasm. Progenitor cells populate the lateral aspects of the deep crypts; endocrine cells are present at the crypt bases. Paneth cells are also scattered in the deep crypts of the ascending and proximal transverse colon but they should not be present in the distal colon (fig. 1-7C). The crypts of the rectal mucosa are shorter and tend to be irregularly dispersed in the lamina propria. They may also show a greater degree of crypt-to-crypt variability and occasional crypt branching.

The colonic lamina propria contains a mixed population of plasma cells, lymphocytes, and eosinophils; inflammatory cells are more numerous in the lamina propria of the proximal colon than the distal colon. The rectal lamina propria is similar, although it frequently contains mucin-filled macrophages that may be prominent in up to 40 percent of patients (23). Intraepithelial lymphocytes are commonly present in small numbers, especially overlying lymphoid aggregates. Small capillaries are normally present at all levels of the lamina propria but lymphovascular channels are limited to the deep mucosa near the crypt bases.

The muscularis mucosae is composed of slender fascicles of smooth muscle cells arranged in inner circular and outer longitudinal layers. It is discontinuous through lymphoid aggregates, often permitting herniation of mucosal elements beyond the level of the muscularis mucosae (fig. 1-7D). The submucosa contains Meissner plexus composed of parasympathetic ganglion cells and sympathetic neurons, arteries, and veins supported by loose connective tissue and fat.

The architecture of the colonic muscularis propria is slightly different than that of the small intestine. Like the small intestinal muscularis propria, it consists of inner circular and outer longitudinal layers between which lies the Auerbach plexus. Although the inner circular layer is continuous throughout the colonic length and circumference, the outer layer is discontinuous. The latter appears as attenuated aggregates of smooth muscle cells that coalesce into three evenly spaced teniae coli. The outer colon is surfaced by a thin layer of loose connective tissue lined by mesothelium on its peritonealized surfaces.

THE NORMAL APPENDIX

Anatomy

Gross Anatomy. The tubular (or vermiform) appendix arises from the medial wall of the cecum. It reaches its maximum diameter by 4 years of age, ultimately averaging 9 cm in length and 0.7 cm in diameter. The teniae coli coalesce at the appendiceal base and completely invest it. The appendix becomes narrower with age, particularly after age 40, as lymphoid tissue decreases and fibrosis increases (24). Its location varies depending on the shape of the cecum and its positioning at the time of embryologic development and rotation (25–27). It most frequently lies 2 to 3 cm below the ileocecal valve posterior to the cecum or ascending colon; other locations include the retroileal space, pre-ileal space, pelvis, and hepatorenal recess. Abnormal positioning of the appendix can explain atypical manifestations of acute appendicitis (28).

Vascular Anatomy. The appendix is supplied by the posterior cecal branch of the ileocolic artery, which is derived from the superior mesenteric artery. Appendiceal venous drainage goes to the superior mesenteric vein. Both arterial and venous structures are supported by the mesoappendix, which is contiguous with the mesentery of the bowel. Small lymph nodes that drain to the pericolic and superior mesenteric lymph nodes are infrequently found within the mesoappendix.

Histology

The mucosa of the appendix is similar to that of the large bowel, although it contains a greater amount of lymphoid tissue, often with germinal centers, and is particularly prominent during childhood and adolescence (fig. 1-8A). The epithelium is composed of tall columnar absorptive cells, goblet cells, Paneth cells, and endocrine cells at the base of the mucosa (fig.

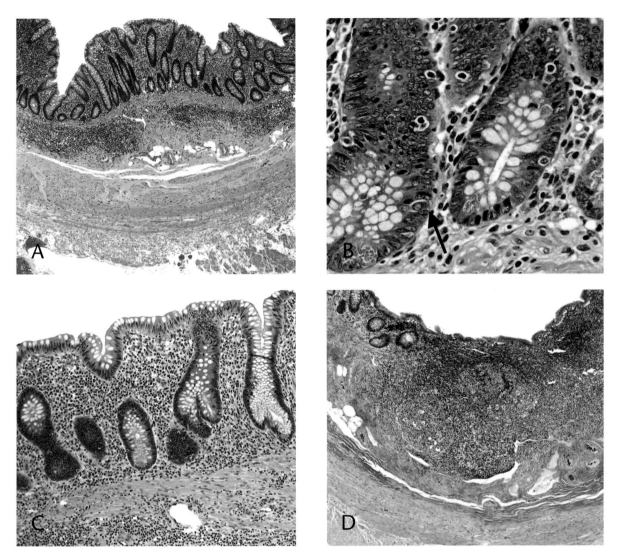

Figure 1-8

NORMAL HISTOLOGIC FEATURES OF THE APPENDIX

The appendiceal mucosa, submucosa, muscularis propria, and serosa are similar to those of the colon, although the appendix contains abundant lymphoid tissue and an irregularly thickened muscularis mucosae (A). The mucosa contains absorptive cells, goblet cells, endocrine cells (arrow), and occasional Paneth cells (B). The crypts are often irregularly distributed and show mild architectural distortion, but these features represent normal variants rather than evidence of appendicitis (C). Lymphoid tissue may be prominent and contains germinal centers with attenuated overlying epithelium; the muscularis mucosae is discontinuous through large lymphoid aggregates (D).

1-8B) (29). The lamina propria normally contains mononuclear cells and occasional eosinophils. The crypts typically display a slightly irregular distribution (fig. 1-8C) (30). Large lymphoid aggregates span the mucosal thickness and extend into the submucosa; disruption of the muscularis mucosae and attenuation of the overlying epithelium are often present (fig. 1-8D) (27,30).

The submucosa, muscularis propria, and serosa are qualitatively similar to analogous structures in the colon. Nerves and ganglion cells are not confined to a myenteric plexus; they are easily identified throughout the inner and outer layers of the muscularis propria (30). Aggregates of smooth muscle cells, particularly those of the inner muscularis propria, may rarely accumulate PAS-D–positive granular material in

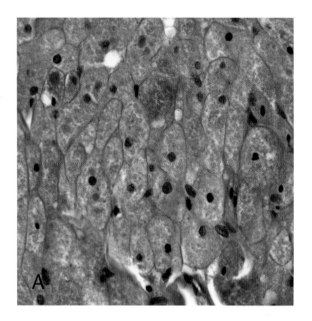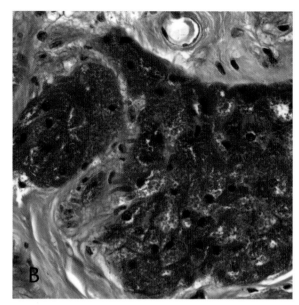

Figure 1-9

GRANULAR DEGENERATION OF THE MUSCULARIS PROPRIA

Some appendices feature abnormal smooth muscle cells in the muscularis propria, particularly its inner layers. Smooth muscle cells are enlarged and round. They contain abundant granular cytoplasm (A) that is strongly positive with PAS-D histochemical stains (B).

their cytoplasm that simulates an inflammatory process or neoplasm (fig. 1-9) (31). Prominent intravascular lymphocytosis in the appendix and meso-appendix is frequently present (fig. 1-10). The serosa is smooth, glistening, and transparent, and a thin layer of peritoneum covers the entire appendix.

THE NORMAL ANUS

Anatomy

Gross Anatomy. The surgical anal canal extends from the anorectal ring to the anal verge and spans approximately 4 cm in the adult. The proximal mucosa gives rise to 8 to 12 longitudinal mucosal folds (i.e., anal columns of Morgagni); pairs of these folds terminate at each of several circumferentially arranged semilunar folds of tissue (i.e. anal valves). The anal valves form the dentate, or pectinate, line and enclose the anal crypts that drain anal glands (32). The dentate line is composed of anorectal mucosa proximally and anodermal mucosa distally in young children, but these types of mucosae are separated by the anal transition zone in adults. The smooth mucosa distal to the dentate line

(i.e., pectin) terminates at the anal verge, which is wrinkled, slightly pigmented, and represents the transition from anoderm to perianal skin.

The internal anal sphincter is continuous with the circular layer of the rectal muscularis propria and terminates proximal to the anal verge. The intrinsic enteric nervous system of the myenteric plexus facilitates rhythmic contractions of the sphincter muscle; extrinsic autonomic control is derived from the hypogastric pelvic nerve plexus. The external anal sphincter is composed of alternating ring-like and elliptical layers of striated skeletal muscle that run from the perineal body to the coccyx. It surrounds the internal anal sphincter and extends caudally, terminating approximately 1 cm distal to the internal anal sphincter. The deep external sphincter is fused with the puborectalis muscle. Fibroelastic septa extend through the external sphincter into the perianal dermis, producing the characteristic folds of the perianal skin (33).

The external anal sphincter is innervated by the inferior rectal branch of the pudendal nerve and the perineal branch of S4. The puborectalis and levator ani form the pelvic diaphragm and provide both sympathetic tonic contraction and voluntary control.

Vascular Anatomy. The anal canal above the dentate line is supplied by branches of the superior hemorrhoidal (rectal) artery. Draining venules coalesce into saccular venous plexuses in the submucosa in the anal cushions, which are most prominent in the right anterior, right posterior, and left lateral positions (34). The anal cushions compress the anal orifice, producing a "Y-shaped" opening and providing nearly 20 percent of the resting anal pressure at the level of the internal anal sphincter (35). The lymphatic vessels of the proximal anus drain to inferior mesenteric and internal iliac lymph nodes.

The anal canal below the dentate line is supplied by the middle and inferior hemorrhoidal arteries and drained by the portal venous system via the inferior mesenteric vein. Lymph flows through inferior rectal lymphatic channels to the superficial inguinal lymph nodes. The upper anal canal is richly innervated by pressure-sensitive fibers from the inferior rectal branch of the pudendal nerve, whereas pain fibers are present below the dentate line.

Histology

The anorectal junction is surfaced by mucosa similar to that of the rectum. A single layer of goblet cells, interspersed colonocytes, and occasional endocrine cells in the crypts are arranged along a basement membrane; the crypts are more irregularly shaped compared with the mucosa of the abdominal colon (36). The lamina propria contains delicate capillaries and venules as well as scattered lymphocytes and plasma cells. Mucin-filled macrophages can be numerous and tend to aggregate in the superficial mucosa (fig. 1-10A). The muscularis mucosae is composed of longitudinally arranged aggregates of smooth muscle cells. The anal transition zone is lined by four to nine cell layers: polarized cuboidal cells are present in the deep layers, whereas surface cells may be flat, cuboidal, or columnar with apical mucin (fig. 1-10B). Histochemical stains demonstrate a predominance of sialomucins in this region (37).

Lobules of mucin-containing anal glands are located in the submucosa and commonly penetrate the internal sphincter. Cells in the neck region have a transitional appearance that gradually gives way to squamous cells at the gland orifice. The anal transition zone epithelium merges with the smooth, nonkeratinizing stratified squamous epithelium at the dentate line (fig. 1-10C). Scattered melanocytes, Langerhans cells, intraepithelial lymphocytes, and Merkel cells are often present (fig. 1-10D).

The perianal skin is surfaced by keratinizing epithelium with a granular cell layer, keratohyalin granules, and a cornified layer of keratin at the anal verge. Dermal papillae, hair follicles, and adnexal structures are present. The submucosa consists of loosely arranged collagen fibrils, fibroblasts, and scattered multinucleated stromal cells above the dentate line. The submucosa of the pectin is rich in elastic tissue and collagen fibrils that tether the mucosa to the underlying muscle. Elastic fibers are most prominent at the anal verge.

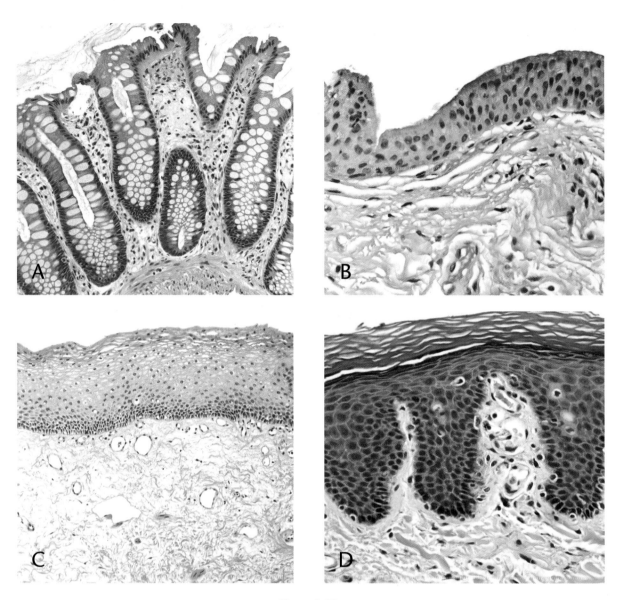

Figure 1-10

NORMAL HISTOLOGIC FEATURES OF THE ANORECTUM

The most distal rectal mucosa contains irregularly distributed colonic crypts with slight surface serration and aggregates of foamy macrophages in the lamina propria (A). Transitional mucosa consists of a multilayered epithelium composed of cuboidal, squamoid, and mucin-containing columnar cells (B). Nonkeratinizing stratified squamous epithelium is supported by loose connective tissue in the anal canal (C). The mucosa near the anal verge is surfaced by basket weave-type keratin with a granular cell layer. Scattered Langerhans cells and melanocytes are present in the epithelium, and basal keratinocytes show pigmentation (D).

REFERENCES

1. El-Zimaity H, Riddell RH. Esophagus. In: Mills SE, ed. Histology for pathologists, 4th ed. Philadelphia: Lippincott Williams & Wilkins; 2012:605-32.
2. Rice TW, Kelsen D, Blackstone SH, et al. Esophagus and esophagogatric junction. In: Amin MB, ed. AJCC cancer staging manual, 8th ed. Chicago: Springer Nature; 2016:185-202.
3. Shaheen NJ, Falk GW, Iyer PG, Gerson LB, American College of Gastroenterology. ACG clinical guideline: diagnosis and management of Barrett's esophagus. Am J Gastroenterol 2016;111:30-51.
4. Putra J, Muller KE, Hussain ZH, et al. Lymphocytic esophagitis in nonachalasia primary esophageal motility disorders: improved criteria, prevalence, strength of association, and natural history. Am J Surg Pathol 2016;40:1679-85.
5. Geboes K, De Wolf-Peeters C, Rutgeerts P, Janssens J, Vantrappen G, Desmet V. Lymphocytes and Langerhans cells in the human oesophageal epithelium. Virchows Arch A Pathol Anat Histopathol 1983;401:45-55.
6. Sharma SS, Venkateswaran S, Chacko A, Mathan M. Melanosis of the esophagus. An endoscopic, histochemical, and ultrastructural study. Gastroenterology 1991;100:13-6.
7. Bogomoletz WV, Lecat M, Amoros F. Melanosis of the oesophagus in a Western patient. Histopathology 1997;30:498-9.
8. Ohashi K, Kato Y, Kanno J, Kasuga T. Melanocytes and melanosis of the oesophagus in Japanese subjects—analysis of factors effecting their increase. Virchows Arch A Pathol Anat Histopathol 1990;417:137-43.
9. Owen DO. Stomach. In: Mills SE, ed. Histology for pathologists, 4th ed. Philadelphia: Lippincott Williams & Wilkins; 2012:633-46.
10. Piasecki C. Blood supply to the human gastroduodenal mucosa with special reference to the ulcer-bearing areas. J Anat 1974;118(Pt 2):295-335.
11. Lirosi MC, Biondi A, Ricci R. Surgical anatomy of gastric lymphatic drainage. Transl Gastroenterol Hepatol 2017;2:14.
12. Choi WT, Lauwers GY. Patterns of gastric injury: beyond Helicobacter pylori. Surg Pathol Clin 2017;10:801-22.
13. Chandrasoma PT, Der R, Ma Y, Dalton P, Taira M. Histology of the gastroesophageal junction: an autopsy study. Am J Surg Pathol 2000;24:402-9.
14. Kamoshida S, Saito E, Fukuda S, Kato K, Iwasaki A, Arakawa Y. Anatomical location of enterochromaffin-like (ECL) cells, parietal cells, and chief cells in the stomach demonstrated by immunocytochemistry and electron microscopy. J Gastroenterol 1999;34:315-20.
15. Mani BK, Zigman JM. A strong stomach for somatostatin. Endocrinology 2015;156:3876-9.
16. Reiner L, Platt R, Rodriguez FL, Jimenez F. Injection studies on the mesenteric arterial circulation. II. Intestinal infarction. Gastroenterology 1960;39:747-57.
17. King SL, Dekaney CM. Small intestinal stem cells. Curr Opin Gastroenterol 2013;29:140-5.
18. Ranganathan S, Schmitt LA, Sindhi R. Tufting enteropathy revisited: the utility of MOC31 (EpCAM) immunohistochemistry in diagnosis. Am J Surg Pathol 2014;38:265-72.
19. Groisman GM, Amar M, Livne E. CD10: a valuable tool for the light microscopic diagnosis of microvillous inclusion disease (familial microvillous atrophy). Am J Surg Pathol 2002;26:902-7.
20. Kucharzik T, Lugering N, Rautenberg K, et al. Role of M cells in intestinal barrier function. Ann N Y Acad Sci 2000;915:171-83.
21. Kucharzik T, Lugering N, Schmid KW, et al. Human intestinal M cells exhibit enterocyte-like intermediate filaments. Gut 1998;42:54-62.
22. Bejarano PA, Aranda-Michel J, Fenoglio-Preiser C. Histochemical and immunohistochemical characterization of foamy histiocytes (muciphages and xanthelasma) of the rectum. Am J Surg Pathol 2000;24:1009-15.
23. Williams R. Development, structure, and function of the appendix. In: Williams RA, Myers P, eds. Pathology of the appendix and its surgical treatment. London: Chapman & Hall Medical; 1994:9-30.
24. Wakeley CP. The position of the vermiform appendix as ascertained by an analysis of 10,000 cases. J Anat 1933;67(Pt 2):277-83.
25. Deshmukh S, Verde F, Johnson PT, Fishman EK, Macura KJ. Anatomical variants and pathologies of the vermix. Emerg Radiol 2014;21:543-52.
26. Gramlich TL, Petras RE. Vermiform appendix. In: Mills SE, ed. Histology for pathologists, 3rd ed. Philadelphia: Lippincott Williams & Wilkins; 2007:649-62.
27. Kim S, Lim HK, Lee JY, Lee J, Kim MJ, Lee AS. Ascending retrocecal appendicitis: clinical and computed tomographic findings. J Comput Assist Tomogr 2006;30:772-6.
28. Millikin PD. Eosinophilic argentaffin cells in the human appendix. Arch Pathol 1974;98:393-5.
29. Lamps LW. Appendix. In: Lamps LW, ed. Diagnostic pathology-normal histology. Park City: Amirsys; 2013:24-7.

30. Fenger C. The anal transitional zone. Acta Pathol Microbiol Immunol Scand Suppl 1987;289:1-42.
31. Lunniss PJ, Phillips RK. Anatomy and function of the anal longitudinal muscle. Br J Surg 1992;79:882-4.
32. Saraswati R, Novelli M. Surgical treatment and pathology: normal histology. In: Cohen R, Windsor A, eds. Anus. London: Springer; 2014:43-7.
33. Lestar B, Penninckx F, Kerremans R. The composition of anal basal pressure. An in vivo and in vitro study in man. Int J Colorectal Dis 1989;4:118-22.
34. Schizas A, Williams A. The normal anus. In: Cohen R, Windsor A, eds. Anus. London: Springer; 2014:1-12.
35. Fenger C, Filipe MI. Pathology of the anal glands with special reference to their mucin histochemistry. Acta Pathol Microbiol Scand A 1977;85:273-85.

2 | DISEASES OF THE ESOPHAGUS

CONGENITAL AND ACQUIRED STRUCTURAL ABNORMALITIES

Esophageal Atresia and Tracheoesophageal Fistula

Definition. *Esophageal atresia* is a blind-ended proximal esophagus. A *fistula* is an abnormal connection between the esophagus, trachea, and/or bronchi.

Clinical Features. Esophageal atresia occurs in approximately 1 in 3,000 live births, and tracheoesophageal fistula affects approximately 1 in 4,000 live births. Both anomalies show a slight male predominance (1). They may be isolated defects, although nearly 50 percent are associated with other congenital anomalies, particularly the VACTERL complex (vertebral, anal, cardiac, tracheal, esophageal, renal, and limb anomalies) and trisomies 13, 18, and 21 (2). Approximately 25 percent of esophageal atresias occur in combination with imperforate anus, pyloric stenosis, duodenal atresia, and other gastrointestinal malformations.

Esophageal atresias and tracheoesophageal fistulas are classified according to the presence and location of communications with the trachea or mainstem bronchi (fig. 2-1) (3). These anomalies can be detected or suspected at the time of fetal ultrasound owing to the presence of polyhydramnios. Esophageal atresia with, or without, tracheoesophageal fistula manifests in infancy with coughing, choking, and vomiting during feeding. Apneic episodes with cyanosis, aspiration, and pneumonia also occur. Imaging reveals a blind, distended pouch in the atretic proximal esophagus and an absence of gas in the stomach and small intestine (4). Resected segments contain the normal wall elements; reactive epithelial changes, inflammation, and fibrosis are variably present (fig. 2-2).

Pathogenesis. The embryonic esophagus and trachea constitute a single tube that divides by lateral wall folding during the 3rd and 4th gestational weeks. Atresia occurs when the lateral walls turn dorsally and cut through the esophageal lumen, whereas fistulas result from failure of the lateral mesodermal walls to meet (5).

Treatment and Prognosis. Surgical restoration of esophageal continuity is the best

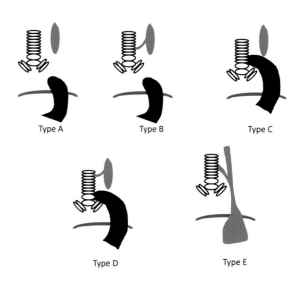

Figure 2-1

ESOPHAGEAL ATRESIAS AND TRACHEOESOPHAGEAL FISTULAE

Type A malformations consist of blind-ended proximal and distal esophageal buds without a tracheobronchial fistula. Type B malformations display a fistula between the proximal esophageal bud and the lower trachea; the distal bud has a blind end. Type C malformations are the most common: the proximal esophagus is a blind-ended pouch that occurs in combination with a fistula connecting the distal esophagus with the trachea/bronchi. Type D malformations show a proximal tracheoesophageal fistula, as well as communication between the distal esophagus and carina. Type E malformations have an "H" configuration with a fistula between the esophagus and trachea.

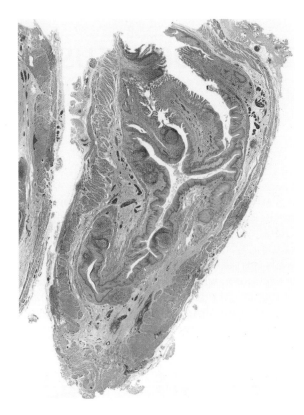

Figure 2-2

TYPE A TRACHEOESOPHAGEAL FISTULA

The blind-ended esophageal pouch is lined by normal squamous epithelium and displays lymphoid nodules in the mucosa.

treatment option, although persistent symptoms related to dysmotility, strictures, and gastroesophageal reflux disease are common (6). Overall prognosis is heavily influenced by the presence of underlying anomalies.

Esophageal Stenosis

Definition. *Esophageal stenosis* is the luminal narrowing of the esophagus.

Clinical Features. Esophageal stenosis is a rare disorder that affects 1 in 50,000 live births, with a slight male predominance. Nearly one-third of cases are associated with other congenital anomalies, particularly tracheoesophageal fistula and esophageal atresia. Esophagram reveals an area of smooth, tapered concentric narrowing that spans 1 to 2 cm (7). Stenosis of the proximal esophagus presents with respiratory symptoms, whereas distal narrowing presents with vomiting. Stenosis may be clinically silent in early infancy and

become symptomatic only when larger liquid or solid meals are consumed (8).

Pathogenesis. Stenosis results from failed recanalization of the embryonic esophagus by the 11th gestational week, fibromuscular malformations in the wall, diaphragms or webs in the mid to distal esophagus, *in utero* ischemia, or occlusion by tracheobronchial remnants (7).

Treatment and Prognosis. Most cases are managed by balloon dilatation, although some require excision of the affected segment and re-anastomosis. Correction allows for normal feeding and appropriate weight gain (8).

Esophageal Rings and Webs

Definition. Fibrous or fibromuscular *rings* in the esophagus may cause focal luminal narrowing. *Webs* are thin, delicate membranes composed of squamous mucosa.

Clinical Features. Esophageal rings show an equal predilection for men and women and are found in 6 to 14 percent of routine barium radiographs. Most esophageal rings are asymptomatic: only 0.5 percent of patients have intermittent dysphagia to solids, gastroesophageal reflux disease, or obstructive symptoms (9).

Webs are described in 5 to 15 percent of patients presenting with dysphagia and are more common in Caucasian women (10). They are associated with celiac disease, bullous dermatologic disorders, graft-versus-host disease, and Plummer-Vinson syndrome (Paterson-Brown-Kelly syndrome) (10). The latter is characterized by esophageal webs, iron deficiency anemia, glossitis, koilonychia, and increased risk of pharyngeal and esophageal cancers, particularly in the proximal esophagus. It occurs in white females in the 4th to 7th decades of life (11).

Pathogenesis. Symptomatic esophageal rings rarely present before the age of 40 years, raising the possibility that they result from chronic injury due to gastroesophageal reflux disease or eosinophilic esophagitis (12). Acquired webs tend to occur in the anterior cervical esophagus and are most likely postinflammatory in nature (10).

Gross Findings. Esophageal rings are thin (2 to 5 mm) diaphragms that show a predilection for the distal esophagus. They are classified in two main groups. Muscular rings (type "A" rings) occur approximately 1.5 cm above the squamocolumnar junction (fig. 2-3A); Schatzki

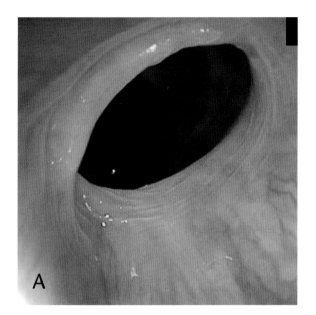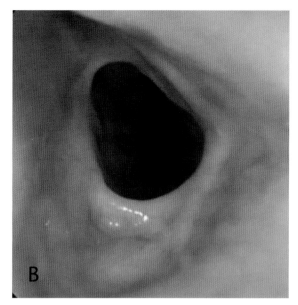

Figure 2-3

RINGS OF THE DISTAL ESOPHAGUS

A thick muscular ring is covered by corrugated-appearing mucosa (A). A Schatzki ring is a thin, circumferential narrowing in the distal esophagus (B).

rings (type "B" rings) are located at the squamocolumnar junction (fig. 2-3B).

Esophageal webs are eccentric, thin, translucent membranes most often located in the proximal esophagus (fig. 2-4) (13). Congenital webs are rare circumferential membranes located in the mid to distal esophagus.

Microscopic Findings. Type A rings contain a prominent muscular component. Schatzki rings consist of mucosa, submucosa, and, in some cases, a minor component of muscularis propria. They are surfaced by squamous mucosa on the proximal side and glandular mucosa on the distal side. The squamous epithelium may be inflamed or show parakeratosis. Webs are composed of variably inflamed squamous mucosa or epithelium.

Treatment and Prognosis. Symptomatic rings and webs can be treated with endoscopic dilatation. Surveillance of the esophagus and pharynx is recommended for patients with Plummer-Vinson syndrome (11).

Esophageal Cysts

Definition. *Esophageal cysts* (also termed *foregut cysts*) are congenital cysts that occasionally communicate with the lumen.

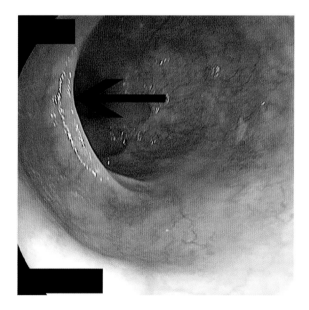

Figure 2-4

ESOPHAGEAL WEB

This web appears as an eccentric, translucent membrane (arrow) in the upper esophagus.

Clinical Features. Esophageal cysts account for 15 to 20 percent of congenital cysts of the gastrointestinal tract (3). They are classified as

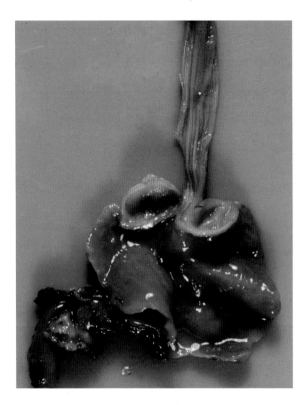

Figure 2-5

ESOPHAGEAL DUPLICATION CYST

An esophagectomy specimen contains a large saccular cyst with a smooth lining arising from the wall of the distal esophagus. (Courtesy of Dr. D. Beneck, New York, NY.)

either *duplication cysts* or *neurenteric remnants*. Duplication cysts contain a muscular wall and various mucosal elements that may or may not have a connection to the lumen. Complete duplication of the esophagus is rare and is usually accompanied by duplication of the stomach (3).

Neurenteric remnants originate in the dorsal midline of the upper esophagus, involving the vertebral column or spinal cord. Most cysts are asymptomatic and detected during imaging performed for unrelated reasons. When lesions do not drain to the lumen, large amounts of fluid can accumulate, causing dysphagia, vomiting, respiratory distress, or retrosternal pain. Neurenteric remnants that communicate with the central nervous system may cause neurologic manifestations (14).

Pathogenesis. The esophageal lumen is occluded by foregut epithelium during the 5th and 6th gestational weeks. This epithelium produces secretions, forming vacuoles that later coalesce to create the new lumen. Duplications form when vacuoles migrate laterally and become surrounded by muscle. Most are located in the distal esophagus slightly to the right of center due to elongation of intrathoracic viscera and dextrorotation of the stomach during embryogenesis (15).

Neurenteric remnants result from adhesions between the endoderm and ectoderm during the 4th gestational week (14). They are usually located in the mediastinum.

Gross Findings. Esophageal cysts can bulge into the lumen and produce endoscopically apparent semispherical impressions (16). The diagnosis is usually established by imaging: endoscopic ultrasound (EUS) demonstrates an intramural cyst within the muscularis propria (17).

Neurenteric remnants appear as diverticula, fistulae, cysts, or fibrous cords. The cysts are thin and translucent with areas of thickening (18).

Microscopic Findings. Esophageal cysts are lined by squamous epithelium as well as other types of gastrointestinal epithelia and ciliated columnar cells supported by loose connective tissue (14). They also contain thick mural bundles of well-organized smooth muscle. Some harbor nodules of cartilage.

Differential Diagnosis. The most problematic diagnostic consideration is a bronchogenic cyst, which is a congenital malformation that occurs in any mediastinal compartment. Bronchogenic cysts are usually associated with the tracheobronchial tree but may involve the esophageal muscularis propria (19). Distinction from esophageal cysts relies on the anatomic location and lack of a well-developed muscularis propria in bronchogenic cysts.

Treatment and Prognosis. Asymptomatic esophageal cysts can be observed, whereas symptomatic lesions are surgically resected (fig. 2-5). Resection may result in a substantially shortened esophagus, recurrent hiatal hernia, and persistent gastroesophageal reflux disease (3).

Diverticula

Definition. *Diverticula* are mucosa-lined outpouchings that communicate with the esophageal lumen.

Clinical Features. Esophageal diverticula are classified by their structure, pathogenesis, and location. Clinical symptoms may be directly attributed to diverticula of the proximal esophagus, or secondary to the underlying conditions that predispose to diverticula of the mid and distal esophagus. Diverticula in the proximal esophagus (*Zenker diverticula*) are the most common acquired diverticula. They show a predilection for the elderly and have an estimated prevalence of less than 0.1 percent (20). Patients with Zenker diverticula present with progressive dysphagia, regurgitation, retrosternal pain, halitosis, or persistent cough. Barium studies readily establish a diagnosis, although diverticula can also be visualized during cross sectional imaging with contrast agents, or during endoscopic examination.

Mid-esophageal and epiphrenic diverticula are usually asymptomatic; clinical manifestations are related to the underlying disorders that predispose to diverticulum development (see below). Mid-esophageal diverticula are regularly encountered in regions where tuberculosis and other mediastinal infections are endemic. Epiphrenic diverticula are more common among patients with esophageal motility disorders. Mid-esophageal and epiphrenic diverticula account for approximately 15 percent of all esophageal diverticula (21).

Pathogenesis. True diverticula contain all layers of the esophageal wall, whereas false diverticula represent herniations of mucosa and submucosa through the muscularis propria. *Congenital diverticula* are true diverticula; they essentially represent duplications that communicate with the lumen through wide orifices. *Acquired diverticula* may be true or false depending on their pathogenesis. *Traction diverticula* represent true diverticula that develop at the level of the tracheal bifurcation in the mid esophagus. They occur when the esophageal adventitia becomes tethered to exuberant fibroinflammatory conditions or neoplasms involving the mediastinal lymph nodes. *Pulsion diverticula* are false diverticula that result from chronically elevated intraluminal pressures. They develop in two locations. *Zenker diverticula* occur in the upper esophagus as a result of discoordinated relaxation of the cricopharyngeus coupled with increased intraluminal pressure that occurs during swallowing (22). *Epiphrenic diverticula* occur immediately proximal to the lower esophageal sphincter in patients with

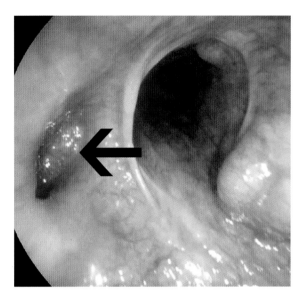

Figure 2-6

EPIPHRENIC DIVERTICULUM

Diverticula appear as wide-mouthed openings (arrow) on the esophageal mucosa. A polyp is present opposite the diverticulum.

peptic strictures or manometric abnormalities, such as achalasia, "nutcracker esophagus," diffuse esophageal spasm, and hypertensive lower esophageal sphincter (23).

Gross Findings. Zenker diverticula are cystic pouches located in the posterior hypopharynx between the cricopharyngeus muscle and pharyngeal constrictor muscles. Mid-esophageal diverticula are tent-shaped defects that tether the esophagus to mediastinal structures. Epiphrenic diverticula are located 1 to 2 cm above the gastroesophageal junction (fig. 2-6).

Microscopic Findings. True diverticula contain all layers of the esophageal wall, whereas false diverticula are composed of mucosa, muscularis mucosae, and submucosa (fig. 2-7). Both true and false diverticula show chronic stasis-related changes with inflammation, fibrosis, squamous hyperplasia, and erosions.

Treatment and Prognosis. Zenker diverticula are repaired by diverticulopexy, or excision of the diverticulum *via* thoracotomy or thoracoscopy. Untreated diverticula may result in recurrent aspiration, fistulization to the bronchial tree, or upper gastrointestinal bleeding (24). Treatment of mid and lower esophageal diverticula is aimed at managing the predisposing condition.

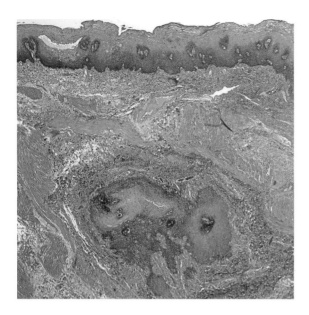

Figure 2-7

FALSE DIVERTICULUM OF THE ESOPHAGUS

Well-circumscribed aggregates of mucosal elements are surrounded by submucosal connective tissue in the muscularis propria.

Intramural Pseudodiverticulosis

Definition. *Intramural pseudodiverticulosis* denotes small, flask-shaped intramural out-pouchings of the submucosal ducts and glands in the esophagus.

Clinical Features. Intramural pseudodiverticulosis is an uncommon, asymptomatic finding that is usually observed in elderly men. It is almost always associated with a stricture of the upper or mid esophagus. Pseudodiverticula can be present above or below the level of the stricture. Patients usually present with dysphagia or obstructive symptoms related to strictures, and many have concurrent *Candida* esophagitis (25). Flask-shaped submucosal lesions are best visualized with a barium swallow; computerized tomography (CT) demonstrates intramural gas-filled cysts.

Pathogenesis. Presumably, strictures result in stasis and inflammation that block the submucosal ducts and cause dilatation of submucosal glands.

Gross Findings. Endoscopic examination reveals linear arrays of small, slightly raised plaques with tiny central ostia (25).

Microscopic Findings. Submucosal cysts are lined by cuboidal and stratified squamous epithelium, similar to native submucosal ducts (fig.

2-8). Associated mucous glands may undergo oncocytic or squamous metaplasia.

Treatment and Prognosis. Pseudodiverticula require no treatment; therapy is aimed at resolving associated strictures and infections. Resolution of underlying disorders results in amelioration of symptoms but pseudodiverticula do not regress (26).

Heterotopias

Definition. A *heterotopia* is ectopic glandular mucosa in the esophagus. Synonyms include *inlet patch* (heterotopic gastric mucosa) and *choristoma*.

Clinical Features. *Gastric heterotopias* are detected in approximately 12 percent of adults who undergo upper endoscopic examination; men and women are equally affected (27). Most are asymptomatic, although large rests of oxyntic-type mucosa can produce enough acid to cause dysphagia, hoarseness, chronic cough, and ear or sinus problems (28). Persistent acid-induced injury can lead to ulcers and strictures (29).

Pancreatic tissue is found in 14 to 24 percent of biopsy samples taken from the gastroesophageal junction. It produces no symptoms and is detected with similar frequencies in men and women (30). *Pancreatic heterotopias* have been reported in association with atresias and duplication cysts, although those relationships likely reflect the high overall prevalence of pancreatic heterotopias in the general population (31).

Sebaceous heterotopias are found in less than 0.005 percent of endoscopic examinations and show a predilection for middle-aged men. Sebaceous heterotopias are asymptomatic and usually occur in the proximal esophagus (32).

Pathogenesis. Squamous mucosa replaces the columnar esophageal lining during the 24th gestational week. This process begins in the mid esophagus. Incomplete re-epithelialization leads to residual islands of glandular mucosa that differentiate into gastric mucosa (33,34). Pancreatic rests presumably result from separation of small portions of the embryonic pancreas during foregut rotation. Recent data fail to support the idea that pancreatic tissue in the distal esophagus reflects inflammation-induced metaplasia (30,35). Sebaceous heterotopias are probably congenital but their pathogenesis is unclear; sebaceous glands are of ectodermal

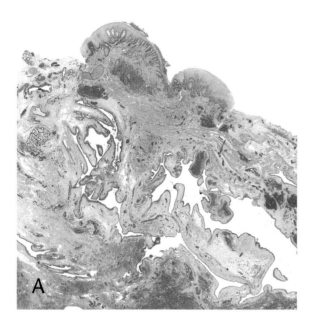 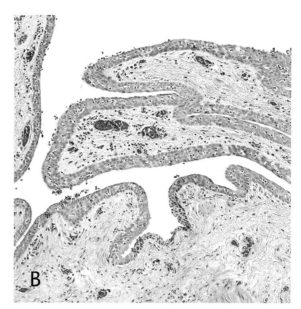

Figure 2-8

INTRAMURAL PSEUDODIVERTICULOSIS

Dilated, epithelium-lined cysts expand the submucosa (A). The cysts are lined by cuboidal and squamous epithelium (B).

origin, whereas the esophagus forms from the embryonic endoderm (36).

Gross Findings. Inlet patches are discrete ovoid islands of pink, velvety mucosa located approximately 15 to 20 cm from the incisors on the lateral aspects of the cervical esophagus (fig. 2-9). They may be flat, elevated, or depressed and are usually solitary, although multifocal heterotopias are occasionally encountered. Gastric heterotopias typically span less than 1 cm but can be up to 5 cm (33). Pancreatic heterotopias are not endoscopically visible (30). Sebaceous heterotopias appear as multiple yellow-white plaques in the upper to mid esophagus (37).

Microscopic Findings. Gastric heterotopias are composed of cardiac, oxyntic, or cardio-oxyntic mucosa (fig. 2-10A). Approximately 3 percent develop foci of intestinal metaplasia unrelated to Barrett esophagus (fig. 2-10B), and patients with *Helicobacter pylori*-associated chronic gastritis can have detectable organisms in heterotopic mucosa (fig. 2-10C,D) (38). Development of dysplasia and adenocarcinoma is exceedingly rare but shows a predilection for men (39).

Pancreatic heterotopias consist of lobules of pancreatic acini; abortive ductal elements are occasionally present. Acinar cells contain

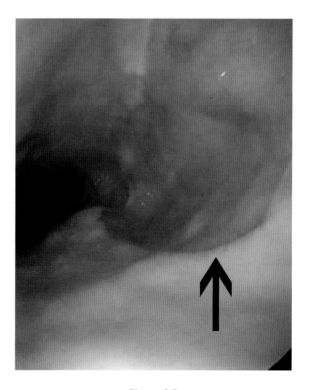

Figure 2-9

GASTRIC HETEROTOPIA OF THE ESOPHAGUS

An inlet patch (arrow) appears as an island of velvety brown mucosa in the proximal esophagus.

25

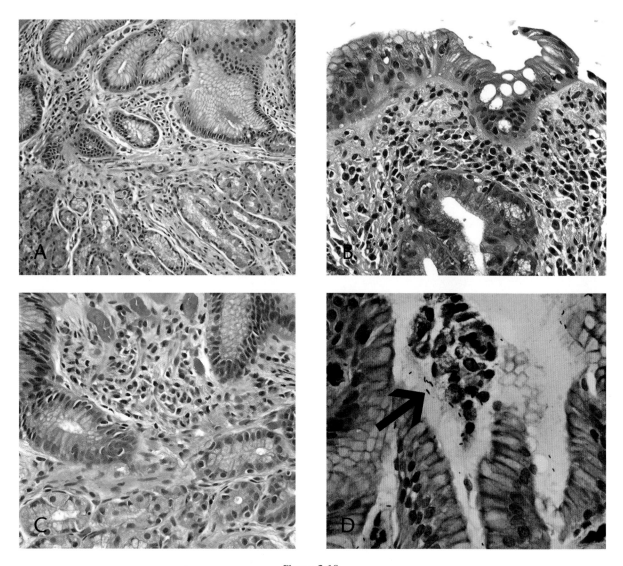

Figure 2-10

GASTRIC HETEROTOPIA OF THE ESOPHAGUS

This inlet patch consists of cardio-oxyntic mucosa with a normal-appearing foveolar surface (A) and a cluster of goblet cells (B). The cardiofundic mucosa of this inlet patch contains plasma cell-rich inflammation (C). A Warthin-Starry silver stain demonstrates *Helicobacter pylori* organisms (arrow), which appear as black curvilinear rods (D).

granular apical cytoplasm and round basally located nuclei (fig. 2-11).

Sebaceous heterotopias contain lobules of lipid-rich cells with foamy, vacuolated cytoplasm. The surface epithelium often shows hyperkeratosis or parakeratosis (fig. 2-12).

Treatment and Prognosis. Treatment of esophageal heterotopias is generally unnecessary, although radiofrequency ablation and argon plasma coagulation can be used for patients with acid-related symptoms due to large inlet patches.

Strictures can occur at ablation sites, particularly when large heterotopias are treated (40).

MOTILITY DISORDERS AND INFILTRATIVE DISEASES

Primary Achalasia

Definition. *Primary achalasia* is an idiopathic condition characterized by incomplete relaxation of the lower esophageal sphincter with decreased or absent esophageal peristalsis.

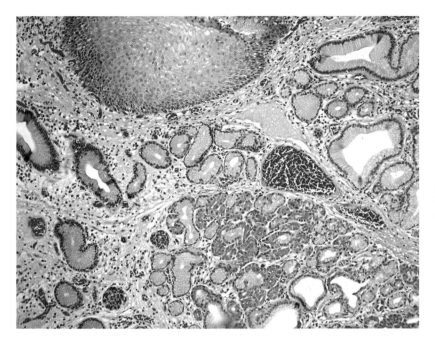

Figure 2-11

PANCREATIC HETEROTOPIA OF THE ESOPHAGUS

Discrete lobules of pancreatic acini and ducts (left) are present in glandular mucosa at the gastro-esophageal junction.

Clinical Features. Primary achalasia is rare, occurring in only 1 per 100,000 persons (41). The disorder usually affects men and women in the 6th decade of life. Primary achalasia is presumably an immune-mediated motility disorder characterized by progressive dysphagia to solids and liquids, regurgitation of undigested food, heartburn, and weight loss. Manometric studies demonstrate aperistalsis after swallowing and incomplete relaxation with elevated pressures in the lower esophageal sphincter (42). Barium esophagram shows impaired esophageal emptying and symmetric tapering of the distal esophagus ("bird beak" sign); the mid and lower esophagus may be dilated and tortuous ("sigmoid esophagus") and display air-fluid levels (43).

Pathogenesis. Primary achalasia results from immune-mediated destruction of the myenteric plexus, including ganglion cells, nerves, and dorsal motor nuclei. These changes result in elevated resting pressures in the lower esophageal sphincter because they predominantly affect intrinsic parasympathetic fibers that normally inhibit contraction (41). The disease likely results from a combination of environmental stimuli in genetically susceptible individuals. It is associated with HLA DQw1, which is prevalent among patients with Sjogren syndrome, Hashimoto thyroiditis, diabetes mellitus, and other autoimmune disorders, as well as HLA

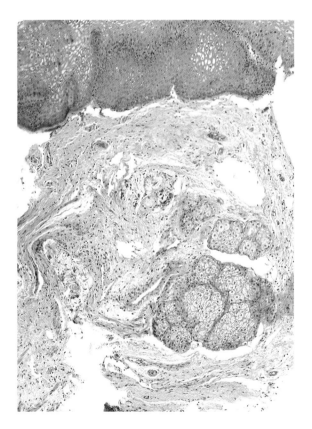

Figure 2-12

SEBACEOUS HETEROTOPIA OF THE ESOPHAGUS

Sebaceous glands are arranged in lobules and contain lipid-rich cells with vacuolated cytoplasm.

DQB*0602 and DRB1*12 alleles in white and black patients, respectively (44,45). Familial cases occur in the setting of Allgrove syndrome (isolated glucocorticoid deficiency, achalasia, alacrima) and have an autosomal recessive inheritance pattern (46).

Gross Findings. The esophagus is markedly dilated and may contain epiphrenic diverticula (fig. 2-13A). The mucosal surface can be normal in early disease, but is often white and scaly or corrugated due to reactive squamous hyperplasia in patients with incomplete esophageal emptying. Patients with severe dysmotility have retained luminal material in the dilated esophagus.

Microscopic Findings. Characteristic features include mononuclear cell-rich inflammation of the myenteric plexus with occasional eosinophils, plasma cells, and mast cells. The nerves may be partially or completely replaced by collagen in later stages, and interstitial cells of Cajal are often absent (47). Ganglion cells, which typically number 1 to 3 per 400X field, are inconspicuous or absent, particularly in the distal and mid esophagus; residual ganglion cells display lymphocytic infiltration ("ganglionitis") or degenerative cytologic features (fig. 2-13B). Hypertrophy of the muscularis propria may be present, although the wall typically shows fibrosis and/or dystrophic calcifications in patients with advanced disease.

Lymphoid aggregates and germinal centers are often numerous in the submucosa, and the mucosa displays stasis-related changes with squamous hyperplasia, parakeratosis, dyskeratosis, edema, and CD4-positive intraepithelial lymphocytes (fig. 2-13C,D). These features should not be considered to be within the spectrum of lymphocytic esophagitis since they reflect mucosal irritation rather than a primary inflammatory condition (48).

Treatment and Prognosis. Pneumatic dilatation of the gastroesophageal junction provides relief for up to 90 percent of patients; those who require further intervention may undergo esophagomyotomy (Heller procedure) or, in some cases, esophagectomy (49). Pharmacologic therapy with botulinum toxin injection is generally reserved for patients who are not candidates for endoscopic or surgical therapy (50). Patients with achalasia are at increased risk for squamous cell carcinoma (51).

Secondary Achalasia

Definition. *Secondary achalasia* (also termed *pseudoachalasia*) is diminished or absent lower esophageal sphincter relaxation and abnormal peristalsis resulting from an identifiable cause.

Clinical Features. Approximately 2 to 4 percent of individuals with esophageal dysmotility have secondary achalasia (52). Affected patients tend to be older, with a variety of comorbid conditions that affect esophageal motility, including carcinoma. Clinical manifestations of secondary achalasia are similar to those of primary achalasia in that patients complain of progressive dysphagia to solids and liquids, vomiting, and/or aspiration. Patients with achalasia resulting from malignancy usually have a shorter duration of symptoms than patients with primary achalasia or dysmotility due to other etiologies, and the former frequently have associated weight loss (53). Manometric findings are similar to those of patients with primary achalasia (49).

Pathogenesis. Secondary achalasia results from destruction of the myenteric plexus by any one of a number of causes. The most frequent cause in the United States is infiltration of the myenteric plexus by invasive adenocarcinoma, particularly, Barrett esophagus-associated adenocarcinoma and carcinomas of the gastric fundus; metastases from the lung, breast, kidney, and other sites produce similar findings (fig. 2-14) (54). Secondary achalasia occasionally occurs as a paraneoplastic manifestation of pulmonary small cell carcinoma among patients with anti-neuronal antibody type 1 (ANNA-1) disease (55).

Amyloidosis, sarcoidosis, mediastinal fibrosis, and a variety connective tissue disorders (e.g., progressive systemic sclerosis, mixed connective tissue disease, Sjogren syndrome, and systemic lupus erythematosus) cause fibrosis and protein deposition in the esophageal wall (56). Less frequent etiologies include increased sympathetic tone in patients with Raynaud phenomenon and segmental parasympathetic demyelination and axonal degeneration among patients with diabetes mellitus (57).

Gross Findings. Similar to patients with primary achalasia, those with secondary achalasia often have proximal esophageal dilation with retained food. Amyloidosis and fibrosis may produce smooth strictures that simulate primary

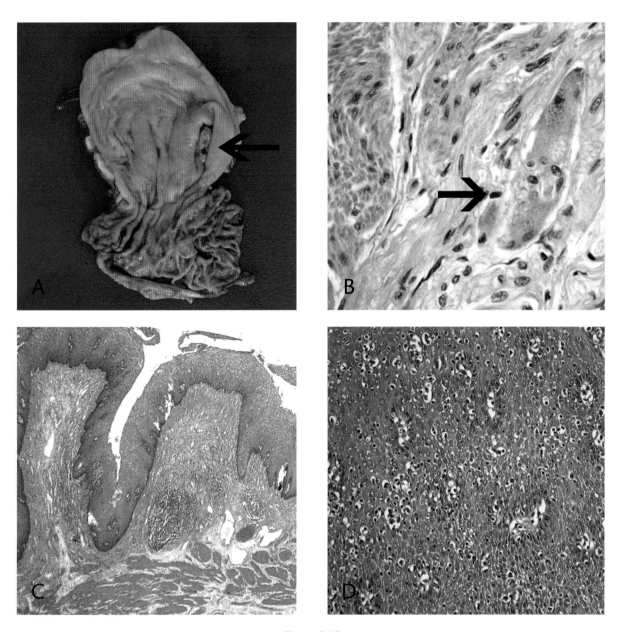

Figure 2-13

PRIMARY ACHALASIA

The esophagus is markedly dilated, with a corrugated appearance owing to squamous hyperplasia. An epiphrenic diverticulum (arrow) is present above the squamocolumnar junction (A). The myenteric plexus contains occasional degenerative ganglion cells (arrow) infiltrated by lymphocytes (B). The undulating surface displays squamous hyperplasia (C) with intraepithelial lymphocytosis resulting from stasis-related mucosal irritation (D).

achalasia, whereas patients with secondary achalasia due to cancer usually have an irregular gastroesophageal junction or malignant-appearing strictures (53). Patients with generalized gastrointestinal dysmotility also have retained food in the stomach. Connective tissue disorders are associated with gastric antral vascular ectasia (GAVE) and gastrointestinal telangiectasias.

Microscopic Findings. Patients with secondary achalasia usually have normal numbers of ganglion cells in the myenteric plexus with the exception of paraneoplastic achalasia (54,55).

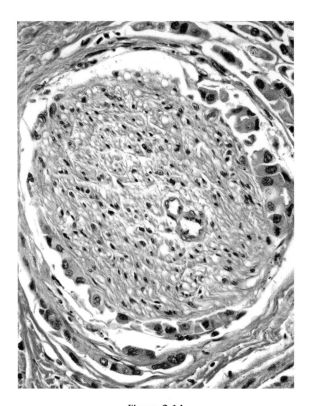

Figure 2-14

**SECONDARY ACHALASIA DUE
TO INFILTRATING CARCINOMA**

This patient with progressive dysphagia died in the emergency department from massive hematemesis. Autopsy revealed extensive infiltration of the myenteric plexus by metastatic mammary carcinoma.

Direct infiltration of the myenteric plexus by tumor cells is characteristic of patients with cancer-related dysmotility. Connective tissue disorders characteristically show mononuclear cell-rich inflammation and fibrosis of the myenteric plexus; granulomas and amyloid deposits are helpful clues when present.

Treatment and Prognosis. The prognosis of patients with secondary achalasia is related to the nature of the underlying disorder. Patients with associated carcinomas or paraneoplastic syndromes usually present with advanced stage disease and have a grim prognosis. Secondary achalasia is often refractory to pneumatic dilatation and requires surgical intervention (49).

Chagas Disease

Definition. *Chagas disease* is secondary achalasia caused by *Trypanosoma cruzi*.

Clinical Features. *Trypanosoma cruzi* is endemic in South and Central America where eight million people are infected (58). Approximately 300,000 persons in the United States are infected, most of whom are immigrants from endemic countries (59). Patients are usually infected during childhood following bites from reduviid insects that carry the parasite, although congenital infection and transmission through blood transfusion or organ transplantation can occur. Most people clear the organisms spontaneously, but 20 to 30 percent develop persistent infection, which can be associated with widespread injury to the gastrointestinal tract, heart, and nervous system (60,61).

Patients with esophageal Chagas disease typically complain of dysphagia to solids and liquids, although delayed gastric emptying, chronic malabsorptive diarrhea due to bacterial overgrowth, and constipation can all occur as a result of generalized dysmotility of the gastrointestinal tract. Chronic constipation and megacolon result from incomplete relaxation of the internal anal sphincter (61). Approximately 25 percent of chronically infected patients develop myocarditis or dilated cardiomyopathy (62). Imaging findings reveal air-fluid levels in the dilated esophagus as well as frequent dilation of the remaining gastrointestinal tract, including the gallbladder and biliary tree.

Pathogenesis. *Trypanosoma cruzi* infects a variety of cell types. Manifestations of chronic disease are related to injury of muscular organs, such as the heart and gastrointestinal tract, and destruction of myenteric neurons. Chronically infected patients have high levels of circulating anti-acetylcholine receptor antibodies (63). It is not clear whether neuronal destruction is directly caused by the parasite, or results from an exuberant inflammatory host response to the organism.

Gross Findings. The esophagus is markedly dilated and tortuous, and contains food, often in association with similar changes in the stomach. Abnormally high anal sphincter tone may be evident upon passage of the endoscope or colonoscope (61).

Microscopic Findings. *Trypanosoma cruzi* are rarely identified in ganglion cells of infected patients; most cases come to clinical attention only after ganglion cells are destroyed. Secondary

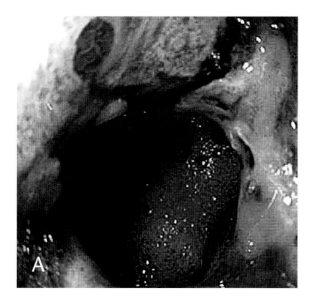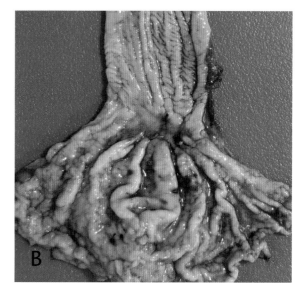

Figure 2-15

SCLERODERMA

Severe acid-related injury and ulcers are present in the distal esophagus (A). An esophagogastrectomy specimen from a patient with scleroderma shows thickened, corrugated squamous mucosa and an indurated ulcer at the gastroesophageal junction (B).

inflammatory changes in the rest of the esophageal wall are similar to those of primary achalasia.

Treatment and Prognosis. Nifurtimox and benznidazole effectively reduce parasitemia. Benzofuran derivatives are active against circulating and intracellular organisms, and cause fewer side effects compared with other agents (64). Unfortunately, none of these agents reverse the cardiac and gastrointestinal sequela of chronic infection; death is usually due to cardiac complications.

Progressive Systemic Sclerosis

Definition. *Progressive systemic sclerosis* (*scleroderma*) is a subtype of collagen vascular disease with a predilection for the esophagus. It is a multi-system immune-mediated disorder characterized by progressive fibrosis and vascular ectasias of the skin, gastrointestinal tract, lungs, and kidneys, often accompanied by vasculitis. The gastrointestinal tract is the most commonly affected organ system; esophageal changes are present in up to 90 percent of patients with scleroderma (65).

Clinical Features. Symptoms include gastroesophageal reflux disease, vomiting, and weight loss. Manometric studies reveal decreased resting tone in the lower esophageal sphincter and low-amplitude peristalsis (66).

Pathogenesis. The etiology of progressive systemic sclerosis is unknown. Affected individuals are more likely to harbor HLA-DRB1, HLA-DQB1, HLA-DPB1, and HLA-DOA1 alleles, as well as alterations in genes that modulate B- and T-cell activation (67). Patients with some other collagen vascular diseases have high titers of anti-U1RNP (68).

Gross Findings. The gastroesophageal junction is usually patulous and displays severe acid-related injury owing to decreased resting tone of the lower esophageal sphincter (fig. 2-15A). The remaining esophagus is often dilated, particularly in advanced stages of disease. The hyperplastic mucosa has a corrugated appearance, reflecting chronic irritation due to stasis (fig. 2-15B).

Microscopic Findings. Diffuse collagen deposition is characteristically present in all layers of the esophagus but is most pronounced in the inner circular layer of the muscularis propria, particularly in the distal two thirds of the esophagus (fig. 2-16) (69). Mural inflammation is minimal to absent. The myenteric plexus is uninflamed and ganglion cells are preserved.

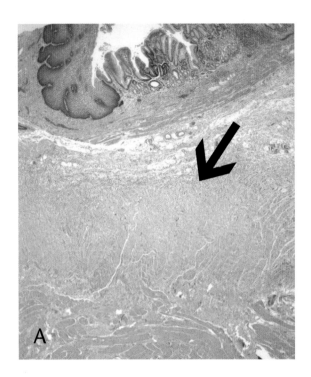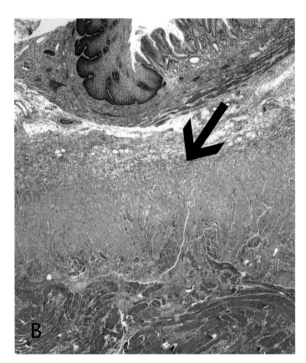

Figure 2-16

SCLERODERMA

Collagen deposition is present in all layers of the esophageal wall, particularly the inner layer of the muscularis propria (arrow) (A). A trichrome stain highlights collagen in the inner muscular layer (arrow) with relative sparing of the outer muscularis propria (B).

Arterioles of the submucosa and adventitia often show intimal proliferation. Reflux-related ulcers, erosions, and inflammation are usually present in the distal esophagus.

Treatment and Prognosis. Treatment consists of anti-inflammatory and immunosuppressive agents. Complications include stricture, perforation, fistulae, and superimposed candidiasis (70). Patients with progressive systemic sclerosis are at increased risk for Barrett esophagus (71).

Other Disorders with Abnormal Manometric Findings

Diffuse esophageal spasm, idiopathic muscular hypertrophy (nutcracker esophagus), and *isolated hypertensive lower esophageal sphincter* are clinically defined motility disorders based on imaging and manometric studies. Their gross and histologic features remain poorly characterized. The best studied is idiopathic muscular hypertrophy, which displays concentric thickening of the distal two thirds of the esophagus, producing a "funnel shaped" deformity and a

"grasping" sensation upon instrumentation with an endoscope or nasogastric tube (72).

CAUSES OF ESOPHAGEAL HEMORRHAGE

Varices

Definition. *Varices* are dilated collateral veins resulting from portosystemic shunting in the setting of portal venous hypertension.

Clinical Features. The demographic features of esophageal varices parallel those of chronic liver diseases and cirrhosis; approximately 50 percent of cirrhotic patients develop varices (73). Parasitic infections of the biliary tree, such as *Schistosoma* species, *Clonorchis sinensis*, and *Opisthorchis viverrini*, can cause portal hypertension and varices, especially in endemic regions (74). Esophageal varices develop at a rate of 8 percent per year among cirrhotic patients. They occur in the deep and superficial layers of the esophagus and stomach, in the pelvis (hemorrhoids), and in the epigastric veins of the periumbilical area ("caput medusae"). Those of

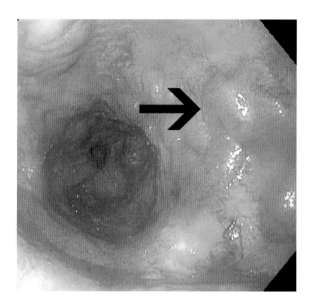

Figure 2-17

ESOPHAGEAL VARICES

Tortuous blue-tinged varices (arrow) are oriented parallel to the long axis of the esophagus.

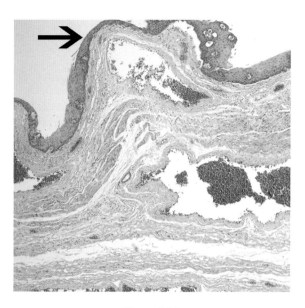

Figure 2-18

ESOPHAGEAL VARICES

Sections taken at autopsy from a patient with variceal bleeding show dilated, thin-walled veins in the mucosa and submucosa. The overlying squamous epithelial layers are attenuated (arrow).

the distal esophagus and stomach are at highest risk for rupture and bleeding.

Varices are asymptomatic until bleeding occurs. Minor bleeding episodes may be subclinical or produce melena, whereas massive bleeding results in hematemesis. Variceal bleeding occurs at a rate of 5 to 15 percent annually (75).

Pathogenesis. Chronic liver disease leads to fibrosis, architectural distortion of the parenchyma, and decreased endogenous nitric oxide production, all of which increase resistance to intrahepatic blood flow. Compensatory portosystemic collateral venous channels develop, but are insufficient to relieve elevated portal pressures. As a result, pressures in the portal venous system that normally range from 3 to 5 mmHg increase to more than 10 to 12 mmHg (76). Intraluminal pressures are further elevated as esophageal veins cross the muscularis propria, causing them to dilate and herniate into the mucosa (77).

Gross Findings. Endoscopic examination is the gold standard for diagnosing varices. Bleeding risk is related to vessel diameter, which is graded as small (5 mm or less) or large (more than 5 mm). Varices are longitudinally oriented and often tortuous. They may resemble large folds when surfaced by normal mucosa, or are blue and shiny when distended (fig. 2-17). Red wales are longitudinal,

whip-like markings of the variceal surfaces that are considered to reflect high bleeding risk (78). Varices may be apparent at autopsy: they are longitudinally oriented flat areas of blue discoloration that are best appreciated when the esophagus is everted and formalin-fixed prior to sectioning.

Microscopic Features. Cross sections demonstrate thin, ectatic veins that expand the submucosa and are surfaced by eroded, inflamed, or normal squamous mucosa (fig. 2-18). They may contain thrombi or show perivenular hemorrhage, particularly when patients undergo endoscopic therapy (77).

Treatment and Prognosis. Vasopressin, somatostatin analogues, and β-blockers can be used to decrease overall blood flow through the portal venous system. Patients at high risk for variceal bleeding may undergo variceal ligation. Those who experience multiple bleeding episodes despite these treatments are candidates for transjugular intrahepatic portosystemic shunt (TIPS), which is considered a bridge to liver transplantation (73).

The mortality risk during the first episode of variceal bleeding is 15 to 20 percent and rises to 50 percent after 1 year, despite aggressive

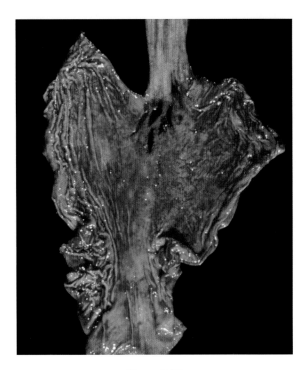

Figure 2-19

MALLORY-WEISS LACERATIONS

Mucosal tears are usually located on the lesser curvature of the proximal stomach. They occasional cross the gastroesophageal junction and emanate into the esophagus.

management (79). Patients who undergo shunt procedures are at risk for hepatic encephalopathy.

Mucosal Tears and Esophageal Rupture

Definition. *Mucosal tear* (also termed *Mallory-Weiss tear*) is a superficial laceration in the distal esophagus and proximal stomach. *Esophageal rupture* (also termed *Boerhaave syndrome*) is a transmural laceration of the esophagus.

Clinical Features. Mucosal tears account for up to 15 percent of all cases of acute upper gastrointestinal bleeding, and most patients present with hemoptysis or hematemesis (80). They usually develop in patients who experience rapidly increased pressure gradients across the gastroesophageal junction. Esophageal rupture is extremely rare. It is heralded by the sudden onset of severe chest pain and results in massive hemorrhage with hypovolemic shock. Both types of injury tend to occur in elderly patients and are reported more often in men (80). Mucosal lacerations are more common among alcoholic patients and others who have episodes of violent retching,

but can also occur in pregnant patients during labor and victims of traumatic abdominal injury.

Iatrogenic tears develop as a result of endoscopy or transesophageal echocardiogram, particularly among patients with low body mass indices. Mucosal tears complicate 0.007 to 0.49 percent of upper endoscopic procedures (81).

Pathogenesis. Vomiting, retching, severe coughing, or even forceful hiccups can result in mucosal tears or esophageal rupture (82). Shearing forces due to powerful contractions of the diaphragm can tear the mucosa and deeper layers, especially when a hiatal hernia is present (83).

Gross Findings. Mucosal tears are longitudinal rents in the lesser curvature of the proximal stomach that extend along the right lateral aspect of the esophagus (fig. 2-19) (80). Esophageal ruptures are most common in the distal esophagus, approximately 3 to 6 cm above the diaphragm. They usually span 2 to 3 cm and elicit a striking inflammatory reaction in periesophageal soft tissues.

Microscopic Findings. Mucosal tears extend into submucosa where hemorrhage, organizing fibrin, and neutrophil-rich inflammation are encountered immediately after the injury. These changes become progressively organized with granulation tissue, chronic inflammation, and fibrosis. Esophageal rupture is characterized by transmural hemorrhage with little or no inflammation in the acute setting.

Treatment and Prognosis. Most mucosal tears resolve spontaneously and can be managed conservatively; endoscopic clip placement, epinephrine injection, or argon plasma coagulation can be used in cases of persistent bleeding (80). Esophageal rupture requires immediate intervention. Patients may undergo endoscopic stent placement with drains in the pleural space, although surgical repair is usually required. Esophageal rupture is a catastrophic event that is fatal in up to 40 percent of cases (84).

INFLAMMATORY CONDITIONS OF THE ESOPHAGUS

Corrosive Esophagitis

Definition. *Corrosive esophagitis* (also termed *caustic esophagitis*) is an esophageal injury caused by the ingestion of chemicals, usually household cleaners.

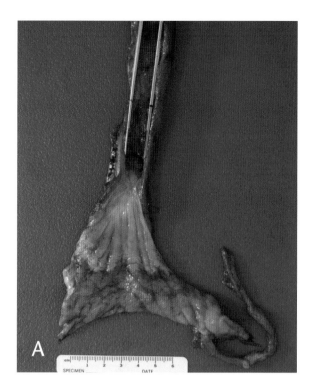 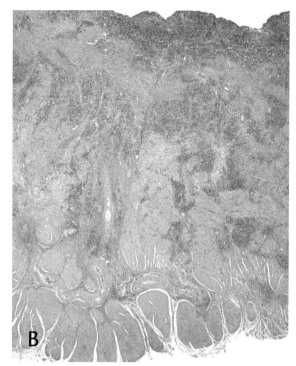

Figure 2-20

CORROSIVE ESOPHAGITIS WITH STRICTURE

Esophagogastrectomy was required after a patient developed a long-segment stricture following ingestion of a combination of sodium hydroxide and sodium hypochlorite (A). Fibrosis of the muscularis propria and dense, patchy chronic inflammation are present in the stricture (B).

Clinical Features. Up to 80 percent of cases of caustic esophagitis occur in children who accidentally ingest household cleaners. Affected adults may ingest harmful substances in attempted suicides or under the effects of alcohol and other agents that impair judgment. Caustic ingestion is more common in developing countries due to lack of education and regulation of potentially harmful agents (85).

Dysphagia, abdominal pain, and vomiting or hematemesis occur within hours of contact with the esophagus and stomach. Pain with swallowing, drooling, and respiratory distress reflect burns in the mouth and upper airways. Patients should be monitored for increasingly severe pain within the first 2 weeks of ingestion, as perforations may develop within that time. Progressive dysphagia results from strictures at sites of mural injury.

Pathogenesis. Many alkaline household cleaners contain potassium hydroxide and penetrate deeply into tissues where they combine with proteins to cause liquefactive necrosis and vascular thrombosis. Lye is another metal hydroxide compound that has been used by those attempting suicide and causes a similar injury. Acid burns produce eschars that may limit their penetration beyond that of the initial insult (85). For this reason, acids tend to cause less severe injury than alkaline compounds.

Gross Findings. Endoscopy is often delayed due to the risk of perforation. Tissue friability and black eschars are surrounded by striking edema. Long segment strictures and mucosal thickening occur after healing. Resection specimens from patients with obstructing strictures feature a short, thickened esophagus with luminal narrowing (fig. 2-20A)

Microscopic Findings. Early injury is marked by necrosis, hemorrhage, and edema. Mucosal sloughing and granulation tissue formation occur within days of ingestion. Healed segments show re-epithelialization and mural collagen deposition, often accompanied by chronic inflammatory cell infiltrates (fig. 2-20B) (86).

Treatment and Prognosis. Patients with perforation or massive bleeding require emergent surgery. Those who are amenable to conservative management are at risk for severe gastroesophageal reflux disease. Mucosal healing may be accompanied by mural scarring with impaired motility or obstruction (85). Lye ingestion is associated with an increased risk of squamous cell carcinoma (86).

Gastroesophageal Reflux Disease

Definition. *Gastroesophageal reflux disease* (GERD) is a type of esophageal injury resulting from retrograde flow of gastric or duodenal contents into the esophagus.

Clinical Features. GERD is an increasingly common disorder among adults and children and is the most important risk factor for developing Barrett esophagus. It is more common among individuals who consume alcohol and use tobacco products (87). Obesity, pregnancy, hiatal hernia, scleroderma and related connective tissue diseases, and neuromuscular dysfunction are important risk factors. Its prevalence is estimated at 18 to 28 percent in North America and 9 to 26 percent in Europe compared with less than 10 percent in Asia and the Middle East (88). The incidence is approximately 5 per 1,000 persons in the United States and United Kingdom (89).

GERD equally affects men and women, and blacks and whites, although white men are more likely to develop erosive esophagitis, Barrett esophagus, and adenocarcinoma than other groups (90). Rising rates of obesity and central adiposity are partly responsible for the increasing incidence of GERD (91). Some evidence suggests that widespread *Helicobacter pylori* eradication also plays a role: chronic gastritis due to *H. pylori* decreases the acidity of gastric contents, thereby protecting the distal esophagus from acid-related injury (92). Seventy to 85 percent of infants experience gastroesophageal reflux in the first year of life, and premature infants are at even higher risk due to ineffective peristalsis (93).

GERD produces endoscopically or histologically appreciable esophageal injury as well as a variety of clinical manifestations (94). Symptoms usually result from reflux of gastric acid, although retrograde flow of bilious duodenal contents into the esophagus causes similar changes. Common presenting symptoms include epigastric burning, regurgitation, dysphagia, and abdominal fullness. Some patients complain of chest pain that simulates angina pectoris, whereas others develop chronic cough, hoarseness, laryngitis, and dental erosions. Infants may present with vomiting, gagging, failure to thrive, or poor weight gain. Symptoms tend to be more severe after meals due to postprandial pooling of acid, and they may be aggravated by recumbency (95).

Most patients are diagnosed based on clinical features and endoscopic findings. pH monitoring can help establish the diagnosis in symptomatic patients who have normal endoscopic findings (94).

Pathogenesis. The lower esophageal sphincter muscles and diaphragmatic crus normally work synergistically to prevent retrograde flow of gastroduodenal contents. Prolonged relaxation of the lower esophageal sphincter and weakening of the diaphragmatic crus lead to retrograde flow of gastric and duodenal contents. Factors that decrease resting tone of the lower esophageal sphincter or increase pressure on the gastroesophageal junction promote reflux into the distal esophagus and exacerbate GERD.

Reflux-related mucosal injury was previously believed to result from the direct effects of acid and pepsin on the squamous mucosa. However, recent data suggest injured squamous epithelial cells elaborate cytokines that incite an inflammatory response and induce epithelial cell proliferation (96). Inflammatory mediators, such as interleukin (IL)-8, IL-6, and platelet activating factor, recruit leukocytes from the peripheral blood and stimulate production of other molecules, including IL-1β, tumor necrosis factor-alpha (TNF-α), and eotaxins. The net effect of these changes is a self-sustaining cycle of inflammation and repair that causes mucosal damage and remodeling (97,98).

Gross Findings. Endoscopic alterations are most pronounced in the distal 5 to 10 cm of the esophagus. Although historical data suggested that 50 percent of patients with GERD symptoms lack endoscopic evidence of injury, most patients with nonerosive reflux disease (NERD) do have endoscopic abnormalities when high-resolution endoscopic techniques are used. However, erosive esophagitis is present in only 30 percent of patients with heartburn, and approximately 20 percent of patients with clinical

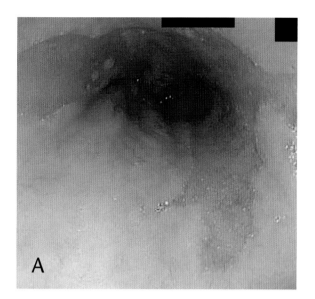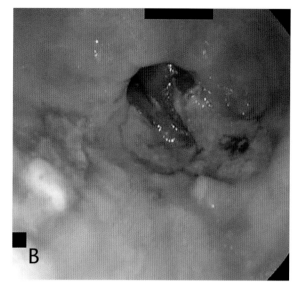

Figure 2-21

GASTROESOPHAGEAL REFLUX DISEASE

Mild reflux-related injury produces linear areas of erythema emanating from the gastroesophageal junction (A). More severe injury causes ulcers surfaced by yellow-white exudates near the gastroesophageal junction (B).

symptoms have normal endoscopic examinations (99). Mild changes include erythema and increased vascularity.

Erosive esophagitis is defined by loss of mucosal integrity, or "breaks" in the mucosa that appear as erosions, ulcers, and exudates (fig. 2-21A). It is endoscopically classified as low- or high-grade depending upon the linear and circumferential extent of mucosal defects (fig. 2-21B) (100).

Microscopic Findings. Acid and bile reflux induce variably severe epithelial and inflammatory changes in the squamous mucosa. The basal proliferative zone is often expanded to 10 to 15 percent of the mucosal thickness (fig. 2-22A). Papillae are elongated, occupying more than two-thirds of the total mucosal thickness (101). Dilated papillary blood vessels, or vascular lakes, may be present but are not specific features of GERD (fig. 2-22B).

Other common findings include swollen squamous epithelial cells with pale cytoplasm and multinucleated squamous cells with prominent nucleoli (fig. 2-22C,D). Unlike squamous cells infected by herpesvirus, these multinucleated cells lack nuclear molding, marginated chromatin, and intranuclear inclusions (102). Intercellular bridges are usually prominent and reflect intra-

mucosal edema; this finding has been termed "dilated intercellular spaces" and is a sensitive marker of GERD-related injury (103). Severe injury may be marked by erosions and ulcers.

GERD features intraepithelial eosinophils, neutrophils, and lymphocytes (fig. 2-23). Cytotoxic T-lymphocytes are universally present in symptomatic patients and may outnumber other cell types, including eosinophils (104). They are believed to propagate mucosal injury through the elaboration of cytokines and, in fact, are the first inflammatory cells to infiltrate the squamous epithelium in patients with GERD symptoms (105,106). Eosinophils are present in 20 to 40 percent of patients with symptomatic GERD and tend to be evenly distributed throughout the mucosa, or more concentrated in the peripapillary epithelium (107,108). Neutrophils are rarely present in nonerosive GERD but can be numerous when ulcers or erosions are identified endoscopically (101). Biopsy samples from patients who undergo photodynamic therapy, radiofrequency ablation, or cryotherapy for Barrett esophagus-related neoplasia often display mildly increased eosinophils in the re-epithelialized squamous mucosa (109).

Differential Diagnosis. The differential diagnosis of GERD includes a variety of immune-mediated, medication-related, and infectious

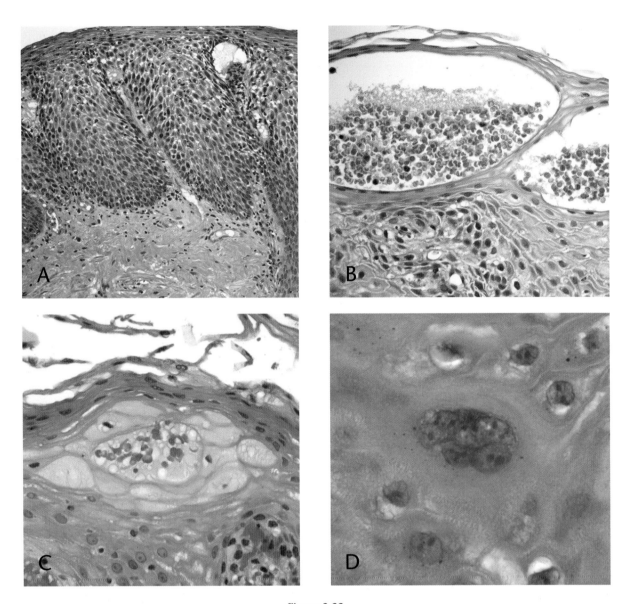

Figure 2-22

GASTROESOPHAGEAL REFLUX DISEASE

Gastroesophageal reflux causes hyperplasia of the squamous mucosa with expansion of the basal layers and elongated papillae (A). Dilated papillary blood vessels are nonspecific, but frequently present (B). Balloon cells are present in the upper two thirds of the mucosa (C). Multinucleated squamous epithelial cells are usually seen in the deeper cell layers; they contain prominent nucleoli and coarse chromatin (D).

etiologies. Most of these show characteristic clinical, endoscopic, and histologic features that readily allow their distinction, as discussed in subsequent sections. The two most problematic entities in the differential diagnosis are eosinophilic esophagitis and lymphocytic esophagitis. Although most cases of eosinophilic esophagitis feature high numbers of intraepithelial eosin-ophils (over 50 per high-power field), some show fewer eosinophils, overlapping with the spectrum of eosinophilia seen in GERD (110). Findings more typical of eosinophilic esopha-gitis include eosinophil-rich inflammation at multiple sites in the esophagus, eosinophils in superficial epithelium and keratin debris, eosinophil microabscesses, and pronounced

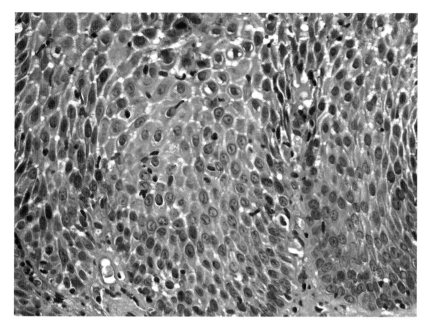

Figure 2-23

GASTROESOPHAGEAL REFLUX DISEASE

Mixed inflammation is present throughout the mucosal thickness. Small, mature T-lymphocytes with irregular nuclear contours ("squiggle cells") are present in high numbers, accompanying singly dispersed eosinophils, most of which are intact. Intercellular bridges are prominent.

Table 2-1

CLINICAL AND HISTOLOGIC FEATURES OF EOSINOPHILIC ESOPHAGITIS AND GASTROESOPHAGEAL REFLUX DISEASE

Feature	Eosinophilic Esophagitis	Gastroesophageal Reflux Disease
Clinical Presentation	Any age group	Any age group
	Men more than women	Men and women equally affected
	Atopic disorders, including asthma	Heartburn, epigastric pain, bloating, regurgitation
	Dysphagia to solids, impaction	
	Nausea and vomiting in children	Chronic cough, hoarseness
Endoscopic Findings	Rings, linear furrows, plaques anywhere in esophagus	Mucosal erythema, ulcers, strictures distally
Distribution of Disease	Patchy, often spares distal esophagus	More severe in distal esophagus
Histologic Features		
Numbers of eosinophils	Often >15 per high-power field	Usually <15 per high-power field
Distribution of eosinophils	More numerous in superficial epithelium	Evenly distributed in epithelium or more numerous in peri-papillary areas
Eosinophil microabscesses	Common	Absent
Degranulated eosinophils	Frequent, may be in aggregates	Rare, isolated cells
Eosinophil-rich parakeratosis	Common, highly specific	Absent
Lymphocytes	Present, fewer than eosinophils	Present, often outnumber eosinophils
Mucosal injury		
Basal zone hyperplasia	Often 50% of mucosal thickness	Up to 15% of mucosal thickness
Papillary elongation	Usually mild	Prominent
Intercellular edema	Present, often marked	Present
Hyalinized lamellar fibrosis	Present	Irregular fibrosis limited to strictures

eosinophil degranulation. Eosinophilic esophagitis also features a greater degree of basal zone hyperplasia, intercellular edema, and hyalinized fibrosis of the lamina propria (Table 2-1). Typical endoscopic features of eosinophilic esophagitis (e.g. furrows, multiple rings, plaques) are not seen in patients with GERD.

Intraepithelial lymphocytes are often prominent in cases of GERD and can simulate the features of lymphocytic esophagitis, especially

Figure 2-24

GASTROESOPHAGEAL REFLUX DISEASE

Gastroesophageal reflux disease features mucosal edema and prominent intraepithelial lymphocytes evenly dispersed throughout the mucosa. In fact, intraepithelial lymphocytosis confined to the gastroesophageal junction almost always reflects reflux esophagitis, rather than lymphocytic esophagitis.

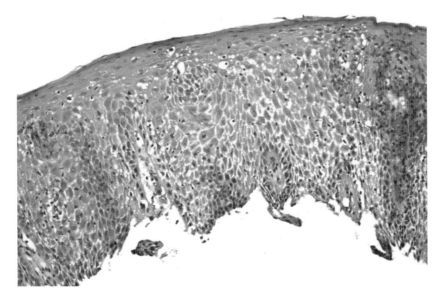

when granulocytic infiltrates are inconspicuous in the latter. The distribution of lymphocytes in GERD is similar to that of lymphocytic esophagitis, and GERD may feature both intercellular edema and single necrotic keratinocytes (48). As a general rule, intraepithelial lymphocytosis confined to the gastroesophageal junction or distal esophagus is far more likely to represent GERD than lymphocytic esophagitis (fig. 2-24).

Cases of GERD that feature erosions and ulcers can show striking regenerative changes that simulate squamous dysplasia or even carcinoma, especially when basal zone expansion, mitotic activity, and nuclear enlargement are prominent. Dysplasia shows an abrupt transition from the adjacent, non-neoplastic epithelium with partial or full-thickness architectural distortion and cytologic abnormalities (fig. 2-25). Abnormal keratinization with prominent parakeratosis, development of a granular cell layer (epidermoid metaplasia), and hyperkeratosis are more common in dysplasia than non-neoplastic, regenerative mucosa (fig. 2-26). Reactive squamous mucosa shows orderly architecture with a uniform interface between basal epithelial cells and the lamina propria. Proliferating squamous epithelial cells and mitotic figures are confined to the basal layers (fig. 2-27A,B). Regenerating squamous mucosa adjacent to ulcers may show pseudoepitheliomatous hyperplasia (fig. 2-27C) with an irregular interface between the epithelium and lamina propria; bizarre fibroblasts in ulcers can simulate invasive malignancy (fig. 2-27D).

Treatment and Prognosis. Proton pump inhibitors (PPIs) block acid secretion by gastric parietal cells and are first-line agents in the management of GERD symptoms (111). Antacids and histamine-2 receptor blockers may be used to control milder symptoms or as adjuncts to PPI therapy. Lifestyle modification and weight loss can also help control symptoms.

Patients who do not experience relief with medical therapy or have alkaline reflux may require surgical or endoscopic intervention. Laparoscopic fundoplication, banding of the gastroesophageal junction, and electrical stimulation of the lower esophageal sphincter are effective strategies (112,113).

Longstanding GERD can cause peptic strictures, although the most important consequence of GERD is development of Barrett esophagus. Barrett esophagus is a premalignant condition with low risk (0.2 to 0.5 percent per year) for progression to adenocarcinoma (114). Risk factors for development of Barrett esophagus include more than 5 years of GERD, age over 50 years, male gender, obesity, and tobacco use (114).

Eosinophilic Esophagitis

Definition. *Eosinophilic esophagitis* is a hypersensitivity disorder characterized by esophageal eosinophilia. It is more appropriately considered to represent *allergic esophagitis*.

Clinical Features. Eosinophilic esophagitis is most common in Western Europe, North America, and Australia, but relatively rare in

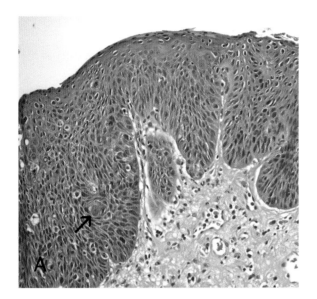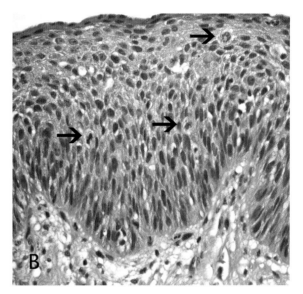

Figure 2-25

SQUAMOUS DYSPLASIA

Squamous dysplasia shows architectural abnormalities with irregular buds of dysplastic epithelium protruding into the lamina propria. Papillae project into the mucosa at irregular heights and angles. Deep keratinization is present (arrow) (A). Atypical epithelial cells with large nuclei and prominent nucleoli are present throughout the mucosa. Mitotic figures (arrows) are present in the deep and superficial layers (B).

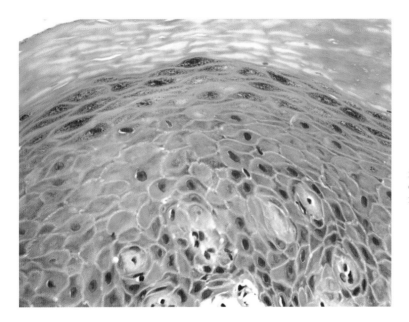

Figure 2-26

EPIDERMOID METAPLASIA

Hyperorthokeratosis overlies a prominent granular cell layer. Mature squamous cells show slight disorganization but are not overtly dysplastic.

the Middle East, Asia, and Africa (115). Its incidence is estimated at 2 to 12 per 100,000 patients who undergo upper endoscopy annually, with peaks in the 4th to 5th decades of life (116,117). The incidence of eosinophilic esophagitis has risen rapidly in recent years, largely reflecting heightened awareness, improved sanitation, and altered tolerance to antigens among Western population (118). Eradication of *H. pylori* is inversely associated with eosinophilic esophagitis, and the disease occurs with greater frequency among patients with celiac disease, inflammatory bowel disease, and other autoimmune disorders (119–122). Exposure to

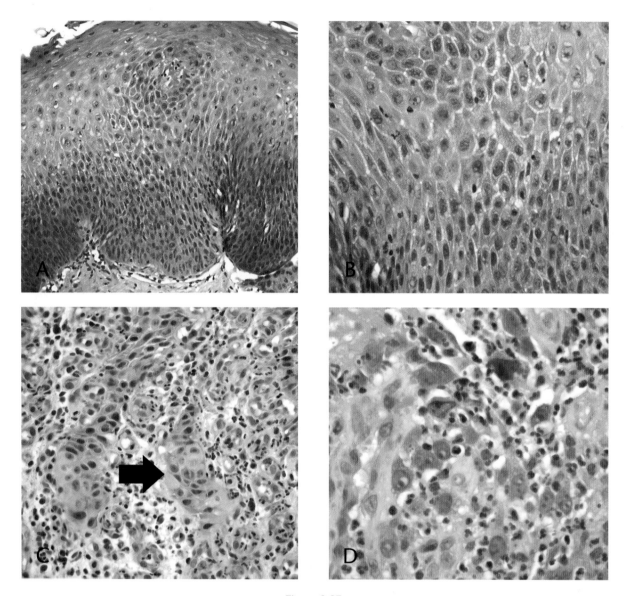

Figure 2-27

GASTROESOPHAGEAL REFLUX DISEASE

The squamous epithelium displays a smooth interface with the underlying lamina propria. Proliferating cells are confined to the deep epithelium (A). Cells in the basal zone contain nuclei with fine chromatin, inconspicuous nucleoli, and occasional mitotic figures (B). Irregular nests of squamous cells (arrow) extend into granulation tissue adjacent to an ulcer, simulating invasive carcinoma. Lesional cells contain slightly enlarged nuclei without nuclear overlapping or atypical mitotic figures (C). Reactive fibroblasts in granulation tissue contain enlarged, hyperchromatic nuclei and abundant cytoplasm (D).

antibiotics early in life and preterm birth are likely predisposing factors (123,124).

Eosinophilic esophagitis is an important and increasingly recognized cause of esophageal dysfunction in adults and children. The diagnosis is based on a constellation of clinical, endoscopic, and pathologic findings, and is defined by an absence of other causes for esophageal eosinophilia, such as GERD and idiopathic eosinophilic gastroenteritis (125,126).

Typical patients are young adults or children, particularly males, with food allergies, asthma, eczema, chronic rhinitis, environmental allergies, and other atopic disorders. Many patients have peripheral eosinophilia. The most common presenting symptom in adults is dysphagia to solids, which may be accompanied by food impaction. Infants and toddlers present with difficult feedings, and children are more likely to have vomiting and abdominal pain. Persistent inflammation and progressive remodeling of subepithelial connective tissue can cause esophageal stenosis and produce obstructive symptoms (127).

The diagnosis is usually established during upper endoscopic examination. Peripheral eosinophil counts, cytokine levels, and eosinophil granule proteins may be measured to monitor response to therapy (128).

Pathogenesis. Eosinophilic esophagitis is probably triggered by an aberrant immune response to environmental stimuli in genetically susceptible individuals. The relative risk ranges from 10- to 60-fold among family members of patients with the disorder (129). Many patients have allelic polymorphisms at 5q22 of *TSLP* which cause abnormal sensitization of type 2 T-helper (Th2) cells (130). Presumably, Th2 lymphocytes are stimulated by allergens to produce IL-13 and IL-5 as well as other pro-inflammatory cytokines (131,132). These cytokines upregulate *CCL26*, which encodes eotaxin-3, a chemotactic factor for eosinophils in the esophagus (133). Recruitment of eosinophils and mast cells damages the mucosa and promotes fibrosis through excess production of TGF-β (134). Mutations at 2p23 of *CAPN14* that affect cytoskeletal dynamics and impair epithelial barrier function are also common (135). These effects are compounded by overproduction of IL-13, which downregulates production of desmoglein, cadherin-1, and filaggrin; these cell adhesion molecules play important roles in maintaining intercellular junctions between keratinocytes (136,137).

Gross Findings. Typical endoscopic features include linear furrows, concentric rings throughout the length of the esophagus, and plaque-like white patches (fig. 2-28). Patients with longstanding disease frequently develop strictures or diaphragm-like rings with smooth edges. The findings may be patchy, and the endoscopic examination is normal in up to 25 percent of patients (138). Diagnostic histologic changes are often present in both endoscopically normal and abnormal mucosae (139,140).

The sensitivity for a histologic diagnosis improves with increasing numbers of specimens, and approaches 100 percent when five or six samples are examined (141). Endoscopists are encouraged to obtain multiple biopsy samples from all levels of the esophagus and include tissue from normal and abnormal areas to optimize diagnostic yield (126).

Microscopic Findings. Eosinophilic esophagitis features eosinophil-rich inflammation in biopsy samples from multiple levels of the esophagus. Intraepithelial eosinophilia is highly variable; eosinophils typically number at least 15 per 400X field but can range up to several hundred in a single high-power field (fig. 2-29A,B) (110). Well-oriented mucosal samples display a predominantly superficial distribution of eosinophils in the mid and upper epithelium.

Eosinophil microabscesses are accompanied by extensive eosinophil degranulation; granules often surround individual keratinocytes. Degranulated and intact eosinophils in parakeratosis account for endoscopically apparent plaques. This "scale crust" is far more commonly encountered in cases of eosinophilic esophagitis than GERD. Intraepithelial T-cells are usually present and may be numerous.

The background mucosa typically shows striking expansion of the basal zone, often accounting for 25 to 50 percent of the mucosal thickness (fig. 2-29C). Intercellular edema accentuates intercellular bridges (fig. 2-29D). Parallel arrays of hyalinized, faintly eosinophilic collagen are commonly encountered in the lamina propria, especially in patients with longstanding disease (fig. 2-29A).

Differential Diagnosis. A diagnosis of eosinophilic esophagitis should only be rendered when patients lack mucosal eosinophilia at other gastrointestinal sites; the combination of mucosal eosinophilia in the esophagus and elsewhere suggests a diagnosis of eosinophilic gastroenteritis. Eosinophilic gastroenteritis is closely related to, but more severe than, eosinophilic esophagitis. It is also a hypersensitivity disorder that shows a predilection for young males, and it is histologically indistinguishable from eosinophilic esophagitis based on esophageal biopsy analysis alone. Patients usually present with malabsorptive symptoms that reflect intestinal involvement (142).

Eosinophilic esophagitis may be indistinguishable from GERD when mucosal

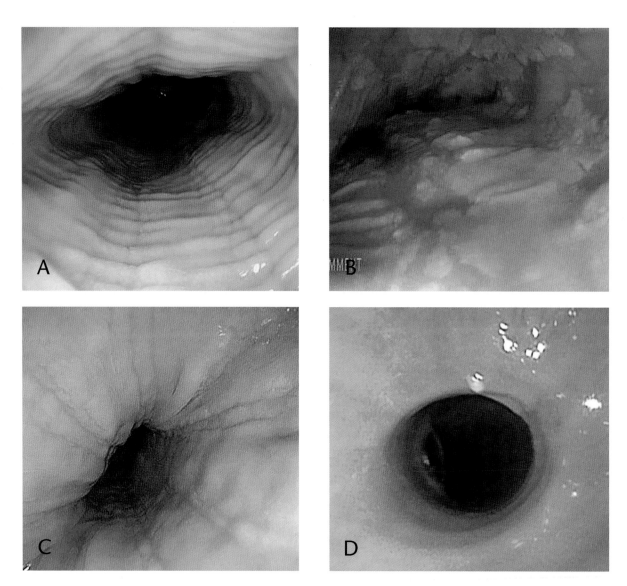

Figure 2-28

EOSINOPHILIC ESOPHAGITIS

Multiple concentric rings are characteristic of eosinophilic esophagitis. This case also shows a hint of longitudinal furrows (A). White plaques reflecting desquamated eosinophil-rich parakeratosis are apparent in another example (B). Linear furrows involve the entire circumference of the mucosa (C). Smooth diaphragm-like strictures are occasionally present (D).

eosinophilia is mild and sampling is limited to the distal esophagus (Table 2-1). Rare patients with severe GERD have far more than 15 eosinophils per high-power field in mucosal samples; their samples usually also show basal zone hyperplasia, papillary elongation, and intercellular edema (143). Distinguishing features of eosinophilic esophagitis include luminal orientation of eosinophils, eosinophil microabscesses, extensively degranulated eosinophils, and eosino-

phils in detached keratin (138,144). Lamellated, hyalinized collagen in the lamina propria favors a diagnosis of eosinophilic esophagitis, particularly in pediatric patients (145,146).

Some patients with clinical, endoscopic, and histologic features of eosinophilic esophagitis respond to PPI therapy (PPI-responsive esophageal eosinophilia) (147). These patients have gene expression profiles in esophageal biopsy samples similar to those of patients

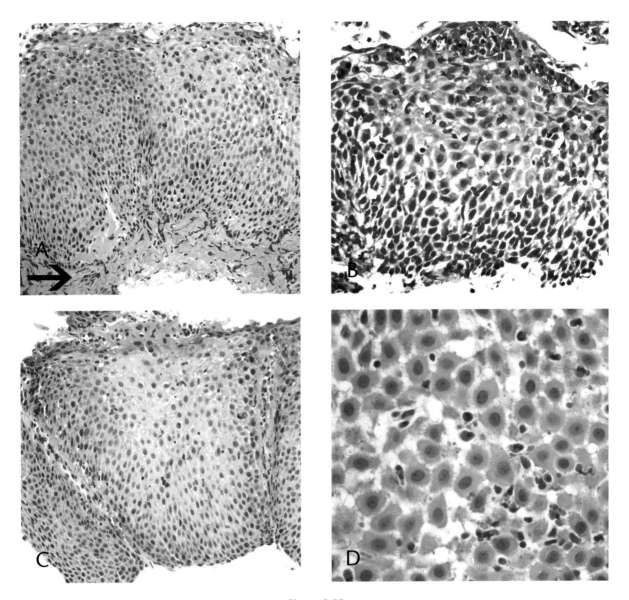

Figure 2-29

EOSINOPHILIC ESOPHAGITIS

Numerous, superficially distributed eosinophils are present in the epithelium. Hyalinized fibrosis (arrow) obliterates the lamina propria (A). Eosinophil microabscesses and degranulated eosinophils at the surface are highly specific features of eosinophilic esophagitis (B). Basal zone hyperplasia and elongated papillae simulate gastroesophageal reflux disease, although the presence of numerous degranulated eosinophils in parakeratosis is a helpful clue to the diagnosis of eosinophilic esophagitis (C). Marked mucosal edema separates squamous epithelial cells; the intercellular bridges are visible (D).

with eosinophilic esophagitis (148). Some of these patients probably have GERD, or injury triggered by GERD. Presumably, acid-induced damage exposes the deep mucosa to luminal allergens that incite an inflammatory response, which is reversed when acid suppression restores the mucosal barrier (149). On the other hand, PPIs also have anti-inflammatory prop-erties that provide symptomatic relief for many patients with eosinophilic esophagitis. For this reason, the American College of Gastroenterology recommends PPIs as one first-line therapy in the management of eosinophilic esophagitis; treatment response is no longer used to distinguish patients with eosinophilic esophagitis from those with GERD (150).

Treatment and Prognosis. Spontaneous resolution of symptoms does not occur in most patients with eosinophilic esophagitis. Treatment options include several approaches. Some patients respond to PPI therapy, elimination of dietary allergens, and intake of liquids with meals (151). Topical corticosteroids are used to induce a symptomatic response followed by budesonide for maintenance therapy; systemic corticosteroids are reserved for refractory symptoms (152,153). Although leukotriene inhibitors (montelukast) and monoclonal antibodies to IL-5 (mepolizumab and reslizumab) showed promise in early studies, their roles in managing patients with eosinophilic esophagitis are not clearly established (154). Patients with strictures can be treated with esophageal dilatation (155). Almost all patients with eosinophilic esophagitis develop recurrent symptoms upon withdrawal of treatment.

Lymphocytic Esophagitis

Definition. *Lymphocytic esophagitis (lymphocytic esophagitis pattern)* is a lymphocyte-rich inflammatory condition of the squamous mucosa with few or absent granulocytes.

Clinical Features. Lymphocytic esophagitis is a histologic pattern of injury that can be seen in association with a variety of disorders including GERD, candidiasis, esophageal dysmotility, and immune-mediated conditions. It shows a predilection for women in the 5th to 6th decades and has been increasingly reported since its description in 2006 (156,157). Approximately two-thirds of patients present with dysphagia (156–159).

Most pediatric patients with lymphocytic esophagitis have underlying Crohn disease, although the converse is not true; only 25 percent of children with Crohn disease have lymphocytic esophagitis (160,161). Unfortunately, esophageal lymphocytosis is not a specific finding in adult patients. A high percentage of adult cases reported in the literature are associated with GERD, achalasia, or candidiasis. Once these etiologies are excluded, however, a substantial number of cases are associated with celiac disease, Crohn disease, thyroiditis, collagen vascular disease, common variable immunodeficiency, and several medications (162,162a).

Pathogenesis. The etiology of lymphocytic esophagitis is unknown. Early reports that it rep-

resented a form of allergic contact injury proved to be inaccurate (158). Some authors have suggested relationships between CD8-positive T-cells in the esophageal mucosa and alcohol or tobacco use, medications, and immune-mediated injury (163,164). Esophageal lymphocytosis featuring predominantly CD4-positive T-cells occurs in association with motility disorders. At least two-thirds of patients with achalasia, 40 percent of patients with nutcracker esophagus, and 20 percent of those with diffuse esophageal spasm have intraepithelial lymphocytosis (48,165). Increased mucosal lymphocytes in the setting of esophageal dysmotility likely represents a secondary alteration related to luminal stasis rather than a pathologic process; samples obtained early in the disease course are often normal.

Gross Findings. Once GERD, infection, and esophageal motility disorders are excluded, approximately one-third of patients with lymphocytic esophagitis have a normal endoscopic examination and a similar proportion have endoscopic features that simulate the appearance of eosinophilic esophagitis with multiple rings, furrows, plaques, and strictures (fig. 2-30) (156,158).

Microscopic Findings. Lymphocytic esophagitis is defined by the presence of increased intraepithelial lymphocytes, particularly in the peripapillary epithelium, with rare or absent granulocytes (fig. 2-31) (157). Reported diagnostic criteria have focused on assessing lymphocyte number and vary from 12 to over 50 intraepithelial lymphocytes per 400X field (156, 160,161,166). Similar to eosinophilic esophagitis, however, most cases feature mucosal injury in addition to lymphocytosis.

Intraepithelial lymphocytes are accompanied by intercellular edema and dyskeratosis, and these changes are usually evident at multiple levels in the esophagus. The presence of readily apparent eosinophils or neutrophils should prompt considerations for infection, GERD, or a drug-related injury.

Differential Diagnosis. Lichen planus is an immune-mediated disorder affecting the skin and mucous membranes of middle-aged adults. Esophageal involvement is rare and almost always associated with mucocutaneous lesions. Unlike lymphocytic esophagitis, which generally displays diffuse esophageal involvement, lichen planus produces webs or strictures in the upper to mid esophagus but spares the distal esophagus. Biopsy samples show features similar to those of lymphocytic esophagitis, although there are some differences. Lichen planus features dense, band-like lymphocytic infiltrates in the lamina propria with degeneration of basal keratinocytes (fig. 2-32). Direct immunofluorescence reveals globular IgM deposits along the basement membrane and complement staining of apoptotic keratinocytes. The term "lichenoid esophagitis pattern" has been proposed to describe cases that share histologic features with lichen planus but lack supportive immunofluorescent evidence. Most of these cases could probably be classified as lymphocytic esophagitis (167). In fact, distinction between involvement of the esophagus by lichen planus and lymphocytic esophagitis may be impossible based on histologic features alone. Knowledge of the clinical and endoscopic findings, as well as the presence of band-like inflammation in the lamina propria and degeneration of basal keratinocytes, are helpful diagnostic clues.

Lymphocytes in other Types of Esophagitis. Biopsy samples from patients with GERD contain increased intraepithelial lymphocytes that often outnumber eosinophils (105,106,168). GERD usually displays mixed inflammation with scattered eosinophils and elicits changes limited to the distal esophagus (fig. 2-33). Candidiasis

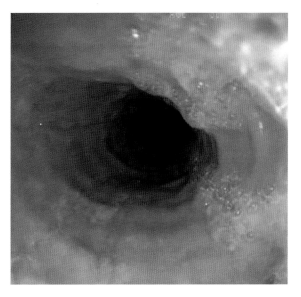

Figure 2-30

LYMPHOCYTIC ESOPHAGITIS

Concentric rings and logitudinal furrows simulate the endoscopic appearance of eosinophilic esophagitis.

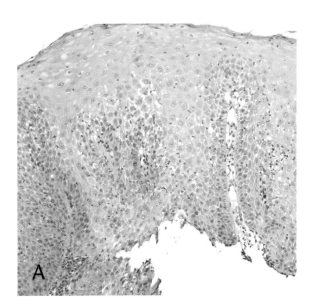
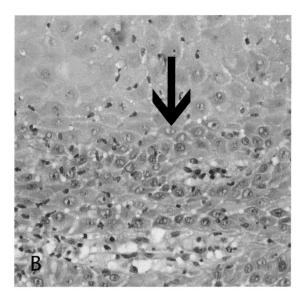

Figure 2-31

LYMPHOCYTIC ESOPHAGITIS

Squamous hyperplasia is accompanied by elongated papillae and intraepithelial lymphocytosis (A). The inflammatory infiltrate is denser in the peripapillary region (arrow). Prominent intercellular bridges reflect mucosal edema (B).

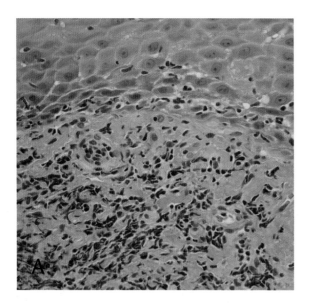
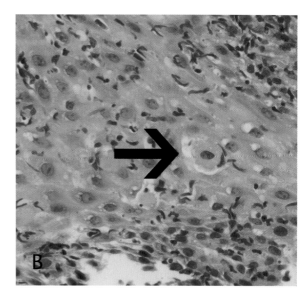

Figure 2-32

ESOPHAGEAL LICHEN PLANUS

Subepithelial lymphocytic-rich inflammation is associated with injured basal keratinocytes and infiltrating lymphocytes along the base of the epithelium (A). Numerous lymphocytes and scattered dyskeratotic cells (arrow) are present at all levels in the epithelium (B).

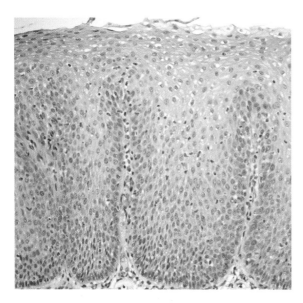

Figure 2-33

GASTROESOPHAGEAL REFLUX DISEASE

Lymphocytes outnumber eosinophils and are more numerous in the peripapillary epithelium, similar to their distribution in lymphocytic esophagitis.

elicits intraepithelial lymphocytosis and simulates lymphocytic esophagitis, especially when granulocytes are sparse. Intraepithelial lympho-

cytes are also increased in the squamous mucosa adjacent to Barrett esophagus, particularly in patients who experience frequent reflux-related symptoms or have undergone cryotherapy (164,166). Lymphocytosis in combination with striking dyskeratosis and neutrophils can be seen in drug-related injury. Ipilimumab causes this type of immune-mediated alteration and other checkpoint inhibitors produce similar, although possibly milder, changes (fig. 2-34). Given the wide range of entities that may feature intraepithelial lymphocytosis, a diagnosis of lymphocytic esophagitis should be reserved for situations in which other causes have been excluded and the findings are correlated with clinical and endoscopic information.

Treatment and Prognosis. Most studies regarding lymphocytic esophagitis are retrospective and include large numbers of patients with achalasia and GERD (156). Available data suggest that symptoms often resolve with PPI therapy or oral corticosteroids (156,163).

Drug-Induced Injury

Definition. *Drug-induced esophagitis* results from injury due to medication.

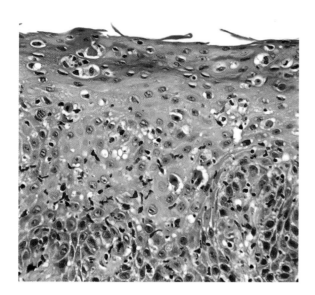

Figure 2-34

IPILIMUMAB-INDUCED ESOPHAGITIS

Numerous lymphocytes and apoptotic keratinocytes are characteristic of ipilimumab-induced injury.

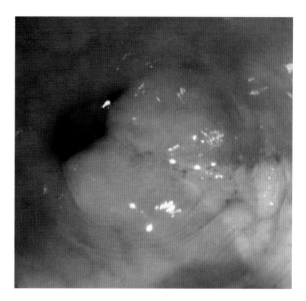

Figure 2-35

DRUG-INDUCED ESOPHAGITIS

A discrete ulcer in the distal esophagus is surfaced by yellow-white exudate and surrounded by normal squamous mucosa.

Clinical Features. Medication-related esophagitis can result from the expected therapeutic action of a drug, secondary systemic or immune-mediated effects of an agent, or direct mucosal contact with a swallowed medication. It shows a predilection for areas of esophageal narrowing or compression, including where the esophagus rests on the left mainstem bronchus and is crossed by the aorta, the gastroesophageal junction, sites of previous injury, and over an enlarged left atrium.

Almost any medication can cause esophageal injury upon prolonged contact with the squamous mucosa and, thus, patients of any age and gender may develop drug-induced esophagitis. Drug-induced esophagitis is more likely when medications are ingested while in the recumbent position or without adequate water (169). Elderly patients who take multiple medications are at higher risk, especially if they are debilitated. Common offending agents include antibiotics, nonsteroidal anti-inflammatory drugs (NSAIDs), emepronium bromide, alendronate, ferrous sulfate, phenytoin, and, most recently, crizotinib (170–172). Drugs that alter the local pH, have cytotoxic effects, or decrease tissue perfusion produce characteristic patterns of injury, discussed below. Drug-induced esophagitis is heralded by the sudden onset of retrosternal pain, odyno-phagia, dysphagia, or vomiting. Bleeding from esophageal ulcers may result in melena.

Gross Findings. Medications that exert their therapeutic effects in the esophagus produce diffuse mucosal injury. Chemotherapeutic agents cause focal or extensive desquamation as a result of their effects on proliferative epithelium. Targeted therapies, such as ipilimumab, cause immune-mediated ulcers and erythema.

Endoscopic features of drug-induced esophagitis include erosions or ulcers that are often discontinuous with the gastroesophageal junction. Impacted pill fragments may be present at sites of luminal narrowing. Most ulcers are discrete lesions surrounded by normal-appearing mucosa (fig. 2-35). "Kissing" ulcers on opposite sides of the lumen are characteristic of a drug-related injury reflecting contact of the agent with the mucosa at multiple points (169).

Microscopic Findings. Drug-induced esophagitis is associated with erosions, ulcers, and fibrinous exudates (fig. 2-36). Fragments of microcrystalline cellulose and crospovidone, two common pharmaceutical fillers, may be seen in ulcer beds or ulcer debris, although they are not, themselves, topically corrosive. Microcrystalline cellulose appears as clear, rod-shaped or chunky crystals that are birefringent

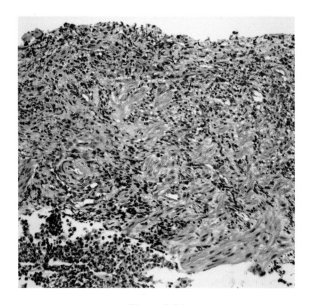

Figure 2-36

DRUG-INDUCED ESOPHAGITIS

Inflammed granulation tissue is present in a mid-esophageal ulcer.

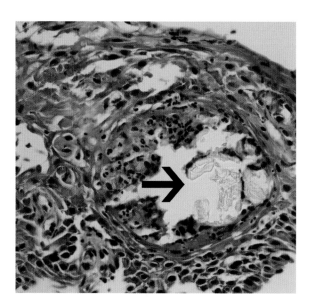

Figure 2-37

MICROCRYSTALLINE CELLULOSE

Microcrystalline cellulose appears as irregular and rod-shaped, clear, refractile fragments (arrow) embedded in inflammation.

in polarized light (fig. 2-37) (173). Crospovidone crystals are irregular, coral-shaped fragments with a pink core and purple outer rim (fig. 2-38) (173,174).

Some medications, particularly immuno-modulatory agents, cause keratinocyte necrosis, which can be a clue to a drug-related injury (175). The combination of apoptotic squamous cells in the mid and superficial epithelium, intraepithelial lymphocytes, and neutrophilic inflammation is characteristic of checkpoint inhibitors, as previously described. Specific features associated with other agents are described below.

Alendronate. Alendronate is an amino-bis-phosphonate that inhibits osteoclast-mediated bone resorption (176). It causes a severe corrosive injury when its amino acid side chain is oxidized and elaborates free radicals (177). Biopsy findings include coagulative necrosis of the squamous mucosa that resembles a caustic injury. Although alendronate has been described as a cause of esophagitis dissecans superficialis; it is not. Rather it causes mucosal necrosis and luminal casts; this extent of tissue necrosis is not within the spectrum of sloughing esophagitis (fig. 2-39).

Doxycycline. Doxycycline is commonly used in the treatment of infections, acne, and acne

rosacea. This drug acidifies its local environment to a pH of less than 3 upon dissolution, and can cause an acid burn when in direct contact with the squamous mucosa. Lesions appear as circumferential ulcers and localized areas of desquamation (178). Striking edema and neutrophil-rich inflammation in the deep and mid squamous mucosa is characteristic (fig. 2-40) (179). These layers can separate from the superficial epithelium, which undergoes coagulative necrosis and sloughs into the lumen.

Ferrous Sulfate. Oral iron supplements are widely used to treat iron-deficiency anemia and can damage mucosae through multiple mechanisms. Iron catalyzes the formation of reactive oxygen metabolites. Therapeutic iron doses generally cause mild injury, whereas high doses diffuse into cells in a concentration-dependent manner and cause direct toxicity with necrosis, perforation, and strictures. Iron deposits appear as extracellular brown crystals that are incorporated into fibroinflammatory debris and granulation tissue of the ulcer bed, and can be seen in keratinocytes (fig. 2-41A,B) (180). They are refractile, nonpolarizing, and highlighted with Prussian blue stains (fig. 2-41C).

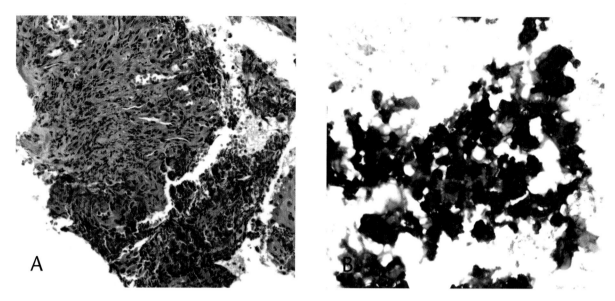

Figure 2-38

CROSPOVIDONE PILL FRAGMENTS

Crospovidone crystals are present in granulation tissue of an esophageal ulcer (A). This component of many medications contains crystals with pink cores and peripheral basophilia (B).

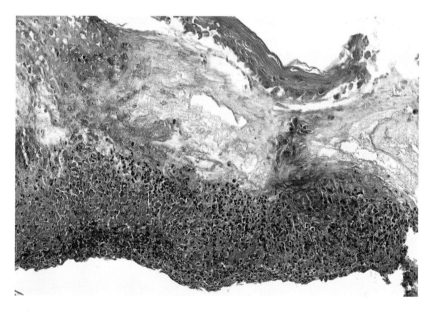

Figure 2-39

BISPHOSPHONATE-INDUCED INJURY

Full thickness coagulative necrosis of the squamous mucosa is caused by contact with bisphosphonate pills, producing the endoscopic appearance of desquamation.

Sodium Polystyrene (Kayexalate). Sodium polystyrene is a cation exchange resin used to treat hyperkalemia in renal transplant patients. In the past, the resin was suspended in a concentrated sorbitol solution, which caused severe gastrointestinal injury due to the osmotic effects of sorbitol. For this reason, sodium polystyrene is now delivered in a powder form or water-based suspension, and kayexalate-related esophageal injury has become vanishingly rare in the United States (181). Similar to all binding resins, however, kayexalate crystals can adhere to mucosal surfaces, particularly ulcers. Thus, detection of kayexalate crystals in ulcerated gastrointestinal biopsy samples should not be interpreted as pathogenic unless the drug formulation is known. Kayexalate crystals are rhomboidal or triangular, deeply basophilic,

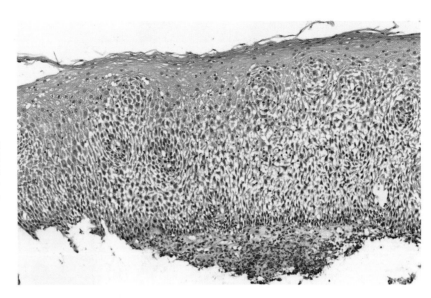

Figure 2-40

DOXYCYCLINE-INDUCED INJURY

Striking intercellular edema in the deep mucosa is accompanied by relative sparing of the superficial epithelium. A neutrophil-rich inflammatory infiltrate is also present.

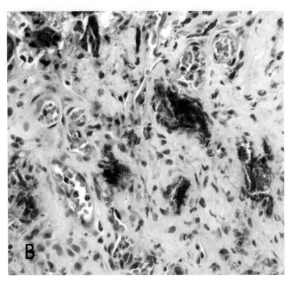

Figure 2-41

IRON PILL ESOPHAGITIS

Golden brown iron crystals are incorporated into the granulation tissue of an esophageal erosion (A) and impart a golden brown appearance to squamous cells (B). The crystals are blue with a Prussian blue stain (C).

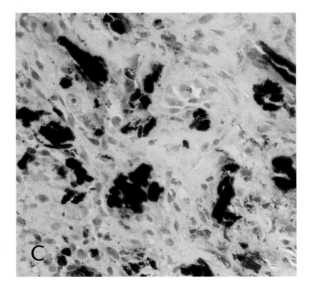

and have a characteristic internal mosaic pattern that resembles stacked bricks or fish scales. They are refractile, but do not polarize (fig. 2-42) (182).

Treatment and Prognosis. Drug-induced esophagitis is usually self-limited and symptoms resolve with supportive care. Cessation of the offending drug or PPI therapy can facilitate mucosal healing (169).

INFECTIOUS ESOPHAGITIS

Candida Esophagitis

Definition. *Candida esophagitis* (*moniliasis*) occurs secondary to infection by fungi of the *Candida* genus.

Clinical Features. *C. albicans* is the most common cause of infectious esophagitis (183). *C. glabrata* (formerly *C. torulopsis*) and *C. tropicalis* are responsible for a substantial minority of infections (184). All of these organisms tend to cause injury in immunocompromised individuals, although the nature of the immunodeficiency is highly variable and occasional patients are immunocompetent. *Candida* may proliferate in esophageal ulcers or colonize necrotic tumors.

Prior to the development of excellent antiviral therapy, *Candida* accounted for more than 50 percent of symptomatic esophagitis cases among patients with human immunodeficiency virus (HIV) infection (185). Other risk factors in the modern era include diabetes mellitus, recent antimicrobial therapy, malignancy, chemotherapy, and immunosuppressive therapy (186). Up to 30 percent of patients with eosinophilic esophagitis who receive oral corticosteroids develop *Candida* esophagitis (187). Longstanding PPI therapy is also a risk factor for candidiasis, presumably due to decreased sterilization of gastric contents (188).

Infected patients present with dysphagia, odynophagia, or epigastric pain, and often have concomitant oral thrush (189). Patients with infection elsewhere in the gastrointestinal tract are usually severely ill; they may have fungal septicemia, diarrhea, or gastrointestinal bleeding.

Pathogenesis. *Candida* are commensal inhabitants of mucocutaneous tissues. They can superficially invade the squamous epithelium when local defenses are altered or when T-cell

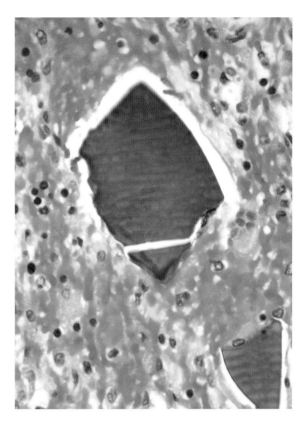

Figure 2-42

KAYEXALATE CRYSTALS

Kayexalate crystals are rhomboid and basophilic with a distinct internal mosaic pattern that resembles stacked bricks.

function is impaired. Deeper invasion of the lamina propria and hematogenous dissemination occur in extremely sick patients (183).

Gross Findings. Candidiasis elicits epithelial hyperplasia with exuberant hyperkeratosis that produces fluffy white-yellow, often confluent plaques (fig. 2-43). Insufflation of the esophagus during endoscopy separates the plaques, imparting a linear appearance. The intervening mucosa may be normal, erythematous, or edematous, and that underlying the plaques is often friable.

Microscopic Findings. *Candida* sp. are dimorphic, existing as yeast and pseudohyphae. Yeast are ovoid and span 3 to 5 μm, whereas pseudohyphae are elongated with incomplete septa; pseudohyphae are only present when the organisms are proliferating; their detection usually implies infection rather than swallowed, commensal organisms (184).

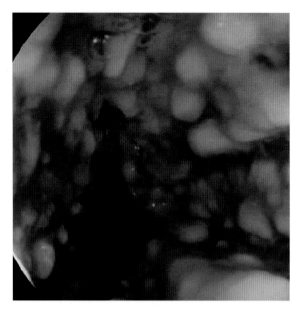

Figure 2-43

CANDIDA **ESOPHAGITIS**

Confluent yellow-white plaques are present on a background of hyperemic squamous mucosa.

Candidiasis causes squamous hyperplasia, hyperkeratosis, and parakeratosis. The mucosa is mildly edematous and contains a mixed inflammatory infiltrate featuring numerous lymphocytes and scattered neutrophils, as well as superficial microabscesses and occasional eosinophils (fig. 2-44A). Detection of neutrophilic aggregates at the mucosal surface should prompt evaluation for fungal infection, especially if associated with brightly eosinophilic parakeratosis (fig. 2-44B). However, the inflammatory infiltrate is not consistently present; it may be diminished in severely immunocompromised individuals. Pseudohyphae are usually oriented perpendicular to squamous cells (fig. 2-44B). Single detached keratinocytes and keratin debris often contain numerous organisms and can be a helpful clue to the diagnosis (fig. 2-44C).

Organisms are apparent in hematoxylin and eosin (H&E)-stained sections but can be highlighted with both periodic acid–Schiff with diastase (PAS-D) and Grocott methenamine silver (GMS) stains (fig. 2-44D).

Differential Diagnosis. The morphologic features of *Candida* are morphologically distinct from those of rarer fungal infections, such as *Aspergillus*, *Blastomyces*, and *Cryptococcus* sp. Desquamative disorders including graft-versus-host disease, radiation-induced injury, sloughing esophagitis, eosinophilic esophagitis, and even sebaceous heterotopias can produce endoscopically visible white plaques, but are readily distinguished from candidiasis based on clinical features and biopsy analysis.

Treatment and Prognosis. *Candida* esophagitis responds well to antifungal treatment with fluconazole. Intravenous amphotericin B is required to treat disseminated candidiasis. The overall prognosis is related to the nature of underlying comorbid conditions.

Herpesvirus Esophagitis

Definition. *Herpesvirus esophagitis* is infection caused by herpes simplex virus (HSV)-1 or HSV-2 (human herpes virus-1 or -2).

Clinical Features. HSV-1 has a worldwide seroprevalence of 80 to 90 percent and is more common in communities of lower socioeconomic status. HSV-2 infection is less common, with an estimated seroprevalence of 22 percent in the United States (190). *Herpes simplex viruses* infect mucous membranes, mucosae, and parenchymal organs in immunocompetent and immunocompromised hosts (191). Esophageal disease is identified in approximately 2 percent of patients at autopsy; it is usually caused by HSV-1, but HSV-2 infection is well described (192,193). It is more common in men, particularly those under 40 years of age, and occurs in up to 30 percent of patients with HIV infection and AIDS (194).

Serologic tests for HSV-associated glycoproteins help establish the diagnosis but do not distinguish between active infection and the asymptomatic carrier state (195). Presenting symptoms include odynophagia, retrosternal pain, heartburn, and fever. Concomitant oral ulcers and skin rash may be present (194).

Pathogenesis. Herpes simplex viruses are members of the Herpesviridae family. They contain linear double-stranded DNA within a protein capsid surrounded by a glycoprotein matrix (196). Viruses reside in dorsal ganglia after primary infection and travel along sensory neurons to replicate in target tissues when reactivated (190). The virus is shed in secretions from infected individuals and transmitted *via* contact with mucous membranes.

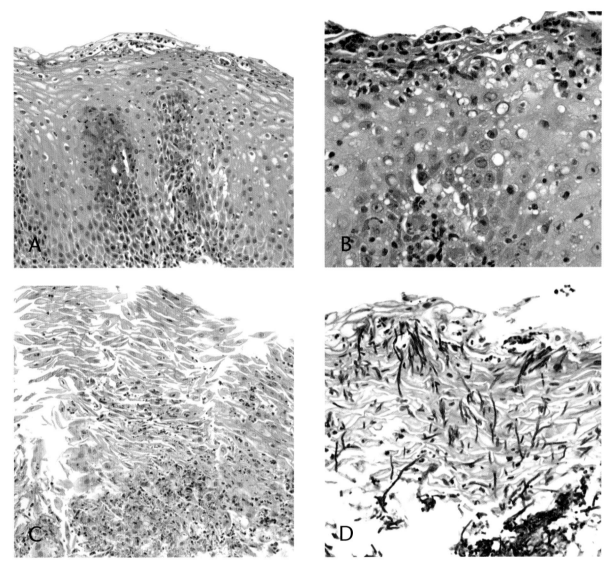

Figure 2-44

CANDIDA **ESOPHAGITIS**

Esophageal candidiasis elicits mucosal hyperplasia with lymphocytosis (A) and superficial neutrophilic microabscesses (B). Organisms are present in "shredded wheat" luminal keratin debris (C). Pseudohyphae and yeast are highlighted by a periodic acid–Schiff diastase (PAS-D) stain (D).

Gross Findings. Ulcers show a predilection for the distal esophagus where they appear as round shallow lesions (fig. 2-45). Severe infection results in large, confluent ulcers with irregular borders. The adjacent mucosa may be normal or friable.

Microscopic Findings. HSV esophagitis causes markedly inflamed ulcers with a mixed inflammatory exudate rich in macrophages (fig. 2-46A) (197). Virus-infected epithelial cells are most numerous in the superficial mucosa adjacent to the ulcers and in detached necrotic keratinocytes which display brightly eosinophilic cytoplasm. They contain single or multiple enlarged nuclei with irregular contours and nuclear molding. Nucleoli and chromatin are obscured by viral inclusions. There are two types of inclusions: Cowdry A inclusions are glassy, eosinophilic, and surrounded by rarified chromatin, whereas Cowdry B inclusions are

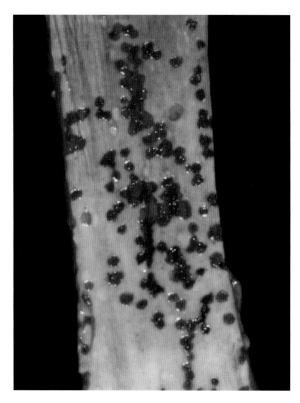

Figure 2-45

HERPES ESOPHAGITIS

Shallow, discrete ulcers are present in the mid and distal esophagus.

basophilic and powdery with a rim of condensed chromatin (fig. 2-46B,C).

Immunohistochemical stains directed against HSV-1 and HSV-2 are widely available. They do cross-react with both viruses and, thus, are not reliable for subclassifying viruses (fig. 2-46B) (198). Culture and PCR are more reliable for purposes of viral subtyping (199).

Differential Diagnosis. Varicella zoster virus (VZV) can cause esophagitis and nuclear inclusions that closely mimic the features of HSV. However, VSV inclusions are distributed throughout the mucosal thickness and tend to be more numerous in the peripapillary epithelium. Varicella is also accompanied by hemorrhagic, fibrinous exudates and less macrophage-rich inflammation (fig. 2-47). Immunohistochemistry directed against VZV detects far more numerous infected cells than are evident in routinely stained sections (fig. 2-47D) (200). Distinction from HSV infection

is clinically important, as patients with VZV esophagitis are often systemically ill and can die of disseminated disease.

Multinucleated squamous epithelial cells can be seen in association with any type of esophagitis and generally reflect a reparative change (fig. 2-48). In contrast to virally infected epithelial cells, reactive cells lack nuclear molding and viral cytopathic changes. They contain even chromatin and prominent, often multiple, nucleoli.

Treatment and Prognosis. Outbreaks of HSV esophagitis are usually self-limited in immunocompetent patients and do not require therapy. Immunocompromised individuals should be treated with antiviral agents since they are more likely to experience complications, such as bleeding and perforation (192). Infected patients harbor latent virus and are at risk for disease reactivation.

Cytomegalovirus Esophagitis

Definition. *Cytomegalovirus esophagitis* is an ulcerative esophagitis resulting from primary cytomegalovirus (CMV) infection or viral reactivation.

Clinical Features. The seroprevalence of CMV approaches 50 percent in the United States, although acute CMV infection is asymptomatic in 90 percent of immunocompetent individuals (201). Approximately 10 percent of immunocompromised patients develop reactivated infection, particularly those with T-cell deficiencies, transplant recipients, and those with acquired immunodeficiency syndrome (AIDS) (202). Reactivation of CMV among immunocompetent patients is far less common (203). Infection can damage virtually all organs in immunosuppressed patients; severe complications result from CMV-related hepatitis, gastroenteritis, pneumonia, and retinitis (204).

Affected patients present with odynophagia, nausea, vomiting, and abdominal pain. Acute infection is associated with detectable CMV-specific IgM antibodies within 2 to 6 weeks of exposure; these titers decline within 2 to 3 months in immunocompetent individuals. Viral reactivation is signaled by rising anti-CMV IgG antibody titers (204). The virus is usually detected by PCR in the urine, blood, and stool of patients with viremia. Although PCR-based assays are rapid and highly sensitive, they have

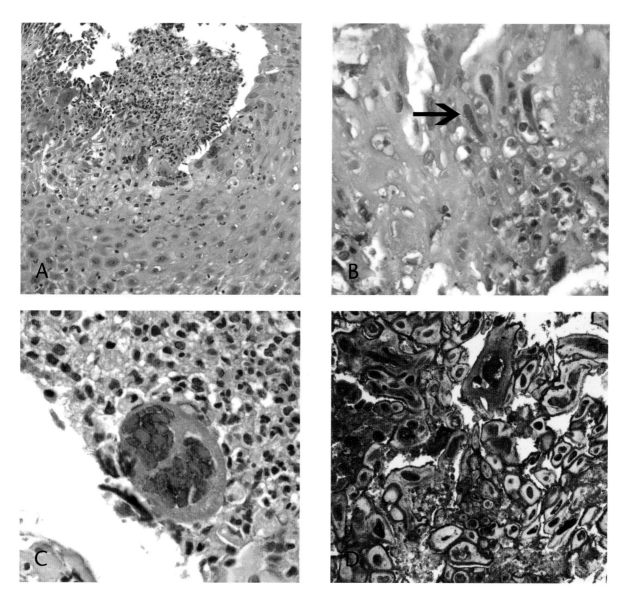

Figure 2-46

HERPES ESOPHAGITIS

Viral cytopathic changes are present in enlarged squamous cells that contain multiple, molded nuclei. Superficial erosions are accompanied by macrophage-rich exudates (A). Cowdry A nuclear inclusions are red (arrow) and surrounded by chromatin clearing (B). Cowdry B inclusions are powdery blue with a prominent rim of condensed chromatin (C). An immunostain confirms the diagnosis of herpes esophagitis (D).

low specificity for clinically significant active infection; low DNA copy numbers can still result in a positive test (205).

Pathogenesis. CMV is a β-herpesvirus shed in secretions of carriers. It establishes latent infection in lymphocytes and endothelial cells after primary exposure. Reactivation of infection can occur as a result of transient or persistent immunosuppression, at which time CMV enters the circulation and causes end organ damage through a combination of inflammatory and ischemic mechanisms (206,207).

Gross Findings. Typical CMV-related esophageal ulcers are large, serpiginous lesions in the mid and distal esophagus (fig. 2-49). The background mucosa may be normal or erythematous.

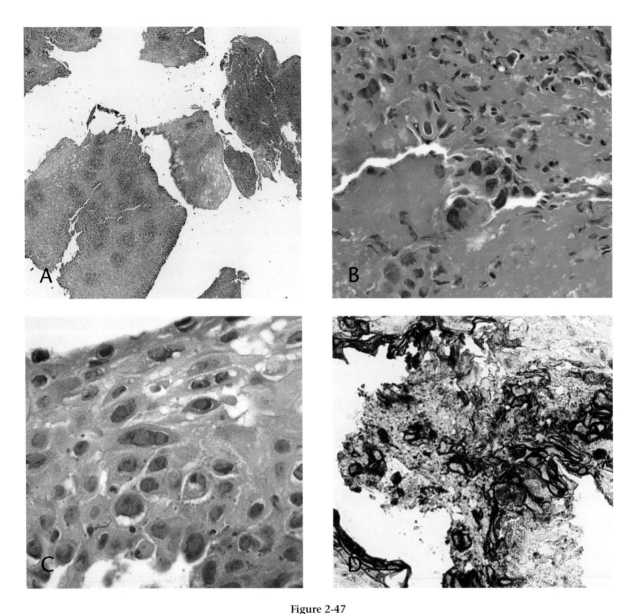

Figure 2-47

VARICELLA ZOSTER ESOPHAGITIS

Varicella-associated esophagitis tends to be more hemorrhagic than herpes simplex virus (HSV)-associated injury (A); scattered infected cells are embedded in fibrin (B). Multinucleated epithelial cells with basophilic inclusions and marginated chromatin resemble those of HSV, and are evenly distributed throughout the mucosal thickness (C). Dyskeratotic cells and necrotic cellular debris are readily identified. An immunostain for varicella zoster virus (VZV) shows strong, diffuse staining of infected cells (D).

Microscopic Findings. CMV infects endothelial cells and glandular epithelial cells, but it does not infect squamous epithelial cells. As the name implies, infected cells are frequently enlarged, with eccentric nuclei and abundant amphophilic or eosinophilic cytoplasm. Cytoplasmic viral inclusions appear as multiple, brightly eosinophilic, slightly refractile granules (fig. 2-50A). Nuclear inclusions resemble Cowdry A inclusions: they are amphophilic or eosinophilic and surrounded by rarified chromatin that imparts an "owl's eye" appearance.

Infected endothelial cells are often associated with perivascular neutrophil-rich infiltrates or luminal thrombi, both of which represent clues to the diagnosis that warrant careful evaluation,

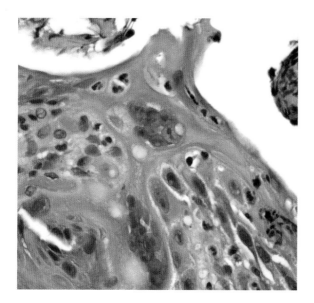

Figure 2-48

REACTIVE SQUAMOUS CELL ATYPIA

Multinucleated squamous epithelial cells can result from esophageal injury. Prominent nucleoli and a lack of both nuclear molding and peripheral chromatin condensation help distinguish them from viral inclusions.

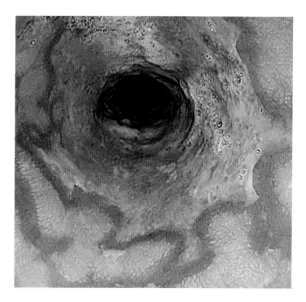

Figure 2-49

CYTOMEGALOVIRUS (CMV) ESOPHAGITIS

Circumferential ulcers with a serpiginous contour are present in the mid esophagus of a patient with CMV infection.

especially when exuberant inflammation obscures viral inclusions (fig. 2-50B,C). Similar to HSV esophagitis, CMV infection often elicits a macrophage-rich inflammatory response (fig. 2-50D) (197). Classic cytologic features may not be prominent when detected in patients receiving antiviral prophylaxis (fig. 2-51).

Immunohistochemical stains against CMV are highly sensitive and widely available, although they regularly label granulocytes and plasma cells. Only strong staining of large, morphologically compatible cells should be considered a positive result. Immunohistochemical stains occasionally detect isolated CMV inclusions, unaccompanied by inflammation. The significance of this finding is not entirely clear, but some patients experience symptomatic relief following antiviral therapy (208).

Differential Diagnosis. Activated fibroblasts can display cytomegaly and nuclear atypia that simulate CMV-associated cytopathic changes, especially in patients who receive radiation therapy (fig. 2-52). These cells generally contain dispersed chromatin and one or more nucleoli, and lack viral inclusions. Immunohistochemical stains for CMV are negative in these cases.

Treatment and Prognosis. Most patients are treated with intravenous ganciclovir. Orally administered valganciclovir can be used for those who have gastrointestinal disease. Patients who do not respond to ganciclovir may be treated with oral foscarnet (202).

Idiopathic HIV-Associated Ulcers

Some patients with advanced HIV disease or AIDS develop large esophageal ulcers in the absence of an identifiable cause. *Idiopathic HIV-associated ulcers* are more common in patients with CD4-positive T-cell counts of less than 100/μL and they show a predilection for the mid esophagus (209). Idiopathic HIV-associated ulcers may be quite large, spanning up to 10 cm, and have sharply circumscribed margins with clean bases. Histologic features are not specific: the ulcers display mixed inflammation associated with granulation tissue, as well as a sparse infiltrate in the background squamous mucosa.

A substantial proportion (50 to 70 percent) of cases harbor known pathogens, most commonly CMV and HSV, when molecular techniques are employed (210). The remainder likely result from either unidentified opportunistic pathogens or

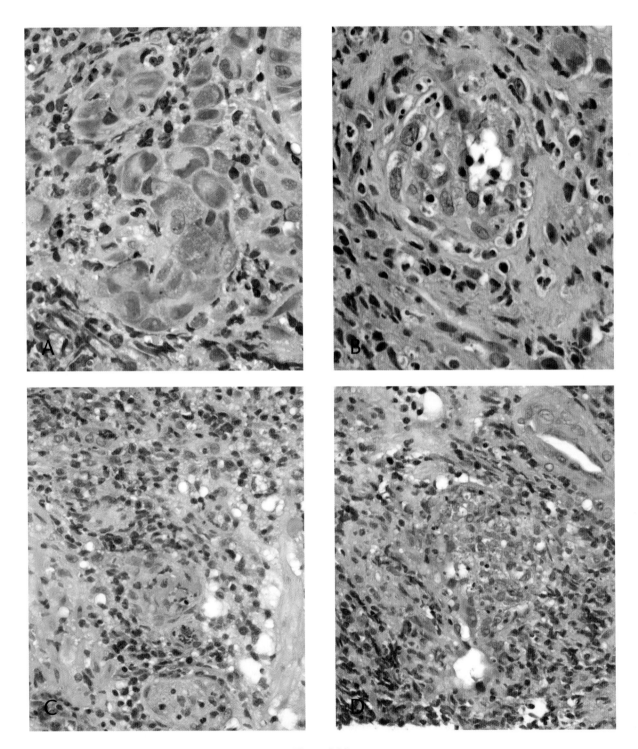

Figure 2-50

CYTOMEGALOVIRUS ESOPHAGITIS

Large CMV-infected endothelial cells are present in granulation tissue at the base of an ulcer. Infected cells contain abundant amphophilic cytoplasm with red, granular inclusions. Eccentric basophilic nuclear inclusions are also present (A). Viral infection causes endothelial injury associated with neutrophil-rich inflammation (B) and occasional fibrin thrombi (C). Cytomegalovirus also elicits a macrophage-rich infiltrate around small vessels, which is helpful clue to the diagnosis (D).

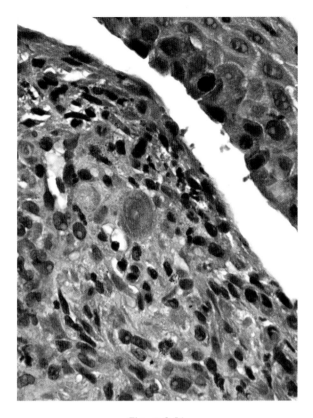

Figure 2-51

CYTOMEGALOVIRUS ESOPHAGITIS

Virally infected cells show less atypical features when detected in patients receiving antiviral prophylaxis. The cells are not as large and contain less amphophilic cytoplasm with smaller nuclear inclusions.

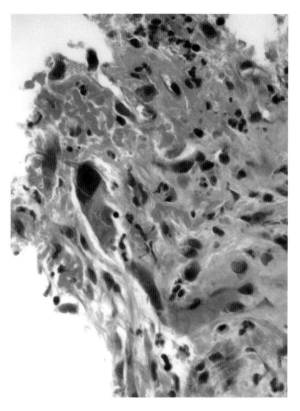

Figure 2-52

RADIATION ESOPHAGITIS

Bizarre fibroblasts simulate CMV inclusions. They are enlarged with eccentric nuclei and abundant cytoplasm, but they have prominent, often multiple nucleoli.

HIV itself. The latter may directly harm the mucosa or alter local immunity, rendering the esophagus more susceptible to injury or infection. Indeed, some cases resolve after treatment with antiretroviral therapy alone (211).

DESQUAMATING DISORDERS

Esophagitis Dissecans Superficialis

Definition. *Esophagitis dissecans superficialis* is a noninflammatory desquamative disorder characterized by the separation of parakeratosis or superficial epithelium from the rest of the squamous mucosa. It is also called *sloughing esophagitis*.

Clinical Features. Esophagitis dissecans superficialis is defined by a combination of endoscopic and histologic features. It shows a predilection for women. The disorder is uncommon but likely underreported in the literature.

The largest series included 41 patients identified during a 13-year period (212).

Sloughing esophagitis is a self-limited disorder characterized by minimal or mild symptoms, and typically occurs in the setting of polypharmacy among elderly, debilitated patients. A substantial proportion of cases are detected in asymptomatic patients who undergo endoscopy for unrelated reasons. Some patients have GERD-type symptoms with dysphagia or heartburn, whereas others present dramatically with regurgitation of tubular casts or esophageal obstruction (212–215).

Pathogenesis. The cause of esophagitis dissecans superficialis is not known, although it is most likely related to a medication-induced injury. More than 70 percent of affected patients use opioids or psychoactive drugs that cause dry mouth, including selective serotonin and norepinephrine reuptake inhibitors (213).

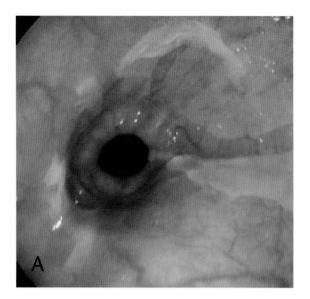
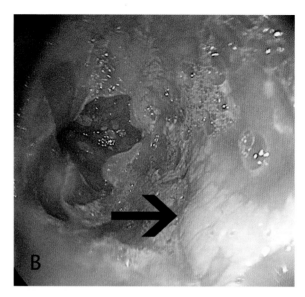

Figure 2-53

ESOPHAGITIS DISSECANS SUPERFICIALIS

Longitudinal casts of sloughed squamous epithelium peel away from the underlying esophageal mucosa, which is essentially normal (A). Some casts are plaque-like (arrow), simulating candidiasis (B).

Gross Findings. The endoscopic features are characteristic: long casts composed of detached parakeratotic material or partial-thickness mucosa are present in the lumen (fig. 2-53A) (213). The mucosa underlying sloughed material is normal or shows only minimal inflammatory changes. Plaques of desquamated material resembling esophageal candidiasis are occasionally encountered (fig. 2-53B). Collapsed casts can also simulate the rings and furrows of eosinophilic esophagitis.

Microscopic Findings. The characteristic histologic features of esophagitis dissecans superficialis are best appreciated at low magnification. Layers of parakeratosis have a two-toned appearance: hypereosinophilic superficial layers contain pyknotic nuclei and overlie viable parakeratosis that may or may not be attached to the squamous mucosa (fig. 2-54, left). Superficial sloughing is due to separation within the parakeratotic layer or in the superficial viable epithelium. The squamous mucosa is generally uninflamed, although some cases show collections of granulocytes within the area of separation between the superficial and deep layers (fig. 2-54, right). Detached strips of parakeratotic material and squamous epithelium show coagulative necrosis of the superficial parakeratotic layers, particularly at the edges

(fig. 2-55). Bacterial and fungal colonies are sometimes associated with sloughed epithelium.

Differential Diagnosis. Medications that cause drug-induced esophagitis (e.g., iron, bisphosphonates, potassium chloride, doxycycline, and NSAIDs), mucocutaneous bullous diseases, radiation injury, and graft-versus-host disease have all been implicated as causes of esophagitis dissecans superficialis due to their potential to cause desquamation. However, all of these disorders cause mucosal injury with endoscopically or histologically evident inflammatory changes and, unlike esophagitis dissecans superficialis, are unlikely to resolve spontaneously. Artifactual disruption of the squamous epithelium due to mucosal instrumentation may simulate the features of sloughing esophagitis dissecans superficialis (fig. 2-56).

Treatment and Prognosis. Strictly defined, esophagus dissecans superficialis resolves spontaneously without sequela. Reported development of strictures or perforation likely reflects misclassification of other desquamating disorders as esophagitis dissecans superficialis.

Acute Esophageal Necrosis

Definition. *Acute esophageal necrosis (black esophagus)* is acute segmental esophageal ischemia.

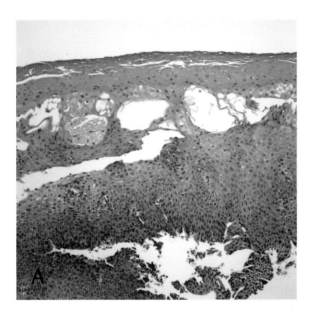 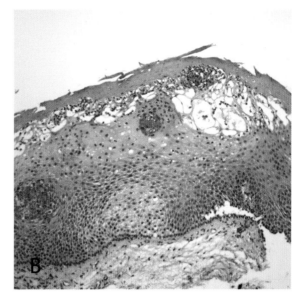

Figure 2-54

ESOPHAGITIS DISSECANS SUPERFICIALIS

Biopsy samples show separation between a compact layer of squamous epithelium and parakeratosis; the most superficial layers of parakeratosis are necrotic, imparting a two-toned appearance (A). Some cases display neutrophil-rich aggregates in the area of separation between the squamous epithelium and sloughed layers, although the viable squamous mucosa is uninflamed (B).

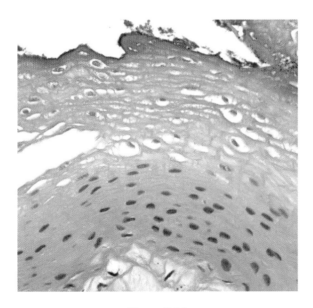 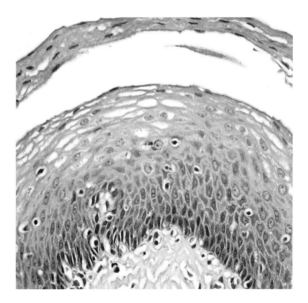

Figure 2-55

ESOPHAGITIS DISSECANS SUPERFICIALIS

The sloughed layer of parakeratotic material has a two-toned appearance, with superficial coagulative necrosis.

Figure 2-56

ARTIFACTUAL INTRAEPITHELIAL SEPARATION

Instrumentation during endoscopy or grossing procedures can separate superficial squamous cell layers from the rest of the epithelium. Mechanically induced separation in the epithelium does not display parakeratosis, necrosis, or an inflammatory response.

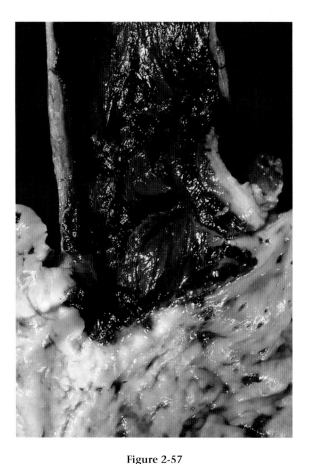

Figure 2-57

ACUTE ESOPHAGEAL NECROSIS

The esophageal mucosa shows brown-black discoloration. (Courtesy of Dr. G. Aristi-Urista, Mexico City, Mexico.)

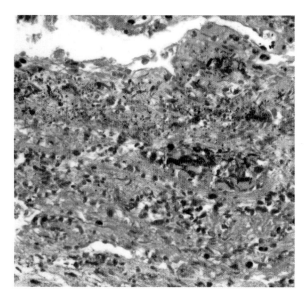

Figure 2-58

ACUTE ESOPHAGEAL NECROSIS

Brown-black discoloration of the mucosa reflects extensive necrosis and extracellular pigment that simulates the appearance of iron.

Clinical Features. Fewer than 100 cases of acute esophageal necrosis have been reported (216). Most occur in men after the 6th decade of life, many of whom are debilitated. Patients present with abdominal pain, hematemesis, or syncope secondary to hypovolemia (217). Luminal narrowing in areas of edematous or necrotic mucosa and healed strictures produce a "string sign" on barium esophagram (217).

Pathogenesis. Acute esophageal necrosis likely reflects esophageal ischemia resulting from profound hypotension due to hypovolemia or sepsis, or in the setting of thromboembolic disorders. Some cases are explained by mechanical obstruction from a gastric volvulus, postsurgical vascular compromise, or segmental devascularization following radiofrequency ablation for atrial fibrillation (217,218,218a). Necrosis shows a predilection for the distal third of the esophagus (219).

Gross Findings. Acute esophageal necrosis is marked by black discoloration of the esophagus, accompanied by mucosal hemorrhage and friability (fig. 2-57).

Microscopic Findings. Acute esophageal ischemia results in coagulative necrosis accompanied by minimal inflammation. Necrotic tissue often contains abundant golden brown pigment that resembles extracellular iron, although Prussian blue stains are negative (fig. 2-58). Cases in which surgical reconstruction is delayed may display mural fibrosis and chronic inflammatory infiltrates.

Differential Diagnosis. Corrosive esophagitis due to caustic ingestion of acid or alkaline substances shows extensive necrosis, although injury is generally accompanied by striking edema, ulcers, neutrophil-rich inflammation, and exuberant granulation tissue (220).

Treatment and Prognosis. Acute esophageal necrosis is a life-threatening condition with a mortality rate of 32 to 36 percent (218,221,222). It may resolve with supportive measures, antibiotic therapy, and nasogastric tube feeding.

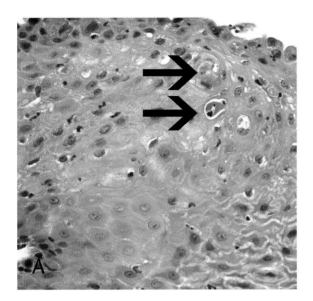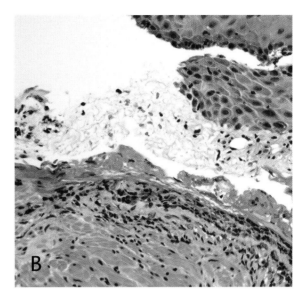

Figure 2-59

GRAFT-VERSUS-HOST DISEASE

Necrotic squamous epithelial cells (arrows) are scattered throughout the mucosa (A). A denuded portion of mucosa displays lymphocyte-rich inflammation in the superficial lamina propria (B).

Patients who survive the acute episode frequently develop strictures at sites of injury. Surgical reconstruction may be required when esophageal perforation occurs (223).

Other Pauci-Inflammatory Conditions that Cause Esophageal Desquamation

Graft-versus-Host Disease. Acute graft-versus-host disease is an important cause of morbidity and mortality in hematopoietic stem cell transplant patients: it occurs in 30 to 70 percent of allogeneic transplant recipients (224). This disorder is less common, but well-described, in those who receive autologous grafts, particularly for the treatment of multiple myeloma (225). Common sites of involvement include the gastrointestinal tract, skin, liver, and lungs.

The frequency of esophageal graft-versus-host disease is difficult to estimate because the diagnostic features are often subtle, but it is less common than involvement of other gastrointestinal sites. Esophageal biopsy samples display abnormalities in approximately one-third of patients (226). Dysphagia and odynophagia are manifestations of esophageal disease.

Endoscopic examination reveals desquamation accompanied by ulcers and erythema (227). Some patients develop webs in the proximal esophagus, which tends to be more severely affected than other areas of the esophagus (228). Key histologic features include necrotic squamous cells at all levels in the mucosa, apoptotic debris and vacuolization in the basal region, and lymphocytic interface inflammation (fig. 2-59). Strictures secondary to subepithelial fibrosis can develop in chronic cases (86).

The differential diagnosis includes mycophenolate mofetil-associated injury, which produces similar histologic changes in the esophagus. Distinction between these entities is usually based on review of material obtained from other sites in the gastrointestinal tract (see chapter 5) (175).

Radiation Esophagitis. Approximately 30 percent of patients with lung cancer who undergo thoracic radiotherapy develop radiation esophagitis (229,230). Symptoms usually develop within 14 to 90 days of treatment initiation and include odynophagia, retrosternal pain, and weight loss (231). Endoscopic examination reveals desquamation, granular edematous mucosa, and ulcers (fig. 2-60). Histologic alterations are not specific but feature patchy dyskeratosis, keratinocytes with vacuolated cytoplasm scattered throughout the mucosal thickness, and disorganization of basal keratinocytes that show

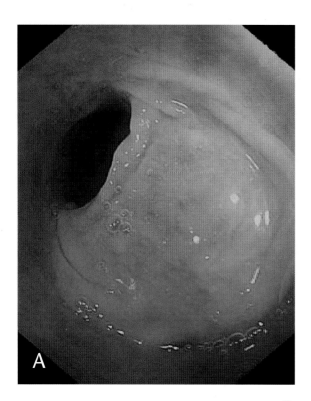
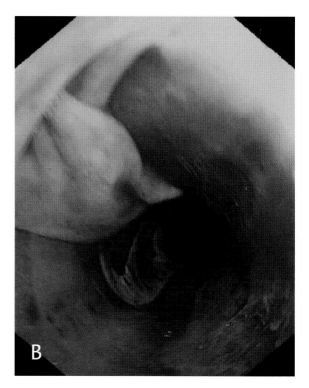

Figure 2-60

RADIATION ESOPHAGITIS

Ionizing radiation causes direct injury to proliferating squamous epithelium, producing webs (A) or desquamation with casts of sloughed epithelium (B).

abnormal keratinization. The intact squamous mucosa may be thin and atrophic (fig. 2-61A,B). Hyalinized lamina propria with vascular ectasias can develop over time (fig. 2-61C). Radiation-induced squamous and stromal cell atypia is common. Affected cells display cytomegaly, nucleomegaly, and multinucleation (fig. 2-61D). Changes may persist for decades following the cessation of therapy (86).

Concurrent chemotherapy nearly doubles the risk of radiation esophagitis (232). Platinum-based therapy sensitizes the esophageal mucosa to the ionizing effects of radiation (230). Chemotherapy alone can also cause desquamating esophagitis with squamous cell atypia, nuclear enlargement, hyperchromasia, and nucleolar prominence that simulate the features of dysplasia (fig. 2-62). However, the atypia occurs in an attenuated, nonproliferative epithelium, and tends to affect single or clustered cells on a background of less atypical epithelial cells. Nuclei are enlarged and hyperchromatic, but degenerative in appearance.

Mucocutaneous Bullous Diseases Involving the Esophagus

Inherited and acquired immune-mediated disorders affecting intercellular adhesion can involve the esophagus. Most patients have an established diagnosis prior to developing esophageal symptoms, although disease onset may be heralded by odynophagia, dysphagia, or upper gastrointestinal bleeding in some cases. Intact, flaccid bullae are rarely encountered; endoscopy usually reveals variably sized ulcers or desquamation.

Pemphigus Vulgaris. Pemphigus vulgaris is an autoimmune disorder caused by IgG antibodies against adhesion proteins, desmoglein 1 and desmoglein 3, present in the basal layers of the squamous epithelium. Antibody and complement deposition results in separation between basal keratinocytes and the more superficial squamous epithelium, producing superficial bullae and erosions. Affected individuals often harbor HLA-DRB1 and HLA-DQB1 alleles (233). The disorder manifests in the 4th to 6th decades,

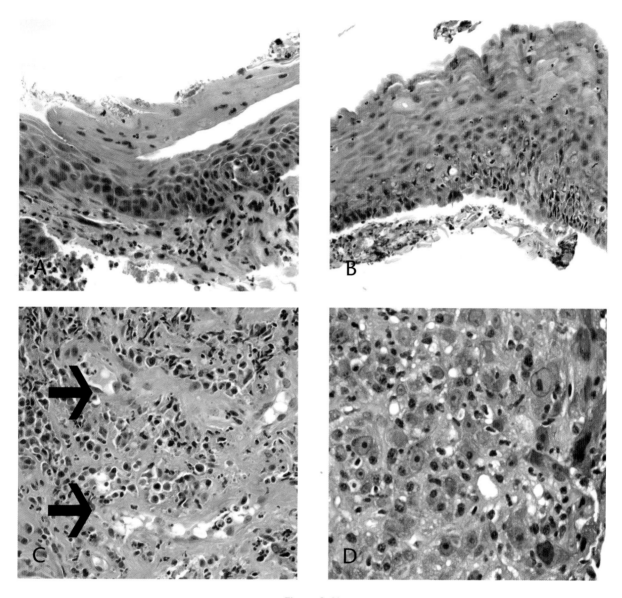

Figure 2-61

RADIATION ESOPHAGITIS

Radiation causes attenuation of the squamous mucosa (A) with vacuolated, squamoid cells in the basal layer (B). Blood vessels (arrows) in an ulcer bed show prominent endothelial cells and are surrounded by cellular debris (C). Atypical fibroblasts contain abundant cytoplasm and large nuclei with multiple nucleoli (D).

affects men and women equally, and tends to be more common among patients of Jewish and Middle Eastern descent (233). Esophageal disease develops in up to 40 percent of affected patients (234). Endoscopy reveals large shallow ulcers, desquamation, and luminal casts of denuded mucosa and fibrin (fig. 2-63).

Histologic features include fragments of mildly inflamed squamous epithelium with rounded keratinocytes, as well as separate fragments of inflamed or fibrotic lamina propria with residual basal keratinocytes (fig. 2-64, left). These cells protude into the lumen, resembling hobnail cells or "tombstones" (fig. 2-64, right). Direct immunofluorescence reveals intercellular IgG and C3 deposits.

Bullous Pemphigoid. Bullous pemphigoid is caused by IgG autoantibodies to the

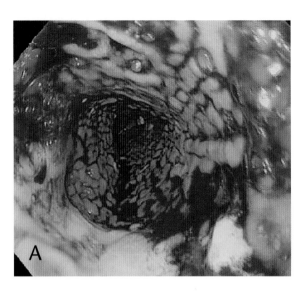
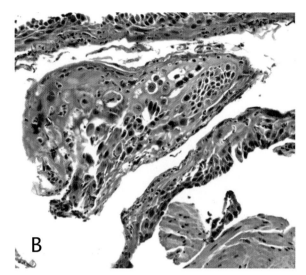

Figure 2-62

CHEMOTHERAPY-RELATED INJURY

Chemotherapy can cause severe esophagitis with extensive desquamation (A). The squamous mucosa is attenuated with striking cytologic atypia. Injured cells contain nuclei with prominent nucleoli and hyperchromasia. Necrotic keratinocytes are present (B).

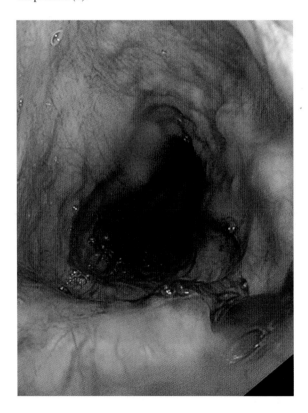

Figure 2-63

PEMPHIGUS VULGARIS

Flaccid bullae and shallow erosions are present throughout the esophagus.

hemidesmosomal components BP180 and BP230. The disease manifests with subepithelial bullae and affects the elderly with a female predominance; it is more common in the setting of polypharmacy among debilitated patients (235). Esophageal involvement occurs in approximately 5 percent of cases (236). Biopsy samples feature desquamation and attenuated, injured squamous epithelium with eosinophil-rich infiltrates, and inflamed lamina propria (fig. 2-65). Direct immunofluorescence demonstrates linear IgG and C3 deposition in detached epithelial fragments or along the basement membrane (237).

Epidermolysis Bullosa. Inherited epidermolysis bullosa is caused by mutations in *COL7A1*, which encodes type VII collagen (238). Patients present in childhood with mucocutaneous fragility, severe dysphagia, and strictures that require dilatation (239). The junctional and simplex forms produce intraepithelial bullae, whereas the dystrophic form causes blisters at the epithelial-subepithelial junction. Direct immunofluorescence demonstrates linear IgG deposits in the desquamated epithelium in the junctional and dystrophic forms, and lamina propria deposits in epidermolysis bullosa simplex (237).

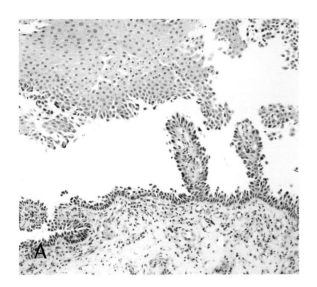
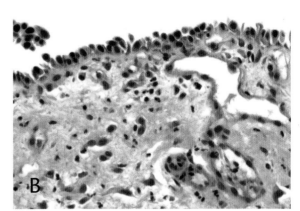

Figure 2-64

PEMPHIGUS VULGARIS

An intraepithelial bulla is seen in the esophagus of a patient with pemphigus vulgaris. The cells above the split are rounded and those below the split appear to be "clinging" to the basement membrane (A). (Courtesy of Dr. E. Montgomery, Baltimore, MD.) Basal keratinocytes attached to the basement membrane protrude into the lumen (B).

Epidermolysis bullosa acquisita is a similar disorder caused by autoantibodies to type VII collagen. It features linear IgG and C3 deposits along the basement membrane (240).

Erythema Multiforme and Related Conditions. Erythema multiforme minor, erythema multiforme major (Stevens-Johnson syndrome), and toxic epidermal necrolysis comprise a spectrum of related bullous disorders that are usually related to drug hypersensitivity. The latter two forms of the disease can involve the esophagus, resulting in desquamation and friability secondary to epithelial necrosis (241,242).

BARRETT ESOPHAGUS

Definition. *Barrett esophagus* is a premalignant condition characterized by replacement of the distal esophageal squamous epithelium by columnar mucosa. The American College of Gastroenterology defines it as intestinal metaplasia with goblet cells present in an endoscopically visible segment that spans at least 1 cm (243). Others define it as columnar metaplasia in the tubal esophagus, regardless of the presence of goblet cells (244). *Columnar-lined esophagus* is a synonym.

Clinical Features. The prevalence of Barrett esophagus is estimated to be approximately 5 percent in the United States; it affects 10 to 15

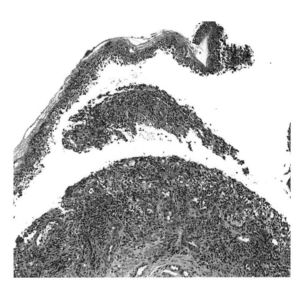

Figure 2-65

BULLOUS PEMPHIGOID

Subepithelial bullae are associated with marked inflammation in the detached lamina propria. The squamous epithelium is attenuated and inflamed.

percent of patients with longstanding GERD (245,246). Nonsteroidal anti-inflammatory drugs, PPI therapy, statins, and infection with *H. pylori* are inversely related to Barrett esophagus (247–249). Patients with Barrett esophagus tend to be older

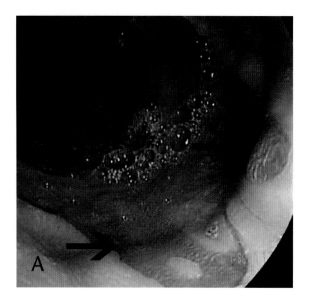
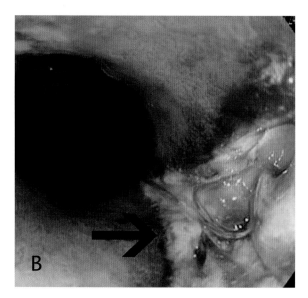

Figure 2-66

BARRETT ESOPHAGUS AND RELATED NEOPLASIA

Tongues of salmon-colored mucosa (arrows) project into the squamous lining in a patient with Barrett esophagus (A). An ulcer (arrow) in a Barrett segment proved to harbor invasive adenocarcinoma (B).

(over 50 years of age) white men with central obesity (250). Additional risk factors include prior esophageal manipulation and hiatal hernia. Barrett esophagus is clinically silent, but many patients have a history of GERD symptoms, including heartburn, regurgitation, and dysphagia.

Pathogenesis. Barrett esophagus is an adaptive response to chronic inflammation induced by the reflux of gastroduodenal contents into the distal esophagus. Exposure to acid or bile salts alters expression of transcription factors that determine epithelial cell differentiation. Intestinal-type transcription factors, including SOX9 and CDX2, are upregulated, whereas expression of transcription factors driving squamous differentiation, such as SOX2, is decreased (251,252). Columnar epithelium may develop from undifferentiated progenitor cells of the esophagus or submucosal glands (253).

Dysplasia develops when metaplastic mucosa accumulates molecular alterations that promote development of dysplasia and adenocarcinoma. Aneuploidy and other cytogenetic abnormalities are often detected in Barrett esophagus and increase with progressive neoplasia; DNA methylation and loss of heterozygosity affecting *CDKN2A* and *TP53* are frequently detected in dysplastic mucosae (254,255).

Gross Findings. The squamocolumnar junction, or Z-line, corresponds to the gastroesophageal junction in the uninflamed esophagus but is proximally displaced in Barrett esophagus. Barrett mucosa appears as salmon-colored, tongue-like projections of glandular mucosa that extend from the tips of the rugal folds into the tubular esophagus.

Columnar metaplasia may be circumferential or appear as islands surrounded by squamous epithelium (fig. 2-66A). It can be classified according to the length of affected mucosa as short- (1 to 3 cm) and long- (over 3 cm) segment disease, or by the Prague C&M criteria that estimate affected surface area according to circumferential extent and maximum length of columnar-lined esophagus (256).

The likelihood of detecting goblet cells increases with the number of endoscopic biopsies obtained. Sampling with approximately eight tissue fragments from the columnar-lined esophagus and across the squamocolumnar junction is generally adequate to detect goblet cells when they are present (257). Approximately two-thirds of cases of Barrett-related neoplasia are not endoscopically appreciable, and up to 18 tissue samples per centimeter of Barrett mucosa may be required to detect them (258). Endoscopically

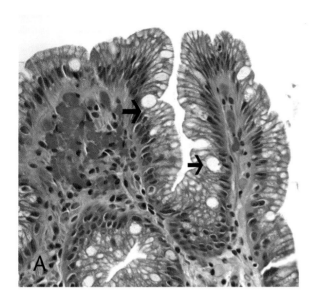
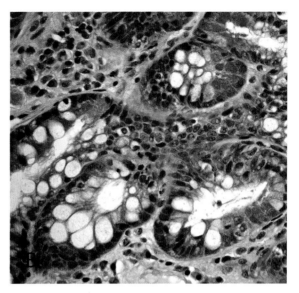

Figure 2-67

BARRETT ESOPHAGUS

Goblet cells are interspersed among foveolar-type mucinous epithelial cells. Individual goblet cells (arrows) contain pale blue, round mucin vacuoles and basal nuclei (A). Other types of specialized epithelia, including Paneth cells and endocrine cells, may be present (B).

evident nodules, plaques, and ulcers are more likely to represent adenocarcinomas than dysplasia (fig. 2-66B) (259).

Microscopic Findings. Barrett esophagus displays goblet cells with round, faintly basophilic mucin vacuoles interspersed among non-goblet columnar cells that are similar to gastric foveolar lining cells (fig. 2-67A). Clusters of oxyntic glands are commonly detected near the gastroesophageal junction, and Paneth cells and endocrine cells may also be present (fig. 2-67B). Mixed inflammation is usually found in the lamina propria, which is frequently supported by a thickened, duplicated muscularis mucosae (fig. 2-68) (260). The deepest layer of muscularis mucosae represents the boundary between the mucosa and submucosa.

Argon plasma coagulation, radiofrequency ablation, and photodynamic therapy can cause interpretive challenges when evaluating samples from patients with Barrett esophagus. These methods devitalize targeted tissue, which re-epithelializes with squamous mucosa (261, 262). Previously ablated mucosa may contain metaplastic or dysplastic glands under the newly epithelialized surface, concealing it from endoscopic view (263).

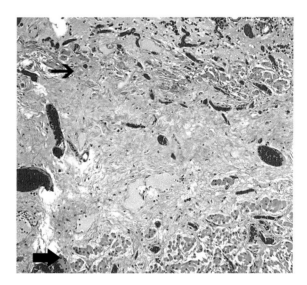

Figure 2-68

BARRETT ESOPHAGUS

The inner duplicated layer of muscularis mucosae is thin and discontinuous (arrow), whereas the original outer layer is thicker (block arrow). The lamina propria tissue in between should not be mistaken for submucosa.

The presence or absence of dysplasia in biopsy samples is the most important element in determining surveillance and treatment protocols

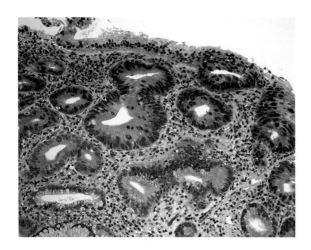

Figure 2-69

**BARRETT ESOPHAGUS:
LOW-GRADE GLANDULAR DYSPLASIA**

Foci of low-grade dysplasia contain slightly crowded glands with minimal variability in size and shape. Atypical cells contain enlarged, hyperchromatic nuclei and show an abrupt transition to non-neoplastic Barrett mucosa.

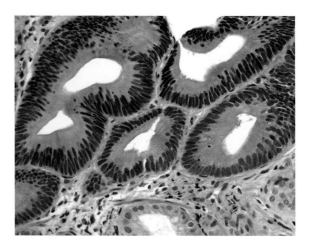

Figure 2-70

**BARRETT ESOPHAGUS:
LOW-GRADE GLANDULAR DYSPLASIA**

Intestinal-type dysplasia resembles a colonic adenoma. The nuclei are elongated and hyperchromatic, but polarized to the basement membrane.

for patients with Barrett esophagus. Barrett mucosa is classified as negative or positive for dysplasia; dysplasia is further classified as either low- or high-grade (264). Samples negative for dysplasia display evenly spaced glands with abundant intervening stroma. Cells contain uniform basally oriented nuclei and abundant apical mucin. Mitotic figures are limited to the deep gland regions.

The general features of dysplasia include increased density of glands and lack of surface maturation in foci that show an abrupt transition to adjacent non-neoplastic Barrett mucosa (fig. 2-69). Intestinal-type low-grade dysplasia features hyperchromatic, elongated, and pseudostratified nuclei that maintain their orientation to the basement membrane (fig. 2-70). The glands of high-grade dysplasia are more crowded with complex architectural abnormalities, including branched or budding glands, secondary lumens, and intraluminal papillae (fig. 2-71A). Nuclei show a greater degree of variability in size and shape; some have prominent nucleoli (fig. 2-71B). Mitotic figures are often numerous and may be abnormal. Cases that display cytologic atypia, but fall short of criteria for low-grade dysplasia, may be provisionally classified as indefinite for dysplasia. For example, some cases show features of low-grade dysplasia in glands accompanied

by surface maturation, or cytologic abnormalities in association with active inflammation or erosions (fig. 2-72).

Morphologic variants of dysplasia include "non-adenomatous," or "foveolar-type," dysplasia and crypt dysplasia (265,266). The former refers to closely packed glands with round cells that contain vesicular nuclei and prominent nucleoli (fig. 2-73). Crypt dysplasia refers to overtly dysplastic cytologic abnormalities limited to deep crypt regions; these foci may harbor *TP53* mutations and display proliferative abnormalities in some cases (fig. 2-74). However, the diagnosis of crypt dysplasia is controversial owing to poor interobserver agreement and overlapping cytologic features with those of reactive cytologic atypia (267).

For practical purposes, most low-grade atypia limited to deep glands is regarded as negative or indefinite for dysplasia. High-grade atypia in the deep glands likely constitutes dysplasia, regardless of the presence, or absence, of surface maturation.

Immunohistochemical Findings. Goblet cells contain acidic sialomucins and sulfomucins and, thus, are bright blue with Alcian blue histochemical stains (pH 2.5). The neutral mucins of non-goblet columnar epithelial cells are magenta when stained with period acid–Schiff (PAS). The combination of these histochemical

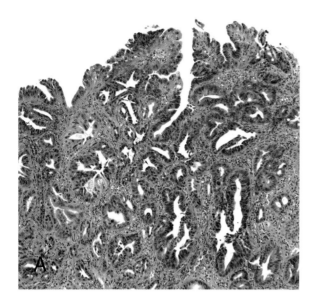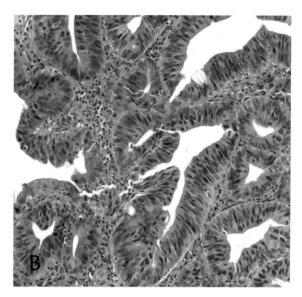

Figure 2-71

BARRETT ESOPHAGUS: HIGH-GRADE GLANDULAR DYSPLASIA

Glands are crowded and show complex architecture with intraluminal buds and papillae (A). Nuclei are round with prominent nucleoli and frequent mitotic figures (B).

stains distinguish goblet cells from other mucinous epithelia, although Alcian blue positivity is not specific for goblet cells (fig. 2-75A,B). Pseudogoblet cells, columnar blues, normal-appearing non-goblet columnar cells, and esophageal submucosal glands all show variable Alcian blue staining (fig. 2-75C,D) (268).

Goblet cells stain with immunohistochemical markers of intestinal differentiation, namely CDX2, MUC2, MUC1, DAS1, BMP4, SHH, and 45M1, but non-goblet columnar epithelia also stain with these markers (251,269–273). Immunopositivity of non-goblet epithelia for these markers does not predict ultimate development of intestinal metaplasia or dysplasia; they have no role in the routine evaluation of clinical cases of Barrett esophagus (274).

Molecular Genetic Findings. Common genetic abnormalities in Barrett esophagus-related dysplasia include abnormal DNA content, loss of heterozygosity at cancer-related gene loci, and methylation-induced gene silencing. Flow cytometry and fluorescence *in situ* hybridization (FISH) have been used to detect these abnormalities and risk stratify patients with non-dysplastic Barrett esophagus. Patients with aneuploid and tetraploid DNA content detected by flow cytometry are at increased risk of

neoplastic progression (275). Those with loss of heterozygosity for *TP53* are at higher cancer risk than those with two intact *TP53* alleles (276,277). Multi-probe FISH panels may identify at-risk patients (278). Increased numbers of methylated genes, such as *CDKN2a*, *HPP1*, and *RUNX3* correlate with disease progression (279). These and other molecular assays are likely to have a role in the management of Barrett esophagus patients in the future, but are not yet used in routine practice.

Differential Diagnosis. Inflammation-induced alterations in non-goblet columnar cells can simulate goblet cells. Pseudogoblet cells are distended foveolar epithelial cells that contain a small amount of acid mucin, imparting a blue tinge to the cytoplasm and weak Alcian blue positivity (fig. 2-76). Columnar blues are barrel-shaped columnar epithelial cells that contain blue-tinged mucin without a well-delineated mucin vacuole; these cells are most prominent in ducts draining mucosal and submucosal glands (fig. 2-77). Multilayered epithelium is a hybrid epithelium containing several layers of immature-appearing squamous epithelial cells surfaced by acid mucin-containing columnar cells (fig. 2-78). Multilayered epithelium is often found adjacent to the squamocolumnar

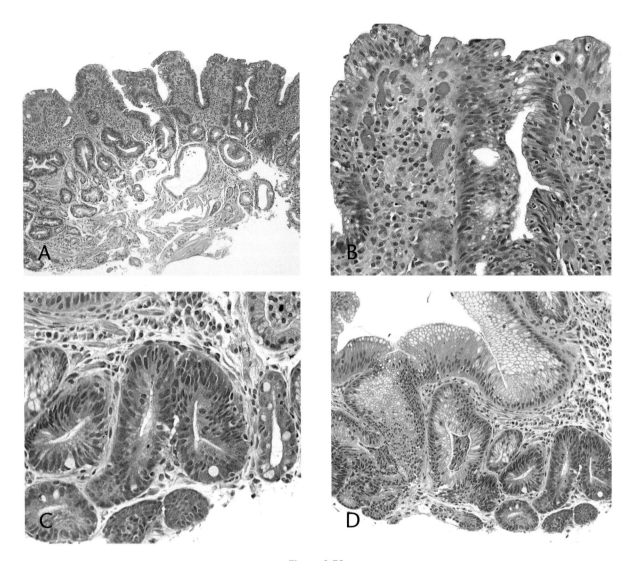

Figure 2-72

BARRETT ESOPHAGUS: INDEFINITE FOR DYSPLASIA

Glands within Barrett mucosa show low-grade cytologic abnormalities but surface maturation is present (A). Mild cytologic atypia extends to the surface but neutrophils are scattered throughout the epithelium (B). A crowded cluster of metaplastic glands contains cells with dark, enlarged nuclei (C). The surface epithelium overlying the same area is mature. Cells contain ample cytoplasm with small nuclei (D). (Courtesy of Dr. E. Montgomery, Baltimore, MD.)

junction or lining ducts that drain to the surface, as well as in combination with well-developed goblet cells. It is widely considered a precursor to intestinal metaplasia (280).

Goblet cells in samples taken near the gastroesophageal junction may represent intestinal metaplasia of the gastric cardia, which is associated with negligible cancer risk (281). Current guidelines discourage sampling of a normal or slightly irregular Z-line for this reason. However, some histologic features favor an esophageal, rather than gastric, origin when sampling near the gastroesophageal junction reveals goblet cells. These include comingling of columnar epithelium and squamous mucosa, and columnar epithelium overlying esophageal submucosal glands and ducts (282). Immunohistochemical stains have no role in the distinction between goblet cells derived from the gastric cardia and tubular esophagus (274).

Inflammation-mediated injury can induce regenerative atypia in Barrett mucosa that simulates features of glandular dysplasia. Reactive changes include mild gland crowding with surface maturation and gradual transitions to obviously non-neoplastic areas (fig. 2-79A). Cytologic atypia is generally mild or moderate (fig. 2-79B). In contrast, low-grade dysplasia is sharply demarcated from adjacent non-neoplastic mucosa and shows a lack of maturation with abnormal proliferation, as discussed previously.

Immunohistochemistry has been proposed as an adjunct in the distinction between reparative atypia and dysplasia in some cases of Barrett esophagus. Staining for p53 is normally limited to the deep glands; mutations may result in diffuse nuclear accumulation of the abnormal protein or a null phenotype with absent staining. Although aberrant p53 expression is common in high-grade dysplasia and adenocarcinomas, it does not reliably distinguish low-grade dysplasia from non-dysplastic Barrett mucosa (283). Some data suggest that p53 staining improves interobserver agreement with respect to the diagnosis of low-grade dysplasia, and that the presence of p53 positivity increases the likelihood of neoplastic progression in patients with low-grade dysplasia (284). On the other hand, data are insufficient to support the use of p53 as a predictive marker independent of morphologic diagnosis (274). Immunohistochemical staining for alpha-methylacyl-CoA racemase (AMACR)

increases in extent and intensity with progressively severe neoplasia, but false negative and false positive results are common (285).

Treatment and Prognosis. Patients with non-dysplastic Barrett mucosa are at increased

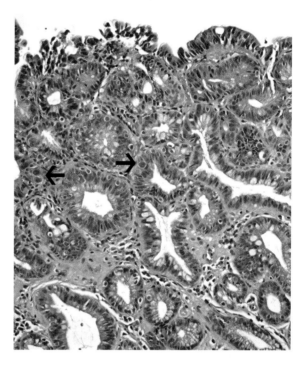

Figure 2-73

NON-ADENOMATOUS BARRETT-RELATED DYSPLASIA

Dysplastic epithelial cells contain round nuclei with vesicular chromatin and prominent nucleoli. Scattered endocrine cells (arrows) are also present.

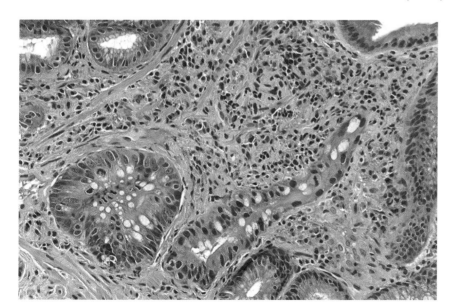

Figure 2-74

BARRETT ESOPHAGUS: CRYPT DYSPLASIA

The deep glands contain cells with marked cytologic atypia. Scattered mitotic figures, and apoptotic debris are present. The overlying surface is mature.

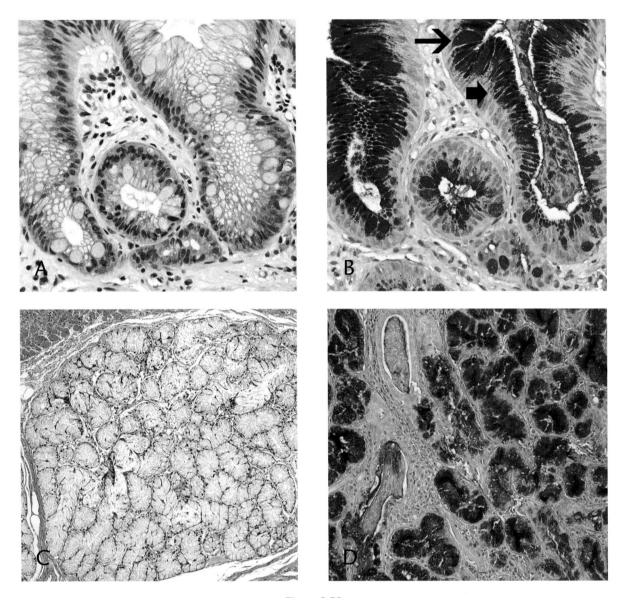

Figure 2-75

GOBLET CELLS

Goblet cells contain faintly basophilic acid mucin compared with foveolar-type epithelial cells (A). An Alcian blue/PAS stain highlights blue goblet cells (arrow) and magenta foveolar cells (block arrow) (B). Any cell type that contains acid mucin can show strong Alcian blue positivity; pale blue submucosal glands (C) stain similarly to goblet cells with Alcian blue (D). (A,B: courtesy of Dr. E. Montgomery, Baltimore, MD.)

risk for the development of esophageal adenocarcinoma, which occurs at a rate of 0.2 to 0.5 percent annually (114,286,287). The length of Barrett esophagus correlates with progression risk (288). Patients with Barrett esophagus who lack dysplasia undergo endoscopic surveillance at 3- to 5-year intervals indefinitely. Carcinoma develops at an annual rate of approximately 0.7 percent among patients with low-grade dysplasia (289). High-grade dysplasia progresses to invasive adenocarcinoma at a rate of approximately 7 percent per year (290,291). When detected, foci of dysplasia are endoscopically treated with a combination of modalities, including ablation and local excision.

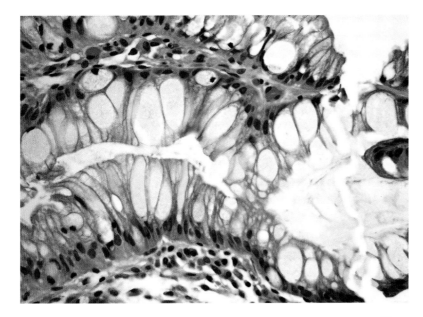

Figure 2-76

**PSEUDOGOBLET CELLS
AT THE
GASTROESOPHAGEAL JUNCTION**

Pseudogoblet cells are distended by pale pink, neutral mucin.

Figure 2-77

**COLUMNAR BLUES
IN ESOPHAGEAL DUCTS**

Columnar blues contain acid mucin but lack distinct mucin vacuoles. These cells are not present in the surface epithelium.

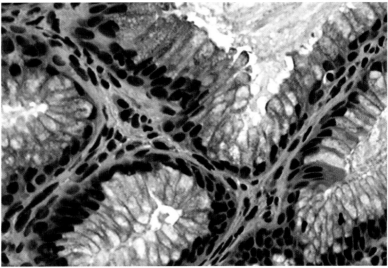

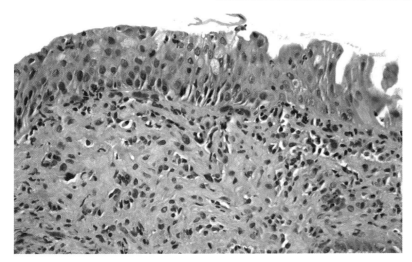

Figure 2-78

MULTILAYERED EPITHELIUM

Multilayered epithelium contains admixed mucinous epithelial cells and immature squamous cells.

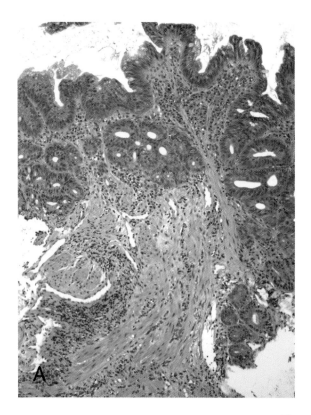
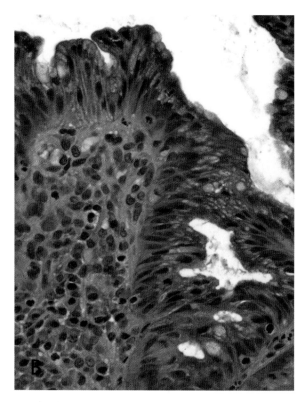

Figure 2-79

BARRETT ESOPHAGUS: REACTIVE CYTOLOGIC ABNORMALITIES

Inflammation can cause gland crowding and mild cytologic abnormalities in the glands (A). The surface epithelial cells in the same area show preserved polarity and minimal cytologic atypia without increased mitotic activity (B).

POLYPS OF THE ESOPHAGUS

Glycogenic Acanthosis

Definition. *Glycogenic acanthosis* is hyperplastic squamous mucosa with intracytoplasmic accumulation of glycogen. Synonyms include *pachydermia nodosa* and *esophageal leukoplakia*.

Clinical Features. Glycogenic acanthosis is found in approximately 3.5 percent of adults who undergo upper endoscopic examination (292). It is a non-neoplastic lesion unrelated to leukoplakia or squamous cell carcinoma. It is usually an incidental finding in adult patients, but occurs in up to 80 percent of patients with PTEN hamartoma-tumor (Cowden) syndrome as discussed in chapter 6 (293). It does not require therapy.

Pathogenesis. The etiology of glycogenic acanthosis is not clear. Isolated lesions may represent a reparative change observed in association with GERD, although they do not regress following PPI therapy (292).

Gross Findings. Glycogenic acanthosis forms solitary or multiple, pearly white plaques or nodules on a background of normal squamous mucosa (fig. 2-80). Solitary lesions are usually incidental findings, whereas numerous lesions raise concern for PTEN hamartoma-tumor syndrome. In fact, the presence of numerous lesions is a highly specific marker of this polyposis disorder.

Microscopic Findings. Glycogenic acanthosis is composed of thickened squamous mucosa that contains enlarged cells with pale cytoplasm and abundant glycogen (fig. 2-81A). Enlarged cells are more numerous in the superficial epithelium; they lack nuclear atypia and are unaccompanied by increased inflammation (fig. 2-81B).

Treatment and Prognosis. No treatment is necessary for glycogenic acanthosis and it has no malignant potential.

Hyperplastic Polyp

Definition. *Hyperplastic polyp* is an inflammatory polyp composed of cardiac-type or squamous mucosa. Synonyms include *inflammatory polyp, regenerative polyp,* and *endophytic squamous papilloma.*

Clinical Features. Hyperplastic polyps usually arise on a background of GERD, and thus, tend to be more common among middle-aged men (294). They can also result from medication-induced injury and infection. Some large polyps may bleed.

Gross Findings. Hyperplastic polyps occur throughout the esophagus but most are found in the distal esophagus near the gastroesophageal junction. Polyps tend to be small and may be sessile or pedunculated.

Microscopic Findings. Hyperplastic polyps are reparative in nature. Most near the gastroesophageal junction contain cardiac-type mucinous glands and foveolar surface epithelium, with or without admixed oxyntic glands (fig. 2-82) (294). They often display frond-like projections of edematous lamina propria with dilated glands lined by mucin-depleted or hypermucinous epithelium. Intestinal metaplasia may be present, particularly when occurring in patients with Barrett esophagus. Lesions obtained from the gastroesophageal junction may be associated with chronic gastritis. Polyps located above the gastroesophageal junction are partially or completely surfaced by squamous mucosa (295). They share overlapping morphologic features with endophytic squamous papillomas and probably represent the same entity, as described below.

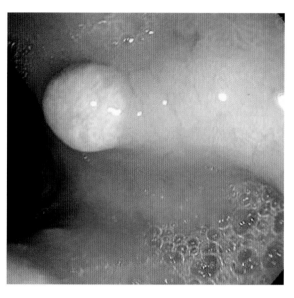

Figure 2-80

GLYCOGENIC ACANTHOSIS

A smooth yellow nodule is present on a background of normal squamous mucosa.

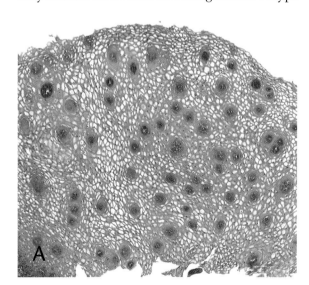

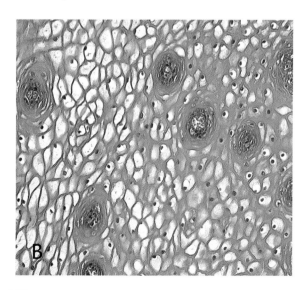

Figure 2-81

GLYCOGENIC ACANTHOSIS

Marked expansion of the squamous mucosa creates a dome-shaped protuberance (A). The squamous epithelial cells contain abundant clear cytoplasm and small, uniform nuclei (B).

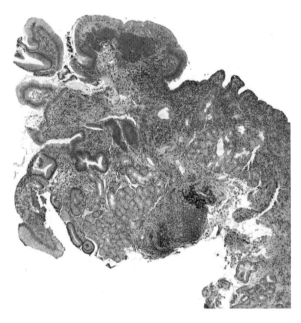

Figure 2-82

**HYPERPLASTIC POLYP OF THE
GASTROESOPHAGEAL JUNCTION**

An exuberant proliferation of gastric-type epithelium displays crowded, somewhat dilated glands supported by inflamed lamina propria.

Treatment and Prognosis. Hyperplastic polyps are benign. Recurrence and neoplastic progression are not reported.

Squamous Papilloma

Definition. *Squamous papilloma* is a non-neoplastic proliferation of squamous epithelium supported by fibrovascular stroma. Synonyms include *inflammatory polyp* and *hyperplastic polyp*.

Clinical Features. Squamous papillomas are detected in less than 0.5 percent of adults who undergo upper endoscopy (296,297). Most are reparative lesions unassociated with high-risk HPV infection. Patients tend to be older adults and men are more frequently affected than women. Isolated lesions do not cause symptoms. Patients with squamous papillomatosis of the respiratory tree may develop esophageal disease and present with dysphagia, hoarseness, coughing, or dyspnea.

Pathogenesis. Most squamous papillomas are postinflammatory lesions associated with GERD (296). A few are caused by infection by HPV and most of these occur in patients with squamous papillomatosis. Reported HPV infection rates range from 5 to 50 percent, likely reflecting regional variability of HPV prevalence, differences in methods used to detect the virus, and contamination of PCR reactions. Detected HPV is usually a low-risk strain (6 and 11); high-risk serovars are rarely identified (298).

Squamous papillomatosis affecting the respiratory tree can rarely involve the esophagus and is almost always caused by HPV types 6 and 11 (299,300). Multiple esophageal papillomas are reported in patients with focal dermal hypoplasia (Goltz-Gorlin syndrome) (301,302). This is a rare disorder caused by X-linked mutations in *PORCN* that result in abnormalities affecting skin, hair, nails, and teeth, as well as ocular and limb formation (303).

Gross Findings. Solitary papillomas are usually found in the mid to lower esophagus. Well-demarcated, sub-centimeter lesions are present on a background of normal-appearing squamous mucosa or esophagitis. They are usually round, sessile nodules or display numerous papillary projections (fig. 2-83) (304). Esophageal papillomatosis carpets the entire esophagus with wart-like growths, particularly the cervical esophagus (300).

Microscopic Findings. Squamous papillomas are classified as exophytic, endophytic, or spiked (305). *Exophytic papillomas* contain finger-like fibrovascular cores lined by hyperplastic squamous epithelium (fig. 2-84). *Endophytic papillomas* show inverted growth of hyperplastic squamous epithelium into the supporting lamina propria (fig. 2-85). *Spiked papillomas* show verrucous growth with a granular cell layer subjacent to hyperkeratosis (fig. 2-86). Squamous maturation is orderly; cytologic atypia is minimal or absent.

Differential Diagnosis. Superficial samples of squamous cell carcinoma may simulate the features of a papilloma, although even well-differentiated carcinomas display cytologic atypia and disorderly maturation.

Treatment and Prognosis. Squamous papillomas are benign and can be removed endoscopically. Completely removed papillomas do not recur and are not associated with the development of invasive squamous cell carcinoma (306). Development of squamous cell carcinoma has been reported in rare patients with squamous papillomatosis managed by observation, but the histologic features of these cases are not well-documented (307).

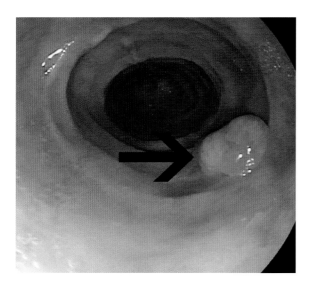

Figure 2-83

SQUAMOUS PAPILLOMA OF THE ESOPHAGUS

This squamous papilloma forms a sessile nodule (arrow) in the distal esophagus. The surface is similar to the background mucosa.

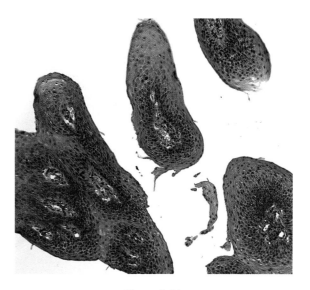

Figure 2-84

EXOPHYTIC PAPILLOMA OF THE ESOPHAGUS

Multiple frond-like projections are surfaced by squamous mucosa and supported by fibrovascular cores.

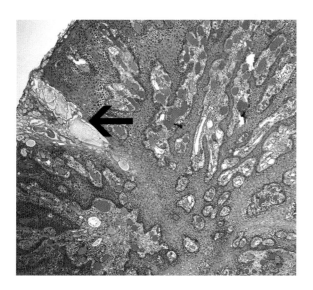

Figure 2-85

SQUAMOUS PAPILLOMA OF THE ESOPHAGUS

A nodular proliferation of squamous cells displays intracellular edema at the surface (arrow) and dilated subepithelial blood vessels.

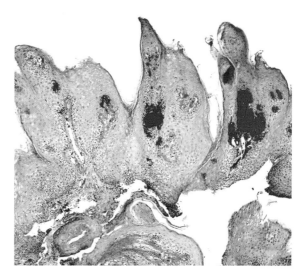

Figure 2-86

SPIKED PAPILLOMA OF THE ESOPHAGUS

A spiked papilloma has a wart-like growth pattern with a thin layer of parakeratosis at the surface.

Polypoid Fibroadipose Tumors of the Esophagus

Definition. *Polypoid fibroadipose tumors* are fibrovascular polyps of the proximal esophagus or pharynx. Synonyms include *giant fibrovas-cular polyp, fibrolipoma*, and *atypical lipomatous tumor/well-differentiated liposarcoma*.

Clinical Features. Fibroadipose tumors in the esophagus are rare: the largest series included 16 cases (308). Most patients are middle-aged to elderly men who present with dysphagia. Rare

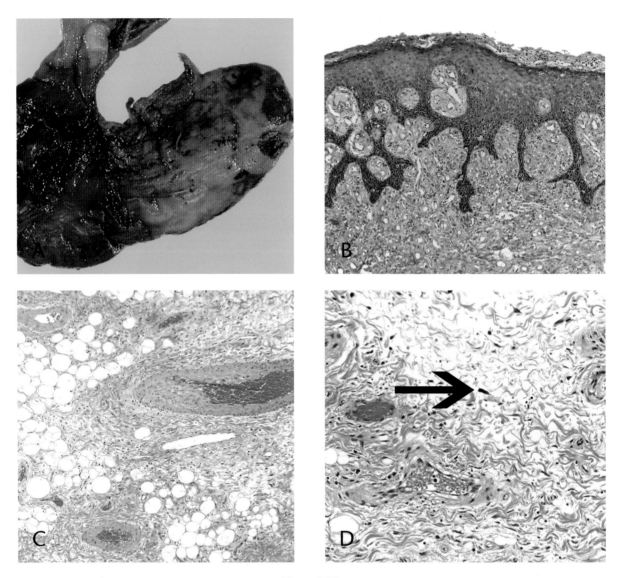

Figure 2-87

POLYPOID FIBROADIPOSE TUMOR OF ESOPHAGUS

A resected polypoid fibroadipose tumor appears as a sausage-shaped fatty protuberance with multiple erosions (A). The polyp is surfaced by squamous mucosa with pseudoepitheliomatous hyperplasia (B). The core of the lesion consists of lobules of mature adipose tissue and fibrous bands (C). Occasional bizarre stromal cells with hyperchromatic nuclei (arrow) are present, similar to those of well-differentiated lipomatous neoplasms (D). (Courtesy of Dr. J. G. Mantilla, Seattle, WA.)

patients regurgitate the mass into the mouth, develop intermittent airway obstruction, or present with asphyxia (309).

Pathogenesis. Polypoid fibroadipose tumors were once thought to be non-neoplastic lesions that developed as a result of traction on redundant esophageal folds, particularly in the relatively weak region of Laimer triangle below the cricopharyngeal muscle (310). However, emerging data suggest that many, if not all, of these lesions are atypical lipomatous tumors/well-differentiated liposarcomas. They often show immunohistochemical overexpression of *MDM2* and CDK4, as well as MDM2 amplification by FISH (311–313).

Gross Findings. Lesions are large and smooth, sausage-shaped masses spanning 10 to 25 cm (fig. 2-87A) (310). Cut sections show lobules of yellow adipose tissue traversed by irregular fibrous bands.

Microscopic Findings. Polypoid fibroadipose tumors are surfaced by squamous epithelium that may be eroded or show pseudoepitheliomatous hyperplasia (fig. 2-87B). They contain dilated subepithelial blood vessels overlying a core of mature adipose tissue (fig. 2-87C). Fat lobules are separated by collagenous or myxoid septa that contain occasional enlarged cells with slightly hyperchromatic nuclei (fig. 2-87D). The relative proportions of fat and fibrous tissue are highly variable. Tumors with abundant adipose tissue contain scattered hyperchromatic stromal cells. Rare examples contain sheets of mitotically active, pleomorphic spindle cells that may represent areas of dedifferentiated liposarcoma (313).

FISH for amplified *MDM2* is the most reliable ancillary study, although immunohistochemistry for MDM2 or CDK4 can also be used. Some authors suggest that a diagnosis of fibrovascular polyp should only be made when these studies are negative (313).

Treatment and Prognosis. Polypoid fibroadipose tumors should be resected, particularly since many likely represent fatty neoplasms that have potential for local recurrence or dedifferentiation (313). Treatment consists of endoscopic resection or subtotal esophagectomy (314–316).

REFERENCES

1. Shaw-Smith C. Oesophageal atresia, tracheo-oesophageal fistula, and the vacterl association: review of genetics and epidemiology. J Med Genet 2006;43:545-54.
2. Carli D, Garagnani L, Lando M, et al. VACTERL (vertebral defects, anal atresia, tracheoesophageal fistula with esophageal atresia, cardiac defects, renal and limb anomalies) association: disease spectrum in 25 patients ascertained for their upper limb involvement. J Pediatr 2014; 164:458-62.
3. Achildi O, Grewal H. Congenital anomalies of the esophagus. Otolaryngol Clin North Am 2007;40:219-44.
4. Kunisaki SM, Bruch SW, Hirschl RB, Mychaliska GB, Treadwell MC, Coran AG. The diagnosis of fetal esophageal atresia and its implications on perinatal outcome. Pediatr Surg Int 2014;30:971-7.
5. Dunkley ME, Zalewska KM, Shi E, Stalewski H. Management of esophageal atresia and tracheoesophageal fistula in North Queensland. Int Surg 2014;99:276-9.
6. Slater BJ, Rothenberg SS. Tracheoesophageal fistula. Semin Pediatr Surg 2016;25:176-8.
7. McCann F, Michaud L, Aspirot A, Levesque D, Gottrand F, Faure C. Congenital esophageal stenosis associated with esophageal atresia. Dis Esophagus 2015;28:211-5.
8. Serrao E, Santos A, Gaivao A, Tavares A, Ferreira S. Congenital esophageal stenosis: a rare case of dysphagia. J Radiol Case Rep 2010;4:8-14.
9. Muller M, Gockel I, Hedwig P, et al. Is the Schatzki ring a unique esophageal entity? World J Gastroenterol 2011;17:2838-43.
10. Smith MS. Diagnosis and management of esophageal rings and webs. Gastroenterol Hepatol (N Y) 2010;6:701-4.
11. Novacek G. Plummer-vinson syndrome. Orphanet J Rare Dis 2006;1:36.
12. Mann NS, Leung JW. Pathogenesis of esophageal rings in eosinophilic esophagitis. Med Hypotheses 2005;64:520-3.
13. Changela K, Haeri NS, Krishnaiah M, Reddy M. Plummer-vinson syndrome with proximal esophageal web. J Gastrointest Surg 2016;20:1074-5.
14. Chen CT, Lai HY, Jung SM, Lee CY, Wu CT, Lee ST. Neurenteric cyst or neuroendodermal cyst? Immunohistochemical study and pathogenesis. World Neurosurg 2016;96:85-90.
15. Rathod J, Disawal A, Taori K, et al. Communicating tubular duplication of upper esophagus-a rare occurrence. J Clin Imaging Sci 2011;1:33.
16. Wiechowska-Kozlowska A, Wunsch E, Majewski M, Milkiewicz P. Esophageal duplication cysts: endosonographic findings in asymptomatic patients. World J Gastroenterol 2012;18:1270-2.
17. Somani P, Sharma M. Endoscopic ultrasound of esophageal duplication cyst. Indian J Gastroenterol. 2016;35:497-8.

18. Kapoor V, Johnson DR, Fukui MB, Rothfus WE, Jho HD. Neuroradiologic-pathologic correlation in a neurenteric cyst of the clivus. AJNR Am J Neuroradiol 2002;23:476-9.

19. Han C, Lin R, Yu J, et al. A case report of esophageal bronchogenic cyst and review of the literature with an emphasis on endoscopic ultrasonography appearance. Medicine (Baltimore) 2016;95:e3111.

20. Achkar E. Esophageal diverticula. Gastroenterol Hepatol (N Y) 2008;4:691-3.

21. Michael H, Fisher RS. Treatment of epiphrenic and mid-esophageal diverticula. Curr Treat Options Gastroenterol 2004;7:41-52.

22. Le Mouel JP, Fumery M. Zenker's diverticulum. N Engl J Med 2017;377:e31.

23. Tapias LF, Morse CR, Mathisen DJ, et al. Surgical management of esophageal epiphrenic diverticula: a transthoracic approach over four decades. Ann Thorac Surg 2017;104:1123 30.

24. Ballehaninna UK, Shaw JP, Brichkov I. Traction esophageal diverticulum: a rare cause of gastro-intestinal bleeding. Springerplus 2012;1:50.

25. Sinha SK, Nain CK, Udawat HP, et al. Cervical esophageal web and celiac disease. J Gastroenterol Hepatol 2008;23(Pt 1):1149-52.

26. de Oliveira LL, Carneiro FO, Baba ER, et al. Esophageal intramural pseudodiverticulosis: a rare endoscopic finding. Case Rep Med 2013;2013:154767.

27. Peitz U, Vieth M, Evert M, Arand J, Roessner A, Malfertheiner P. The prevalence of gastric heterotopia of the proximal esophagus is underestimated, but preneoplasia is rare—correlation with Barrett's esophagus. BMC Gastroenterol 2017;17:87.

28. Chong VH, Jalihal A. Heterotopic gastric mucosal patch of the esophagus is associated with higher prevalence of laryngopharyngeal reflux symptoms. Eur Arch Otorhinolaryngol 2010;267:1793-9.

29. Shimamura Y, Winer S, Marcon N. A giant circumferential inlet patch with acid secretion causing stricture. Clin Gastroenterol Hepatol 2017;15:A22-3.

30. Schneider NI, Plieschnegger W, Geppert M, et al. Pancreatic acinar cells—a normal finding at the gastroesophageal junction? Data from a prospective central European multicenter study. Virchows Arch 2013;463:643-50.

31. Trifan A, Tarcoveanu E, Danciu M, Hutanasu C, Cojocariu C, Stanciu C. Gastric heterotopic pancreas: an unusual case and review of the literature. J Gastrointestin Liver Dis 2012;21:209-12.

32. Chiu KW, Wu CK, Lu LS, Eng HL, Chiou SS. Diagnostic pitfall of sebaceous gland metaplasia of the esophagus. World J Clin Cases 2014;2:311-5.

33. Chong VH. Clinical significance of heterotopic gastric mucosal patch of the proximal esophagus. World J Gastroenterol 2013;19:331-8.

34. von Rahden BH, Stein HJ, Becker K, Liebermann-Meffert D, Siewert JR. Heterotopic gastric mucosa of the esophagus: literature-review and proposal of a clinicopathologic classification. Am J Gastroenterol 2004;99:543-51.

35. Johansson J, Hakansson HO, Mellblom L, et al. Prevalence of precancerous and other metaplasia in the distal oesophagus and gastro-oesophageal junction. Scand J Gastroenterol 2005;40:893-902.

36. Montalvo N, Tapia V, Padilla H, Redroban L. Heterotopic sebaceous glands in the esophagus, a very rare histopathological diagnosis: a case report and review of the literature. Clin Case Rep 2017;5:89-92.

37. Fukuchi M, Tsukagoshi R, Sakurai S, et al. Ectopic sebaceous glands in the esophagus: endoscopic findings over three years. Case Rep Gastroenterol 2012;6:217-22.

38. Fang Y, Chen L, Chen DF, et al. Prevalence, histologic and clinical characteristics of heterotopic gastric mucosa in chinese patients. World J Gastroenterol 2014;20:17588-94.

39. Riddiough GE, Hornby ST, Asadi K, Aly A. Gastric adenocarinoma of the upper oesophagus: a literature review and case report. Int J Surg Case Rep 2017;30:205-14.

40. Dunn JM, Sui G, Anggiansah A, Wong T. Radiofrequency ablation of symptomatic cervical inlet patch using a through-the-scope device: a pilot study. Gastrointest Endosc 2016;84:1022-6.

41. O'Neill OM, Johnston BT, Coleman HG. Achalasia: a review of clinical diagnosis, epidemiology, treatment and outcomes. World J Gastroenterol 2013;19:5806-12.

42. Sato H, Takahashi K, Mizuno KI, et al. Esophageal motility disorders: new perspectives from high-resolution manometry and histopathology. J Gastroenterol 2018;53:484-93.

43. El-Takli I, O'Brien P, Paterson WG. Clinical diagnosis of achalasia: how reliable is the barium x-ray? Can J Gastroenterol 2006;20:335-7.

44. Wong RK, Maydonovitch CL, Metz SJ, Baker JR Jr. Significant dqw1 association in achalasia. Dig Dis Sci 1989;34:349-52.

45. Verne GN, Hahn AB, Pineau BC, Hoffman BJ, Wojciechowski BW, Wu WC. Association of HLA-DR and -DQ alleles with idiopathic achalasia. Gastroenterology 1999;117:26-31.

46. Kilicli F, Acibucu F, Senel S, Dokmetas HS. Allgrove syndrome. Singapore Med J 2012;53:e92-94.

47. Goldblum JR, Rice TW, Richter JE. Histopathologic features in esophagomyotomy specimens from patients with achalasia. Gastroenterology 1996;111:648-54.

48. Xue Y, Suriawinata A, Liu X, et al. Lymphocytic esophagitis with CD4 t-cell-predominant intraepithelial lymphocytes and primary esophageal motility abnormalities: a potential novel clinicopathologic entity. Am J Surg Pathol 2015;39:1558-67.

49. Jia Y, McCallum RW. Pseudoachalasia: still a tough clinical challenge. Am J Case Rep 2015;16:768-73.

50. Ates F, Vaezi MF. The pathogenesis and management of achalasia: current status and future directions. Gut Liver 2015;9:449-63.

51. Rios-Galvez S, Meixueiro-Daza A, Remes-Troche JM. Achalasia: a risk factor that must not be forgotten for esophageal squamous cell carcinoma. BMJ Case Rep 2015;2015.

52. Stone ML, Kilic A, Jones DR, Lau CL, Kozower BD. A diagnostic consideration for all ages: pseudoachalasia in a 22-year-old male. Ann Thorac Surg 2012;93:e11-2.

53. Ponds FA, van Raath MI, Mohamed SM, Smout AJ, Bredenoord AJ. Diagnostic features of malignancy-associated pseudoachalasia. Aliment Pharmacol Ther 2017;45:1449-58.

54. Gockel I, Eckardt VF, Schmitt T, Junginger T. Pseudoachalasia: a case series and analysis of the literature. Scand J Gastroenterol 2005;40:378-85.

55. Liu W, Fackler W, Rice TW, Richter JE, Achkar E, Goldblum JR. The pathogenesis of pseudoachalasia: a clinicopathologic study of 13 cases of a rare entity. Am J Surg Pathol 2002;26:784-8.

56. Arif T, Masood Q, Singh J, Hassan I. Assessment of esophageal involvement in systemic sclerosis and morphea (localized scleroderma) by clinical, endoscopic, manometric and ph metric features: a prospective comparative hospital based study. BMC Gastroenterol 2015;15:24.

57. Kahaleh, MB. Raynaud phenomenon and the vascular disease in scleroderma. Curr Opin Rheumatol 2004;16:718-22.

58. Bennett C, Straily A, Haselow D, et al. Chagas disease surveillance activities—seven states, 2017. MMWR Morb Mortal Wkly Rep 2018;67:738-41.

59. Kirchhoff LV. Epidemiology of American trypanosomiasis (Chagas disease). Adv Parasitol 2011;75:1-18.

60. Liu, Q, Zhou, XN. Preventing the transmission of American trypanosomiasis and its spread into non-endemic countries. Infect Dis Poverty 2015;4:60.

61. Matsuda NM, Miller SM, Evora PR. The chronic gastrointestinal manifestations of Chagas disease. Clinics (Sao Paulo) 2009;64:1219-24.

62. Sabino EC, Ribeiro AL, Salemi VM, et al. Ten-year incidence of chagas cardiomyopathy among asymptomatic trypanosoma cruzi-seropositive former blood donors. Circulation 2013;127:1105-15.

63. Lages-Silva E, Crema E, Ramirez LE, et al. Relationship between trypanosoma cruzi and human chagasic megaesophagus: blood and tissue parasitism. Am J Trop Med Hyg 2001;65:435-41.

64. Pinto-Martinez A, Hernandez-Rodriguez V, Rodriguez-Duran J, Hejchman E, Benaim G. Anti-trypanosoma cruzi action of a new benzofuran derivative based on amiodarone structure. Exp Parasitol 2018;189:8-15.

65. Capobianco J, Grimberg A, Thompson BM, Antunes VB, Jasinowodolinski D, Meirelles GS. Thoracic manifestations of collagen vascular diseases. Radiographics 2012;32:33-50.

66. Gyger G, Baron M. Systemic sclerosis: gastrointestinal disease and its management. Rheum Dis Clin North Am 2015;41:459-73.

67. Tsou PS, Sawalha AH. Unfolding the pathogenesis of scleroderma through genomics and epigenomics. J Autoimmun 2017;83:73-94.

68. Habash-Bseiso DE, Yale SH, Glurich I, Goldberg JW. Serologic testing in connective tissue diseases. Clin Med Res 2005;3:190-3.

69. Roberts CG, Hummers LK, Ravich WJ, Wigley FM, Hutchins GM. A case-control study of the pathology of oesophageal disease in systemic sclerosis (scleroderma). Gut 2006;55:1697-703.

70. Forbes A, Marie I. Gastrointestinal complications: the most frequent internal complications of systemic sclerosis. Rheumatology (Oxford) 2009;48(Suppl 3):iii36-9.

71. Wipff J, Coriat R, Masciocchi M, et al. Outcomes of Barrett's oesophagus related to systemic sclerosis: a 3-year eular scleroderma trials and research prospective follow-up study. Rheumatology (Oxford) 2011;50:1440-4.

72. Shimada H, Kise Y, Chino O, et al. A case of superficial esophageal cancer complicated with idiopathic muscular hypertrophy of the esophagus. Tokai J Exp Clin Med 2003;28:103-8.

73. Garcia-Tsao G, Sanyal AJ, Grace ND, et al. Prevention and management of gastroesophageal varices and variceal hemorrhage in cirrhosis. Hepatology 2007;46:922-38.

74. Sayasone S, Rasphone O, Vanmany M, et al. Severe morbidity due to opisthorchis viverrini and schistosoma mekongi infection in lao people's democratic republic. Clin Infect Dis 2012;55:e54-7.

75. Cardenas A. Management of acute variceal bleeding: emphasis on endoscopic therapy. Clin Liver Dis 2010;14:251-62.

76. Groszmann RJ, Garcia-Tsao G, Bosch J, et al. Beta-blockers to prevent gastroesophageal varices in patients with cirrhosis. N Engl J Med 2005;353:2254-61.

77. Arakawa M, Masuzaki T, Okuda K. Pathomorphology of esophageal and gastric varices. Semin Liver Dis 2002;22:73-82.

78. Abby Philips C, Sahney A. Oesophageal and gastric varices: historical aspects, classification and grading: everything in one place. Gastroenterol Rep (Oxf) 2016;4:186-95.

79. Mallet M, Rudler M, Thabut D. Variceal bleeding in cirrhotic patients. Gastroenterol Rep (Oxf) 2017;5:185-92.

80. Okada M, Ishimura N, Shimura S, et al. Circumferential distribution and location of mallory-weiss tears: recent trends. Endosc Int Open 2015;3:E418-24.

81. Cappell MS, Dass K, Manickam P. Characterization of the syndrome of ugi bleeding from a mallory-weiss tear associated with transesophageal echocardiography. Dig Dis Sci 2014;59:2381-9.

82. Brown JD. Hiccups: an unappreciated cause of the Mallory-Weiss syndrome. Am J Med 2015;128:e19-20.

83. Kortas DY, Haas LS, Simpson WG, Nickl NJ 3rd, Gates LK Jr. Mallory-Weiss tear: predisposing factors and predictors of a complicated course. Am J Gastroenterol 2001;96:2863-5.

84. de Schipper JP, Pull ter Gunne AF, Oostvogel HJ, van Laarhoven CJ. Spontaneous rupture of the oesophagus: Boerhaave's syndrome in 2008. Literature review and treatment algorithm. Dig Surg 2009;26:1-6.

85. Contini S, Scarpignato C. Caustic injury of the upper gastrointestinal tract: comprehensive review. World J Gastroenterol 2013;19:3918-30.

86. Almashat SJ, Duan L, Goldsmith JD. Non-reflux esophagitis: a review of inflammatory diseases of the esophagus exclusive of reflux esophagitis. Semin Diagn Pathol 2014;31:89-99.

87. Vakil N. Disease definition, clinical manifestations, epidemiology and natural history of GERD. Best Pract Res Clin Gastroenterol 2010;24:759-64.

88. Boeckxstaens G, El-Serag HB, Smout AJ, Kahrilas PJ. Republished: symptomatic reflux disease: the present, the past and the future. Postgrad Med J 2015;91:46-54.

89. El-Serag HB, Sweet S, Winchester CC, Dent J. Update on the epidemiology of gastro-oesophageal reflux disease: a systematic review. Gut 2014;63:871-80.

90. Cook MB, Chow WH, Devesa SS. Oesophageal cancer incidence in the United States by race, sex, and histologic type, 1977-2005. Br J Cancer 2009;101:855-9.

91. Kramer JR, Fischbach LA, Richardson P, et al. Waist-to-hip ratio, but not body mass index, is associated with an increased risk of Barrett's esophagus in white men. Clin Gastroenterol Hepatol 2013;11:373-81.

92. Fischbach LA, Graham DY, Kramer JR, et al. Association between Helicobacter pylori and Barrett's esophagus: a case-control study. Am J Gastroenterol 2014;109:357-68.

93. Czinn SJ, Blanchard S. Gastroesophageal reflux disease in neonates and infants: when and how to treat. Paediatr Drugs 2013;15:19-27.

94. Hirano I, Richter JE, Practice Parameters Committee of the American College of Gastroenterology. ACG practice guidelines: esophageal reflux testing. Am J Gastroenterol 2007;102:668-85.

95. Furuta K, Kushiyama Y, Kawashima K, et al. Comparisons of symptoms reported by elderly and non-elderly patients with GERD. J Gastroenterol 2012;47:144-9.

96. Souza RF, Huo X, Mittal V, et al. Gastroesophageal reflux might cause esophagitis through a cytokine-mediated mechanism rather than caustic acid injury. Gastroenterology 2009;137:1776-84.

97. Isomoto H, Wang A, Mizuta Y, et al. Elevated levels of chemokines in esophageal mucosa of patients with reflux esophagitis. Am J Gastroenterol 2003;98:551-6.

98. Altomare A, Ma J, Guarino MP, et al. Platelet-activating factor and distinct chemokines are elevated in mucosal biopsies of erosive compared with non-erosive reflux disease patients and controls. Neurogastroenterol Motil 2012;24:943-e463.

99. Gyawali CP, Kahrilas PJ, Savarino E, et al. Modern diagnosis of GERD: the Lyon Consensus. Gut 2018;67:1351-62.

100. Rath HC, Timmer A, Kunkel C, et al. Comparison of interobserver agreement for different scoring systems for reflux esophagitis: impact of level of experience. Gastrointest Endosc 2004;60:44-9.

101. Haggitt RC. Histopathology of reflux-induced esophageal and supraesophageal injuries. Am J Med 2000;108(Suppl 1):109-11.

102. Singh SP, Odze RD. Multinucleated epithelial giant cell changes in esophagitis: a clinicopathologic study of 14 cases. Am J Surg Pathol 1998;22:93-9.

103. Vieth M, Fiocca R, Haringsma J, et al. Radial distribution of dilated intercellular spaces of the esophageal squamous epithelium in patients with reflux disease exhibiting discrete endoscopic lesions. Dig Dis 2004;22:208-12.

104. Basseri B, Levy M, Wang HL, et al. Redefining the role of lymphocytes in gastroesophageal reflux disease and eosinophilic esophagitis. Dis Esophagus 2010;23:368-76.

105. Ronkainen J, Aro P, Storskrubb T, et al. High prevalence of gastroesophageal reflux symptoms and esophagitis with or without symptoms in the general adult swedish population: a Kalixanda study report. Scand J Gastroenterol 2005;40:275-85.

106. Dunbar KB, Agoston AT, Odze RD, et al. Association of acute gastroesophageal reflux disease with esophageal histologic changes. JAMA 2016;315:2104-12.

107. Zentilin P, Savarino V, Mastracci L, et al. Reassessment of the diagnostic value of histology in patients with gerd, using multiple biopsy sites and an appropriate control group. Am J Gastroenterol 2005;100:2299-306.

108. Furuta GT, Liacouras CA, Collins MH, et al. Eosinophilic esophagitis in children and adults: a systematic review and consensus recommendations for diagnosis and treatment. Gastroenterology 2007;133:1342-63.

109. Halsey KD, Arora M, Bulsiewicz WJ, et al. Eosinophilic infiltration of the esophagus following endoscopic ablation of Barrett's neoplasia. Dis Esophagus 2013;26:113-6.

110. Shah A, Kagalwalla AF, Gonsalves N, Melin-Aldana H, Li BU, Hirano I. Histopathologic variability in children with eosinophilic esophagitis. Am J Gastroenterol 2009;104:716-21.

111. Kahrilas PJ, Shaheen NJ, Vaezi MF, American Gastroenterological Association Institute; Clinical Practice and Quality Management Committee. American gastroenterological association medical position statement on the management of gastroesophageal reflux disease. Gastroenterology 2008;135:1383-91.

112. Ganz RA, Peters JH, Horgan S. Esophageal sphincter device for gastroesophageal reflux disease. N Engl J Med 2013;368:2039-40.

113. Rodriguez L, Rodriguez P, Gomez B, et al. Long-term results of electrical stimulation of the lower esophageal sphincter for the treatment of gastroesophageal reflux disease. Endoscopy 2013;45:595-604.

114. Hvid-Jensen F, Pedersen L, Drewes AM, Sørensen HT, Funch-Jensen P. Incidence of adenocarcinoma among patients with Barrett's esophagus. N Engl J Med 2011;365:1375-83.

115. Dellon ES, Hirano I. Epidemiology and natural history of eosinophilic esophagitis. Gastroenterology 2018;154:319-32.

116. Warners MJ, de Rooij W, van Rhijn BD, et al. Incidence of eosinophilic esophagitis in the Netherlands continues to rise: 20-year results from a nationwide pathology database. Neurogastroenterol Motil 2018;30:13165.

117. van Rhijn BD, Verheij J, Smout AJ, Bredenoord AJ. Rapidly increasing incidence of eosinophilic esophagitis in a large cohort. Neurogastroenterol Motil 2013;25:47-52.e45.

118. Dellon ES, Erichsen R, Baron JA, et al. The increasing incidence and prevalence of eosinophilic oesophagitis outpaces changes in endoscopic and biopsy practice: national population-based estimates from Denmark. Aliment Pharmacol Ther 2015;41:662-70.

119. von Arnim U, Wex T, Link A, et al. Helicobacter pylori infection is associated with a reduced risk of developing eosinophilic oesophagitis. Aliment Pharmacol Ther 2016;43:825-30.

120. Dellon ES, Peery AF, Shaheen NJ, et al. Inverse association of esophageal eosinophilia with helicobacter pylori based on analysis of a us pathology database. Gastroenterology 2011;141:1586-92.

121. Jensen ET, Eluri S, Lebwohl B, Genta RM, Dellon ES. Increased risk of esophageal eosinophilia and eosinophilic esophagitis in patients with active celiac disease on biopsy. Clin Gastroenterol Hepatol 2015;13:1426-31.

122. Peterson K, Firszt R, Fang J, Wong J, Smith KR, Brady KA. Risk of autoimmunity in EoE and families: a population-based cohort study. Am J Gastroenterol 2016;111:926-32.

123. Jensen ET, Kappelman MD, Kim HP, Ringel-Kulka T, Dellon ES. Early life exposures as risk factors for pediatric eosinophilic esophagitis. J Pediatr Gastroenterol Nutr 2013;57:67-71.

124. Jensen ET, Bertelsen RJ. Assessing early life factors for eosinophilic esophagitis: lessons from other allergic diseases. Curr Treat Options Gastroenterol 2016;14:39-50.

125. Liacouras CA, Furuta GT, Hirano I, et al. Eosinophilic esophagitis: updated consensus recommendations for children and adults. J Allergy Clin Immunol 2011;128:3-22.

126. Dellon ES, Gonsalves N, Hirano I, et al. ACG clinical guideline: evidenced based approach to the diagnosis and management of esophageal eosinophilia and eosinophilic esophagitis (EoE). Am J Gastroenterol 2013;108:679-93.

127. Straumann A, Conus S, Degen L, et al. Long-term budesonide maintenance treatment is partially effective for patients with eosinophilic esophagitis. Clin Gastroenterol Hepatol 2011;9:400-409.e401.

128. Menard-Katcher C, Furuta GT. Non- and semi-invasive methods of monitoring eosinophilic esophagitis. Dig Dis 2014;32:102-6.

129. Alexander ES, Martin LJ, Collins MH, et al. Twin and family studies reveal strong environmental and weaker genetic cues explaining heritability of eosinophilic esophagitis. J Allergy Clin Immunol 2014;134:1084-92.

130. Rothenberg ME, Spergel JM, Sherrill JD, et al. Common variants at 5q22 associate with pediatric eosinophilic esophagitis. Nat Genet 2010;42:289-91.

131. Mishra A, Hogan SP, Brandt EB, Rothenberg ME. Il-5 promotes eosinophil trafficking to the esophagus. J Immunol 2002;168:2464-9.

132. Zuo L, Fulkerson PC, Finkelman FD, et al. Il-13 induces esophageal remodeling and gene expression by an eosinophil-independent, il-13r alpha 2-inhibited pathway. J Immunol 2010;185:660-9.

133. Blanchard C, Mishra A, Saito-Akei H, Monk P, Anderson I, Rothenberg ME. Inhibition of human interleukin-13-induced respiratory and oesophageal inflammation by anti-human-interleukin-13 antibody (CAT-354). Clin Exp Allergy 2005;35:1096-103.

134. Aceves SS, Chen D, Newbury RO, Dohil R, Bastian JF, Broide DH. Mast cells infiltrate the esophageal smooth muscle in patients with eosinophilic esophagitis, express tgf-beta1, and increase esophageal smooth muscle contraction. J Allergy Clin Immunol 2010;126:1198-204.e1194.

135. Kottyan LC, Davis BP, Sherrill JD, et al. Genome-wide association analysis of eosinophilic esophagitis provides insight into the tissue specificity of this allergic disease. Nat Genet 2014;46:895-900.

136. Sherrill JD, Kc K, Wu D, et al. Desmoglein-1 regulates esophageal epithelial barrier function and immune responses in eosinophilic esophagitis. Mucosal Immunol 2014;7:718-29.

137. Fallon PG, Sasaki T, Sandilands A, et al. A homozygous frameshift mutation in the mouse flg gene facilitates enhanced percutaneous allergen priming. Nat Genet 2009;41:602-8.

138. Dellon ES, Gibbs WB, Fritchie KJ, et al. Clinical, endoscopic, and histologic findings distinguish eosinophilic esophagitis from gastroesophageal reflux disease. Clin Gastroenterol Hepatol 2009;7:1305-13.

139. Salek J, Clayton F, Vinson L, et al. Endoscopic appearance and location dictate diagnostic yield of biopsies in eosinophilic oesophagitis. Aliment Pharmacol Ther 2015;41:1288-95.

140. Hori K, Watari J, Fukui H, et al. Do endoscopic features suggesting eosinophilic esophagitis represent histological eosinophilia? Dig Endosc 2014;26:156-63.

141. Nielsen JA, Lager DJ, Lewin M, Rendon G, Roberts CA. The optimal number of biopsy fragments to establish a morphologic diagnosis of eosinophilic esophagitis. Am J Gastroenterol 2014;109:515-20.

142. Yantiss RK. Eosinophils in the GI tract: how many is too many and what do they mean? Mod Pathol 2015;28(Suppl 1):S7-21.

143. Rodrigo S, Abboud G, Oh D, et al. High intraepithelial eosinophil counts in esophageal squamous epithelium are not specific for eosinophilic esophagitis in adults. Am J Gastroenterol 2008;103:435-42.

144. Parfitt JR, Gregor JC, Suskin NG, Jawa HA, Driman DK. Eosinophilic esophagitis in adults: distinguishing features from gastroesophageal reflux disease: a study of 41 patients. Mod Pathol 2006;19:90-6.

145. Li-Kim-Moy JP, Tobias V, Day AS, Leach S, Lemberg DA. Esophageal subepithelial fibrosis and hyalinization are features of eosinophilic esophagitis. J Pediatr Gastroenterol Nutr 2011;52:147-53.

146. Chehade M, Sampson HA, Morotti RA, Magid MS. Esophageal subepithelial fibrosis in children with eosinophilic esophagitis. J Pediatr Gastroenterol Nutr 2007;45:319-28.

147. Molina-Infante J, Ferrando-Lamana L, Ripoll C, et al. Esophageal eosinophilic infiltration responds to proton pump inhibition in most adults. Clin Gastroenterol Hepatol 2011;9:110-7.

148. Wen T, Dellon ES, Moawad FJ, Furuta GT, Aceves SS, Rothenberg ME. Transcriptome analysis of proton pump inhibitor-responsive esophageal eosinophilia reveals proton pump inhibitor-reversible allergic inflammation. J Allergy Clin Immunol 2015;135:187-97.

149. Molina-Infante J, Bredenoord AJ, Cheng E, et al. Proton pump inhibitor-responsive oesophageal eosinophilia: an entity challenging current diagnostic criteria for eosinophilic oesophagitis. Gut 2016;65:524-31.

150. Dellon ES, Gonsalves N, Hirano I, et al. ACG clinical guideline: evidenced based approach to the diagnosis and management of esophageal eosinophilia and eosinophilic esophagitis (EoE). Am J Gastroenterol 2013;108:679-93.

151. Spergel JM, Brown-Whitehorn TF, Beausoleil JL, et al. 14 years of eosinophilic esophagitis: clinical features and prognosis. J Pediatr Gastroenterol Nutr 2009;48:30-6.

152. Butz BK, Wen T, Gleich GJ, et al. Efficacy, dose reduction, and resistance to high-dose fluticasone in patients with eosinophilic esophagitis. Gastroenterology 2014;147:324-33.

153. Miehlke S, Hruz P, Vieth M, et al. A randomised, double-blind trial comparing budesonide formulations and dosages for short-term treatment of eosinophilic oesophagitis. Gut 2016;65:390-9.

154. Dougherty T Jr, Stephen S, Borum ML, Doman DB. Emerging therapeutic options for eosinophilic esophagitis. Gastroenterol Hepatol (N Y) 2014;10:106-16.

155. Schoepfer AM, Gonsalves N, Bussmann C, et al. Esophageal dilation in eosinophilic esophagitis: effectiveness, safety, and impact on the underlying inflammation. Am J Gastroenterol 2010;105:1062-70.

156. Cohen S, Saxena A, Waljee AK, et al. Lymphocytic esophagitis: a diagnosis of increasing frequency. J Clin Gastroenterol 2012;46:828-32.

157. Rubio CA, Sjodahl K, Lagergren J. Lymphocytic esophagitis: a histologic subset of chronic esophagitis. Am J Clin Pathol 2006;125:432-7.

158. Purdy JK, Appelman HD, Golembeski CP, McKenna BJ. Lymphocytic esophagitis: a chronic or recurring pattern of esophagitis resembling allergic contact dermatitis. Am J Clin Pathol 2008;130:508-13.

159. Haque S, Genta RM. Lymphocytic oesophagitis: clinicopathological aspects of an emerging condition. Gut 2012;61:1108-14.

160. Ebach DR, Vanderheyden AD, Ellison JM, Jensen CS. Lymphocytic esophagitis: a possible manifestation of pediatric upper gastrointestinal crohn's disease. Inflamm Bowel Dis 2011;17:45-9.

161. Sutton LM, Heintz DD, Patel AS, Weinberg AG. Lymphocytic esophagitis in children. Inflamm Bowel Dis 2014;20:1324-8.

162. Daniels JA, Lederman HM, Maitra A, Montgomery EA. Gastrointestinal tract pathology in patients with common variable immunodeficiency (CVID): a clinicopathologic study and review. Am J Surg Pathol 2007;31:1800-12.

162a. Pittman ME, Hissong E, Katz PO, Yantiss RK. Lymphocyte-predominant esophagitis: a distinct and likely immune-mediated disorder encompassing lymphocytic and lichenoid esophagitis. Am J Surg Pathol 2020;44:198-205.

163. Pasricha S, Gupta A, Reed CC, Speck O, Woosley JT, Dellon ES. Lymphocytic esophagitis: an emerging clinicopathologic disease associated with dysphagia. Dig Dis Sci 2016;61:2935-41.

164. Kissiedu J, Thota PN, Gohel T, Lopez R, Gordon IO. Post-ablation lymphocytic esophagitis in Barrett esophagus with high grade dysplasia or intramucosal carcinoma. Mod Pathol 2016;29:599-606.

165. Putra J, Muller KE, Hussain ZH, et al. Lymphocytic esophagitis in nonachalasia primary esophageal motility disorders: improved criteria, prevalence, strength of association, and natural history. Am J Surg Pathol 2016;40:1679-85.

166. Connor J, Sanchez C, Reid B, et al. Lymphocytic esophagitis in Barrett's esophagus: correlation with patient symptoms and risk factors. Mod Pathol 2014;27:169A.

167. Salaria SN, Abu Alfa AK, Cruise MW, Wood LD, Montgomery EA. Lichenoid esophagitis: clinicopathologic overlap with established esophageal lichen planus. Am J Surg Pathol 2013;37:1889-94.

168. Basseri B, Vasiliauskas EA, Chan O, et al. Evaluation of peripapillary lymphocytosis and lymphocytic esophagitis in adult inflammatory bowel disease. Gastroenterol Hepatol (N Y) 2013;9:505-11.

169. Kim SH, Jeong JB, Kim JW, et al. Clinical and endoscopic characteristics of drug-induced esophagitis. World J Gastroenterol 2014;20:10994-9.

170. Jung P, Fortinsky KJ, Gallinger ZR, Tartaro P. Severe erosive pill esophagitis induced by crizotinib therapy: a case report and literature review. Case Rep Gastrointest Med 2016; 2016:3562820.

171. Kadayifci A, Gulsen MT, Koruk M, Savas MC. Doxycycline-induced pill esophagitis. Dis Esophagus 2004;17:168-71.

172. Zezos P, Harel Z, Saibil F. Cloxacillin: a new cause of pill-induced esophagitis. Can J Gastroenterol Hepatol 2016;2016:2904256.

173. Shaddy SM, Arnold MA, Shilo K, et al. Crospovidone and microcrystalline cellulose: a novel description of pharmaceutical fillers in the gastrointestinal tract. Am J Surg Pathol 2017;41:564-9.

174. Findeis-Hosey JJ, Gonzalez RS. Crospovidone: pharmaceutical filler found commonly in gastrointestinal pathology specimens. Histopathology 2017;71:331-3.

175. Nguyen T, Park JY, Scudiere JR, Montgomery E. Mycophenolic acid (cellcept and myofortic) induced injury of the upper gi tract. Am J Surg Pathol 2009;33:1355-63.

176. Abraham SC, Cruz-Correa M, Lee LA, Yardley JH, Wu TT. Alendronate-associated esophageal injury: pathologic and endoscopic features. Mod Pathol 1999;12:1152-7.

177. Nagano Y, Matsui H, Shimokawa O, et al. Bisphosphonate-induced gastrointestinal mucosal injury is mediated by mitochondrial superoxide production and lipid peroxidation. J Clin Biochem Nutr 2012;51:196-203.

178. Morris TJ, Davis TP. Doxycycline-induced esophageal ulceration in the U.S. military service. Mil Med 2000;165:316-9.

179. Banisaeed N, Truding RM, Chang CH. Tetracycline-induced spongiotic esophagitis: a new endoscopic and histopathologic finding. Gastrointest Endosc 2003;58:292-4.

180. Abraham SC, Yardley JH, Wu TT. Erosive injury to the upper gastrointestinal tract in patients receiving iron medication: an underrecognized entity. Am J Surg Pathol 1999;23:1241-7.

181. Chaitman M, Dixit D, Bridgeman MB. Potassium-binding agents for the clinical management of hyperkalemia. P T 2016;41:43-50.

182. Abraham SC, Bhagavan BS, Lee LA, Rashid A, WU TT. Upper gastrointestinal tract injury in patients receiving kayexalate (sodium polystyrene sulfonate) in sorbitol: clinical, endoscopic, and histopathologic findings. Am J Surg Pathol 2001;25:637-44.

183. van de Veerdonk FL, Kullberg BJ, Netea MG. Pathogenesis of invasive candidiasis. Curr Opin Crit Care 2010;16:453-9.

184. Antinori S, Milazzo L, Sollima S, Galli M, Corbellino M. Candidemia and invasive candidiasis in adults: a narrative review. Eur J Intern Med 2016;34:21-8.

185. Patel PK, Erlandsen JE, Kirkpatrick WR, et al. The changing epidemiology of oropharyngeal candidiasis in patients with HIV/AIDS in the era of antiretroviral therapy. AIDS Res Treat 2012;2012:262471.

186. Wilson A, Delport J, Ponich T. Candida glabrata esophagitis: are we seeing the emergence of a new azole-resistant pathogen? Int J Microbiol 2014;2014:371631.

187. von Arnim U, Malfertheiner P. Eosinophilic esophagitis—treatment of eosinophilic esophagitis with drugs: corticosteroids. Dig Dis 2014;32:126-9.

188. Daniell HW. Acid suppressing therapy as a risk factor for Candida esophagitis. Dis Esophagus 2016;29:479-83.

189. Asayama N, Nagata N, Shimbo T, et al. Relationship between clinical factors and severity of esophageal candidiasis according to Kodsi's classification. Dis Esophagus 2014;27:214-9.

190. Steiner I, Kennedy PG, Pachner AR. The neurotropic herpes viruses: herpes simplex and varicella-zoster. Lancet Neurol 2007;6:1015-28.

191. Geraci G, Pisello F, Modica G, Sciume C. Herpes simplex esophagitis in immunocompetent host: a case report. Diagn Ther Endosc 2009;2009:717183.

192. Canalejo Castrillero E, Garcia Duran F, Cabello N, Garcia Martinez J. Herpes esophagitis in healthy adults and adolescents: report of 3 cases and review of the literature. Medicine (Baltimore) 2010;89:204-10.

193. Itoh T, Takahashi T, Kusaka K, et al. Herpes simplex esophagitis from 1307 autopsy cases. J Gastroenterol Hepatol 2003;18:1407-11.

194. Ramanathan J, Rammouni M, Baran J Jr, Khatib R. Herpes simplex virus esophagitis in the immunocompetent host: an overview. Am J Gastroenterol 2000;95:2171-6.

195. Wald A, Ashley-Morrow R. Serological testing for herpes simplex virus (HSV)-1 and HSV-2 infection. Clin Infect Dis 2002;35(Suppl 2):S173-82.

196. Fatahzadeh M, Schwartz RA. Human herpes simplex virus infections: epidemiology, pathogenesis, symptomatology, diagnosis, and management. J Am Acad Dermatol 2007;57:737-64.

197. Greenson JK, Beschorner WE, Boitnott JK, Yardley JH. Prominent mononuclear cell infiltrate is characteristic of herpes esophagitis. Hum Pathol 1991;22:541-9.

198. Balachandran N, Oba DE, Hutt-Fletcher LM. Antigenic cross-reactions among herpes simplex virus types 1 and 2, Epstein-Barr virus, and cytomegalovirus. J Virol 1987;61:1125-35.

199. Strick LB, Wald A. Diagnostics for herpes simplex virus: is PCR the new gold standard? Mol Diagn Ther 2006;10:17-28.

200. Mostyka M, Shia J, Neumann WL, Whitney-Miller CL, Feely M, Yantiss RK. Clinicopathologic features of varicella zoster virus infection of the upper gastrointestinal tract. Am J Surg Pathol 2020. [Online ahead of print]

201. Staras SA, Dollard SC, Radford KW, Flanders WD, Pass RF, Cannon MJ. Seroprevalence of cytomegalovirus infection in the United States, 1988-1994. Clin Infect Dis 2006;43:1143-51.

202. You DM, Johnson MD. Cytomegalovirus infection and the gastrointestinal tract. Curr Gastroenterol Rep 2012;14:334-42.

203. Rafailidis PI, Mourtzoukou EG, Varbobitis IC, Falagas ME. Severe cytomegalovirus infection in apparently immunocompetent patients: a systematic review. Virol J 2008;5:47.

204. Nakase H, Herfarth H. Cytomegalovirus colitis, cytomegalovirus hepatitis and systemic cytomegalovirus infection: common features and differences. Inflamm Intest Dis 2016;1:15-23.

205. Lawlor G, Moss AC. Cytomegalovirus in inflammatory bowel disease: pathogen or innocent bystander? Inflamm Bowel Dis 2010;16:1620-7.

206. Cook CH, Trgovcich J, Zimmerman PD, Zhang Y, Sedmak DD. Lipopolysaccharide, tumor necrosis factor alpha, or interleukin-1beta triggers reactivation of latent cytomegalovirus in immunocompetent mice. J Virol 2006;80:9151-8.

207. Adler B, Sinzger C. Endothelial cells in human cytomegalovirus infection: one host cell out of many or a crucial target for virus spread? Thromb Haemost 2009;102:1057-63.

208. Yan Z, Wang L, Dennis J, Doern C, Baker J, Park JY. Clinical significance of isolated cytomegalovirus-infected gastrointestinal cells. Int J Surg Pathol 2014;22:492-8.

209. Lv B, Cheng X, Gao J, et al. Human immunodeficiency virus (HIV) is highly associated with giant idiopathic esophageal ulcers in acquired immunodeficiency syndrome (AIDS) patients. Am J Transl Res 2016;8:4464-71.

210. Borges MC, Colares JK, Lima DM, Fonseca BA. Advantages and pitfalls of the polymerase chain reaction in the diagnosis of esophageal ulcers in aids patients. Dig Dis Sci 2009;54:1933-9.

211. Nishijima T, Tsukada K, Nagata N, et al. Antiretroviral therapy alone resulted in successful resolution of large idiopathic esophageal ulcers in a patient with acute retroviral syndrome. AIDS 2011;25:1677-9.

212. Hart PA, Romano RC, Moreira RK, et al. Esophagitis dissecans superficialis: clinical, endoscopic, and histologic features. Dig Dis Sci 2015;60:2049-57.

213. Purdy JK, Appelman HD, McKenna BJ. Sloughing esophagitis is associated with chronic debilitation and medications that injure the esophageal mucosa. Mod Pathol 2012;25:767-75.

214. Albert DM, Ally MR, Moawad FJ. The sloughing esophagus: a report of five cases. Am J Gastroenterol 2013;108:1816-7.

215. Carmack SW, Vemulapalli R, Spechler SJ, Genta RM. Esophagitis dissecans superficialis ("sloughing esophagitis"): a clinicopathologic study of 12 cases. Am J Surg Pathol 2009;33:1789-94.

216. Ben Soussan E, Savoye G, Hochain P, et al. Acute esophageal necrosis: a 1-year prospective study. Gastrointest Endosc 2002;56:213-7.

217. Kim DB, Bowers S, Thomas M. Black and white esophagus: rare presentations of severe esophageal ischemia. Semin Thorac Cardiovasc Surg 2017;29:256-9.

218. Gurvits GE, Shapsis A, Lau N, Gualtieri N, Robilotti JG. Acute esophageal necrosis: a rare syndrome. J Gastroenterol 2007;42:29-38.

218a. Jessurun J, Cui I, Aristi-Urista G. Acute (gangrenous) esophageal necrosis (black esophagus). A rare form of injury with specific histologic features and diverse clinical associations with a common pathogenesis. Hum Pathol 2019;87:44-50.

219. Worrell SG, Oh DS, Greene CL, DeMeester SR, Hagen JA. Acute esophageal necrosis: a case series and long-term follow-up. Ann Thorac Surg 2014;98:341-2.

220. Chibishev A, Pereska Z, Simonovska N, Chibisheva V, Glasnovic M, Chitkushev LT. Conservative therapeutic approach to corrosive poisonings in adults. J Gastrointest Surg 2013;17:1044-9.

221. Grudell AB, Mueller PS, Viggiano TR. Black esophagus: report of six cases and review of the literature, 1963-2003. Dis Esophagus 2006;19:105-10.

222. Augusto F, Fernandes V, Cremers MI, et al. Acute necrotizing esophagitis: a large retrospective case series. Endoscopy 2004;36:411-5.

223. McLaughlin CW, Person TD, Denlinger CE. Management of acute esophageal necrosis syndrome. J Thorac Cardiovasc Surg 2011;141:e23-4.

224. Holtan SG, Pasquini M, Weisdorf DJ. Acute graft-versus-host disease: a bench-to-bedside update. Blood 2014;124:363-73.

225. Lazarus HM, Sommers SR, Arfons LM, et al. Spontaneous autologous graft-versus-host disease in plasma cell myeloma autograft recipients: flow cytometric analysis of hematopoietic progenitor cell grafts. Biol Blood Marrow Transplant 2011;17:970-8.

226. Ip S, Marquez V, Schaeffer DF, Donnellan F. Sensitivities of biopsy sites in the endoscopic evaluation of graft-versus-host disease: retrospective review from a tertiary center. Dig Dis Sci 2016;61:2351-6.

227. Sodhi SS, Srinivasan R, Thomas RM. Esophageal graft versus host disease. Gastrointest Endosc 2000;52:235.

228. Trabulo D, Ferreira S, Lage P, Rego RL, Teixeira G, Pereira AD. Esophageal stenosis with sloughing esophagitis: a curious manifestation of graft-vs-host disease. World J Gastroenterol 2015;21:9217-22.

229. Simone CB 2nd. Thoracic radiation normal tissue injury. Semin Radiat Oncol 2017;27:370-7.

230. Yazbeck VY, Villaruz L, Haley M, Socinski MA. Management of normal tissue toxicity associated with chemoradiation (primary skin, esophagus, and lung). Cancer J 2013;19:231-7.

231. Werner-Wasik M, Yorke E, Deasy J, Nam J, Marks LB. Radiation dose-volume effects in the esophagus. Int J Radiat Oncol Biol Phys 2010;76(Suppl):S86-93.

232. Palma DA, Senan S, Oberije C, et al. Predicting esophagitis after chemoradiation therapy for non-small cell lung cancer: an individual patient data meta-analysis. Int J Radiat Oncol Biol Phys 2013;87:690-6.

233. Kneisel A, Hertl M. Autoimmune bullous skin diseases. Part 1: clinical manifestations. J Dtsch Dermatol Ges 2011;9:844-57.

234. Trattner A, Lurie R, Leiser A, et al. Esophageal involvement in pemphigus vulgaris: a clinical, histologic, and immunopathologic study. J Am Acad Dermatol 1991;24(Pt 1):223-6.

235. Joly P, Baricault S, Sparsa A, et al. Incidence and mortality of bullous pemphigoid in France. J Invest Dermatol 2012;132:1998-2004.

236. Zehou O, Raynaud JJ, Le Roux-Villet C, et al. Oesophageal involvement in 26 consecutive patients with mucous membrane pemphigoid. Br J Dermatol 2017;177:1074-85.

237. Smoller BR, Woodley DT. Differences in direct immunofluorescence staining patterns in epidermolysis bullosa acquisita and bullous pemphigoid. J Am Acad Dermatol 1992;27(Pt 1):674-8.

238. Fine JD, Bruckner-Tuderman L, Eady RA, et al. Inherited epidermolysis bullosa: updated recommendations on diagnosis and classification. J Am Acad Dermatol 2014;70:1103-26.

239. Gottschalk A, Venherm S, Vowinkel T, Tübergen D, Frosch M, Hahnenkamp K. Anesthesia for balloon dilatation of esophageal strictures in children with epidermolysis bullosa dystrophica: from intubation to sedation. Curr Opin Anaesthesiol 2010;23:518-22.

240. Delgado L, Aoki V, Santi C, Gabbi T, Sotto M, Maruta C. Clinical and immunopathological evaluation of epidermolysis bullosa acquisita. Clin Exp Dermatol 2011;36:12-8.

241. Brown CS, Defazio JR, An G, et al. Toxic epidermal necrolysis with gastrointestinal involvement: a case report and review of the literature. J Burn Care Res 2017;38:e450-5.

242. Belafsky PC, Postma GN, Koufman JA, Bach KK. Stevens-Johnson syndrome with diffuse esophageal involvement. Ear Nose Throat J 2002;81:220.

243. Shaheen NJ, Falk GW, Iyer PG, Gerson LB, American College of Gastroenterology. ACG clinical guideline: diagnosis and management of Barrett's esophagus. Am J Gastroenterol 2016;111:30-51.

244. Fitzgerald RC, di Pietro M, Ragunath K, et al. British Society of Gastroenterology guidelines on the diagnosis and management of Barrett's oesophagus. Gut 2014;63:7-42.

245. Ronkainen J, Aro P, Storskrubb T, et al. Prevalence of Barrett's esophagus in the general population: an endoscopic study. Gastroenterology 2005;129:1825-31.

246. Rex DK, Cummings OW, Shaw M, et al. Screening for Barrett's esophagus in colonoscopy patients with and without heartburn. Gastroenterology 2003;125:1670-7.

247. Zhang S, Zhang XQ, Ding XW, et al. Cyclooxygenase inhibitors use is associated with reduced risk of esophageal adenocarcinoma in patients with Barrett's esophagus: a meta-analysis. Br J Cancer 2014;110:2378-88.

248. Singh S, Garg SK, Singh PP, et al. Acid-suppressive medications and risk of oesophageal adenocarcinoma in patients with Barrett's oesophagus: a systematic review and meta-analysis. Gut 2014;63:1229-37.

249. Singh S, Singh AG, Singh PP, Murad MH, Iyer PG. Statins are associated with reduced risk of esophageal cancer, particularly in patients with Barrett's esophagus: a systematic review and meta-analysis. Clin Gastroenterol Hepatol 2013;11:620-9.

250. Runge TM, Abrams JA, Shaheen NJ. Epidemiology of Barrett's esophagus and esophageal adenocarcinoma. Gastroenterol Clin North Am 2015;44:203-31.

251. Zhang X, Westerhoff M, Hart J. Expression of SOX9 and CDX2 in nongoblet columnar-lined esophagus predicts the detection of Barrett's esophagus during follow-up. Mod Pathol 2015;28:654-61.

252. Asanuma K, Huo X, Agoston A, et al. In oesophageal squamous cells, nitric oxide causes S-nitrosylation of Akt and blocks SOX2 (sex determining region Y-box 2) expression. Gut 2016;65:1416-26.

253. Wang DH. The esophageal squamous epithelial cell-still a reasonable candidate for the Barrett's esophagus cell of origin? Cell Mol Gastroenterol Hepatol 2017;4:157-60.

254. Stachler MD, Taylor-Weiner A, Peng S, et al. Paired exome analysis of Barrett's esophagus and adenocarcinoma. Nat Genet 2015;47:1047-55.

255. Galipeau PC, Prevo LJ, Sanchez CA, Longton GM, Reid BJ. Clonal expansion and loss of heterozygosity at chromosomes 9p and 17p in premalignant esophageal (Barrett's) tissue. J Natl Cancer Inst 1999;91:2087-95.

256. Sharma P, Dent J, Armstrong D, et al. The development and validation of an endoscopic grading system for Barrett's esophagus: the Prague C & M criteria. Gastroenterology 2006;131:1392-9.

257. Panarelli NC, Yantiss RK. The importance of biopsy sampling practices in the pathologic evaluation of gastrointestinal disorders. Curr Opin Gastroenterol 2016;32:374-81.

258. Reid BJ, Blount PL, Feng Z, Levine DS. Optimizing endoscopic biopsy detection of early cancers in Barrett's high-grade dysplasia. Am J Gastroenterol 2000;95:3089-96.

259. Montgomery E, Bronner MP, Greenson JK, et al. Are ulcers a marker for invasive carcinoma in Barrett's esophagus? Data from a diagnostic variability study with clinical follow-up. Am J Gastroenterol 2002;97:27-31.

260. Lewis JT, Wang KK, Abraham SC. Muscularis mucosae duplication and the musculo-fibrous anomaly in endoscopic mucosal resections for Barrett esophagus: implications for staging of adenocarcinoma. Am J Surg Pathol 2008;32:566-71.

261. Franchimont D, Van Laethem JL, Deviere J. Argon plasma coagulation in Barrett's esophagus. Gastrointest Endosc Clin N Am 2003;13:457-66.

262. Dulai GS, Jensen DM, Cortina G, Fontana L, Ippoliti A. Randomized trial of argon plasma coagulation vs. multipolar electrocoagulation for ablation of Barrett's esophagus. Gastrointest Endosc 2005;61:232-40.

263. Hornick JL, Blount PL, Sanchez CA, et al. Biologic properties of columnar epithelium underneath reepithelialized squamous mucosa in Barrett's esophagus. Am J Surg Pathol 2005;29:372-80.

264. Reid BJ, Haggitt RC, Rubin CE, et al. Observer variation in the diagnosis of dysplasia in Barrett's esophagus. Hum Pathol 1988;19:166-78.

265. Rucker-Schmidt RL, Sanchez CA, Blount PL, et al. Nonadenomatous dysplasia in Barrett esophagus: a clinical, pathologic, and DNA content flow cytometric study. Am J Surg Pathol 2009;33:886-93.

266. Lomo LC, Blount PL, Sanchez CA, et al. Crypt dysplasia with surface maturation: a clinical, pathologic, and molecular study of a Barrett's esophagus cohort. Am J Surg Pathol 2006;30:423-35.

267. Coco DP, Goldblum JR, Hornick JL, et al. Interobserver variability in the diagnosis of crypt dysplasia in Barrett esophagus. Am J Surg Pathol 2011;35:45-54.

268. Johnson DR, Abdelbaqui M, Tahmasbi M, et al. CDX2 protein expression compared to alcian blue staining in the evaluation of esophageal intestinal metaplasia. World J Gastroenterol 2015;21:2770-6.

269. Phillips RW, Frierson HF Jr, Moskaluk CA. CDX2 as a marker of epithelial intestinal differentiation in the esophagus. Am J Surg Pathol 2003;27:1442-7.

270. Steininger H, Pfofe DA, Muller H, Haag-Sunjic G, Fratianu V. Expression of CDX2 and MUC2 in Barrett's mucosa. Pathol Res Pract 2005;201:573-7.

271. McIntire MG, Soucy G, Vaughan TL, Shahsafaei A, Odze RD. MUC2 is a highly specific marker of goblet cell metaplasia in the distal esophagus and gastroesophageal junction. Am J Surg Pathol 2011;35:1007-13.

272. Hahn HP, Blount PL, Ayub K, et al. Intestinal differentiation in metaplastic, nongoblet columnar epithelium in the esophagus. Am J Surg Pathol 2009;33:1006-15.

273. Groisman GM, Amar M, Meir A. Expression of the intestinal marker Cdx2 in the columnar-lined esophagus with and without intestinal (Barrett's) metaplasia. Mod Pathol 2004;17:1282-8.

274. Srivastava A, Appelman H, Goldsmith JD, Davison JM, Hart J, Krasinskas AM. The use of ancillary stains in the diagnosis of Barrett esophagus and Barrett esophagus-associated dysplasia: recommendations from the Rodger C. Haggitt Gastrointestinal Pathology Society. Am J Surg Pathol 2017;41:e8-21.

275. Reid BJ, Levine DS, Longton G, Blount PL, Rabinovitch PS. Predictors of progression to cancer in Barrett's esophagus: baseline histology and flow cytometry identify low- and high-risk patient subsets. Am J Gastroenterol 2000;95:1669-76.

276. Reid BJ, Prevo LJ, Galipeau PC, et al. Predictors of progression in Barrett's esophagus II: baseline 17p (p53) loss of heterozygosity identifies a patient subset at increased risk for neoplastic progression. Am J Gastroenterol 2001;96:2839-48.

277. Fahmy M, Skacel M, Gramlich TL, et al. Chromosomal gains and genomic loss of p53 and p16 genes in Barrett's esophagus detected by fluorescence in situ hybridization of cytology specimens. Mod Pathol 2004;17:588-96.

278. Fritcher EG, Brankley SM, Kipp BR, et al. A comparison of conventional cytology, DNA ploidy analysis, and fluorescence in situ hybridization for the detection of dysplasia and adenocarcinoma in patients with Barrett's esophagus. Hum Pathol 2008;39:1128-35.

279. Sato F, Jin Z, Schulmann K, et al. Three-tiered risk stratification model to predict progression in Barrett's esophagus using epigenetic and clinical features. PLoS One 2008;3:e1890.

280. Glickman JN, Spechler SJ, Souza RF, Lunsford T, Lee E, Odze RD. Multilayered epithelium in mucosal biopsy specimens from the gastroesophageal junction region is a histologic marker of gastroesophageal reflux disease. Am J Surg Pathol 2009;33:818-25.

281. Zaninotto G, Avellini C, Barbazza R, et al. Prevalence of intestinal metaplasia in the distal oesophagus, oesophagogastric junction and gastric cardia in symptomatic patients in north-east Italy: a prospective, descriptive survey. The Italian Ulcer Study Group "GISU." Dig Liver Dis 2001;33:316-21.

282. Srivastava A, Hornick JL, Li X, et al. Extent of low-grade dysplasia is a risk factor for the development of esophageal adenocarcinoma in Barrett's esophagus. Am J Gastroenterol 2007;102:483-94.

283. Kastelein F, Biermann K, Steyerberg EW, et al. Aberrant p53 protein expression is associated with an increased risk of neoplastic progression in patients with Barrett's oesophagus. Gut 2013;62:1676-83.

284. Kaye PV, Haider SA, Ilyas M, et al. Barrett's dysplasia and the Vienna classification: reproducibility, prediction of progression and impact of consensus reporting and p53 immunohistochemistry. Histopathology 2009;54:699-712.

285. Kastelein F, Biermann K, Steyerberg EW, et al. Value of alpha-methylacyl-CoA racemase immunochemistry for predicting neoplastic progression in Barrett's oesophagus. Histopathology 2013;63:630-9.

286. Bhat S, Coleman HG, Yousef F, et al. Risk of malignant progression in Barrett's esophagus patients: results from a large population-based study. J Natl Cancer Inst 2011;103:1049-57.

287. Salemme M, Villanacci V, Cengia G, Cestari R, Missale G, Bassotti G. Intestinal metaplasia in Barrett's oesophagus: an essential factor to predict the risk of dysplasia and cancer development. Dig Liver Dis 2016;48:144-7.

288. Anaparthy R, Gaddam S, Kanakadandi V, et al. Association between length of Barrett's esophagus and risk of high-grade dysplasia or adenocarcinoma in patients without dysplasia. Clin Gastroenterol Hepatol 2013;11:1430-6.

289. Singh S, Manickam P, Amin AV, et al. Incidence of esophageal adenocarcinoma in Barrett's esophagus with low-grade dysplasia: a systematic review and meta-analysis. Gastrointest Endosc 2014;79:897-909.

290. Rastogi A, Puli S, El-Serag HB, Bansal A, Wani S, Sharma P. Incidence of esophageal adenocarcinoma in patients with Barrett's esophagus and high-grade dysplasia: a meta-analysis. Gastrointest Endosc 2008;67:394-8.

291. Shaheen NJ, Sharma P, Overholt BF, et al. Radiofrequency ablation in Barrett's esophagus with dysplasia. N Engl J Med 2009;360:2277-88.

292. Lee JK, Kum J, Ghosh P. Education and imaging. Gastrointestinal: glycogenic acanthosis. J Gastroenterol Hepatol 2007;22:1550.

293. Pilarski R, Burt R, Kohlman W, Pho L, Shannon KM, Swisher E. Cowden syndrome and the pten hamartoma tumor syndrome: systematic review and revised diagnostic criteria. J Natl Cancer Inst 2013;105:1607-16.

294. Long KB, Odze RD. Gastroesophageal junction hyperplastic (inflammatory) polyps: a clinical and pathologic study of 46 cases. Am J Surg Pathol 2011;35:1038-44.

295. Abraham SC, Singh VK, Yardley JH, WU TT. Hyperplastic polyps of the esophagus and esophagogastric junction: histologic and clinicopathologic findings. Am J Surg Pathol 2001;25:1180-7.

296. Jideh B, Weltman M, Wu Y, Chan CH. Esophageal squamous papilloma lacks clear clinicopathological associations. World J Clin Cases 2017;5:134-9.

297. Takeshita K, Murata S, Mitsufuji S, et al. Clinicopathological characteristics of esophageal squamous papillomas in Japanese patients—with comparison of findings from western countries. Acta Histochem Cytochem 2006;39:23-30.

298. Szentirmay Z, Szanto I, Balint I, et al. [Causal association between human papilloma virus infection and head and neck and esophageal squamous cell carcinoma.] Magy Onkol 2002;46:35-41. [Hungarian]

299. Fortes HR, von Ranke FM, Escuissato DL, et al. Recurrent respiratory papillomatosis: a state-of-the-art review. Respir Med 2017;126:116-21.

300. Batra PS, Hebert RL 2nd, Haines GK 3rd, Holinger LD. Recurrent respiratory papillomatosis with esophageal involvement. Int J Pediatr Otorhinolaryngol 2001;58:233-8.

301. Pasman EA, Heifert TA, Nylund CM. Esophageal squamous papillomas with focal dermal hypoplasia and eosinophilic esophagitis. World J Gastroenterol 2017;23:2246-50.

302. Kashyap P, Sweetser S, Farrugia G. Esophageal papillomas and skin abnormalities. Focal dermal hypoplasia (goltz syndrome) manifesting with esophageal papillomatosis. Gastroenterology 2011;140:784, 1111.

303. Motil KJ, Fete M, Fete TJ. Growth, nutritional, and gastrointestinal aspects of focal dermal hypoplasia (Goltz-Gorlin syndrome). Am J Med Genet C Semin Med Genet 2016;172C:29-33.

304. Nakamura M, Okamoto T, Kiyotoki S, et al. Esophageal squamous papilloma with tentacular processes. Gastrointest Endosc 2011;74:1143-4.

305. Odze R, Antonioli D, Shocket D, Noble-Topham S, Goldman H, Upton M. Esophageal squamous papillomas. A clinicopathologic study of 38 lesions and analysis for human papillomavirus by the polymerase chain reaction. Am J Surg Pathol 1993;17:803-12.

306. Mosca S, Manes G, Monaco R, Bellomo PF, Bottino V, Balzano A. Squamous papilloma of the esophagus: long-term follow up. J Gastroenterol Hepatol 2001;16:857-61.

307. Attila T, Fu A, Gopinath N, Streutker CJ, Marcon NE. Esophageal papillomatosis complicated by squamous cell carcinoma. Can J Gastroenterol 2009;23:415-9.

308. Levine MS, Buck JL, Pantongrag-Brown L, Buetow PC, Hallman JR, Sobin LH. Fibrovascular polyps of the esophagus: clinical, radiographic, and pathologic findings in 16 patients. AJR Am J Roentgenol 1996;166:781-7.

309. Sargent RL, Hood IC. Asphyxiation caused by giant fibrovascular polyp of the esophagus. Arch Pathol Lab Med 2006;130:725-7.

310. Fries MR, Galindo RL, Flint PW, Abraham SC. Giant fibrovascular polyp of the esophagus. A lesion causing upper airway obstruction and syncope. Arch Pathol Lab Med 2003;127:485-7.

311. Boni A, Lisovsky M, Dal Cin P, Rosenberg AE, Srivastava A. Atypical lipomatous tumor mimicking giant fibrovascular polyp of the esophagus: report of a case and a critical review of literature. Hum Pathol 2013;44:1165-70.

312. Jakowski JD, Wakely PE Jr. Rhabdomyomatous well-differentiated liposarcoma arising in giant fibrovascular polyp of the esophagus. Ann Diagn Pathol 2009;13:263-8.

313. Graham RP, Yasir S, Fritchie KJ, Reid MD, Greipp PT, Folpe AL. Polypoid fibroadipose tumors of the esophagus: 'giant fibrovascular polyp' or liposarcoma? A clinicopathological and molecular cytogenetic study of 13 cases. Mod Pathol 2018;31:337-42.

314. Aloraini A, Nahal A, Ferri LE. Transoral endoscopic resection of esophageal liposarcoma. Ann Thorac Surg 2012;94:e121-2.

315. Will U, Lorenz P, Urban H, Meyer F. Curative endoscopic resection of a huge pedunculated esophageal liposarcoma. Endoscopy 2007;39(Suppl 1):E15-6.

316. Lin ZC, Chang XZ, Huang XF, et al. Giant liposarcoma of the esophagus: a case report. World J Gastroenterol 2015;21:9827-32.

3 DISEASES OF THE STOMACH

CONGENITAL AND ACQUIRED STRUCTURAL ABNORMALITIES

Gastric Atresia

Gastric atresia is the complete occlusion of the pylorus. It is a rare event, affecting 1 in 100,000 live births and accounting for 1 percent of gastrointestinal atresias (1). Patients present with abdominal distention and forceful, non-bilious vomiting. Imaging reveals a dilated, air-filled stomach accompanied by an absence of gas in the small intestine.

The pathogenesis of pyloric atresia is unknown. Some cases occur sporadically or in association with esophageal atresia. Others develop in patients with epidermolysis bullosa, suggesting they result from *in utero* injury (2).

Atresias are classified based on the nature of the discontinuity between the distal stomach and the duodenum. The least severe lesions (type A) consist of a web or membrane at the pylorus that separates the stomach from the duodenum. Type B atresias appear as a fibrous cord between the stomach and duodenum. Complete lack of any connection between the stomach and the duodenum is classified as a type C atresia (3).

Webs and thin membranes can be endoscopically ruptured or dilated. Complete separation of the duodenal and gastric lumens requires surgical resection with anastomosis. The outcome is generally good, although it may be limited by associated congenital abnormalities.

Pyloric Stenosis

Definition. *Infantile hypertrophic pyloric stenosis* is the complete or near-complete, obstruction of the pyloric sphincter due to muscular hypertrophy. *Acquired pyloric stenosis* is gastric outlet obstruction secondary to inflammation, fibrosis, or neoplasia.

Clinical Features. Infantile hypertrophic pyloric stenosis affects 1 in 500 live births and shows a male predilection, occurring 4 to 5 times more commonly in boys than girls (4). First-born children and family members of affected infants are at increased risk (5). Other risk factors include maternal smoking, maternal alcohol consumption, and *in utero* exposure to macrolide antibiotics (6–8). The deformity is associated with trisomies 18 and 21, as well as neuromuscular, connective tissue, and metabolic syndromes (9). There is a negative association between breast-feeding and hypertrophic pyloric stenosis (10).

Affected infants are usually healthy at birth, but return to clinic at a few weeks of age with projectile, post-prandial, non-bilious vomiting, abdominal distention, electrolyte imbalances, hypokalemia, and alkalosis. A palpable periumbilical olive-like mass may be present (11,12). Ultrasound reveals a thick, elongated pyloric channel ("string sign") and narrow antrum ("beak sign") (13,14).

Acquired pyloric stenosis is much less common than it was prior to the era of *Helicobacter pylori* eradication, reflecting a decreased incidence of peptic ulcer disease. It shows a predilection for middle-aged males and presents with early satiety, post-prandial nausea or vomiting, and epigastric pain. Radiographic imaging typically shows delayed gastric emptying and an elongated, narrow pyloric channel. A mushroom-like deformity may be present when the pylorus bulges into the duodenum (15).

Pathogenesis. The causes of infantile hypertrophic pyloric stenosis are not clear but it likely results from a combination of heritable and environmental factors. The negative correlation between breastfeeding and infantile hypertrophic pyloric stenosis may be related to high levels of vasoactive intestinal peptide in breast milk, which promotes muscle relaxation, whereas increased motilin levels in formula-fed babies may cause chronic pylorospasm (10,16).

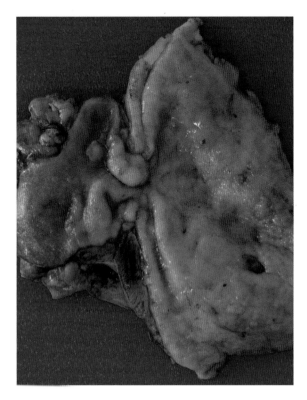

Figure 3-1

ACQUIRED PYLORIC STENOSIS

Circumferential scarring of the pyloric channel causes gastric outlet obstruction. The stomach (right) is dilated.

Most adults with acquired pyloric stenosis have gastric outlet obstruction due to healed gastric and duodenal ulcers, neoplastic infiltration by carcinoma or lymphoma, or postoperative adhesions (15). Some have idiopathic hypertrophic pyloric stenosis, which may represent a mild form of infantile disease, vagal hyperactivity, or prolonged pylorospasm (17).

Gross Findings. Idiopathic hypertrophic pyloric stenosis appears as a markedly narrowed pylorus with a smooth border ("cervix sign") (18). The muscularis propria is prominent and may form a circumferential, fusiform mass more than twice the normal thickness. Acquired stenoses have an irregular contour, reflecting fibrosis or an infiltrative malignancy (fig. 3-1).

Microscopic Findings. Idiopathic hypertrophic pyloric stenosis usually reflects disproportionate hypertrophy of the middle circular layer of the muscularis propria with a normal, or nearly normal, outer layer and inconspicuous inner oblique layer. Disorganized aggregates of smooth muscle cells associated with interstitial collagen deposits are accompanied by a sparse lymphocytic infiltrate. Decreased numbers of interstitial cells of Cajal are occasionally encountered and enteric nerves may be hypertrophic (19).

Pyloric stenosis due to peptic ulcer disease features fibrosis and chronic inflammation with variably severe destruction of the muscularis propria. The submucosa generally shows a greater amount of scarring than the muscularis propria (fig. 3-2). Infiltrating neoplastic cells may be present in the muscularis propria and around nerves when patients present with gastric outlet obstruction secondary to malignancy.

Treatment and Prognosis. Pyloromyotomy is the preferred treatment for both infants and adults with idiopathic hypertrophic pyloric stenosis (20). Infants are able to feed normally within 3 months of surgery, whereas the clinical course of adults is more variable (21). Adults with refractory symptoms may undergo distal gastrectomy or gastroenterostomy. Patients with secondary stenosis due to peptic ulcer disease generally require distal gastrectomy. Those with strictures secondary to malignancies may be surgical candidates. Endoscopic dilatation is mostly ineffective among patients with primary and secondary pyloric stenosis; symptomatic recurrence is common in both groups (22).

Duplication Cysts

Definition. *Duplication cyst* is a congenital duplication of the gastric wall that develops within the muscularis propria. Synonyms include *foregut duplication cyst* and *enterogenous cyst*.

Clinical Features. Gastric duplication cysts account for only 4 percent of all alimentary duplications; they are more common in females (23,24). Up to 50 percent of cases are associated with other developmental anomalies including esophageal duplications, Meckel diverticulum, ventricular septal defects, spinal cord defects, and Turner syndrome (23,24). Approximately two thirds of cases present in infancy with vomiting, difficulty feeding, and a palpable epigastric mass (25). Fewer than 25 percent are detected after 12 years of age, in which case they are usually incidentally discovered by imaging or intraoperatively (26). Large lesions can cause obstructive

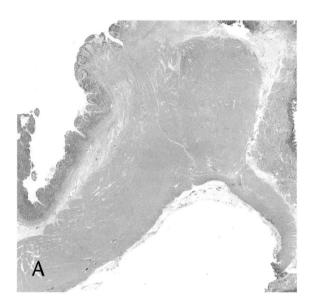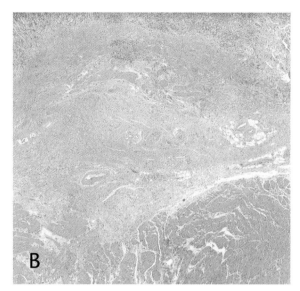

Figure 3-2

ACQUIRED PYLORIC STENOSIS

Marked hypertrophy of the muscularis propria (A) is accompanied by submucosal fibrosis and scarring of the inner muscularis propria (B).

symptoms, bleeding, or pain due to perforation (25,27). Duplications containing ectopic pancreatic tissue may develop pancreatitis-related inflammation that leads to a fistula or mimics a pancreatic pseudocyst (24).

Pathogenesis. Duplications form during the second to third months of embryogenesis. Epithelial proliferation during that time normally occludes the gut lumen; aberrant recanalization lateral to the lumen presumably gives rise to duplication cysts. Duplications may also form as a result of traction between the notochord and embryonic endoderm (28).

Gross Findings. Most duplications occur along the greater curvature of the stomach within the muscularis propria. Approximately 80 percent lack communication with the stomach (28). Endoscopists may note a bulge in the lumen of an otherwise normal-appearing stomach. Ultrasound reveals an intramural cyst with a mucosal lining (25). Cysts contain mucoid material and show variable denudation (fig. 3-3A).

Microscopic Findings. Gastric duplication cysts contain muscularis mucosae, submucosa, and mucosa with a mixed epithelial lining composed of gastric-type mucosa, intestinal epithelium, or ciliated columnar cells that resemble those of the

embryonic foregut (figs. 3-3B–D). Mural aggregates of pancreatic tissue are frequently encountered.

Treatment and Prognosis. Duplications are surgically resected when they are detected because they may bleed, perforate, or rarely, undergo malignant transformation (29). Adenocarcinoma and endocrine tumors have been reported to develop in duplication cysts and usually present at an advanced stage (26,30,31).

Diverticula

Definitions. *Congenital diverticulum* (also called *true diverticulum*) is a mural outpouching containing all layers of the gastric wall. *Acquired diverticulum* (also called *false diverticulum*) is the herniation of mucosa and submucosa through muscularis propria.

Clinical Features. Gastric diverticula are detected in less than 0.1 percent of endoscopic examinations (32). Most are clinically asymptomatic and detected when imaging studies are performed for other reasons. Large diverticula may cause a sensation of fullness or pain owing to compression of other structures. Erosions can result in gastrointestinal hemorrhage.

Pathogenesis. Congenital diverticula are developmental abnormalities that communicate with the gastric lumen through a widely patent

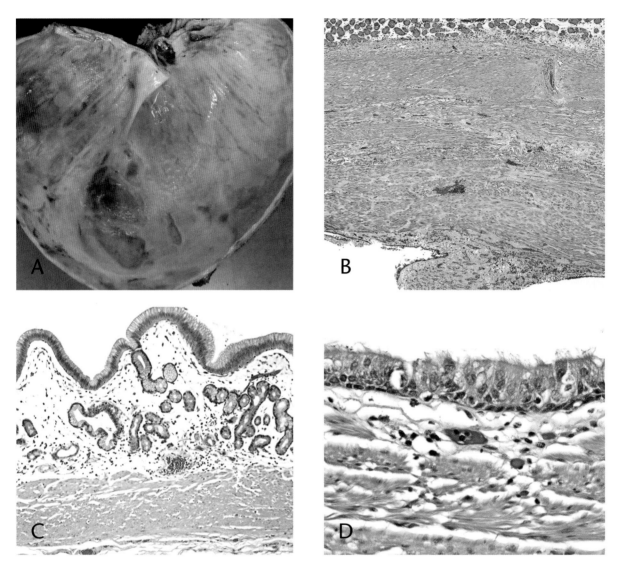

Figure 3-3

GASTRIC DUPLICATION CYST

The cyst has a muscular wall and thin mucosa with prominent submucosal vessels. A small portion of stomach is present in the upper right corner (A). The cyst (bottom) shares a muscular wall with the native stomach (top) (B). The lining is composed of rudimentary gastric-type mucosa (C) and ciliated columnar epithelium (D).

orifice. Their pathogenesis is likely similar to that of duplication cysts. Acquired diverticula develop secondary to increased intragastric pressure; they are more common among patients with gastric outlet obstruction.

Gross Findings. Diverticula appear as sac-like protrusions radiographically, and patulous orifices when viewed endoscopically. Congenital lesions are most commonly located in the posterior fundus, whereas acquired lesions tend to de-

velop in the gastric antrum where large vascular bundles penetrate the muscularis propria (33).

Microscopic Findings. Congenital diverticula contain all layers of the stomach wall. They are lined by variably inflamed gastric mucosa, but may contain pancreatic acini, ductules, or squamous epithelium as well. Acquired diverticula contain inflamed or eroded gastric mucosal elements supported by submucosa. They lack a muscularis propria.

Treatment and Prognosis. Treatment and prognosis are mostly related to the underlying conditions that predispose to diverticulum formation, such as peptic ulcer disease. Management of diverticula is controversial: small lesions of the proximal stomach (i.e. cardia) can probably be clinically followed, but larger lesions of the distal stomach may require surgical resection due to a risk of carcinoma development or persistent bleeding (32).

Pancreatic Heterotopia and Metaplasia

Definition. *Pancreatic heterotopia* is a congenital rest of pancreatic tissue. *Pancreatic metaplasia* is the replacement of glandular mucosa by pancreatic acinar elements. Synonyms include *ectopic pancreas* and *pancreatic rest*.

Clinical Features. Pancreatic acini are present in 18 to 24 percent of biopsy samples from the gastroesophageal junction and are asymptomatic (34–37). Pancreatic glands are also detected in the proximal stomachs of 50 percent of patients with autoimmune gastritis (38). They are much less common in the antrum, where they tend to be murally located, producing abdominal pain, fullness, nausea, and vomiting (39). Localized pancreatitis and pancreatic neoplasia have been reported in large heterotopias of the distal stomach (40).

Pathogenesis. The embryonic pancreas forms from outpouchings in the endodermal lining of the duodenum that fuse during dextrorotation of the foregut. Presumably, pancreatic heterotopias develop when ectopic tissues become entrapped during migration (34,36).

Pancreatic metaplasia in the setting of autoimmune gastritis represents an adaptive response to chronic inflammation. Although some authors have suggested that pancreatic tissue at the gastroesophageal junction is metaplastic in nature, most data indicate that these tissues are congenital rests (34).

Gross Findings. Pancreatic tissue of the gastroesophageal junction and gastric mucosa produces no gross or endoscopically apparent abnormalities. Larger lesions in the muscularis propria and submucosa appear as smooth nodules with an umbilicated center (fig. 3-4).

Microscopic Findings. Pancreatic heterotopias contain variable amounts of pancreatic acini, ductules, and islets of Langerhans. Pan-

creatic tissue in the mucosa consists entirely of acini. Metaplasia occurs on a background of autoimmune gastritis with loss of oxyntic glands, intestinal and pyloric metaplasia, and enterochromaffin-like (ECL)-cell hyperplasia (fig. 3-5). Mural rests form circumscribed nodules of acinar tissue that insinuate between bundles of smooth muscle cells (fig. 3-6). Some are associated with a cuff of lymphoid tissue. Rarely, they consist entirely of dilated ducts accompanied by smooth muscle hyperplasia (fig. 3-6D). In fact, gastric adenomyomas likely represent ductular proliferations in pancreatic heterotopias, similar to those of the ampulla (31).

Treatment and Prognosis. Mucosal heterotopias do not require treatment. Symptomatic large mural lesions are generally resected. Although uncommon, any type of pancreatic neoplasia can develop in a mural heterotopia; ductal neoplasms are the most frequently described (41).

MOTILITY DISORDERS

Gastroparesis

Definition. *Gastroparesis* is delayed gastric emptying in the absence of mechanical obstruction.

Clinical Features. Transient gastroparesis develops in virtually all patients who undergo gastric bypass and gastric fundoplication, and in many patients with viral gastroenteritis (42,43). The prevalence of gastroparesis outside these settings is less than 0.1 percent, with a female predilection (44). Most cases are idiopathic or occur in association with diabetes mellitus (45). In fact, among patients with type I and type II diabetes mellitus, the 10-year risks of gastroparesis development are approximately 5 percent and 1 percent, respectively (46). Other disorders that cause gastroparesis include Parkinson disease, amyloidosis, scleroderma, mesenteric ischemia, and malignant infiltration of the myenteric plexus (47).

Patients with gastroparesis complain of postprandial fullness, nausea, vomiting, bloating, and upper abdominal pain (48). Solid-phase gastric scintigraphy, whereby residual volumes of technetium-labeled meals are measured, is the diagnostic gold standard (49). *Gastroparesis-like syndrome* refers to a situation wherein patients have symptoms of gastroparesis, but normal gastric emptying (50,51).

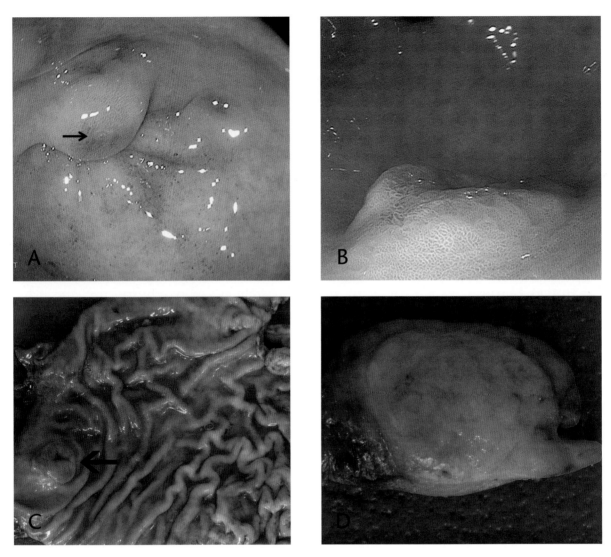

Figure 3-4

PANCREATIC HETEROTOPIA

A pancreatic heterotopia appears as a smooth submucosal nodule with a minute umbilication (arrow) and surrounding mucosal erythema (A). Another heterotopia has a more irregular shape with a larger central depression (B). A resected heterotopia forms a large nodule (arrow) in the distal stomach (C). Cross sections through this area reveal lobulated yellow tissue typical of pancreatic parenchyma (D).

Pathogenesis. The mechanisms underlying gastroparesis depend upon associated conditions. Many patients with progressive gastroparesis have structural alterations in the myenteric plexus that disrupt the balance between cholinergic and adrenergic gastric stimulation (52–54). Destruction of the myenteric plexus and ganglia results from infiltrative disorders, such as amyloidosis (fig. 3-7) and connective tissue diseases, or direct invasion by malignancy.

Damage to the myenteric ganglia and nerves can also result from lymphocytic inflammation, particularly in patients with diabetes mellitus and Parkinson disease.

Gross Findings. The stomach may be distended and often contains retained food. Mucosal ectasias are common in patients with scleroderma (55).

Microscopic Findings. Myenteric ganglia, nerve fibers, and interstitial cells of Cajal are often reduced in patients with gastroparesis compared with controls, but ganglion cells are usually present (54). The myenteric plexus may contain a mild lymphocytic infiltrate, particularly in patients with diabetes mellitus-related gastroparesis. Scleroderma is associated with atrophy of the muscularis propria and fibrosis that tends to be more pronounced in the inner layers (55).

Treatment and Prognosis. Patients are encouraged to consume smaller, more frequent meals to compensate for delayed emptying (48). Diabetic patients require tight glycemic control because high blood glucose levels further diminish antral motor activity (56). Prokinetic dopamine receptor antagonists inhibit the effects of dopamine on gastric emptying and reduce nausea (57). Macrolide antibiotics act on motilin receptors to promote stimulation of smooth muscle cells (58). Non-medical therapeutic options include implanted electrical stimulators and enteral nutrition (59,60).

Bezoar

Definition. *Bezoar* is an undigested agglomeration of swallowed material admixed with gastric secretions.

Clinical Features. Bezoars are detected in 0.5 percent of patients undergoing upper endoscopic examination (61). They are more common in geographic regions where dried fruits are a key dietary component, such as Japan, South Korea, Israel, Spain, Turkey, and the southeastern United States (62–66). Most occur in the stomach, although they may migrate to, or form *de novo* in, the small intestine (67). Bezoars are responsible for up to 3 percent of surgically-managed small bowel obstructions in patients from high-risk regions (68).

Bezoars typically develop in patients with impaired gastric motility, such as those with diabetes mellitus, neurodegenerative disorders, or prior gastric surgery (69,70). They can cause abdominal pain or fullness, melena, hematemesis, and anemia (67). Bleeding complications result from pressure-related mucosal erosions and ulcers (71). Computerized tomography (CT) scans reveal single or multiple heterogeneous luminal masses with internal gas bubbles (72,73).

Pathogenesis. Bezoars are classified by their composition. *Phytobezoars* consist of cellulose- and tannin-rich foods, such as celery, squash, raisins, prunes, and persimmons (74). They

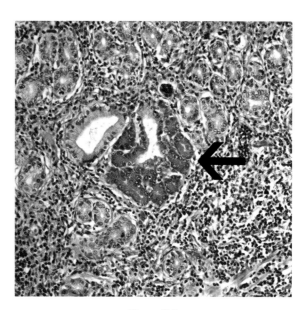

Figure 3-5

PANCREATIC METAPLASIA

A cluster of pancreatic acini (arrow) is present in association with autoimmune gastritis, which is characterized by chronically inflamed mucosa and replacement of oxyntic glands by pyloric glands.

presumably develop as a result of acid-related polymerization of tannins, which creates a matrix that entraps cellulose and its breakdown products (75). *Trichobezoars* are composed of ingested hair held together by food and mucus; they almost always occur in young women with psychiatric conditions linked to hair pulling (trichotillomania) and consumption (trichophagia) (76). *Pharmacobezoars* contain undigested pill fragments and pharmaceutical fillers (77). Bulk-forming laxatives, such as psyllium and guar gum, form masses by absorbing large amounts of water (78). Extended release drug formulations that are coated with cellulose form an insoluble matrix that traps foodstuffs and secretions, similar to phytobezoars. Polymers used to prevent dissolution of enteric-coated drugs in the stomach can also promote bezoar formation (79). *Lactobezoars* develop in infants, particularly premature babies. They are composed of milk and mucus and are more common in infants who are fed synthetic milk products (80).

Gross Findings. Endoscopy reveals single or multiple masses in the gastric lumen. Color and quality depend upon the contents of the bezoar. Those rich in tannins are often black, whereas

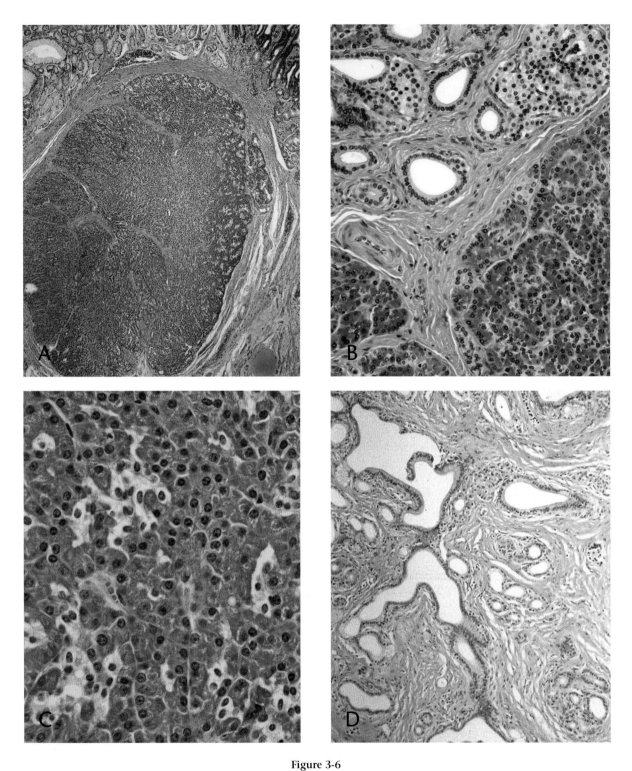

Figure 3-6

PANCREATIC HETEROTOPIA

Lobules of pancreatic tissue consist of ducts and acini within the stomach wall (A). Acini, islets, and ducts are present (B). Acinar cells contain abundant cytoplasmic zymogen granules (C). Some heterotopias are mostly composed of ductules embedded in abundant smooth muscle (D).

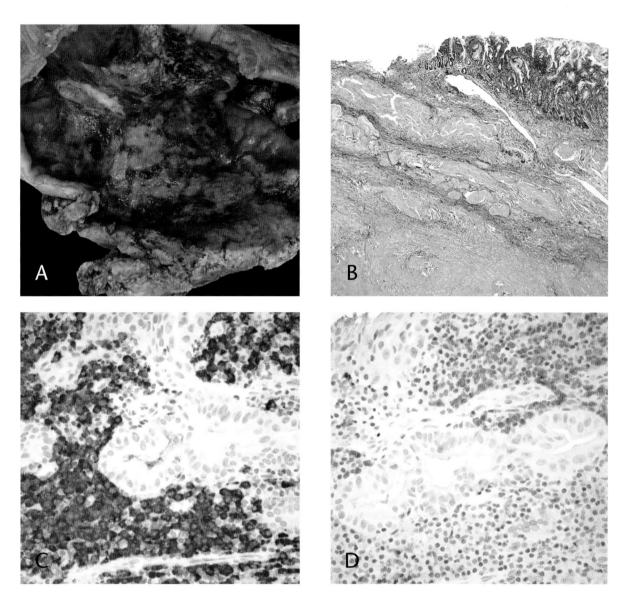

Figure 3-7

AMYLOID-INDUCED GASTROPARESIS

Diffuse amyloid deposition expands the gastric wall and completely effaces the rugal folds (A). The submucosa and muscularis propria contain amorphous faintly eosinophilic amyloid deposits with a cracked, waxy appearance (B). The mucosa is infiltrated by a lambda-restricted plasma cell neoplasm (C). Only rare mucosal plasma cells expression kappa (D).

those with high mucus content are yellow-green (fig. 3-8A) (67). Trichobezoars are readily identified because the hair is not digested by gastric acid (fig. 3-8B). Large bezoars often conform to the shape of the stomach.

Treatment and Prognosis. Bezoars that can be fragmented are removed endoscopically. Some are amenable to dissolution with cola or meat tenderizer (74,81,82). Surgical removal is reserved for bezoars that are refractory to these methods (83).

PAUCI-INFLAMMATORY GASTROPATHIES

Portal Hypertensive Gastropathy

Definition. Engorged gastric mucosal capillaries due to elevated portal venous pressure result in *portal hypertensive gastropathy*.

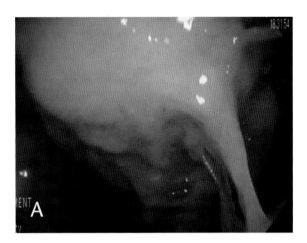 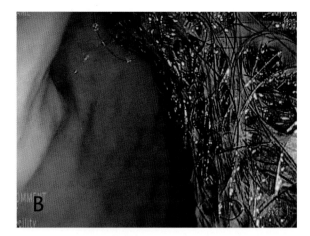

Figure 3-8

BEZOARS

A phytobezoar forms an intraluminal mucus-covered mass (A). A trichobezoar is an aggregate of hair and mucus (B).

Clinical Features. The epidemiology of portal hypertensive gastropathy parallels that of chronic liver disease. Most patients are older males with cirrhosis who have gastric changes during upper endoscopic examination performed to screen for esophageal varices. Vascular engorgement can occur throughout the gastrointestinal mucosae of patients with portal hypertension, although the stomach is most frequently affected. Portal hypertensive gastropathy is implicated as the bleeding source in 3 to 5 percent of patients with chronic gastric bleeding and 2 to 12 percent of patients with acute gastric bleeding secondary to cirrhosis (84,85).

Pathogenesis. Portal hypertensive gastropathy reflects increased blood flow to the gastric mucosa, although there is no consistent correlation with hepatic venous pressure gradients. Release of inflammatory mediators from the liver appears to predispose the gastric mucosa to injury by increasing oxidative stress and impairing healing (86,87).

Gross Findings. Portal hypertensive gastropathy produces a snake skin-like mosaic pattern of mucosal congestion that is usually most pronounced in the proximal stomach (fig. 3-9A). Red-brown spots, edema, petechiae, and erythema are often present (fig. 3-9B). Other features of cirrhosis, such as esophageal varices and spider angiomata, are frequently seen.

Microscopic Findings. Biopsy samples feature mucin-depleted, tortuous pits characteristic of chemical gastropathy, often accompanied by mucosal edema and prominent mucosal blood vessels. Ectatic capillaries are most pronounced at the base of the mucosa (fig. 3-10). Capillaries may be thickened and hyalinized in well-developed cases and are often associated with lamina propria fibrosis.

Differential Diagnosis. The histologic differential diagnosis includes gastric antral vascular ectasia (GAVE) and chemical (i.e., reactive) gastropathy. The former is rarely a consideration in patients with gastric erythema and portal hypertension, and has distinct histologic features. Dilated mucosal capillaries containing fibrin thrombi are typical of gastric antral vascular ectasia and show a predilection for the gastric antrum, rather than the proximal stomach. Chemical gastropathy can simulate the histologic features of portal hypertensive gastropathy, although it also shows a predilection for the antrum and produces less striking endoscopic abnormalities.

Treatment and Prognosis. Portal hypertensive gastropathy is usually asymptomatic or produces only iron deficiency anemia. Acute episodes of hemorrhage are associated with a mortality rate of approximately 9 percent. Up to 16 percent of patients who have one acute hemorrhagic episode experience another bleeding episode (88). Beta-blockers can be used prophylactically to substantially reduce the risk of hemorrhage, whereas octreotide and other vasoactive substances can

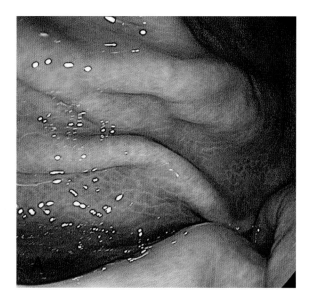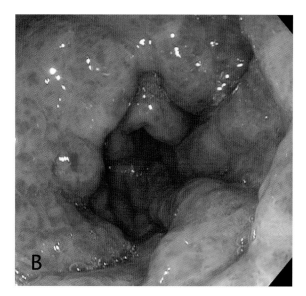

Figure 3-9

PORTAL HYPERTENSIVE GASTROPATHY

The endoscopic hallmark of portal hypertensive gastropathy is enhanced mucosal vascularity in the proximal stomach that imparts a mosaic or "snakeskin" appearance (A). The mottled mucosa is congested and edematous (B).

reduce the severity of acute hemorrhage (89,90). Endoscopic therapy, including argon plasma co-agulation, effectively prevents re-bleeding (91).

Gastric Antral Vascular Ectasia

Definition. *Gastric antral vascular ectasia* is the dilatation of mucosal capillaries in the gastric antrum. It is also known as *watermelon stomach*.

Clinical Features. Gastric antral vascular ectasia is responsible for 4 percent of non-variceal upper gastrointestinal hemorrhage, and tends to occur in the setting of chronic kidney disease, scleroderma, and other connective tissue disorders (92–94). It is more common in elderly women and also occurs in patients with chronic liver disease unassociated with cirrhosis or portal hypertension. Patients typically have iron deficiency anemia, and nearly 90 percent present with melena or hematemesis (95). Gastric antral vascular ectasia is occasionally detected in asymptomatic patients (96).

Pathogenesis. The pathogenesis of gastric antral vascular ectasia is unclear. It is possible that abnormal peristalsis traumatizes mucosal blood vessels in patients with connective tissue disorders (97,98). Other theories suggest that hypergastrinemia increases pyloric sphincter pressure, predisposing the distal gastric mucosa

to injury (99,100). Glucagon, nitric oxide, vaso-active intestinal peptide, and other compounds may cause vascular ectasias in patients with chronic liver disease (101).

Gross Findings. Upper endoscopy shows parallel erythematous streaks that emanate from the pylorus into the proximal antrum, imparting a "watermelon rind" appearance to the mucosa (fig. 3-11). The streaks are most pronounced on the crests of rugae and blanch with pressure.

Microscopic Findings. Antral biopsy samples show chemical gastropathy accompanied by dilated, congested capillaries (fig. 3-12A). Irregularly shaped, thin-walled capillaries are present at all levels in the mucosa. They are frequently surrounded by hyalinized stroma and may contain thrombi (fig. 3-12B).

Differential Diagnosis. The histologic features of gastric antral vascular ectasia simu-late those of portal hypertensive gastropathy. However, the presence of antrum-predominant changes, numerous large vascular spaces, and fibrin thrombi is more typical of gastric antral vascular ectasia than portal hypertensive gas-tropathy. Correlation with clinical and endo-scopic features is usually helpful as well.

Treatment and Prognosis. Intractable hemorrhage due to gastric antral vascular

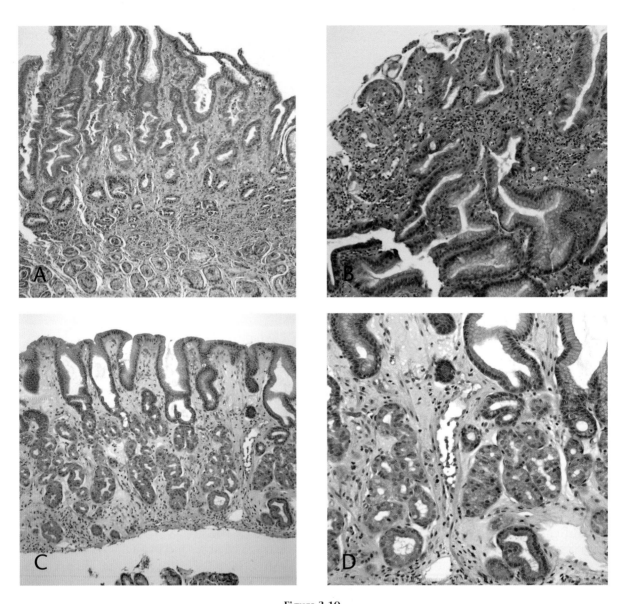

Figure 3-10

PORTAL HYPERTENSIVE GASTROPATHY

Mucosal changes include variably severe chemical gastropathy, vascular engorgement, and fibrosis of the lamina propria (A). Surface erosions, foveolar hyperplasia, and granulation tissue are frequently present in patients with active hemorrhage (B). Milder cases display mucin-depleted foveolar epithelium, regenerative pits with a "corkscrew" configuration, and lamina propria edema (C). Ectatic vessels are most prominent in the deep mucosa (D).

ectasia was historically treated with antrectomy. Modern approaches utilize endoscopic ablation of bleeding vessels with argon plasma or laser coagulation (102–104).

Acute Hemorrhagic Gastropathy

Definition. *Acute hemorrhagic gastropathy* (*acute hemorrhagic gastritis*) is gastric hemorrhage and necrosis in the absence of inflammation.

Clinical Features. Acute hemorrhagic gastropathy accounts for 25 percent of episodes of severe upper gastrointestinal bleeding. It generally occurs in severely ill patients: 2 to 8 percent of patients in intensive care units develop overt gastrointestinal bleeding (105). Patients who take high doses of nonsteroidal anti-inflammatory drugs (NSAIDs) are at increased risk. Presenting symptoms include

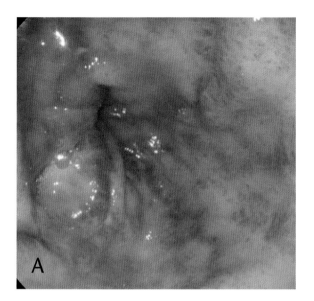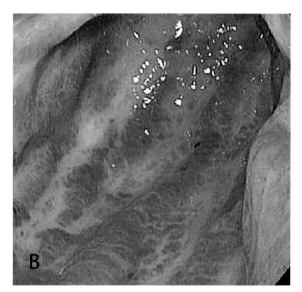

Figure 3-11

GASTRIC ANTRAL VASCULAR ECTASIA

Mucosal hyperemia is most pronounced at the crests of mucosal folds (A). Erythematous streaks radiate from the pylorus and impart a "watermelon rind" appearance to the mucosa (B).

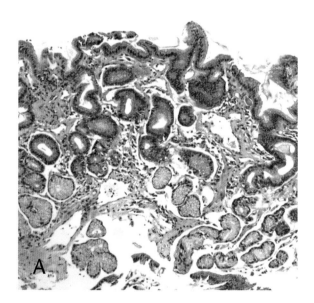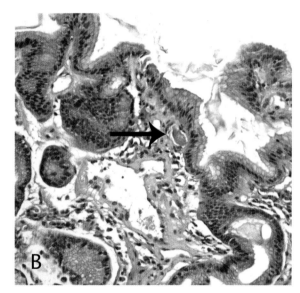

Figure 3-12

GASTRIC ANTRAL VASCULAR ECTASIA

Features of chemical gastropathy, including surface mucin depletion and regenerative pits, are accompanied by dilated mucosal vessels (A). A thrombus (arrow) is present in a subepithelial capillary (B).

severe abdominal pain, hematemesis, and hypovolemia.

Pathogenesis. The rich collateral circulation of the stomach precludes ischemic gastric injury in most instances. However, ischemia contributes to the development of hemorrhagic gastropathy in hypoxic and septic patients (Curling ulcers), as well as those with severe damage to

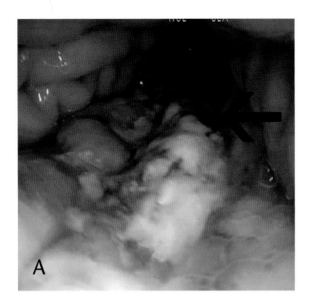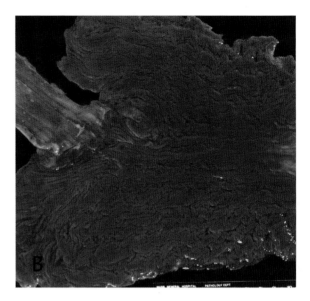

Figure 3-13

ACUTE HEMORRHAGIC GASTROPATHY

A large ulcer with fresh hemorrhage (arrow) is surrounded by edematous and hyperemic rugal folds (A). An autopsy stomach shows edema and congestion of the entire mucosa with several sites of oozing (B).

the central nervous system (Cushing ulcers) (105). NSAIDs inhibit prostaglandin synthesis, which normally maintains mucosal blood flow and mucus secretion (106).

Gross Findings. The mucosa is edematous and hyperemic, with oozing petechiae or diffuse hemorrhage. Ulcers, erosions, and friability are commonly present (fig. 3-13).

Microscopic Findings. Mucosal edema, erosions, fibrin deposition, and hemorrhage are characteristic. Inflammation is absent or limited to areas of erosion. Regenerative glands are mucin depleted, similar to those of chemical gastropathy (fig. 3-14). Severe injury produces deep ulcers and transmural necrosis.

Treatment and Prognosis. Acute hemorrhagic gastropathy is conservatively managed with a combination of broad spectrum antibiotics, vascular support, and intravenous proton pump inhibitor (PPI). Surgical resection is reserved for patients with evidence of gastric perforation. Superficial injury can heal with complete resolution provided the underlying disorder is corrected. Injury that extends into the submucosa or deeper layers heals with fibrosis. The mortality rate of patients with hemorrhagic gastritis approaches 30 percent (107).

Chemical Gastropathy

Definition. *Chemical gastropathy* is mucosal injury due to direct irritation. Synonyms include *reactive gastropathy* and *chemical gastritis*.

Clinical Features. Chemical gastropathy is the most common type of mucosal injury recognized in gastric biopsy samples. It usually results from the direct effects of acid or bile on the mucosa, followed by injury due to a variety of medications. NSAIDs are the most commonly implicated agents, but oral iron supplements and corticosteroids can produce similar changes (106). The overall incidence of chemical gastropathy is difficult to estimate, but it develops in approximately 50 percent of chronic NSAID users (106). Most patients are asymptomatic. Those with symptoms complain of epigastric pain, nausea, and dyspepsia. Erosive injury may lead to iron deficiency anemia.

Pathogenesis. Chemical gastropathy occurs when local irritants disrupt the mucosal barrier and allow hydrochloric acid to directly damage the mucosa. Concurrent histamine release produces mucosal edema while platelet-derived growth factor stimulates smooth muscle cell and fibroblast proliferation (108). Inhibition

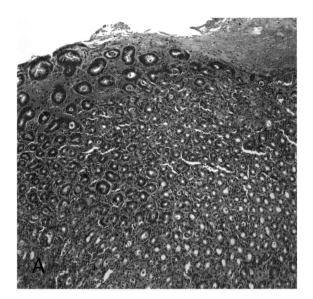 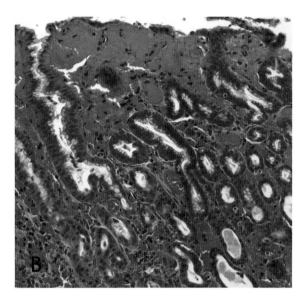

Figure 3-14

ACUTE HEMORRHAGIC GASTROPATHY

Fresh mucosal hemorrhage is associated with adherent organizing blood and sparse inflammation (A). The lamina propria is expanded by extravasated blood and engorged vessels; regenerative epithelial cell changes are also present (B).

of prostaglandin synthesis by NSAIDs results in diminished mucosal blood flow and mucus secretion, the net effect of which increases mucosal susceptibility to surface injury (106).

Gross Findings. Erythema, edema, and hyperemia can occur anywhere in the stomach, but are most severe in the antrum (fig. 3-15). Erosions and hyperplastic/regenerative polyps may also be present.

Microscopic Findings. Chemical gastropathy is characterized by surface epithelial injury and regeneration of the gastric pits on a background of edema without increased inflammation (fig. 3-16A). Surface epithelial cells are mucin depleted, resulting in an increased nuclear to cytoplasmic ratio; the cells appear cuboidal rather than columnar, with hyperchromatic nuclei (fig. 3-16B). The pits are elongated and convoluted ("corkscrew" configuration) and mitotic figures may be detected in the upper pits (fig. 3-16C). Capillary congestion and mucosal edema are often present. Splayed bundles of smooth muscle cells emanate from the muscularis mucosae into the interfoveolar regions; (fig. 3-16D). Inflammation is not prominent unless erosions are present, in which case neutrophils and fibrin are often encountered (fig. 3-17). Patchy intestinal metaplasia may also be identified (108).

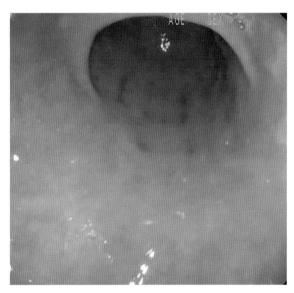

Figure 3-15

CHEMICAL GASTROPATHY

Superficial erosions and patchy hyperemia are most pronounced in the distal stomach.

Differential Diagnosis. Extreme reactive epithelial cell atypia simulates the features of low-grade dysplasia. Clues to a diagnosis of dysplasia include an abrupt transition to adjacent

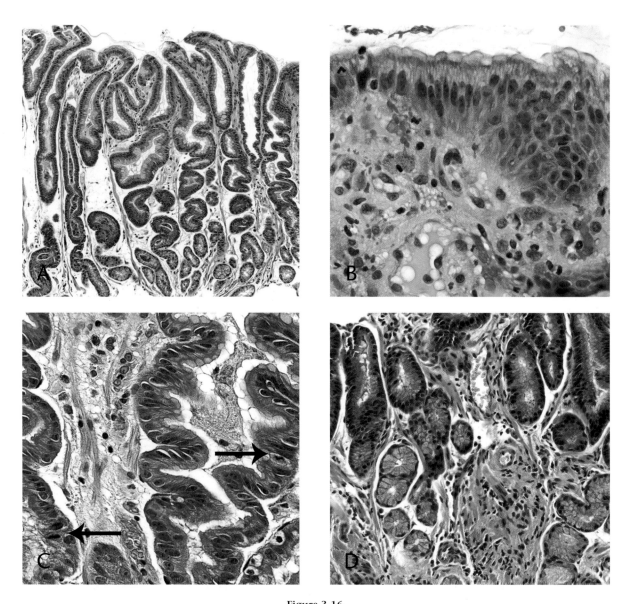

Figure 3-16

CHEMICAL GASTROPATHY

Chemical gastropathy features striking surface epithelial regeneration with corkscrew-shaped pits lined by mucin-depleted cells; the lamina propria is edematous but uninflamed (A). Surface epithelial cells contain hyperchromatic nuclei with prominent nucleoli and tiny apical mucin vacuoles (B). Mitotic figures (arrows) are readily identified in regenerative gastric pits (C). Thin bundles of smooth muscle cells extend into the muscularis mucosae (D).

non-neoplastic epithelium, as well as a greater degree of cytologic atypia, apoptotic debris, and mitotic figures in the surface epithelium. Changes of bile reflux gastropathy are usually indistinguishable from those of acid-related injury, as discussed subsequently.

Treatment and Prognosis. Proton pump inhibitors are used to protect the mucosa from acid-in-duced damage (109). Cessation of the offending agent alleviates symptoms in some patients.

Bile Reflux Gastropathy

Definition. *Bile reflux gastropathy* is injury induced by the retrograde flow of bile into the stomach.

Clinical Features. Bile reflux gastropathy develops in 10 to 30 percent of patients who undergo

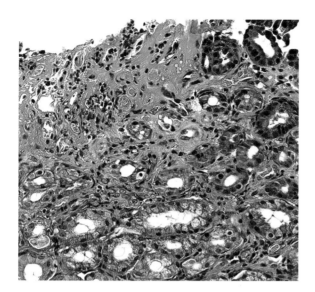

Figure 3-17

CHEMICAL GASTROPATHY

Neutrophils and fibrin are present in association with a surface erosion.

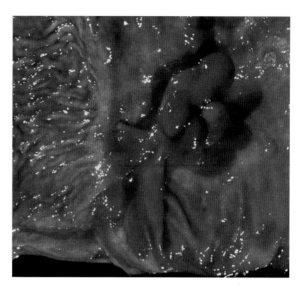

Figure 3-18

GASTRITIS CYSTICA POLYPOSA

A multinodular polyp is present at the anastomosis between the jejunum (left) and the stomach (right).

gastrojejunostomy with antrectomy (Billroth II procedure) for acquired pyloric stenosis due to inflammation or neoplasia (108). This procedure is infrequently performed in an era of *H. pylori* eradication and decreased incidence of peptic ulcer disease and, thus, the disorder is less common than it once was. Retrograde bile flow can also cause gastric injury in non-surgical patients, especially those who smoke or drink alcohol. Duodenal injury frequently occurs following cholecystectomy, ampullectomy, or other procedures that increase mucosal exposure to bile.

Symptoms include abdominal pain and dyspepsia. Erosions and inflammatory polyps at surgical anastomoses occasionally cause bleeding and delayed gastric emptying, respectively (110).

Pathogenesis. Surgical removal, or incompetence, of the pyloric sphincter allows for retrograde flow of bile-containing secretions from the duodenum into the stomach (111). Bile is directly corrosive to the gastric mucosa, causing chemical injury or erosions.

Gross Findings. Bile reflux induces a chemical gastropathy that is most severe in the distal stomach where it causes variably severe erythema and erosions. Post-surgical patients often develop polyps and mural cysts (i.e., *gastritis cystica polyposa* and *gastritis cystica profunda*) at the gastrojejunal anastomosis (fig. 3-18).

Microscopic Findings. Bile reflux causes mucosal edema, mucin depletion of the foveolar epithelium, and glandular regeneration indistinguishable from acid-related chemical gastropathy (fig. 3-19). These changes can be extreme in post-surgical patients, producing masses and ulcers that simulate malignancy. Polyps (i.e., *gastritis cystica polyposa*) consist of hyperplastic, dilated foveolae that are either limited to the mucosa or extend into the submucosa (fig. 3-20). The background oxyntic mucosa is atrophic, with loss of oxyntic glands and pseudopyloric metaplasia (3-21). Foci of intestinal metaplasia are commonly encountered.

Differential Diagnosis. Gastritis cystica polyposa/profunda can feature striking cytologic atypia that simulates invasive adenocarcinoma, particularly when regenerative epithelium expands the submucosa (112). Clues to a benign diagnosis include the lobular low-power appearance of glands, their association with a rim of lamina propria, and gradual transitions between areas of cytologic atypia and those that are more clearly non-neoplastic in nature.

Treatment and Prognosis. The most important complication of bile reflux gastropathy is the development of adenocarcinoma in the gastric remnant (113). The incidence of these "stump carcinomas" is lower than previously believed,

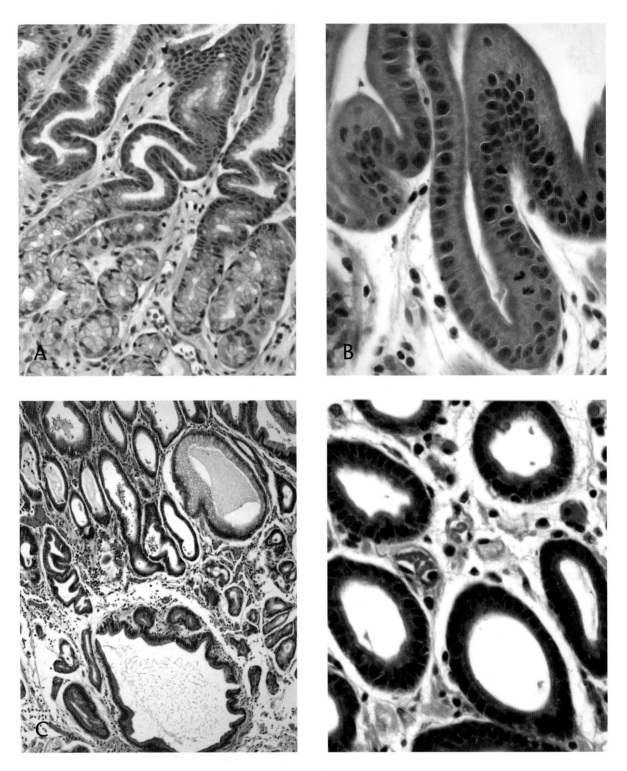

Figure 3-19

BILE REFLUX GASTROPATHY

Corkscrew-shaped, regenerative foveolar glands are present at the mucosal surface (A). They show mucin depletion, mild nuclear enlargement and increased mitotic activity (B). Pits and deeper glands are cystically dilated (C) with mucin depletion and mild cytologic atypia (D).

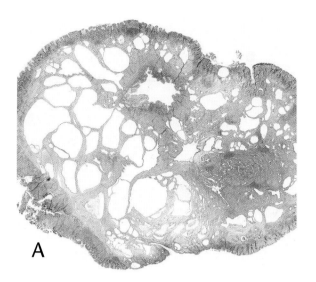
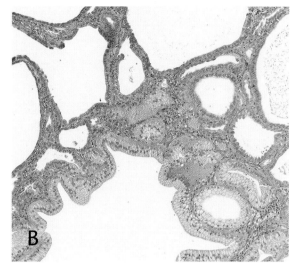

Figure 3-20

GASTRITIS CYSTICA POLYPOSA

A polypoid mass is composed of cystically dilated glands that expand the submucosa and superficial mucosa (A). These cysts are lined by benign gastric epithelium invested with a rim of lamina propria (B).

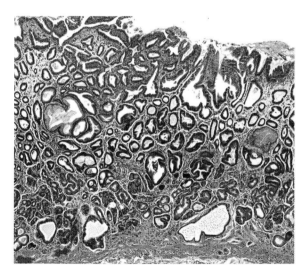
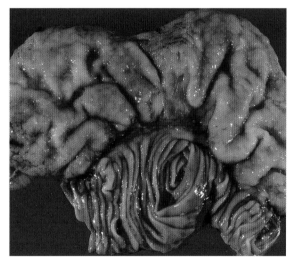

Figure 3-21

BILE REFLUX GASTROPATHY

Oxyntic mucosa at a gastrojejunal anastomosis displays complete loss of oxyntic glands, simulating antral mucosa. Cystically dilated gastric pits are lined by mucin-depleted foveolar epithelium. There is minimal background inflammation.

Figure 3-22

CARCINOMA ARISING IN ASSOCIATION WITH BILE REFLUX GASTROPATHY

Flat, indurated areas are accompanied by markedly thickened gastric folds at the anastomosis, reflecting the presence of infiltrating adenocarcinoma.

occurring in 2 to 5 percent of patients who have undergone gastrojejunal anastomosis (fig. 3-22). For this reason, patients undergo surveillance endoscopy starting 10 to 15 years after gastro-jejunostomy (108).

DRUG-INDUCED GASTRIC INJURY

Mucosal Calcinosis

Definition. *Mucosal calcinosis* is the deposition of calcium and calcium-containing compounds in the gastric mucosa.

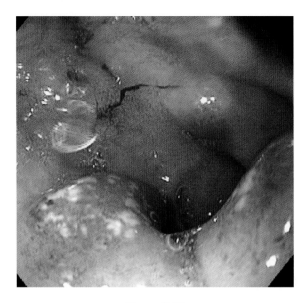

Figure 3-23

MUCOSAL CALCINOSIS

Multiple white plaques are present on the crest of a mucosal fold.

Clinical Features. Gastric mucosal calcinosis is reportedly rare, but its incidence is likely underestimated because it usually does not cause symptoms. It occurs in patients with chronic kidney disease who have hypercalcemia, hyperphosphatemia, and uremia, as well as in solid organ transplant recipients and patients taking aluminum-containing antacids or sucralfate (114). Patients who come to clinical attention present with nausea, vomiting, and abdominal pain due to unrelated causes (115).

Pathogenesis. Mucosal calcinosis is classified as metastatic, dystrophic, or idiopathic. Metastatic calcinosis occurs in dialysis patients with abnormal serum calcium, phosphate, or urea levels (114,116). Dialysis patients also accumulate calcium phosphate deposits in the heart, lung, kidney, and gastrointestinal tract (117). Local inflammation facilitates dystrophic gastric calcification in patients with normal serum calcium levels, particularly those with atrophic gastritis in whom the gastric pH is higher than normal. Organ transplant recipients who take aluminum phosphate-containing antacids or sucralfate can develop calcium-containing deposits in the stomach (118). Citrate-containing blood products can also cause calcium to pre-

cipitate in tissues, particularly in patients who require large volume transfusions (119).

Gross Findings. Mucosal calcinosis appears as multiple white plaques (fig. 3-23) (120). Rare cases produce large, malignant-appearing ulcers (115).

Microscopic Findings. Calcium and calcified deposits form irregular, basophilic clumps in the superficial mucosa that may be associated with macrophages and giant cells (fig. 3-24A) (118). The background mucosa is usually normal, although mucosal calcinosis can occur in the setting of chemical gastropathy, atrophic gastritis, and even adenocarcinoma (114). Phosphates and carbonates within calcium deposits impart dark brown or black coloration with von Kossa stains (fig. 3-24B).

Differential Diagnosis. Kayexalate crystals are basophilic, but are much larger than calcium deposits and are rhomboidal with an internal mosaic pattern. Iron crystals are clumped or fibrillary and golden brown; they stain blue with the Perl iron stain. Some sodium phosphate tablets used for bowel preparations deposit in the gastric mucosa and produce granular purple-black crystals. The crystals do not stain with Prussian blue, but are positive with von Kossa stains, which highlight phosphate or carbonate moieties of calcium salts (121). Lanthanum carbonate can also simulate mucosal calcium deposition, as discussed below.

Treatment and Prognosis. Mucosal calcinosis requires no therapy, although patients with abnormal serum chemistries may need diuresis or dialysis. Discontinuation of antacid agents may also be necessary.

Iron Pill Gastropathy

Definition. *Iron pill gastropathy* is gastric injury secondary to oral supplementation with ferrous sulfate (FeSO4).

Clinical Features. Iron-related erosions are detected in 0.7 percent of upper endoscopic examinations and are more common in elderly patients treated for iron deficiency anemia (122). Some patients complain of dysphagia and vague abdominal pain. Others experience melena or coffee-ground emesis.

Pathogenesis. Oral iron supplements are directly corrosive to the gastric mucosa, particularly at supra-therapeutic doses or when passive uptake of luminal iron exceeds the capacity of absorption mechanisms (122). Ferrous and

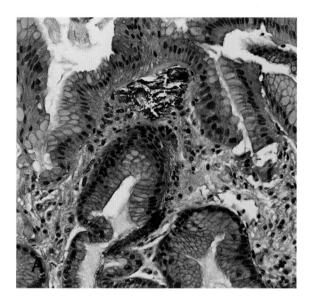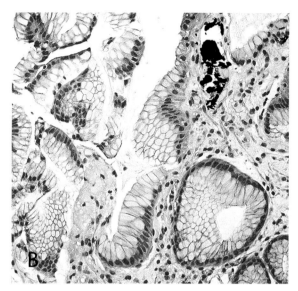

Figure 3-24

MUCOSAL CALCINOSIS

Basophilic crystalline material is present in the lamina propria. The overlying epithelium displays mild reactive changes (A). A von Kossa stain shows dark brown/black staining of phosphates within the deposits (B).

ferric ions catalyze formation of reactive oxygen metabolites that injure the mucosa (122). Iron also promotes thrombosis, causing localized ischemic injury and impaired healing.

Gross Findings. Upper endoscopic exam reveals ulcers and erosions, often with brown-black discoloration (fig. 3-25). Grossly visible crystalline material may be embedded in inflammatory debris (122,123).

Microscopic Findings. Exogenous iron forms extracellular clumps of golden brown crystals in the superficial lamina propria and encrusting blood vessels and collagen fibrils (fig. 3-26A). The background mucosa usually displays features of chemical gastropathy and may be eroded. Hemosiderin accumulation in foveolar epithelial cells and macrophages may be present, but is not prominent in most cases. Prussian blue (i.e., Perl iron) histochemical stains highlight iron deposits and distinguish iron from other crystalline deposits (fig. 3-26B).

Differential Diagnosis. Gastric siderosis can result from systemic iron overload or local hemorrhage, producing intracellular and extracellular hemosiderin granules, respectively. Gastric biopsy samples from patients with elevated circulating iron due to frequent blood transfusions or hereditary hemochromatosis

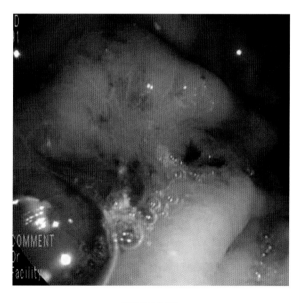

Figure 3-25

IRON PILL GASTROPATHY

Multiple ulcers with brown discoloration are present in the gastric body.

show granular accumulation of iron within glandular epithelial cells (fig. 3-27). Remote hemorrhage manifests with iron accumulation in macrophages, endothelial cells, and other stromal cells (fig. 3-28) (124,125).

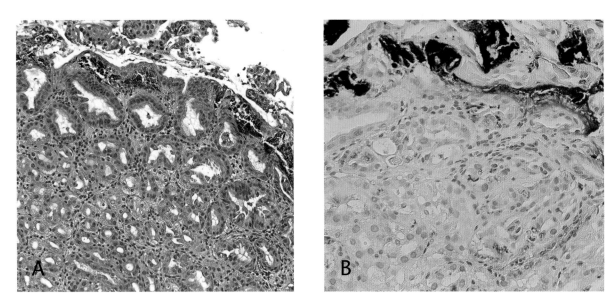

Figure 3-26

IRON PILL GASTROPATHY

The superficial lamina propria contains dark brown crystalline deposits (A). A Prussian blue stain highlights extracellular iron (B).

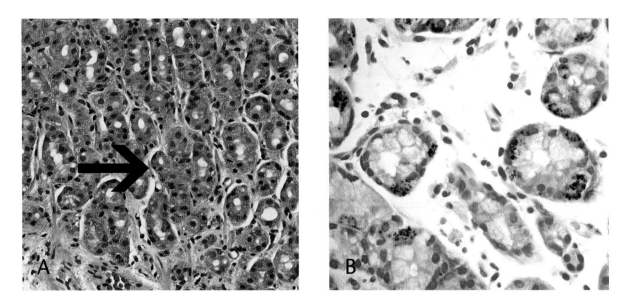

Figure 3-27

GASTRIC SIDEROSIS

Intracellular hemosiderin imparts brown granular discoloration (arrow) to the parietal cell cytoplasm of a patient with hereditary hemochromatosis (A). A Prussian blue stain highlights intracellular iron (B).

Pseudomelanosis can occur in the gastric mucosa, but almost always develops in patients with pseudomelanosis duodeni. It appears as dark brown-black granular deposits unassociated with epithelial cell injury (fig. 3-29).

Lanthanum phosphate is a phosphate binding agent used to prevent hyperphosphatemia in renal dialysis patients. It may deposit in the upper gastrointestinal tract, but, unlike oral iron, appears as coarse, granular, purple-brown material

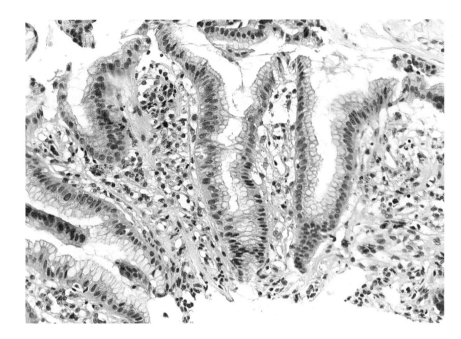

Figure 3-28

REMOTE HEMORRHAGE

Granular iron deposits in lamina propria macrophages reflect resolved hemorrhage. The pigment appears as golden brown coarse granules unassociated with mucosal injury.

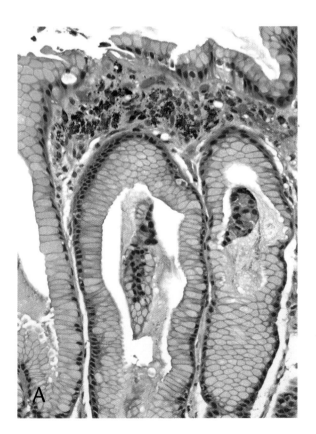

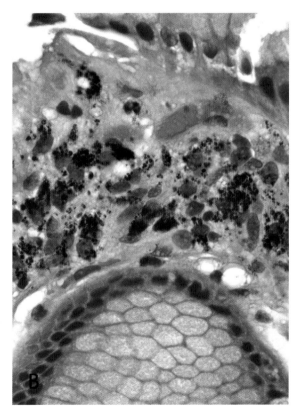

Figure 3-29

PSEUDOMELANOSIS

Pseudomelanosis produces dark brown to black pigment in the superficial lamina propria (A). The granules are darker and finer than iron deposits and only stain weakly with Prussian blue stains (B).

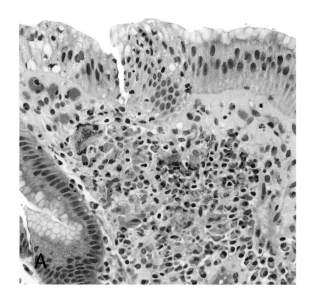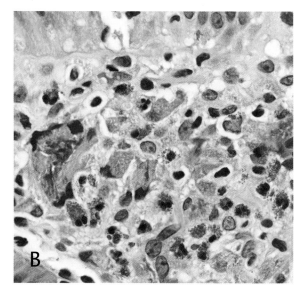

Figure 3-30

LANTHANUM CARBONATE DEPOSITS

Lamina propria macrophages contain basophilic, granular material (A) that forms large cytoplasmic aggregates when present in abundance (B).

in lamina propria macrophages (fig. 3-30) (126). These deposits often show pale staining with Prussian blue, representing a potential diagnostic pitfall (127). Barium deposits appear as golden crystals in lamina propria macrophages; they are generally unassociated with evidence of mucosal injury.

Treatment and Prognosis. Iron pill gastropathy resolves with supportive care. Patients may be advised to drink more water with iron pills to facilitate passage into the small intestine. Liquid iron supplements are not associated with gastropathy and represent an alternative to pill formulations for some patients (128).

Doxycycline-Related Injury

Doxycycline-related injury is an antibiotic-associated gastric injury. The drug causes a contact chemical burn when the agent is hydrolyzed by luminal secretions (106).

Doxycycline is commonly prescribed to adults for treatment of acne and acne rosacea, as well as some bacterial and protozoal infections. It causes direct mucosal injury, resulting in vague abdominal symptoms, epigastric pain, nausea, and hematemesis. Given the frequencies with which this and similar agents are used, it is likely that doxycycline-induced gastric injury is under-recognized (129,130).

Endoscopic findings include white plaques on the rugal crests, erythema, edema, and erosions (129,130). Doxycycline-related injury appears as a chemical gastropathy associated with hypereosinophilic deposits in capillary walls, erosions, and acute inflammation (fig. 3-31A). Capillaries often contain fibrinoid material (fig. 3-31B). Alterations occur throughout the antrum, body, and the proximal duodenum (129). Discontinuation of doxycycline is the only necessary intervention.

THERAPY-RELATED GASTROPATHIES

Graft-versus-Host Disease

Definition. *Graft-versus-host disease* is an injury mediated by donor T-cells following stem cell transplantation. *Acute graft-versus-host disease* occurs within 100 days after stem cell transplant. *Chronic graft-versus-host disease* occurs more than 100 days following stem cell transplant.

Clinical Features. Graft-versus-host disease affects 40 to 80 percent of allogeneic transplant recipients and approximately 5 percent of autologous transplant recipients, particularly those with multiple myeloma (131,132). More than half of patients with acute graft-versus-host disease experience gastrointestinal symptoms,

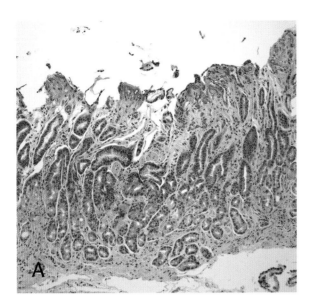 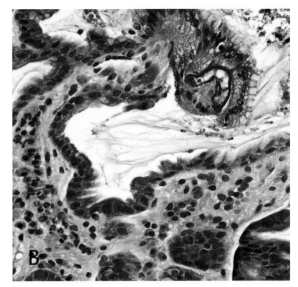

Figure 3-31

DOXYCYCLINE-INDUCED GASTRIC INJURY

Doxycycline causes a chemical gastropathy accompanied by smudgy deposits in mucosal capillaries (A). Deposits are intensely eosinophilic and resemble fibrinoid material (B).

including nausea, vomiting, dyspepsia, diarrhea, and bleeding (133,134). These symptoms usually develop within a few months of stem cell transplant, but can persist for months thereafter. Patients with chronic disease tend to have symptoms related to malabsorption (diarrhea, malnutrition, and weight loss).

Pathogenesis. Induction regimens that ablate recipient bone marrow also up-regulate major histocompatibility (MHC) and minor human leukocyte antigens (HLA) on host tissues. This facilitates their recognition by donor T-cells (135). Activated T-cells promote elaboration of inflammatory mediators, such as IL-1 and TNF-α, resulting in epithelial cell apoptosis and tissue necrosis (136). Many patients also receive prophylactic broad-spectrum antibiotics that alter the gut microbiota and activate local immunity, thereby promoting the development of acute graft-versus-host disease (137).

Gross Findings. Endoscopic findings include edema, erythema, friability, erosions, and ulcers, often with sloughed epithelium (fig. 3-32) (132). The severity of the endoscopic findings shows poor correlation with histologic findings, although patients with bleeding and ulcers often have severe histologic abnormalities (138,139).

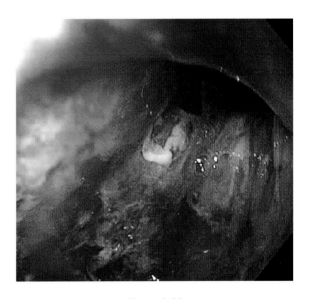

Figure 3-32

GRAFT-VERSUS-HOST DISEASE

The pre-pyloric gastric mucosa is erythematous with decreased mucosal folds. Sloughed mucosa and exudates are present.

Microscopic Findings. The histologic hallmark of acute graft-versus-host disease is epithelial cell apoptosis in the deep mucosa. Epithelial cell apoptosis is most common in the

119

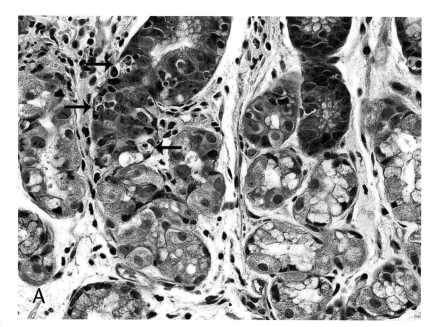

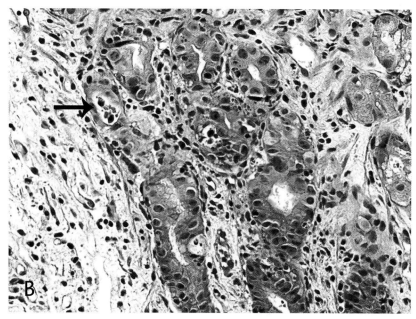

Figure 3-33

GRAFT-VERSUS-HOST DISEASE

Numerous apoptotic epithelial cells (arrows) are present in the deep gastric glands (A). Luminal cellular debris (arrow) and aggregates of karyorrhectic debris signify moderately severe disease (B).

mucous neck cells of the oxyntic mucosa and in the deeper glands in the antrum and cardia (fig. 3-33A). Necrotic cells tend to be smaller and less conspicuous in the stomach than the lower gastrointestinal tract. Cystic dilatation of the glands may be seen in acute graft-versus-host disease, but is not a specific finding. Dilated oxyntic glands often contain apoptotic debris and pyknotic nuclei, reflecting necrotic parietal cells (fig. 3-33B) (140). The background mucosa typically shows minimal, if any, inflammation unless there is a superimposed infection. Severe graft-versus-host disease may feature erosions, ulcers, and neutrophils.

The minimal histologic criteria for graft-versus-host disease are not well established, but examination of multiple serial sections increases the sensitivity of biopsy samples (141,142). Some suggest a diagnosis of graft-versus-host disease when only 1 to 2 apoptotic glandular epithelial cells are present in a single tissue fragment, although PPI therapy can produce similar findings (143). Extensive gland loss, ulcers, and erosions generally correlate with severe disease (138). Biopsy samples from the lower gastrointestinal tract are more sensitive for the detection of graft-versus-host disease than gastric biopsy samples (144).

The features of chronic gastric graft-versus-host disease are nonspecific. They include ulcers, lamina propria fibrosis, and gland loss. Obliterative vascular changes may be present in the submucosa, but are rarely amenable to biopsy (143). Ancillary studies may be employed to exclude other causes of epithelial cell apoptosis, such as cytomegalovirus and adenovirus infection, as discussed subsequently (145).

Differential Diagnosis. Proton pump inhibitor therapy is frequently used to manage upper gastrointestinal symptoms in the immediate post-stem cell transplant period. These medications cause apoptosis of deep glands in both antral and oxyntic mucosae, but the changes are generally mild and consist of only rare apoptotic cells (140). More than occasional necrotic epithelial cells should prompt concern for graft-versus-host disease, especially if viral etiologies have been excluded.

Reactivation of cytomegalovirus or varicella zoster virus and new onset adenovirus infection may complicate recovery of stem cell transplant recipients. All of these viruses cause striking cellular apoptosis that simulates features of graft-versus-host disease (146). Cytomegalovirus produces amphophilic intranuclear inclusions surrounded by halo ("owl's eye" appearance), as well as brightly eosinophilic granular inclusions in the cytoplasm. Inclusions are mostly found in endothelial cells but can also be detected in epithelial cells, particularly neutral mucin-containing glandular cells of the upper gastrointestinal tract (fig. 3-34A). Exuberant granulation tissue can mask rare inclusions, so immunohistochemical stains for cytomegalovirus may be considered when ulcers are present (147). Adenovirus infection can be difficult to detect in routinely stained sections. Clues to the diagnosis include nuclear disarray and cellular debris in the surface epithelium accompanied by smudgy eosinophilic intranuclear inclusions (fig. 3-34C,D)

Mycophenolate mofetil is an immunosuppressive medication used to prevent graft rejection in solid organ and bone marrow transplant recipients. This medication causes a gastroenteritis that shows extensive histologic overlap with graft-versus-host disease, eliciting epithelial apoptosis, ballooned parietal cells with cytoplasmic clearing, and reactive gastropathy (fig. 3-35) (148). Clues to a medication-related injury include the frequent presence of eosinophil infiltrates, mucosal inflammation, and destruction of endocrine cells (see chapter 4) (149).

Treatment and Prognosis. Systemic corticosteroids are the mainstay of therapy for patients with graft-versus-host disease (150). Patients with steroid refractory disease have a poor prognosis with mortality rates approaching 40 percent (151).

Radiation- and Chemotherapy-Related Gastropathy

Definition. This is gastric injury due to external beam radiation or systemic chemotherapy.

Clinical Features. Patients who receive external beam radiation to treat carcinomas of the pancreas and liver, or lymphoma involving retroperitoneal lymph nodes are at highest risk for radiation-induced gastritis. Acute injury occurs within weeks to months of therapy (152). Acute symptoms result from mucosal sloughing and include epigastric pain, early satiety, melena, and hematemesis (153,154). Chronic injury usually manifests within 3 years of radiation treatment (154). Symptoms are related to gastric ischemia resulting from obliterative arteriopathy.

Nontargeted systemic chemotherapeutic agents have cytotoxic effects that alter the proliferation of both neoplastic and non-neoplastic cells. These effects can be quite pronounced in the gastrointestinal tract, resulting in disruption of mucosal integrity. Patients receiving systemic chemotherapy frequently complain of nausea, vomiting, and diarrhea.

Gross Findings. Acute radiation injury results in mucosal edema, friability, and erosions (fig. 3-36A) (155). Chronic injury is associated with atrophy, mucosal pallor, and telangiectasias, similar to radiation-induced injury elsewhere in the gastrointestinal tract (fig. 3-36B). The endoscopic features of chemotherapy-related injury are not specific and include erythema, erosions, and ulcers.

Microscopic Findings. Radiation therapy elicits mucosal edema in combination with mucosal

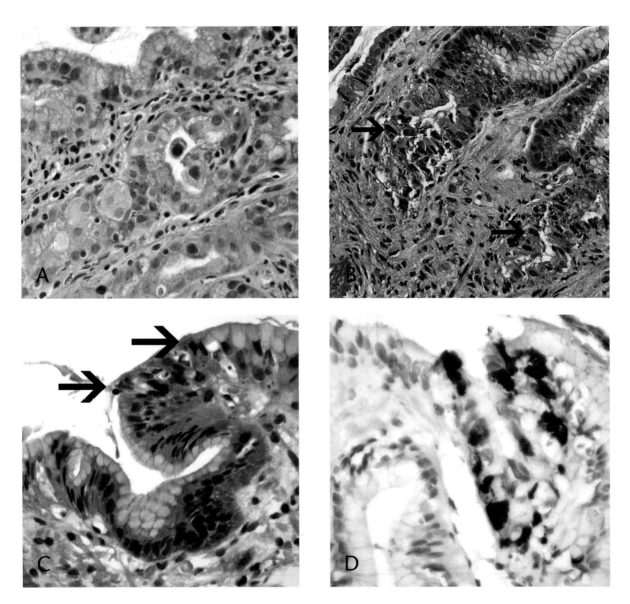

Figure 3-34

VIRAL MIMICS OF GRAFT-VERSUS-HOST DISEASE

Numerous cytomegalovirus inclusions are present in glandular epithelial cells (A). Varicella zoster virus reactivation can cause severe epithelial cell injury in deep gastric glands; viral inclusions (arrows) are difficult to appreciate amidst abundant cellular debris (B). Adenovirus produces smudgy, eosinophilic inclusions that replace epithelial cell nuclei (arrows). Infection imparts a disorganized appearance to the surface epithelial layer (C). Adenovirus-related cytologic changes may be quite subtle, requiring immunohistochemistry for confirmation (D).

fibrin deposits and epithelial injury (156). Dilated gastric glands are lined by attenuated epithelial cells with brightly eosinophilic cytoplasm, hyperchromatic enlarged nuclei, and scattered cellular debris (fig. 3-37). Chronic radiation elicits lamina propria fibrosis and vascular ectasias. The mucosa may contain atypical proliferating fibroblasts that show nuclear enlargement and hyperchromasia. Mucosal capillaries are dilated and hyalinized. Submucosal arterioles display intimal thickening with hyalinization and foamy macrophages (fig. 3-38).

Chemotherapy-related gastritis may display mucin-depleted foveolar epithelium

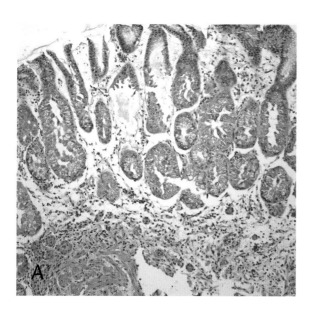
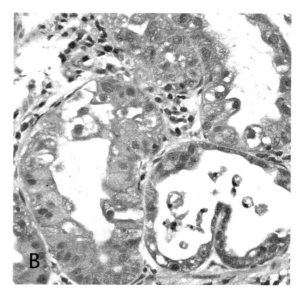

Figure 3-35

MYCOPHENOLATE MOFETIL-ASSOCIATED GASTRIC INJURY

The oxyntic mucosa displays cytoplasmic depletion of the superficial epithelium with patchy mixed inflammation and eosinophils in the deep mucosa (A). Dilated oxyntic glands contain apoptotic debris (B).

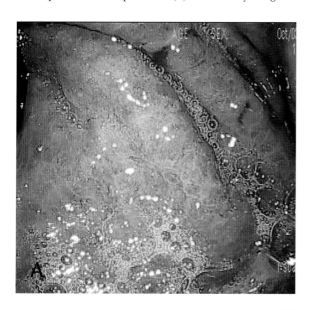
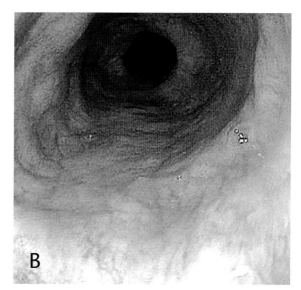

Figure 3-36

RADIATION GASTROPATHY

Diffuse edema, erythema, and patchy petechiae were found in the remnant stomach of a patient undergoing adjuvant chemotherapy and radiation for gastric cancer (A). Chronic radiation causes mucosal atrophy and vascular ectasias (B).

unassociated with lamina propria inflammation or erosive gastropathy with mucosal hemorrhage. Systemic agents inhibit cellular proliferation, resulting in the accumulation of apoptotic debris in gastric glands accompanied by cytologic atypia, nuclear enlargement, and hyperchromasia (fig. 3-39).

Differential Diagnosis. Radiation and chemotherapy can induce cytologic atypia in non-neoplastic epithelium that simulates dysplasia.

123

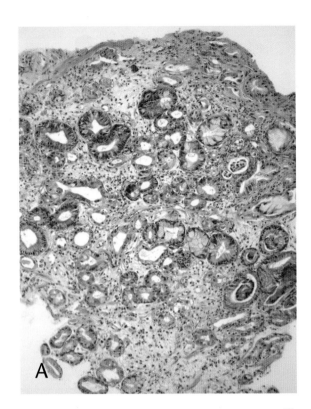 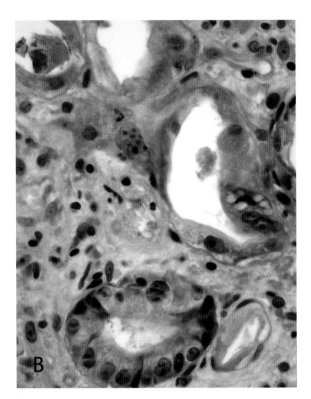

Figure 3-37

ACUTE RADIATION INJURY

Radiation elicits patchy inflammation and edema, as well as cytoplasmic depletion of glandular epithelium (A). Atypical glands show attenuated cytoplasm, nucleomegaly, multinucleation, and nucleolar prominence with preserved nuclear to cytoplasmic ratios (B).

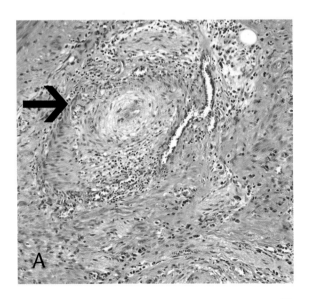 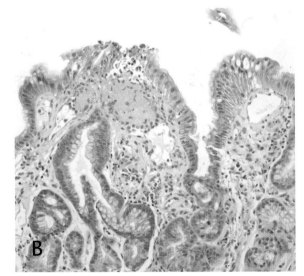

Figure 3-38

CHRONIC RADIATION-INDUCED GASTROPATHY

Myointimal arterial thickening (arrow) leads to chronic ischemic injury (A). Vascular ectasias and lamina propria fibrosis develop months to years after therapy, and may contain fibrin thrombi (B).

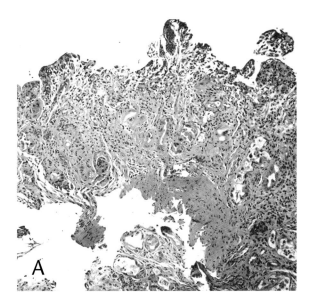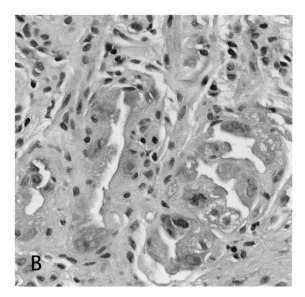

Figure 3-39

CHEMOTHERAPY-INDUCED GASTRIC INJURY

Chemotherapy can cause erosive gastritis with denudation and gland drop-out (A). Regenerative glands are lined by cells with attenuated cytoplasm and enlarged, hyperchromatic nuclei. Necrotic cellular debris is present within disrupted glands (B).

Clues to a diagnosis of reactive cytologic atypia include preserved mucosal architecture, gradual transitions between atypical epithelium and that which is clearly non-neoplastic, a lack of mitotic activity in the atypical epithelium, and a preserved nuclear to cytoplasmic ratio.

Treatment and Prognosis. Patients with therapy-related gastritis are usually treated conservatively with supportive care and nutritional supplementation; those with actively bleeding lesions may require blood transfusions or endoscopic coagulation of bleeding sites (155). Oral prednisolone and proton pump inhibitor therapy alleviate symptoms in some patients (157). Refractory bleeding due to chronic radiation gastritis may be treated with laser coagulation; it rarely requires surgical resection (155).

Selective Internal Radiation Therapy-Related Gastropathy

Definition. *Selective internal radiation therapy (SIRT)-related gastropathy* is gastric injury secondary to embolization with yttrium-90 (^{90}Y)-emitting microspheres.

Clinical Features. ^{90}Y-emitting microspheres are used to treat metastatic colorectal carcinomas, endocrine tumors, and primary hepatocellular carcinomas. Glass or plastic beads are injected into the hepatic arterial circulation, allowing focused delivery of ionizing radiation to hepatic tumors (158–160). Gastrointestinal symptoms after internal radiation therapy are typically mild and include nausea, epigastric discomfort, vomiting, anorexia and occasionally fever (161). However, ^{90}Y beads can travel to the stomach *via* the gastroduodenal artery as well as anomalous connections between the hepatic artery and other arteries that stem from the celiac axis (162,163). Inadvertent embolization of arteries that supply the stomach can cause severe radiation-related gastric injury with epigastric pain, nausea and vomiting, and gastrointestinal hemorrhage.

Pathogenesis. Radioactive beads that embolize feeder arteries become lodged in small gastric and duodenal vessels. Radiation causes localized ischemic injury (164).

Gross Findings. Endoscopy reveals erythema, erosions, and ulcers in areas affected by radiation. Pigmentation of the mucosa and ulcers are occasionally identified, reflecting the presence of ^{90}Y beads (165).

Microscopic Findings. Yttrium microspheres are either clear, refractile, and colorless or basophilic depending on the composition of the beads; both variants measure 20 to 30 µm

125

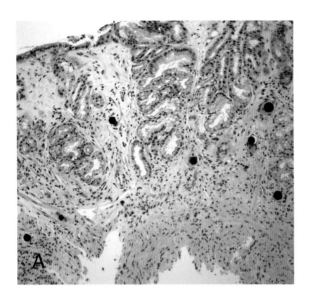
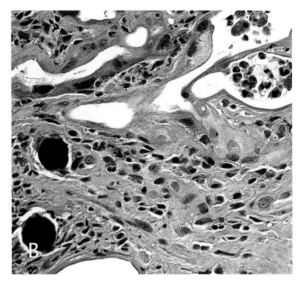

Figure 3-40

SELECTIVE INTERNAL RADIATION THERAPY-INDUCED GASTRITIS

The mucosa is edematous and surfaced by mucin-depleted foveolar epithelial cells; basophilic spheres are lodged in mucosal blood vessels (A). Injured glands contain abundant, slightly eosinophilic cytoplasm and enlarged, hyperchromatic nuclei (B).

in diameter (165). They lodge in mucosal and submucosal blood vessels where they cause severe mucosal injury with erosions or ulcers (fig. 3-40A). Nearby epithelial cells and fibroblasts contain enlarged, hyperchromatic nuclei with prominent nucleoli (fig. 3-40B). Vascular thickening and hyalinization may be seen.

Treatment and Prognosis. Pre-procedural angiograms are widely used to highlight the vascular anatomy of the proximal gastrointestinal tract and prevent inadvertent embolization of the upper gastrointestinal tract (164). Hemostasis is usually achieved with thermocoagulation and endoclips. The effects of local radiation impair wound healing, so multiple endoscopic procedures may be required. NSAIDs exacerbate ulcers and should be withheld. Patients may require a jejunostomy tube for feeding until ulcers heal (166).

INFLAMMATORY DISEASES OF THE STOMACH

Helicobacter-Associated Chronic Gastritis

Definition. *Helicobacter-associated chronic gastritis* is a chronic gastritis caused by the gram-negative bacilli, *H. pylori, H. heilmannii,* and related species.

Clinical Features. Humans are the main reservoir for *H. pylori*, which spreads via the fecal-oral route. At least 50 percent of the global population is infected with *H. pylori*, and most individuals acquire infection during childhood (167). The risk is highest among populations of lower socioeconomic status and in the eastern and southern hemispheres, although the seroprevalence has decreased to approximately 25 percent in the United States in recent decades, likely reflecting improved sanitation (168,169). Infection is slightly more common among men, and is asymptomatic in approximately 80 percent of patients (170). Those with symptoms complain of dyspepsia, nausea, and vomiting; iron deficiency anemia may also be present (171). Peptic ulcers of the stomach and duodenum develop in 10 to 15 percent of symptomatic patients.

Approximately 1 percent of human *Helicobacter* sp. infections are due to *H. heilmannii.* This organism generally causes milder disease with fewer ulcers than *H. pylori*. Infection may be transmitted to humans from animals, particularly household pets (172).

H. pylori is considered a class I carcinogen by the World Health Organization. Although less than 3 percent of infected patients develop gastric cancer, 90 percent of non-cardia gastric cancers are associated with *H. pylori* infection (167). The risk of gastric cancer is increased four-fold among infected patients compared with uninfected individuals, and *H. pylori* eradication decreases this risk by 50 percent (167). Fewer than 1 percent of those infected with *H. pylori* develop lymphoma (173). Nearly all low-grade marginal zone (mucosa-associated lymphoid tissue [MALT]) B-cell lymphomas of the stomach are linked to *H. pylori* infection. Most regress with *H. pylori* eradication, but high-grade transformation can occur.

Pathogenesis. *Helicobacter* organisms employ flagella to localize in the gastric antrum where the pH is higher than that of the proximal stomach. They elaborate urease, which hydrolyzes urea to ammonia and carbon dioxide, thereby neutralizing the local environment between the foveolar epithelium and surface mucus layer (173). Adhesins are important proteins on the outer bacterial membranes that allow them to bind to Lewis blood group antigens on foveolar epithelial cells. Infection elicits a variably severe inflammatory cell infiltrate that elaborates inflammatory mediators, namely, IFN-γ and TNF-α, thereby facilitating the release of reactive oxygen species and inflammatory cytokines that damage the gastric mucosa (173).

Some bacteria contain specific proteins that tend to elicit a more intense inflammatory response and cause a greater degree of mucosal injury. Cytotoxin-associated gene A (CagA)-bearing *H. pylori* strains are particularly virulent because this protein is highly immunogenic, compromises intercellular junctions, and induces DNA damage and apoptosis (173). Vacuolating cytotoxin A (VacA) accumulates within epithelial cells and induces apoptosis. Its release into the lamina propria impairs T-cell function and promotes persistent infection (173).

Gross Findings. Endoscopic features include erythema, erosions, and ulcers that involve the entire stomach or are more severe in the antrum; the examination can also be normal in patients with substantial mucosal inflammation (fig. 3-41). Longstanding infection causes thinning of the rugae, and prominent submucosal vessels (174). Clean-based ulcers may be surrounded by normal-appearing folds or show mural thickening. There is a poor correlation between endo-

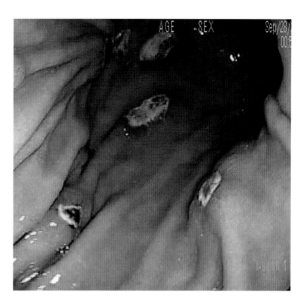

Figure 3-41

HELICOBACTER PYLORI-ASSOCIATED GASTRITIS

Multiple shallow ulcers covered with fibrinous exudate are present in a patient with *H. pylori* infection. The mucosa immediately surrounding the ulcers displays localized erythema with normal rugal folds.

scopic abnormalities and histologic findings unless ulcers are present. Thus, endoscopists should obtain multiple samples from the greater and lesser curvatures of the antrum and corpus (175).

Microscopic Findings. *H. pylori* are slender, curvilinear rods located in gastric mucus and adherent to foveolar epithelium (fig. 3-42A). The organism burden is generally highest in the antrum, unless patients are receiving proton pump inhibitor therapy or the distal stomach displays intestinal metaplasia. Organisms often have a coccoid appearance (fig. 3-42B). Although round bacteria were previously thought to be degenerated in nature, it is now clear that this phenotype represents an adaptive response (176). Occasional organisms can also be found within foveolar and oxyntic cells, although most bacteria in parietal cells are actually trapped in the extracellular canalicular system (fig. 3-42C,D) (177). *H. heilmannii* are longer and thicker than *H. pylori*, and have a spiral configuration (fig. 3-43) (172).

H. pylori infection elicits plasma cell-rich mixed inflammation with variable numbers of neutrophils and erosions, as well as mucin depletion of foveolar epithelial cells and increased

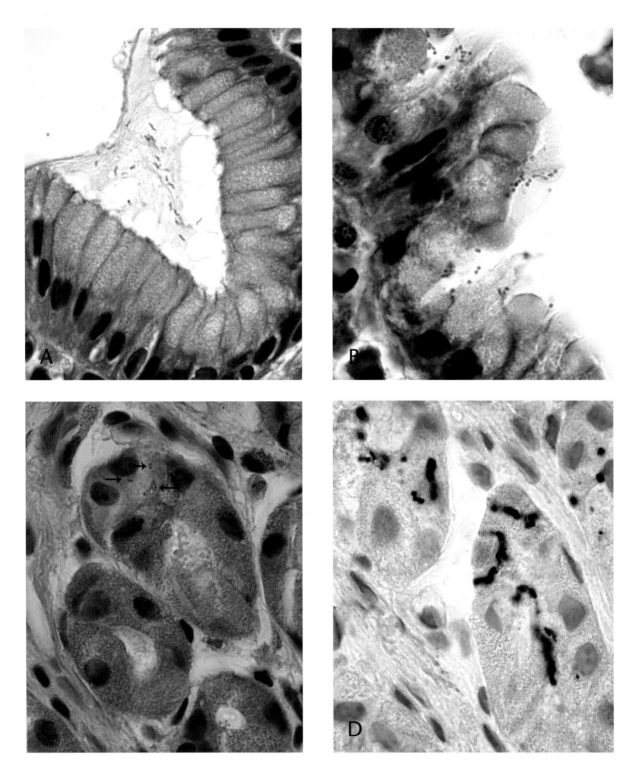

Figure 3-42

HELICOBACTER PYLORI ORGANISMS

Curvilinear bacilli are located in adherent mucus at the foveolar surface (A). Organisms can have a coccoid appearance in some cases (B). Seemingly intracellular *H. pylori* (arrows) are occasionally detected (C). Those that appear to be intracellular in oxyntic glands are usually located in the complex canalicular system of parietal cells, as illustrated with immunohistochemistry (D).

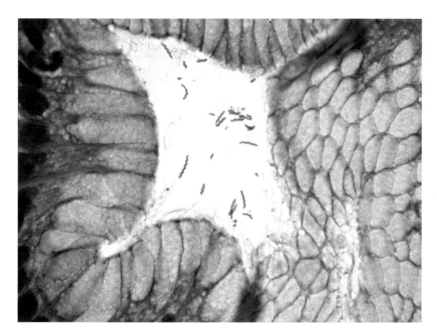

Figure 3-43

HELICOBACTER HEILMANNII

Organisms are longer and thicker than *H. pylori*. They have a distinct tightly coiled corkscrew configuration.

mitotic activity. Lymphoplasmacytic inflammation tends to be most pronounced under the surface epithelium with milder infiltrates in the deep mucosa (fig. 3-44A). Infection of oxyntic mucosa elicits a discrete band of lymphocytes and plasma cells around foveolar epithelium with sparing of oxyntic glands (fig. 3-44B). Neutrophils may be seen but are not the main inflammatory cells in the lamina propria. Neutrophils infiltrate glandular epithelium singly or in clusters, and can form luminal microabscesses, especially in areas with higher numbers of organisms (fig. 3-44C). Lymphoid aggregates and reactive germinal centers are commonly present (fig. 3-44D). Non-necrotic granulomas are occasionally encountered, usually in association with injured glands (fig. 3-45A). Less than 5 percent of infected patients have a lymphocytic gastritis pattern of injury with numerous CD8-positive T-cells in the foveolar epithelium (fig. 3-45B) (178). Inflammatory cell infiltrates tend to be milder in patients with *H. heilmannii* infection as well as those with predominantly intracellular organisms (fig. 3-45C,D).

Neutrophilic inflammation abates rapidly after successful eradication, but chronic inflammatory infiltrates may persist for weeks or months after therapy. Longstanding infection causes mucosal atrophy and intestinal metaplasia of the antrum or entire gastric mucosa; this pattern historically has been referred to as "type B" or "environmental" gastric atrophy (fig. 3-46).

Infection can be clinically detected with a variety of assays. Serologic tests employ enzyme-linked immunosorbent assay (ELISA) technology to detect IgG directed against the organisms; these tests are highly sensitive but do not distinguish active from past infection (179). Antigen tests detect shed bacterial proteins in stool from infected patients. Breath tests detect CO_2 liberated from carbon-labeled urea, reflecting the urease activity of *H. pylori* (180). Urease tests can also be performed on biopsy tissue applied to paper or gel-based kits that indicate altered pH when the organisms hydrolyze urea.

H. pylori organisms are usually readily apparent in routinely stained tissue sections from infected patients; ancillary stains add little value when uninflamed biopsy samples are encountered (181). In fact, organisms are detected in less than 10 percent of patients with chronic inactive gastritis, as defined by clusters of plasma cells expanding the lamina propria (fig. 3-47) (182,183). Ancillary stains may also detect *H. pylori* in a small number of cases with granulomas, lymphocytic gastritis, and increased mucosal eosinophils (181). A number of histochemical stains have been used to highlight the organisms, including Giemsa, Warthin-Starry, and Alcian yellow, but they do not distinguish *Helicobacter* sp. from other bacteria and generally

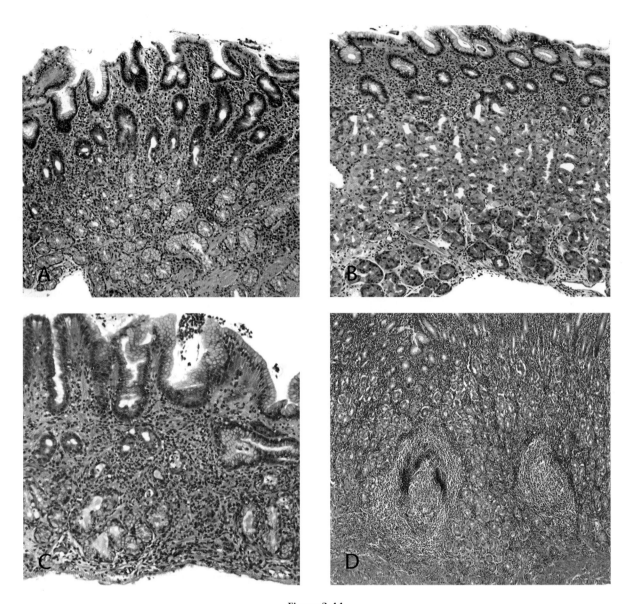

Figure 3-44

HELICOBACTER PYLORI-ASSOCIATED CHRONIC GASTRITIS

The antrum contains a lymphoplasmacytic infiltrate that is more pronounced in the superficial mucosa (A). Infection elicits a similar band of subepithelial mononuclear cell-rich inflammation in the corpus and fundus, but spares the oxyntic glands (B). Neutrophils are present in gastric pits and adjacent lamina propria (C). Reactive lymphoid aggregates are common and, when present, should prompt consideration of *H. pylori* infection (D).

perform no better than hematoxylin and eosin stains when rare organisms are present. Immunohistochemical stains directed against *Helicobacter* demonstrate sensitivity and specificity of nearly 100 percent when bacteria are present, and are most useful when organisms are scarce (181).

Differential Diagnosis. The differential diagnosis of *H. pylori*-associated gastritis includes immune-mediated, infectious, and medication-related disorders. As discussed subsequently, autoimmune gastritis affects oxyntic mucosae and spares the antrum. Infiltrates tend to be more prominent in the deep mucosa and are associated with a greater degree of gland destruction and cellular metaplasia. The stomach is the second most common site of gastrointestinal involvement by syphilis,

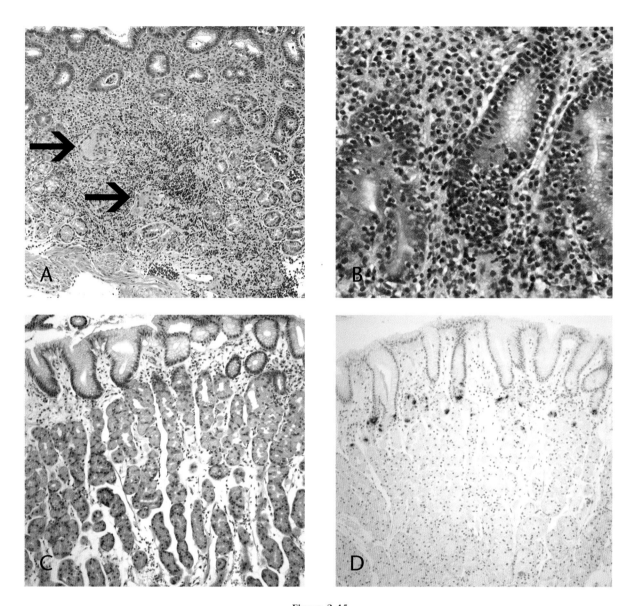

Figure 3-45

***H. PYLORI*-ASSOCIATED GASTRITIS**

Some patients with *H. pylori* infection have unusual features in their gastric biopsy samples. Granulomatous inflammation (arrows) may be present in association with injured glands (A). Occasional cases display striking intraepithelial lymphocytosis (B). Intracellular organisms elicit a minimal inflammatory response (C) despite detection of numerous bacteria by immunohistochemistry (D).

which elicits a plasma cell-rich chronic active gastritis (figs. 3-48, 3-49). Clues to the diagnosis of syphilitic gastritis include the dense nature of lymphoplasmacytic inflammation extending into the deep mucosa, often accompanied by mucosal fibrosis. Medications, particularly targeted agents and sartans, can cause chronic gastritis that simulates the features of *H. pylori* infection.

Approximately 80 percent of gastric marginal zone (MALT) lymphomas arise in association with *H. pylori* infection. They appear as an expansile proliferation of small to medium-sized lymphocytes that effaces the normal mucosal architecture. Lesional cells may have irregular contours resembling centrocytes or abundant pale cytoplasm typical of monocytes. Lymphoepithelial

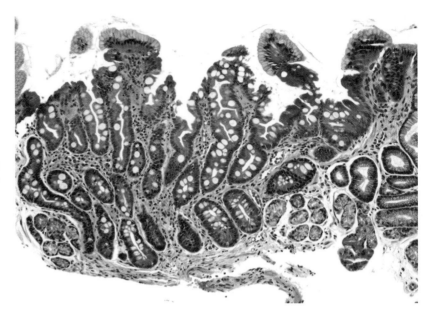

Figure 3-46

ATROPHIC GASTRITIS

Extensive intestinal metaplasia can result from long-standing *H. pylori* infection.

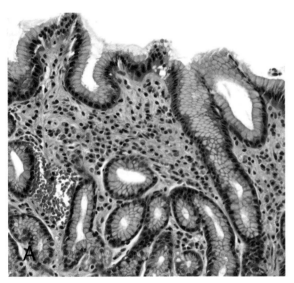

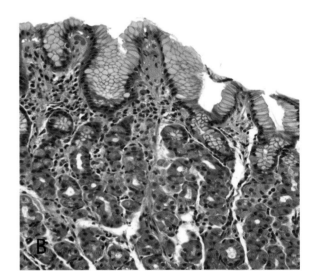

Figure 3-47

CHRONIC INACTIVE GASTRITIS

Clusters of plasma cells expand the superficial lamina propria of the antrum (A) and body (B). This degree of inflammation probably exceeds that normally present and should prompt consideration of *H. pylori* infection.

lesions, or clusters of neoplastic cells infiltrating glandular epithelium, are helpful diagnostic clues. The diagnosis is confirmed by clonal rearrangement of the B-cell receptor gene, detected *via* polymerase chain reaction (PCR) (184).

Patients with infectious mononucleosis may rarely develop Epstein-Barr (EBV) virus-associated gastritis characterized by diffuse polymorphic infiltrates composed of a mixed T- and B-cell population. The disorder may feature focal epithelial infiltration, but lacks the prominent plasma cells typical of *H. pylori* gastritis (fig. 3-50A). *In situ* hybridization for EBV-RNA (fig. 3-50B), highlights infected lymphocytes (185).

Lymphomatoid gastropathy is a rare, self-limited proliferation of benign natural killer (NK) cells that infiltrates the stomach and occasionally involves the gastric epithelium. Lesional cells are large and atypical, but they are not clonal. They express CD56, TIA-1, and granzyme B (186–188).

Treatment and Prognosis. Evaluation for *H. pylori* is recommended when patients have a history of peptic ulcer disease, MALT lymphoma, or endoscopic resection of early gastric cancer. Currently, patients who test positive for *H. pylori* by any means are offered treatment, which consists of a combination of proton pump inhibitors and antibiotics (clarithromycin and amoxicillin or metronidazole) (171). This regimen achieves complete eradication in 90 percent of patients. Treatment failure often reflects non-adherence to therapy or antibiotic resistance. Alternative regimens are also available (171).

Autoimmune Gastritis

Definition. *Autoimmune gastritis* is immune-mediated destruction of oxyntic mucosa. It is also termed *autoimmune metaplastic atrophic gastritis*.

Clinical Features. Autoimmune gastritis shows a predilection for middle-aged women,

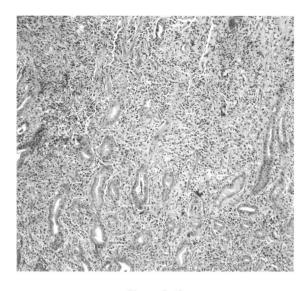

Figure 3-48

SYPHILITIC GASTRITIS

Treponema pallidum infection produces a severe pan-gastritis that features full-thickness mononuclear cell-rich inflammation accompanied by gland destruction.

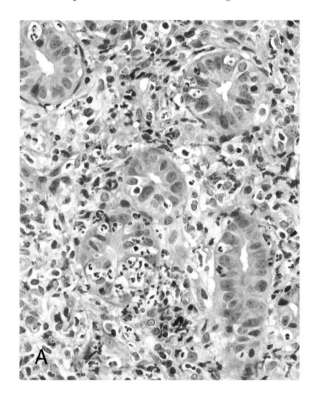
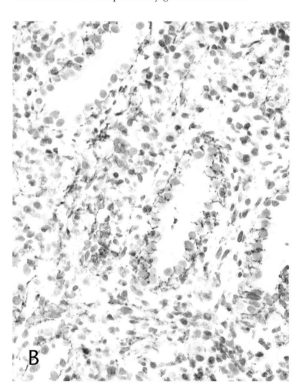

Figure 3-49

SYPHILITIC GASTRITIS

Neutrophilic infiltration of pyloric glands simulates *H. pylori* gastritis, although macrophages are more prominent in the background infiltrate than plasma cells (A). A *T. pallidum* immunostain highlights spirochetes in and around inflamed glands (B).

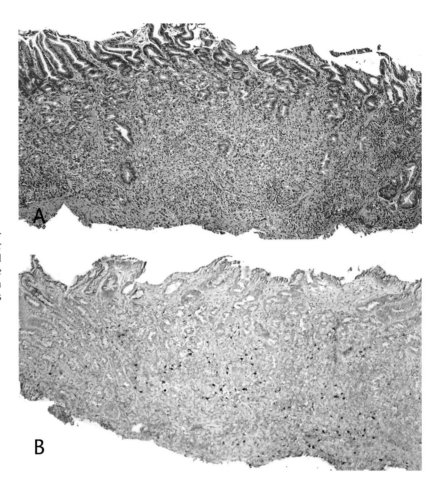

Figure 3-50

EPSTEIN-BARR VIRUS-ASSOCIATED GASTRITIS

Dense lymphoplasmacytic inflammation shows a predilection for the deep mucosa. Lymphoepithelial lesions and gland destruction are prominent (A). *In situ* hybridization for EBV-encoded RNA confirms infection (B).

although Hispanic and African-American women are slightly younger compared with whites (189). Affected patients often have other autoimmune disorders, such as thyroiditis, autoimmune hepatitis, type 1 diabetes mellitus, and systemic lupus erythematosus (190,191). Most affected patients have no, or minimal, upper gastrointestinal symptoms (192). Iron deficiency anemia precedes pernicious anemia due to hypochlorhydria-related impairment of iron absorption. Vitamin B12 deficiency takes years to develop. Manifestations of advanced disease include pernicious anemia, paresthesias, memory impairment, and gait disturbances (193). Typical laboratory findings include elevated serum gastrin levels and circulating autoantibodies to parietal cells and intrinsic factor. These autoantibodies are of limited specificity and may be detected in other autoimmune disorders (194). Autoimmune gastritis is also associated with HLA-B8 and HLA-DR3.

Pathogenesis. Although many patients with autoimmune gastritis have circulating autoantibodies to parietal cells and intrinsic factor, these antibodies are a marker of disease, rather than pathogenic in nature. The disorder is mediated by T-cells that drive oxyntic gland destruction, leading to loss of parietal cell mass and hypochlorhydria. The rising pH of gastric juices results in disrupted acid-mediated inhibition of gastrin elaboration by antral G cells, leading to hypergastrinemia. Gastrin is a trophic hormone that stimulates enterochromaffin-like (ECL) cells to proliferate, resulting in linear and nodular ECL-cell hyperplasia and formation of type I well-differentiated endocrine (carcinoid) tumors. Loss of intrinsic factor impairs vitamin B12 absorption in the ileum (192). *H. pylori* infection may promote the development of autoimmune gastritis in some patients; there are some molecular similarities between bacterial proteins and those of proton pumps on parietal cells (195).

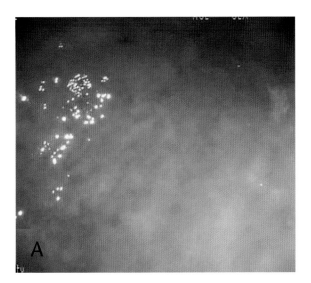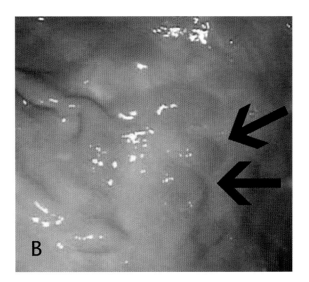

Figure 3-51

AUTOIMMUNE GASTRITIS

Autoimmune gastritis causes mucosal atrophy with loss of rugal folds and prominent submucosal vasculature (A). Raised nodules of residual oxyntic mucosa (arrows) have a polypoid appearance (B).

Gross Findings. Autoimmune gastritis produces no endoscopic abnormalities early in the disease course. Progressive mucosal atrophy leads to effacement of the rugal folds and prominence of submucosal blood vessels (fig. 3-51A). Patients develop hyperplastic polyps, pyloric gland adenomas, intestinal-type adenomas, and "pseudopolyps" of residual oxyntic mucosa (fig. 3-51B).

Microscopic Findings. Early histologic changes of autoimmune gastritis are subtle. Corpus-based chronic gastritis predominantly affects the deep glands or the full-thickness of the mucosa. Lymphoplasmacytic infiltrates feature scattered eosinophils with patchy lymphocytic infiltration of oxyntic glands (fig. 3-52). Scattered glands contain apoptotic cellular debris and others display pyloric, or pseudopyloric, metaplasia characterized by neutral mucin-containing cuboidal epithelial cells (196).

Progressive disease features diffuse lymphoplasmacytic infiltration of the lamina propria with extensive oxyntic gland loss and prominent glandular metaplasia; pyloric, intestinal, and pancreatic cell types are commonly present (fig. 3-53). Complete loss of oxyntic glands may impart the appearance of inflamed antral mucosa ("oxyntic antralization") (192). Extensive intestinal metaplasia with complete oxyntic gland loss and residual pyloric metaplasia has been referred to as "type A" atrophic gastritis (fig. 3-54).

Progressive disease is accompanied by ECL-cell hyperplasia. Linear hyperplasia is arbitrarily defined as at least two groups of five or more adjacent chromogranin-expressing ECL cells in a gland, whereas nodular ECL-cell hyperplasia refers to cell clusters that are less than 150 μm (fig. 3-55). Aggregates of ECL cells may form visible tumors, but are usually smaller than 1 cm (197). They are often multiple and limited to the mucosa or submucosa. They are indolent and non-functional.

Biopsy samples from the antrum are often normal or show features of chemical gastropathy due to bile reflux. The antrum displays G-cell hyperplasia, which can be demonstrated by immunohistochemical stains for gastrin (fig. 3-56).

Immunohistochemistry is a helpful diagnostic adjunct for autoimmune gastritis, particularly in the florid and late stages. Absence of gastrin by immunohistochemistry confirms that biopsy samples were taken from atrophic oxyntic mucosa and did not originate in the antrum. Chromogranin or synaptophysin stains highlight linear and nodular ECL-cell hyperplasia. Stains to rule out *H. pylori* infection should also be considered.

Differential Diagnosis. *H. pylori*-associated gastritis is the main entity in the differential diagnosis of autoimmune gastritis. *H.*

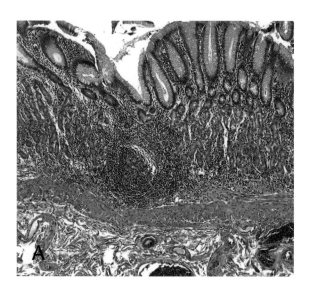
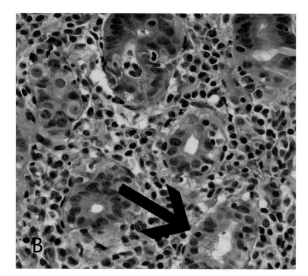

Figure 3-52

AUTOIMMUNE GASTRITIS

The mucosa is expanded by full-thickness chronic inflammation and lymphoid aggregates; oxyntic glands are preserved early in the disease course (A). The inflammatory infiltrates feature numerous eosinophils, plasma cells, and scattered lymphocytes infiltrating oxyntic glands; apoptotic debris and focal pyloric metaplasia (arrow) are also present (B).

pylori-associated gastritis is antrum-based; it often involves the oxyntic mucosa, but does not spare the antrum. Lymphoplasmacytic inflammation is concentrated in the superficial lamina propria in a "band-like" distribution subjacent to the surface epithelium. Neutrophilic infiltration of the pit and surface epithelium is seen, but the oxyntic glands are usually spared.

Treatment and Prognosis. There is no specific treatment for autoimmune gastritis. Patients may undergo endoscopic surveillance, particularly if they have documented intestinal metaplasia. The risk of gastric adenocarcinoma is increased up to three-fold in patients with autoimmune gastritis, depending on the extent of atrophy (198). Vitamin B12 supplementation alleviates symptoms and complications of pernicious anemia. Endocrine tumors (i.e., type 1 carcinoid tumor) are indolent and patients have a greater than 95 percent 5-year survival rate (199). Antrectomy is definitively treats hypergastrinemia but is rarely performed since the overall risk of malignant progression is low.

Collagenous Gastritis

Definition. *Collagenous gastritis* is a type of chronic gastritis that features subepithelial collagen deposition.

Clinical Features. Most cases of collagenous gastritis occur in females and have been historically grouped as pediatric and adult forms (200). The pediatric variant is reportedly limited to the stomach, and presents in adolescence with abdominal pain, anemia, nausea and vomiting, and upper gastrointestinal bleeding. The adult form manifests with abdominal pain, anemia, or chronic watery diarrhea in middle-aged or older adults; many also have collagenous colitis or collagenous sprue. However, more recent data suggest substantial overlap between the clinical features of pediatric and adult patients with collagenous gastritis (201). Both pediatric and adult patients often have other immune-mediated diseases, including Sjogren syndrome, celiac disease, and ulcerative colitis (202).

Pathogenesis. The disorder is usually idiopathic in nature, although an immune-mediated mechanism has been proposed (203). Collagenous gastritis can occur in patients receiving olmesartan and other agents in the class of angiotensin II receptor antagonists used to treat hypertension (201).

Gross Findings. The gastric mucosa tends to be nodular, reflecting retraction in areas of collagen deposition with apparent elevation of relatively spared mucosa (fig. 3-57). Erythema, erosions, and

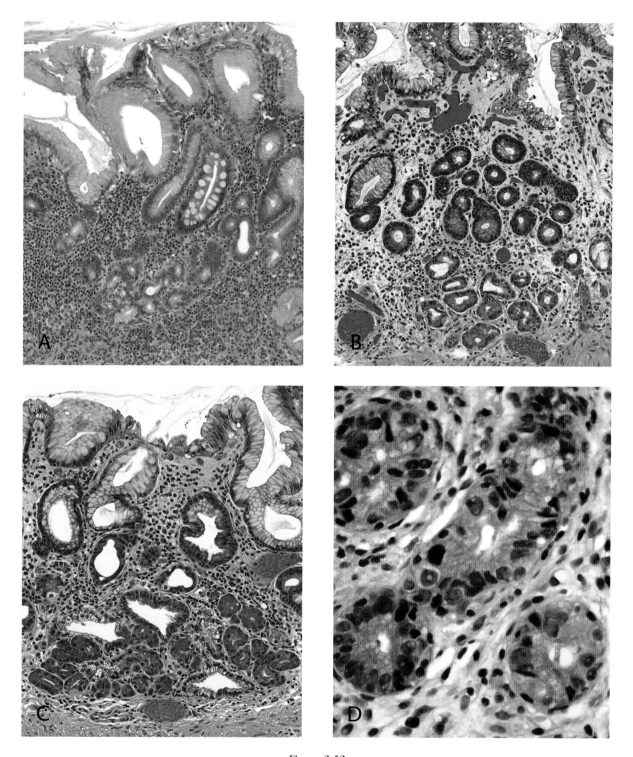

Figure 3-53

AUTOIMMUNE GASTRITIS

Progressive disease features marked chronic inflammation, particularly in the deep mucosa, with replacement of oxyntic glands by pyloric-type glands and foci of intestinal metaplasia (A). Extensive pyloric metaplasia is accompanied by diminished inflammation (B). Lobules of metaplastic pancreatic acini contain eosinophilic granules (C). Samples from patients with megaloblastic anemia may show patchy nuclear enlargement and hyperchromasia, particularly in the deep mucosa (D).

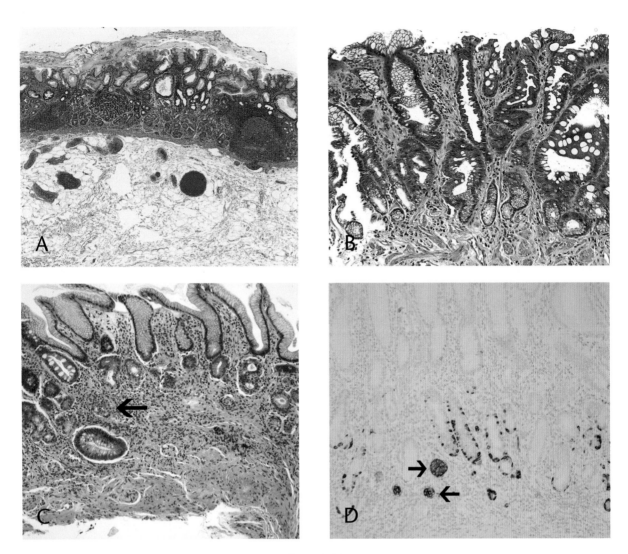

Figure 3-54

AUTOIMMUNE GASTRITIS

Later stages feature a thin mucosa with complete loss of oxyntic glands. Deeply situated lymphoid aggregates are a clue to the diagnosis (A). Complete atrophy is accompanied by minimal inflammation and extensive intestinal metaplasia. A few neutral mucin-containing glands (pyloric metaplasia) are still present in the deep mucosa (B). Atrophic samples display intestinal metaplasia, endocrine cell nodules (arrow), and irregularly distributed pyloric glands (C). A chromogranin immunostain highlights linear and nodular enterochromaffin-like cell (ECL) hyperplasia (arrows) in the gastric body (D).

exudates may be seen, although the stomach is endoscopically normal in some cases (202).

Microscopic Findings. Collagenous gastritis tends to be more severe in the corpus (204). It features irregular subepithelial collagen deposits that measure at least 10 μm in thickness, and range up to 120 μm (205). The collagen layer displays an irregular interface with the underlying lamina propria, and contains entrapped capillaries and inflammatory cells (fig.

3-58A). Artifactual separation of the surface epithelium from the collagen layer can occur. The lamina propria is expanded by lymphoplasmacytic inflammation with variable numbers of eosinophils and intraepithelial neutrophils. Intraepithelial lymphocytosis may be present, but is not prominent. Atrophy of the oxyntic mucosa with pyloric metaplasia, ECL cell hyperplasia, and intestinal metaplasia can simulate autoimmune gastritis (203,206).

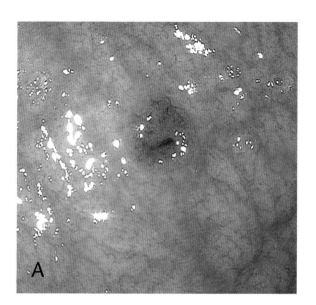
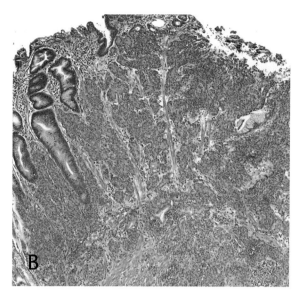

Figure 3-55

ENTEROCHROMAFFIN-LIKE CELL HYPERPLASIA IN AUTOIMMUNE GASTRITIS

Nodules of hyperplastic ECL cells form pale brown nodules (type I gastric carcinoids) accompanied by a background of atrophic oxyntic mucosa (A). These nodules are composed of cellular nests of endocrine cells with minimal atypia (B).

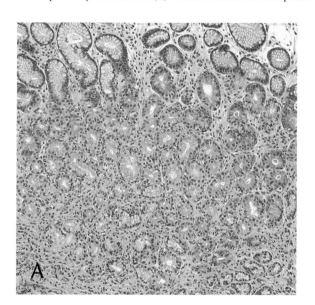
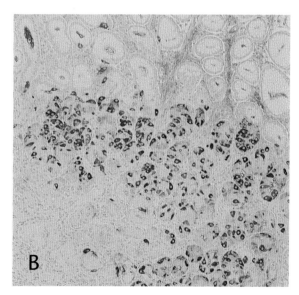

Figure 3-56

ANTRAL ENDOCRINE CELL HYPERPLASIA IN AUTOIMMUNE GASTRITIS

The antral mucosa lacks inflammation, but contains numerous round G cells in deep glands (A). A gastrin immunostain confirms the presence of G-cell hyperplasia (B).

Trichrome stains highlight subepithelial collagen and distinguish it from tangential sections of the basement membrane and amyloid deposits (fig. 3-58B).

Differential Diagnosis. Collagenous gastritis simulates eosinophilic gastroenteritis, lymphocytic gastritis, and autoimmune gastritis, depending on the nature of the inflammatory infiltrate.

None of these disorders features increased subepithelial collagen. Amyloid deposits rarely display a subepithelial distribution with sparing of the lamina propria and blood vessels. As discussed in chapter 4, these deposits are somewhat nodular, display a smooth interface with the lamina propria, and lack entrapped inflammation and capillaries. Amyloid deposits are congophilic and birefringent upon polarization.

Treatment and Prognosis. Patients are treated with a combination of proton pump inhibitors, steroids, and iron supplementation. Available evidence suggests that collagenous gastritis pursues a persistent course in most patients; complete resolution is uncommon even when patients have symptomatic improvement (207). However, some data suggest that cases related to olmesartan can regress following cessation of therapy (208).

Lymphocytic Gastritis

Definition. *Lymphocytic gastritis* is a histologic variant of chronic gastritis featuring intraepithelial lymphocytosis of the foveolar epithelium.

Clinical Features. Lymphocytic gastritis is not a specific disorder. It is a pattern of injury resulting from a variety of etiologies. Lymphocytic gastritis is detected in less than 1 percent of all upper endoscopic examinations and accounts for 2 to 5 percent of chronic gastritis cases (209,

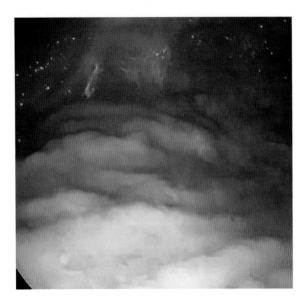

Figure 3-57

COLLAGENOUS GASTRITIS

The rugal folds are effaced and the mucosa is nodular.

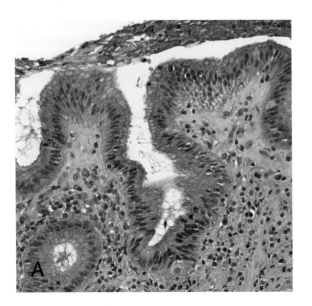
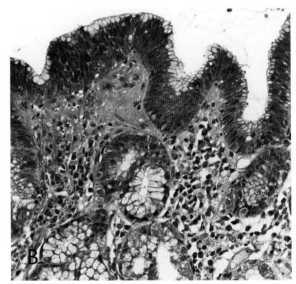

Figure 3-58

COLLAGENOUS GASTRITIS

The thickened subepithelial collagen layer has an irregular interface with the lamina propria. It contains capillaries and inflammatory cells. The background mucosa displays dense lymphoplasmacytic inflammation (A). A trichrome stain highlights thickened collagen (B).

210). It affects adults and children and shows a female predominance (205).

Disease may be confined to the stomach or represent one manifestation of more generalized gastrointestinal lymphocytosis (178). For example, approximately one-third of all patients with celiac disease have lymphocytic gastritis and 40 percent of patients with lymphocytic gastritis have celiac disease, particularly in the pediatric population (211,212).

Chronic gastritis due to *H. pylori* accounts for one-third of cases, although striking intraepithelial lymphocytosis is an uncommon manifestation of *H. pylori* infection overall. Less common associations include concomitant lymphocytic colitis, protein-losing gastropathy reminiscent of Menetrier disease, Crohn disease, and HIV infection (213).

Presenting symptoms are often related to associated disorders such as celiac disease and include diarrhea, abdominal pain, nausea, and vomiting. Almost one-fourth of cases are seemingly idiopathic (178).

Pathogenesis. Most cases of lymphocytic gastritis are related to celiac disease, other immune-mediated disorders, or *H. pylori* infection. Occasional cases occur in association with olmesartan administration. Idiopathic cases are presumably immune-mediated or medication related.

Gross Findings. Approximately 50 percent of cases show normal endoscopic findings. Nearly one third of patients have "varioliform gastritis" characterized by enlarged rugal folds, nodules, and erosions in the corpus (fig. 5-59). This pattern is particularly common in patients with protein-losing gastropathy (214,215).

Microscopic Findings. Lymphocytic gastritis displays at least 30 intraepithelial CD8-positive lymphocytes per 100 foveolar epithelial cells, but counts are often much higher, particularly in idiopathic cases (216). Intraepithelial lymphocytosis is accompanied by variably intense lymphoplasmacytic inflammation in the lamina propria (fig. 3-60). Plasma cell-rich lamina propria inflammation is more prominent in samples from patients with *H. pylori* infection; these cases are also more likely to show neutrophilic inflammation of the gastric pits as well as involvement of oxyntic mucosa. On the other hand, intraepithelial lymphocytosis tends

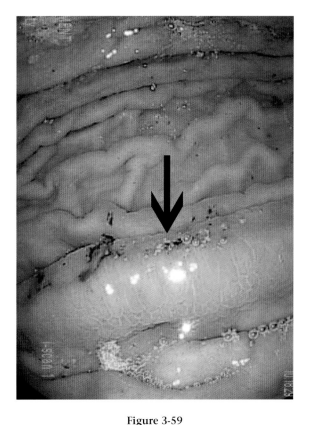

Figure 3-59

VARIOLIFORM GASTRITIS

Markedly enlarged rugae display superficial erosions (arrow).

to be more pronounced in the antrum when associated with celiac disease, often displaying only mild chronic inflammation in the lamina propria. Idiopathic lymphocytic gastritis and protein-losing gastropathy are histologically similar to celiac disease-associated cases, but feature pronounced foveolar hyperplasia (216).

Cases of lymphocytic gastritis should be evaluated with histochemical or immunohistochemical stains to exclude *H. pylori* infection when organisms are not evident in routine sections (181). Immunohistochemical subtyping of intraepithelial lymphocytes is not necessary.

Treatment and Prognosis. Treatment of lymphocytic gastritis is aimed at the underlying causes, such as *H. pylori* eradication and initiation of a gluten-free diet. Intraepithelial lymphocytosis generally resolves after eliminating the offending agent.

141

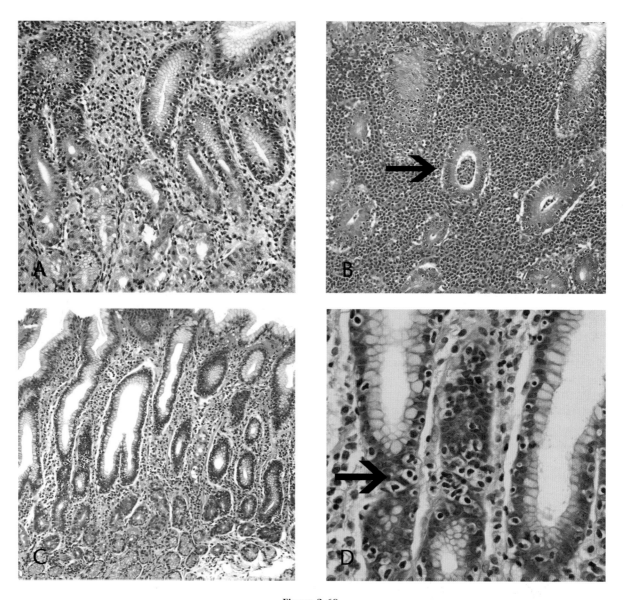

Figure 3-60

LYMPHOCYTIC GASTRITIS

Striking intraepithelial lymphocytosis accompanies plasma cell-rich inflammation in samples from a patient with *H. pylori*-associated gastritis (A). Another case of *H. pylori*-associated lymphocytic gastritis contains neutrophil microabscesses (arrow) and sheets of plasma cells in the lamina propria (B). Evenly distributed mononuclear inflammation is seen in the antral mucosa of a patient with celiac disease (C). Closer examination of the same case demonstrates increased intraepithelial lymphocytes (arrow) (D).

Granulomatous Gastritis

Definition. *Granulomatous gastritis* is a pattern of gastric inflammation featuring epithelioid granulomas.

Clinical Features. Granulomatous gastritis is not a specific entity. Rather, it is a histologic pattern of injury that may occur as a result of several etiologies. Granulomas are occasionally encountered in gastric biopsy samples that are otherwise normal or show chronic gastritis. Crohn disease affects the stomach in 30 to 80 percent of patients with Crohn disease, especially children (217). In this situation, Crohn disease is rarely limited to the stomach; most patients with gastric involvement have intestinal disease. Gastric

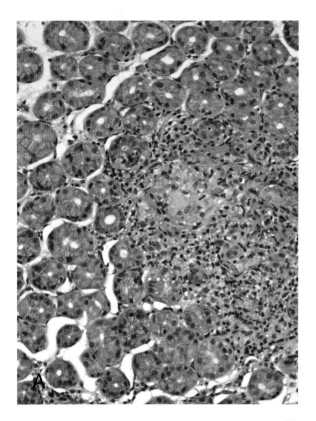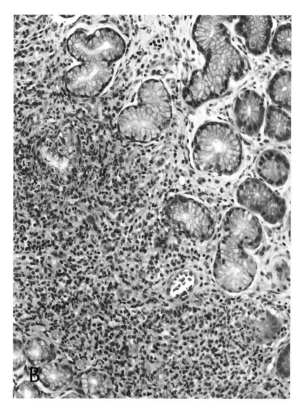

Figure 3-61

GASTRIC CROHN DISEASE

Poorly formed granulomas are accompanied by a focus of increased chronic inflammation (A). An area of mixed inflammation in the lamina propria is associated with gland destruction (B).

manifestations include epigastric pain, vomiting, and delayed gastric emptying.

Sarcoidosis, a systemic disorder with frequent pulmonary symptoms and lymphadenopathy, may involve the stomach; it accounts for 1 to 22 percent of granulomatous gastritis cases. It produces non-specific symptoms such as dyspepsia, early satiety, and weight loss (218). Elevated serum angiotensin converting enzyme levels are highly sensitive and specific for sarcoidosis (219). Granulomatous gastritis also occurs in patients with *Mycobacterium tuberculosis*, fungal, and parasitic infections. Constitutional symptoms such as fever and malaise are common in affected individuals (220). Quantiferon gold tests measure interferon-γ released from macrophages and are highly sensitive and specific for *M. tuberculosis* infection (221).

Gross Findings. The endoscopic features of Crohn disease include nodularity, thickened folds, friability, and aphthous or linear ulcers (218). Sarcoidosis produces nodularity, erosions, and rigidity of the gastric wall (222). Tuberculous gastritis may manifest as an ulcerated mass that simulates carcinoma (223).

Microscopic Findings. Crohn disease-related granulomas are small, non-necrotic, and concentrated in the superficial lamina propria (fig. 3-61A). The background mucosa may show chronic active gastritis or localized pit or gland inflammation (fig. 3-61B) (224). Sarcoidal granulomas are non-necrotic and consist of tight aggregates of epithelioid histiocytes and multinucleated giant cells, often with a peripheral cuff of lymphocytes; they may be found in otherwise unremarkable mucosa or in the setting of chronic gastritis (fig. 3-62). Tuberculosis produces large (approximately 500 μm), confluent granulomas with central necrosis and a peripheral lymphoid cuff. Granulomas are present at all levels in the

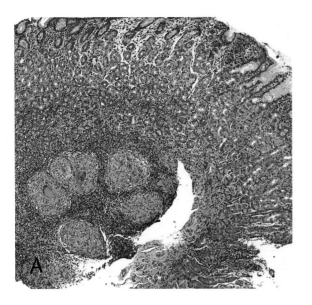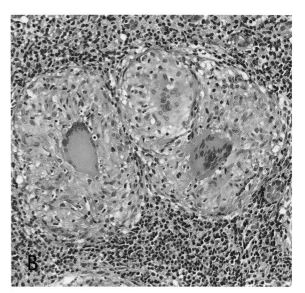

Figure 3-62

GASTRIC SARCOIDOSIS

Multiple large granulomas are associated with dense lymphoid inflammation in the gastric mucosa (A). Tight aggregates of macrophages and multinucleated giant cells are surrounded by a cuff of lymphocytes (B).

gastric wall and are concentrated in the sub-mucosa (225). Other infections that can cause granulomatous gastritis include *Cryptococcus neoformans* and anisakiasis. These infections are discussed further in chapter 4.

Histochemical stains should always be employed to detect organisms when granulomas are found in a patient for the first time. Acid fast bacilli (AFB) stains and immunohistochemistry can be used to highlight *Mycobacteria* sp. Grocott methenamine silver (GMS) and periodic acid–Schiff with diastase (PAS-D) demonstrate fungi. The mucopolysaccharide capsule of *C. neoformans* stains with mucicarmine, although capsule-deficient strains do not take up the stain.

Differential Diagnosis. Virtually any mucosal injury that causes gland disruption can elicit granulomatous inflammation with multinucleated giant cells (fig. 3-63). Granulomas are occasionally encountered in *H. pylori*-associated gastritis. Isolated granulomas are also found in otherwise normal mucosa.

Treatment and Prognosis. Patients with systemic immune-mediated disorders are treated with a variety of immunosuppressive therapies. Antimicrobial regimens are necessary to eradicate infections, as discussed further in chapter 4.

Phlegmonous Gastritis

Definition. *Phlegmonous gastritis* is an acute, purulent gastritis due to non-*H. pylori* bacteria. Synonyms include *acute suppurative gastritis* and *acute necrotizing gastritis*.

Clinical Features. Phlegmonous gastritis is a rare disorder that tends to occur in debilitated patients with achlorhydria, alcoholism, or immunocompromise, although 50 percent of affected patients have no identifiable predisposing condition (226–230). Some cases have been reported after endoscopic resections (231). Presenting symptoms include intense epigastric pain, nausea, vomiting, hematemesis, and diarrhea. Emesis of purulent material is a specific feature of the disorder (232). Imaging fails to demonstrate intramural gas (218).

Pathogenesis. Phlegmonous gastritis is caused by local or systemic bacterial infection that is facilitated by decreased sterilization of gastric contents in the setting of hypochlorhydria. Most cases are attributed to *Streptococcus* sp. particularly S. *pyogenes*. *Staphylococcus* sp., *Haemophilus influenza*, *Klebsiella pneumoniae*, *Enterococcus*, and *Clostridium* sp. have also been implicated (230).

Gross Findings. Phlegmonous gastritis can involve any part of the stomach or cause pangastritis. Typical features include edema, erythema, and copious fibrinopurulent exudates (231).

Microscopic Findings. Most patients do not undergo endoscopic examination and mucosal biopsy. Resection and autopsy specimens feature fibrinopurulent exudates, mucosal necrosis, and neutrophilic abscesses (fig. 3-64). Bacterial colonies in the tissues and luminal contents are characteristic (218).

Differential Diagnosis. Emphysematous gastritis is a more severe form of suppurative gastritis that features intramural gas pockets. It occurs in the setting of systemic infection with gas-forming bacteria, such as *Clostridium* sp. and *Pseudomonas aeruginosa*, or fungemia due to *Candida* or *Mucor* (233–235). Risk factors include alcohol dependence, diabetes mellitus, immunosuppression, or recent gastrointestinal surgery. Caustic ingestion also predisposes to emphysematous gastritis (233).

Treatment and Prognosis. Early intervention with broad-spectrum antibiotics may be curative, but many patients require surgical resection of necrotic tissue. Mortality ranges from 20 to 50 percent despite these measures (230).

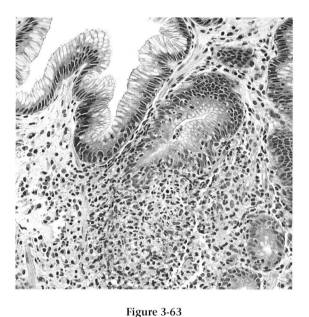

Figure 3-63

PIT RUPTURE-ASSOCIATED INFLAMMATION

Ruptured glands elicit a macrophage-rich inflammatory response when their contents extrude into the lamina propria.

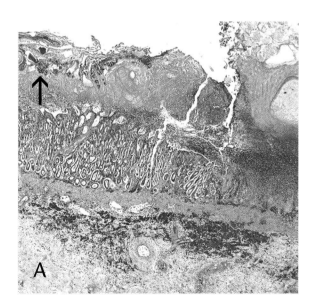
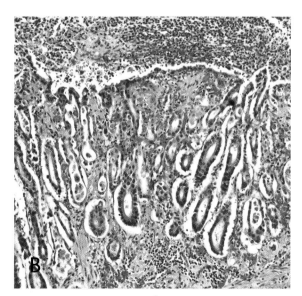

Figure 3-64

PHLEGMONOUS GASTRITIS

Mucosal necrosis and hemorrhage are accompanied by exuberant purulent exudates. Kayexalate crystals (arrow) and other exogenous material (upper right) are present in the ulcer debris (A). Gland destruction is associated with severe mucosal injury and neutrophilic inflammation (B).

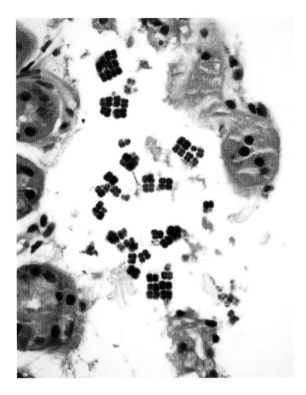

Figure 3-65

SARCINA VENTRICULI

Sarcina ventriculi are cocci arranged in tetrads or multiples of four.

Sarcina Ventriculi and Related Organisms

Definition. *Sarcina ventriculi* are large anaerobic gram-positive cocci arranged in tetrads or multiples of four. They are 1.8 to 3.0 µm in diameter and thrive in an acidic environment.

Clinical Features. The incidence of *Sarcina* sp. infection is difficult to estimate, as data are limited to case reports. Increased awareness has led to more frequent recognition of organisms in gastric samples. *Sarcina* organisms are usually found in gastric biopsies from adults, and more cases have been reported in women than men. Patients often have a history of gastric surgery, delayed gastric emptying, gastric outlet obstruction, ulcers, or gastric adenocarcinoma (236). Patients present with nausea, vomiting, abdominal pain, and melena.

Pathogenesis. The pathogenicity of *Sarcina* organisms is debated. Clinical and imaging studies usually reveal an underlying cause of gastric obstruction, implying that organism de-

tection is a marker of luminal stasis, rather than a pathogen. Its association with rare life-threatening events, including gastric perforation and emphysematous gastritis, raises the possibility that it may be pathogenic in susceptible hosts, although it is likely that such patients are infected with more virulent organisms. *Sarcina* sp. have also been reported in patients who develop complications following bariatric surgery (237).

Gross Findings. The most common endoscopic findings are retained food, bile, and bezoars associated with eroded underlying mucosa.

Microscopic Findings. *Sarcina ventriculi* are round to ovoid organisms that occur in tetrads or multiples of four, reflecting cell division in multiple planes. They have refractile cell walls that resemble vegetable matter (fig. 3-65). They do not invade the mucosa, but are usually found in luminal ulcer debris (238). *Sarcina* organisms are readily visible in hematoxylin and eosin (H&E)-stained sections and are Gram positive with histochemical stains.

Differential Diagnosis. *Micrococcus* organisms are also gram-positive cocci that occur in tetrads, but they are smaller (0.5 µm) than *Sarcina* sp. This environmental bacterium is also a component of normal skin flora, and found in some dairy and meat products. Micrococci are normally commensal organisms, but may produce fatal pneumonia, endocarditis, or meningitis in immunocompromised hosts; gastrointestinal tract infections are not well documented (239).

Treatment and Prognosis. *Sarcina* infection requires no treatment. Therapy is aimed at relieving underlying disorders.

HYPERTROPHIC GASTROPATHIES

Menetrier Disease

Definition. *Menetrier disease* is an acquired hypertrophy of the foveolar compartment of the oxyntic mucosa. It is also termed *hypoproteinemic hypertrophic gastropathy*.

Clinical Features. Menetrier disease can occur in adult and pediatric patients. The adult form shows a predilection for men with a peak incidence in the sixth decade of life (240). Pediatric cases have been reported in combination with cytomegalovirus infection as well as high-dose prostaglandin therapy for congenital heart disease (241,242). Hypertrophic gastritis in pediatric patients generally resolves spontaneously over several weeks, whereas adult disease is a progressive disorder. Clinical symptoms are similar in both populations: patients present with hypoproteinemia, anemia, hypochlorhydria, and peripheral edema; they and are at increased risk for thrombotic events (241). Other symptoms include abdominal pain, nausea, and vomiting.

Pathogenesis. Menetrier disease likely results from localized production of TGF-α, which causes increased epidermal growth factor receptor (EGFR) signaling in the gastric mucosa and abnormal epithelial cell proliferation (243). The etiologic role of cytomegalovirus is unclear, but direct interaction between the virus and EGFR is postulated (244). Decreased parietal cell mass and increased mucus secretion are responsible for the hypochlorhydria, whereas protein-losing enteropathy and peripheral edema result from leakage of proteins across the gastric mucosa.

Gross Findings. Upper endoscopy reveals enlarged rugae in the body and fundus with relative sparing of the antrum. The appearance of the folds has been likened to cerebral convolutions (fig. 3-66). The stomach contains copious, thick mucus (245). Mucosal erosions and ulcers may be present.

Microscopic Findings. The oxyntic mucosa displays foveolar hyperplasia with decreased oxyntic glands (fig. 3-67A). Foveolae are tortuous, with a corkscrew appearance, and often cystic. Their lining cells contain abundant mucin. Inflammation is not prominent, but enlarged rugae are subject to luminal trauma and frequently display superficial erosions and granulation tissue (fig. 3-67B). The muscularis mucosae is thickened and disorganized, reflecting prolapse of hypertrophic mucosal folds (241).

Differential Diagnosis. Superficial samples from Menetrier disease may be indistinguishable from hyperplastic polyps that show expansion of the foveolar compartment and erosions (fig. 3-68). Juvenile polyposis syndrome can also simulate Menetrier disease when it involves the stomach (fig. 3-69). Gastric juvenile polyps contain cystically dilated, tortuous foveolae and affect the antrum, which is mostly spared in cases of Menetrier disease (fig. 3-70). Absence of SMAD4 immunostaining in juvenile polyps helps in their distinction from Menetrier disease (246).

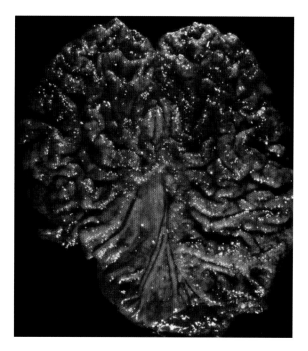

Figure 3-66

MENETRIER DISEASE

Hypertrophic rugal folds are most prominent in the proximal stomach. Several folds are hyperemic or show superficial erosions.

Treatment and Prognosis. There are few effective therapeutic options for patients with Menetrier disease. Partial or total gastrectomy may be necessary for those with intractable symptoms (241). Cetuximab, a monoclonal antibody that blocks ligand binding to EGFR, is effective in some patients (247). Individuals with Menetrier disease are at increased risk for gastric dysplasia and adenocarcinoma (241).

Zollinger-Ellison Syndrome

Definition. *Zollinger-Ellison syndrome* is gastric mucosal hypertrophy caused by autonomous gastrin secretion.

Clinical Features. Zollinger-Ellison syndrome has an estimated annual incidence of 0.2 to 0.4 cases per million. It shows a predilection for middle-aged adults and a slight male predominance. Patients present with signs and symptoms of hyperchlorhydria: heartburn, peptic ulcers, diarrhea, weight loss, and abdominal pain. They often have serum gastrin levels up to 10 times the upper limit of normal (248).

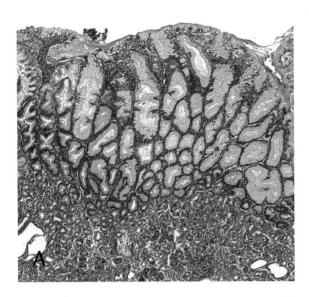 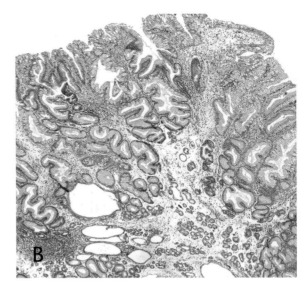

Figure 3-67

MENETRIER DISEASE

The foveolar compartment of the oxyntic mucosa is expanded and comprises more than half of the mucosal thickness. The pits are hypermucinous and convoluted (A). Advanced disease displays markedly decreased oxyntic gland mass with foveolar hyperplasia and edema (B).

Figure 3-68

HYPERPLASTIC POLYP

This hyperplastic polyp displays tortuous gastric pits with few glands in the deep mucosa. Its discrete nature and location in the antrum facilitate a diagnosis.

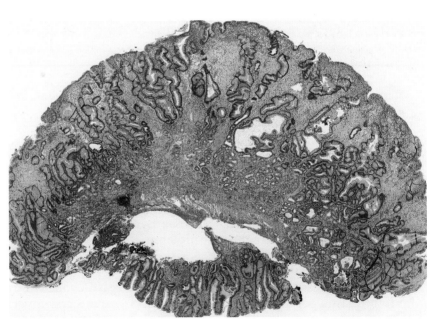

Zollinger-Ellison syndrome usually results from gastrin-producing endocrine tumors that develop sporadically or in the setting of multiple endocrine neoplasia type 1 (MEN1) syndrome. The latter is an autosomal dominant syndrome due to germline *MEN1* mutations on chromosome 11q13, and features parathyroid tumors, pituitary adenomas, and pancreatic endocrine tumors. Most gastrinomas are located in the duodenum (60 percent) or pancreas (30 to 40 percent); they rarely develop in other abdominal sites (249). Imaging modalities that use gallium-labeled somatostatin radiotracers and positron emission tomography provide the best results, although endoscopic ultrasound also detects small pancreatic lesions (250,251).

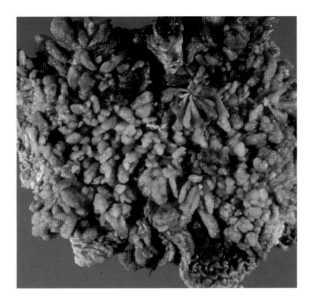

Figure 3-69

JUVENILE POLYPOSIS

Innumerable large polyps carpet the gastric mucosa, simulating a hypertrophic gastropathy. However, the disorder does not spare the antrum, as would be expected of Menetrier disease.

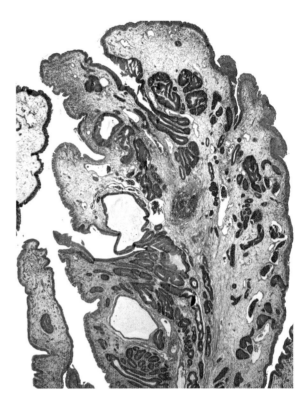

Figure 3-70

JUVENILE POLYPOSIS

Similar to Menetrier disease, juvenile polyps display hyperplastic foveolae and marked lamina propria edema.

Rarely, hypergastrinemia results from primary G-cell hyperplasia (252).

Pathogenesis. Gastrin-producing tumors do not respond to normal feedback inhibition mechanisms that regulate gastric acidity. Persistent hypergastrinemia stimulates parietal cells to proliferate, leading to hyperchlorhydria and expansion of oxyntic gland mass (253). Gastrin also has a trophic effect on ECL cells in the gastric body and fundus, resulting in linear and nodular ECL-cell hyperplasia as well as type II endocrine tumors (248,254).

Gross Findings. Most patients have enlarged, nodular gastric folds associated with erosions and ulcers of the stomach and duodenum (fig. 3-71). Acid-induced strictures in the pyloric channel can cause gastric outlet obstruction and may also be present in the esophagus (255). Gastrin-producing endocrine tumors are usually small; they appear as brown nodules in the duodenum or pancreas.

Microscopic Findings. Gastrin-producing tumors are composed of nests and cords of well-differentiated endocrine cells (fig. 3-72A). Gastrin is a trophic hormone for both parietal cells and ECL cells, so the net effect of marked hypergastrinemia

is expansion of oxyntic gland mass occupying up to 90 percent of the mucosal thickness in combination with nodular ECL-cell hyperplasia (fig. 3-72B,C). Patients with hypergastrinemia due to diffuse G-cell hyperplasia have markedly increased G cells in the antrum (fig. 3-72D).

Differential Diagnosis. Mènètrier disease may simulate the gross appearance of Zollinger-Ellison syndrome, but features expansion of the foveolar compartment and diminished oxyntic gland mass. Hypergastrinemia and tumors composed of ECL cells are encountered in patients with both autoimmune gastritis and Zollinger-Ellison syndrome, although gastrin levels tend to be much higher in the latter situation. Autoimmune gastritis also features ECL cell nodules accompanied by mucosal atrophy. Type II endocrine tumors develop on a background of oxyntic gland hyperplasia in patients with Zollinger-Ellison syndrome.

Treatment and Prognosis. High-dose proton pump inhibitor therapy controls acid-related

149

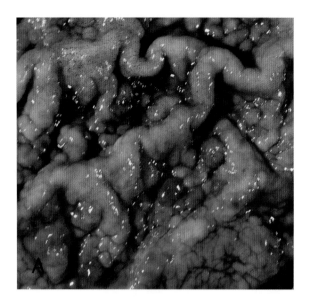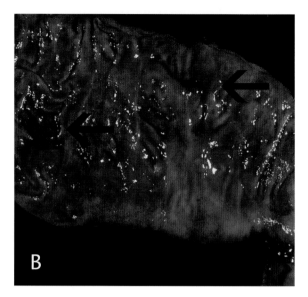

Figure 3-71

ZOLLINGER-ELLISON SYNDROME

The rugal folds are thickened and diffusely nodular (A). Multiple duodenal ulcers (arrows) are present in the same patient (B).

symptoms in some patients, although this treatment may mask detection of diffuse G-cell hyperplasia and result in a delayed diagnosis (248). Complete surgical resection is associated with a greater than 80 percent 15-year survival rate in patients with gastrinomas (256). Outcomes are worse for patients with stage IV disease, who account for nearly 25 percent of patients; survival is approximately 30 percent at 10 years in this patient group (257).

Unlike type I endocrine tumors associated with autoimmune gastritis, type II endocrine tumors due to Zollinger-Ellison syndrome metastasize in 10 to 30 percent of patients, presumably because the trophic effects of gastrin drive proliferation of endocrine cells in patients who often have germline mutations related to MEN syndrome. Metastatic ECL-cell tumors are still associated with a indolent course, with 5-year survival rates ranging from 60 to 90 percent (258). Type II endocrine tumors may regress with somatostatin analogue therapy (248).

GASTRIC POLYPS

Xanthoma

Definition. *Xanthomas* are aggregates of lipid-containing macrophages in the mucosa. Synonyms include *xanthelasma* and *xanthogranuloma*.

Clinical Features. Xanthomas account for less than 1 percent of gastric polyps sampled at endoscopy, and are more commonly detected in elderly women (259). They are asymptomatic. They have been reported in patients with *H. pylori* infection, autoimmune gastritis, and gastric adenocarcinoma. Most are isolated findings.

Pathogenesis. Xanthomas result from the accumulation of lipid-containing macrophages at sites of prior injury. They are not associated with underlying hyperlipidemia or disorders of lipid metabolism (260).

Gross Findings. Xanthomas appear as single or multiple yellow-white plaques or nodules (fig. 3-73). Most are small, spanning 2 to 5 mm (259). They are usually found in the body and fundus.

Microscopic Findings. Ill-defined aggregates of macrophages expand the superficial mucosa (fig. 3-74A). They contain foamy cytoplasm and small nuclei indented by lipid vacuoles (fig. 3-74B). Intervening gastric epithelium may be normal or show features of a hyperplastic/regenerative polyp. The background mucosa is often inflamed.

Histochemical stains for fat, such as oil red O, highlight intracytoplasmic lipid, but require fresh or unprocessed, formalin-fixed tissue. They are seldom used to establish a diagnosis of xanthoma. Immunostains for macrophages,

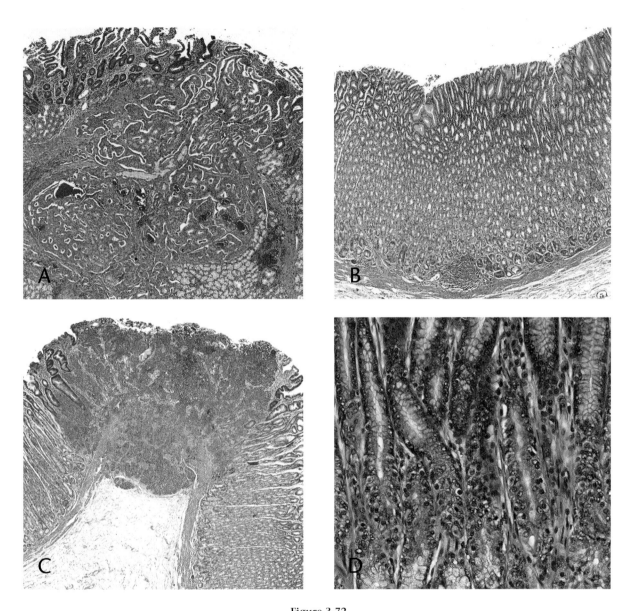

Figure 3-72

ZOLLINGER-ELLISON SYNDROME

A gastrin-producing endocrine tumor of the duodenum displays trabecular and pseudoglandular architecture (A). The same tumor was associated with marked expansion of oxyntic gland mass (B) as well as nodular ECL-cell hyperplasia (C). Rare patients develop hypergastrinemia as a result of diffuse G-cell hyperplasia in the deep glands of the antrum (D).

such as CD68, can facilitate the distinction of xanthoma cells from signet ring cell carcinoma in challenging cases.

Differential Diagnosis. Foamy macrophages superficially resemble signet ring cells, but lack cytologic atypia or mitotic activity. Signet ring cell carcinomas stain for cytokeratins by immunohistochemistry and contain mucin that can be detected with histochemical stains.

Whipple disease, *Mycobacterium avium intracellulare* infection, and histoplasmosis feature macrophage-rich inflammatory cell infiltrates. They show a predilection for the small and large intestine and are discussed in chapter 4.

Crystal-storing histiocytosis is characterized by prominent collections of macrophages that contain abundant eosinophilic cytoplasm and fibrillary cytoplasmic inclusions (fig. 3-75).

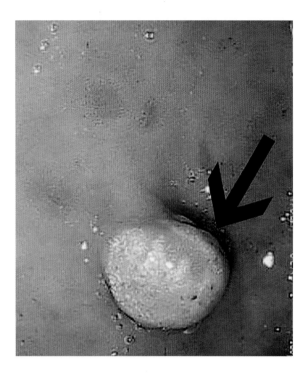

Figure 3-73

GASTRIC XANTHOMA

Most xanthomas are smooth, yellow polyps in the body and fundus (arrow).

This finding is most common in patients with B-cell lymphoproliferative disorders, particularly kappa-restricted plasma cell neoplasms. The inclusions consist of intralysosomal accumulations of monoclonal immunoglobulin light chains (261).

Fundic Gland Polyp

Definition. *Fundic gland polyp* is a polyp composed of dilated oxyntic glands.

Clinical Features. Fundic gland polyps account for 47 percent of all gastric polyps (262). They are detected in approximately 2 percent of patients undergoing upper endoscopic examination (263). Most are sporadic in nature, occur in the fifth to sixth decades, and show a slight female predominance. Fundic gland polyps are detected in nearly 7 percent of patients receiving proton pump inhibitor therapy, but they also develop in patients who do not take these agents. They are less common in patients with *H. pylori*-associated gastritis (264,265). Patients with familial adenomatous polyposis (FAP) develop multiple fundic gland polyps in over 90 percent of cases, as do those with gastric adenocarcinoma and proximal polyposis syndrome (GAPPS)

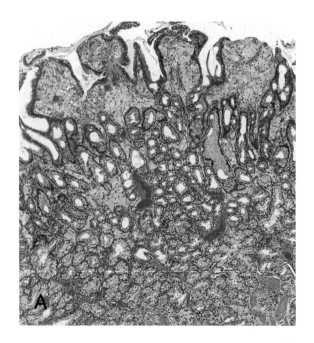
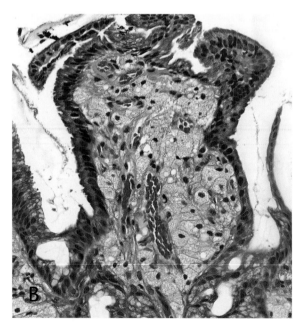

Figure 3-74

GASTRIC XANTHOMA

Foamy macrophages expand the lamina propria (A). They contain tiny cytoplasmic vacuoles and uniform, centrally located nuclei (B).

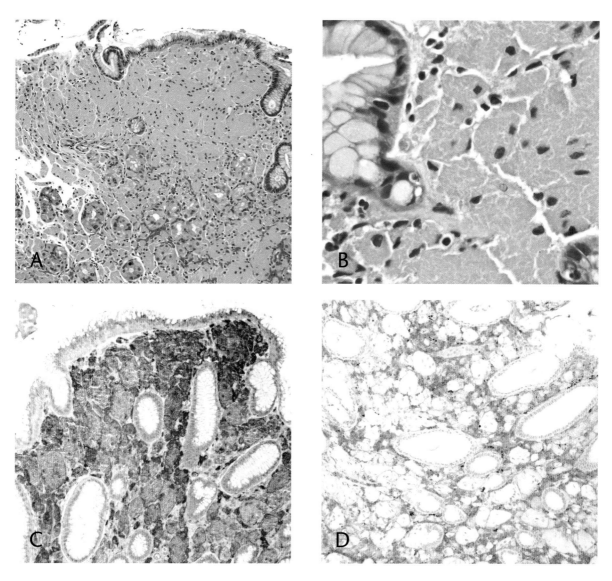

Figure 3-75

CRYSTAL STORING HISTIOCYTOSIS

Collections of macrophages expand the lamina propria and form a polypoid gastric mass (A). They contain linear aggregates of eosinophilic material (B). Macrophages show strong CD68 positivity (C) and their contents are kappa-positive (D) and lambda-negative (not shown).

(266,267). Syndromic polyps affect both sexes equally and manifest in young adulthood (266).

Pathogenesis. Although prior reports described a causal role for proton pump inhibitor therapy in the development of fundic gland polyps, most data do not support this hypothesis and suggest that fundic gland polyps are neoplasms that result from Wnt signaling abnormalities (266). Sporadic fundic gland polyps harbor activating mutations in *CTNNB1*, which

encodes β-catenin (268, 269). Less than 1 percent of these polyps develop low-grade dysplasia but they do not progress to high-grade dysplasia or carcinoma (266). Patients with familial adenomatous polyposis, gastric adenocarcinoma, and GAPPS have germline inactivating mutations in one *APC* allele and develop somatic mutations in the second allele of their fundic gland polyps (270,271). Low-grade dysplasia develops at a higher rate (25 to 60 percent) in

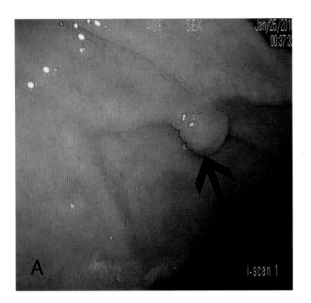
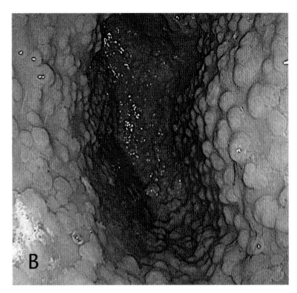

Figure 3-76

FUNDIC GLAND POLYPS

A small sporadic fundic gland polyp (arrow) has a smooth surface that is similar to that of the background mucosa (A). Fundic gland polyps carpet the proximal stomach of a patient with familial adenomatous polyposis (B).

polyps from these patients, but rarely progresses to high-grade dysplasia (272). Most gastric adenocarcinomas that develop in patients with polyposis disorders likely arise from adenomas.

Gross Findings. Sporadic fundic gland polyps are single or multiple and appear as dome-shaped sessile polyps in the body and fundus (fig. 3-76A). Patients with polyposis disorders often have innumerable polyps that carpet the mucosa (fig. 3-76B).

Microscopic Findings. Fundic gland polyps contain cystically dilated oxyntic glands lined by attenuated chief, parietal, and mucin-containing cells (fig. 3-77). Parietal cells may be hypertrophic and project into the lumen with a "snouted" or "hobnail" appearance. The overlying foveolar epithelium and background mucosa are generally normal. When present, dysplasia occurs in the foveolar and mucous neck cells and features low-grade cytologic abnormalities with crowded, slightly hyperchromatic nuclei (fig. 3-78).

Patients with polyposis disorders may have other types of polyps, including gastric foveolar adenomas and pyloric gland adenomas (273). Gastric adenomas, flat dysplasia, and proliferating oxyntic glands within attenuated foveolae ("hyperproliferative aberrant pits") may be seen

in patients with gastric adenocarcinoma and proximal polyposis syndrome (267).

Differential Diagnosis. Oxyntic glands occasionally dilate and show parietal cell hypertrophy, a change that has been termed "proton pump inhibitor effect" (fig. 3-79), but also occurs in other types of gastric injury, such as *H. pylori*-associated gastritis (264). Zollinger-Ellison syndrome features expanded and cystically dilated oxyntic glands, but causes diffuse hypertrophy of the rugae rather than discrete polyps.

Treatment and Prognosis. Sporadic fundic gland polyps do not have malignant potential and can be managed conservatively, even in the presence of low-grade dysplasia (274). Those that develop in patients who take acid suppressive agents may regress upon cessation of therapy (275). Patients with familial adenomatous polyposis undergo regular surveillance of the upper gastrointestinal tract due to the risk of carcinoma development in gastric and duodenal adenomas; large polyps are removed during those procedures, but prophylactic gastrectomy is not indicated for patients who have fundic gland polyps with dysplasia (276). On the other hand, patients with gastric adenocarcinoma and proximal polyposis syndrome have a much higher cancer risk and are generally treated with prophylactic gastrectomy (277).

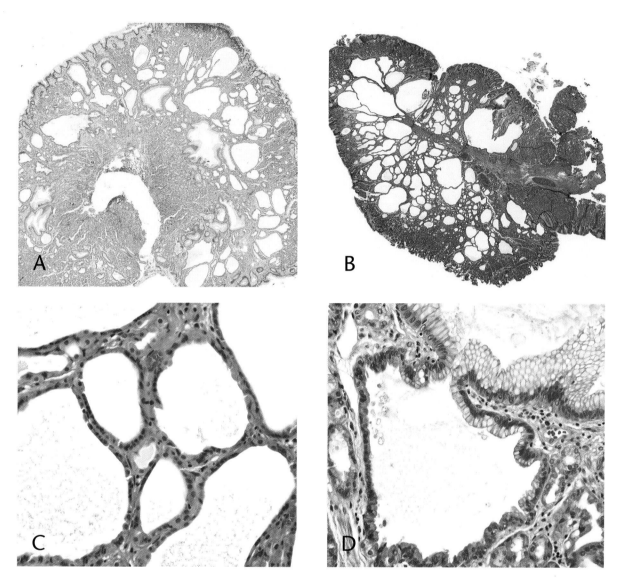

Figure 3-77

FUNDIC GLAND POLYPS

A fundic gland polyp consists of cystically dilated oxyntic and foveolar glands within uninflamed mucosa (A). Large lesions may contain slender groups of smooth muscle cells. Most of the dilated glands are located in the deep mucosa with superficial sparing (B). Lesional glands are lined by attenuated chief and parietal cells (C). Some glands are partially lined by foveolar epithelium (D).

Hyperplastic Polyp

Definition. *Hyperplastic polyp* is a regenerative polyp of the gastric mucosa. Synonyms include *regenerative polyp* and *polypoid foveolar hyperplasia*.

Clinical Features. Hyperplastic polyps account for 14 percent of gastric polyps and tend to occur in older adults with a slight female predilection (275). Most lesions develop in patients with chronic gastritis, although they are also seen in association with chemical gastropathy, peptic ulcers, gastrostomies, and anastomotic sites (278). Hyperplastic polyps are typically asymptomatic. Large lesions that bleed can cause iron deficiency anemia.

Pathogenesis. Most hyperplastic polyps represent an exuberant regenerative response to mucosal injury. Approximately 2 percent of hyperplastic polyps, particularly large lesions,

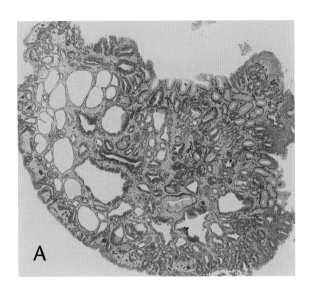
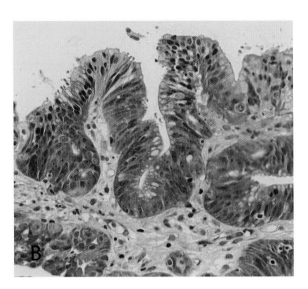

Figure 3-78

FUNDIC GLAND POLYP WITH DYSPLASIA

Multiple foci of crowded glands show nuclear hyperchromasia in the foveolar epithelium (A). The focus of dysplasia is sharply demarcated from reactive foveolar epithelium (B).

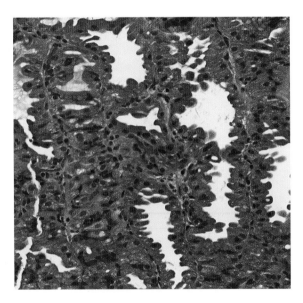

Figure 3-79

PARIETAL CELL HYPERTROPHY

Dilated oxyntic glands are lined by hypertrophic parietal cells with a "snouted" or "hobnail" appearance. Extruded cytoplasmic granules are present in the lumen.

develop foci of dysplasia that may harbor *TP53* alterations, chromosomal aberrations, and microsatellite instability (279,280).

Gross Findings. Hyperplastic polyps show a predilection for the antrum, reflecting the anatomic distributions of chronic gastritis and chemical gastropathy. They appear as single, or multiple, dome-shaped protuberances that are red or slightly yellow, reflecting inflammation and macrophage accumulation, respectively (fig. 3-80). Large (greater than 2 cm) polyps are usually pedunculated and may have a lobulated appearance (275). The background mucosa is often erythematous.

Microscopic Findings. Hyperplastic polyps contain elongated, tortuous, and cystically dilated pits lined by foveolar epithelium. Epithelial cells may show mucin depletion or distention by large mucin vacuoles. Epithelial elements are supported by edematous lamina propria contain variable inflammation and congested capillaries (fig. 3-81). Eroded polyps are partially surfaced by inflamed granulation tissue. Some hyperplastic polyps contain prominent bundles of smooth muscle cells as well as pyloric or oxyntic glands; these features have prompted some authors to term them "mucosal prolapse polyps" (fig. 3-82) (278).

Differential Diagnosis. Regenerative atypia in hyperplastic polyps may simulate the features of dysplasia, although the former generally shows a gradual transition between atypical foci and areas that are clearly reparative in nature (fig. 3-83). Hamartomatous gastric polyps that feature prominent foveolar epithelial components may

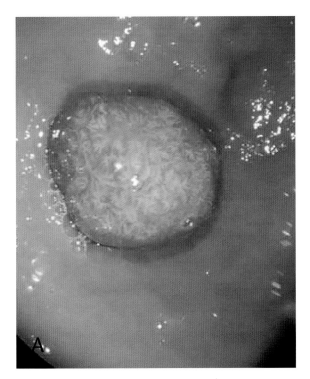 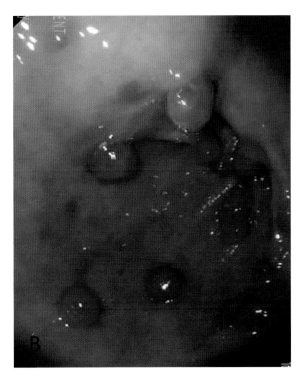

Figure 3-80

HYPERPLASTIC POLYPS

A large hyperplastic polyp is sessile and has prominent vasculature (A). Multiple broad-based erythematous nodules are present on a background of atrophic gastritis (B).

simulate hyperplastic polyps, particularly in superficial samples. Juvenile polyps contain cystically dilated, non-dysplastic glands supported by inflamed, edematous stroma. Peutz-Jeghers polyps contain hyperplastic foveolar epithelium associated with smooth muscle cells, although the latter may not be as prominent in gastric polyps as it is in lesions of the intestines.

Treatment and Prognosis. Hyperplastic polyps that develop in association with *H. pylori*-associated chronic gastritis often regress upon eradication of infection. Although most hyperplastic polyps require no specific therapy, large (greater than 2 cm) or bleeding polyps may be endoscopically resected (275).

NON-NEOPLASTIC MIMICS OF DIFFUSE-TYPE GASTRIC CARCINOMA

Signet Ring Cell Change (Pseudosignet Ring Cells)

Mucosal biopsy samples are prone to fragmentation and artifactual distortion. Injured glands throughout the gastrointestinal tract may degenerate and slough mucin-filled epithelial cells into the lumen, and signet ring-type cells can be seen in the lamina propria surrounding disrupted glands. This finding, termed *signet ring cell change* simulates the appearance of invasive carcinoma.

Signet ring cell change is likely a degenerative phenomenon and has been described in association with various types of injury, including chemical gastropathy, gastritis, ulcers, and various types of ischemic injury, including pseudomembranous colitis. Most commonly, cases of severe chemical gastropathy feature an abnormal population of mucin-containing cells arranged in nests or clusters in the lamina propria (fig. 3-84). Infarcted polyps may contain aggregates of signet ring cells embedded in hemorrhagic lamina propria, reflecting residual mucinous cells from the pit and neck regions that are no longer supported by the basement membrane (fig. 3-85) (281). Striking cytoplasmic vacuolization of oxyntic glands can also occur

157

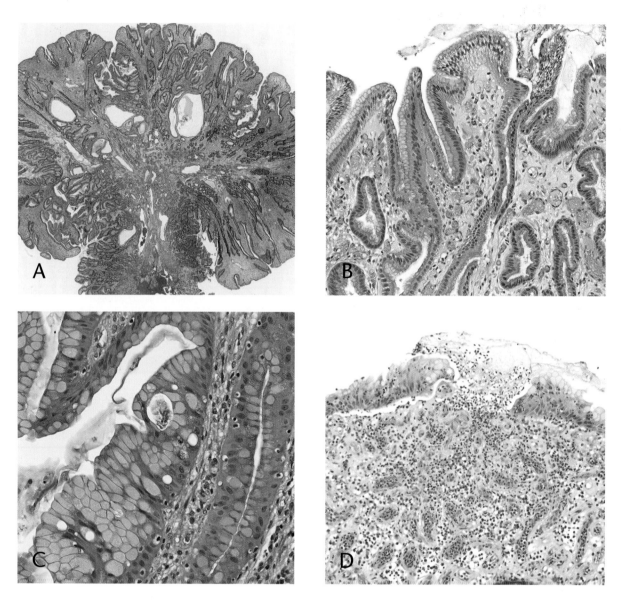

Figure 3-81

HYPERPLASTIC POLYPS

Hyperplastic polyps contain regenerative-appearing mucinous glands supported by edematous lamina propria (A). The surface epithelium is often mucin-depleted and lamina propria capillaries are congested (B). Some foveolar cells are distended by abundant cytoplasmic mucin (C). A large hyperplastic polyp shows surface erosion with inflamed granulation tissue and reactive atypia in the epithelium (D).

in patients receiving proton pump inhibitor therapy (fig. 3-86). This finding can simulate the appearance of signet ring cell carcinoma or signet ring cell carcinoma *in situ* (282).

Helpful clues to a benign diagnosis include an absence of nuclear atypia and mitotic activity in the atypical cell population, as well as confinement of the lesional cells to detached epithelium unsupported by lamina propria. Although detached fragments of malignant epithelium are common in biopsy samples from gland-forming adenocarcinomas, signet ring cell carcinomas always infiltrate the lamina propria or deeper tissues. Thus, care should be taken when considering a malignant diagnosis based solely on the presence of poorly cohesive cells in the lumen.

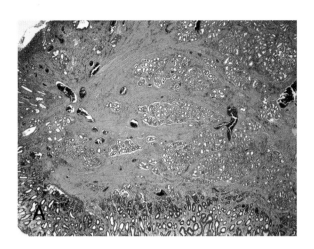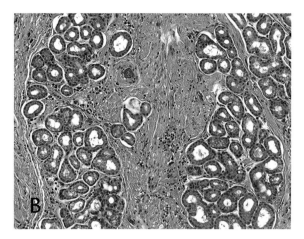

Figure 3-82

HYPERPLASTIC POLYP

Bundles of smooth muscle cells extend toward the surface of a hyperplastic polyp (A) and entrap pyloric glands (B).

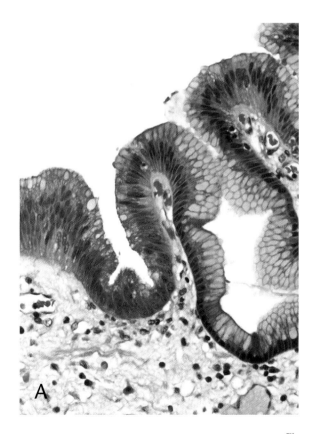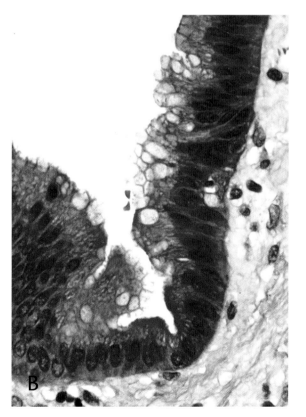

Figure 3-83

HYPERPLASTIC POLYP

An inflamed hyperplastic polyp shows a gradual transition between clearly non-neoplastic epithelium and areas of mild cytologic atypia (A) that show nuclear enlargement and hyperchromasia (B).

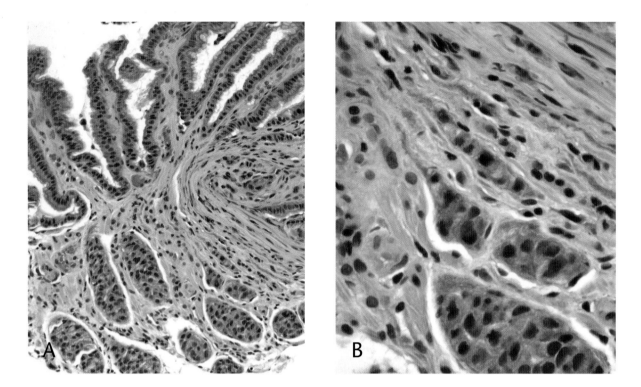

Figure 3-84

CHEMICAL GASTROPATHY WITH ARTIFACTS THAT SIMULATE A NEOPLASM

Chemical gastropathy features mucin depleted surface epithelium and lamina propria fibrosis. Aggregates of mucinous epithelial cells have a seemingly nested architecture that may simulate adenocarcinoma or an endocrine neoplasm (A). Closer examination of the same area reveals a lack of substantial atypia and mitotic activity (B).

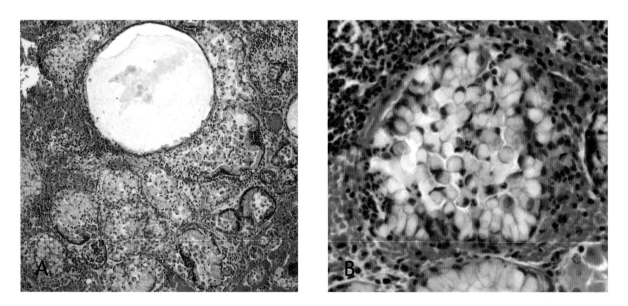

Figure 3-85

INFARCTED POLYP WITH PSEUDOSIGNET RING CELLS

Sloughed epithelial cells in a background of hemorrhagic necrosis simulate signet ring cells (A). Their lobular arrangement is not typical of signet ring cell carcinoma and suggests a benign process (B).

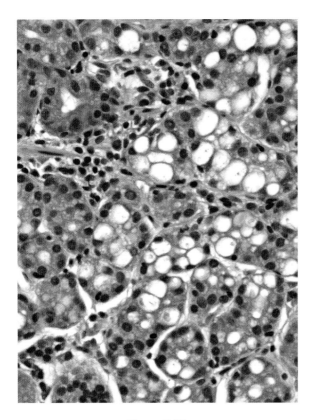

Figure 3-86

PROTON PUMP INHIBITOR EFFECT SIMULATING SIGNET RING CELLS

Cytoplasmic vacuolization of oxyntic glands may be prominent in samples from patients taking proton pump inhibitors. The vacuoles do not contain mucin. This growth pattern is not typical of signet ring cell carcinoma or signet ring cell carcinoma *in situ*.

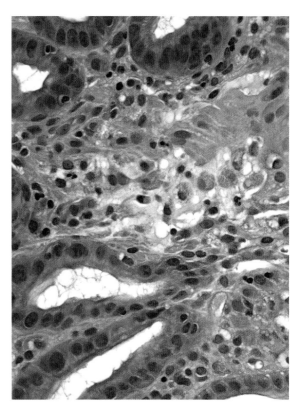

Figure 3-87

MACROPHAGES SIMULATING SIGNET RING CELLS

Lamina propria macrophages in areas of gland destruction simulate signet ring cell carcinoma. They are typically associated with disrupted glands or pits and extruded mucin, which would not be expected in examples of carcinoma.

Immunostains and histochemical stains are of limited value in the distinction between signet ring cell carcinoma and benign epithelial cell mimics. Degenerated or sloughed epithelial cells contain mucin and express keratins, similar to carcinomas. However, degenerated and detached benign epithelial cells show strong membranous staining for E-cadherin and lack p53 staining, whereas many signet ring cell carcinomas show decreased or absent E-cadherin staining and some show increased nuclear p53 positivity (283). Reticulin stains can also be helpful when they demonstrate confinement of atypical cells to glands (284).

Macrophages

Macrophages are frequently present in association with gastritis, gastric erosions, and inflammatory polyps. They are usually readily distinguished from diffuse-type gastric carcinoma but may pose diagnostic challenges when they contain abundant cytoplasmic mucin as a result of mucosal injury (fig. 3-87). Features that support a benign diagnosis include close proximity of the atypical cells to injured or disrupted glands, atypical cells present in extruded mucin, and an isolated finding affecting only rare glands in a background of mucosal injury. Immunohistochemical stains are extremely helpful; macrophages are negative for cytokeratins and show strong diffuse staining for CD68.

REFERENCES

1. Ilce Z, Erdogan E, Kara C, et al. Pyloric atresia: 15-year review from a single institution. J Pediatr Surg 2003;38:1581-4.
2. Agarwala S, Goswami JK, Mitra DK. Pyloric atresia associated with epidermolysis bullosa, malrotation, and high anorectal malformation with recto-urethral fistula: a report of successful management. Pediatr Surg Int 1999;15:264-5.
3. Parelkar SV, Kapadnis SP, Sanghvi BV, et al. Pyloric atresia—three cases and review of literature. Afr J Paediatr Surg 2014;11:362-5.
4. El-Gohary Y, Abdelhafeez A, Paton E, Gosain A, Murphy AJ. Pyloric stenosis: an enigma more than a century after the first successful treatment. Pediatr Surg Int 2018;34:21-7.
5. Lisonkova S, Joseph KS. Similarities and differences in the epidemiology of pyloric stenosis and sids. Matern Child Health J 2014;18:1721-7.
6. Cooper WO, Ray WA, Griffin MR. Prenatal prescription of macrolide antibiotics and infantile hypertrophic pyloric stenosis. Obstet Gynecol 2002;100:101-6.
7. Sorensen HT, Norgard B, Pedersen L, Larsen H, Johnsen SP. Maternal smoking and risk of hypertrophic infantile pyloric stenosis: 10 year population based cohort study. BMJ 2002;325:1011-2.
8. Lodha AK, Satodia P, Whyte H. Fetal alcohol syndrome and pyloric stenosis: alcohol induced or an association? J Perinat Med 2005;33:262-3.
9. Peeters B, Benninga MA, Hennekam RC. Infantile hypertrophic pyloric stenosis—genetics and syndromes. Nat Rev Gastroenterol Hepatol 2012;9:646-60.
10. Werner H, Koch Y, Fridkin M, Fahrenkrug J, Gozes I. High levels of vasoactive intestinal peptide in human milk. Biochem Biophys Res Commun 1985;133:228-32.
11. Smith GA, Mihalov L, Shields BJ. Diagnostic aids in the differentiation of pyloric stenosis from severe gastroesophageal reflux during early infancy: the utility of serum bicarbonate and serum chloride. Am J Emerg Med 1999;17:28-31.
12. Taylor ND, Cass DT, Holland AJ. Infantile hypertrophic pyloric stenosis: has anything changed? J Paediatr Child Health 2013;49:33-7.
13. Mullassery D, Mallappa S, Shariff R, et al. Negative exploration for pyloric stenosis—is it preventable? BMC Pediatr 2008;8:37.
14. Forster N, Haddad RL, Choroomi S, Dilley AV, Pereira J. Use of ultrasound in 187 infants with suspected infantile hypertrophic pyloric stenosis. Australas Radiol 2007;51:560-3.
15. Lin HP, Lin YC, Kuo CY. Adult idiopathic hypertrophic pyloric stenosis. J Formos Med Assoc 2015;114:659-62.
16. Lucas A, Sarson DL, Blackburn AM, Adrian TE, Aynsley-Green A, Bloom SR. Breast vs bottle: endocrine responses are different with formula feeding. Lancet 1980;1:1267-9.
17. Ikenaga T, Honmyo U, Takano S, et al. Primary hypertrophic pyloric stenosis in the adult. J Gastroenterol Hepatol 1992;7:524-6.
18. Schuster MM, Smith VM. The pyloric "cervix sign" in adult hypertrophic pyloric stenosis. Gastrointest Endosc 1970;16:210-1.
19. Bateson EM, Talerman A, Walrond ER. Radiological and pathological observations in a series of seventeen cases of hypertrophic pyloric stenosis of adults. Br J Radiol 1969;42:1-8.
20. Sun WM, Doran SM, Jones KL, Davidson G, Dent J, Horowitz M. Long-term effects of pyloromyotomy on pyloric motility and gastric emptying in humans. Am J Gastroenterol 2000;95:92-100.
21. Peters B, Oomen MW, Bakx R, Benninga MA. Advances in infantile hypertrophic pyloric stenosis. Expert Rev Gastroenterol Hepatol 2014;8:533-41.
22. Kuwada SK, Alexander GL. Long-term outcome of endoscopic dilation of nonmalignant pyloric stenosis. Gastrointest Endosc 1995;41:15-7.
23. Blinder G, Hiller N, Adler SN. A double stomach in an adult. Am J Gastroenterol 1999;94:1100-2.
24. D'Journo XB, Moutardier V, Turrini O, et al. Gastric duplication in an adult mimicking mucinous cystadenoma of the pancreas. J Clin Pathol 2004;57:1215-8.
25. Singh JP, Rajdeo H, Bhuta K, Savino JA. Gastric duplication cyst: two case reports and review of the literature. Case Rep Surg 2013;2013:605059.
26. Johnston J, Wheatley GH 3rd, El Sayed HF, Marsh WB, Ellison EC, Bloomston M. Gastric duplication cysts expressing carcinoembryonic antigen mimicking cystic pancreatic neoplasms in two adults. Am Surg 2008;74:91-4.
27. Mardi K, Kaushal V, Gupta S. Foregut duplication cysts of stomach masquerading as leiomyoma. Indian J Pathol Microbiol 2010;53:160-1.
28. Kim DH, Kim JS, Nam ES, Shin HS. Foregut duplication cyst of the stomach. Pathol Int 2000;50:142-5.
29. Donkervoort SC, Baak LC, Blaauwgeers JL, Gerhards MF. Laparoscopic resection of a symptomatic gastric diverticulum: a minimally invasive solution. JSLS 2006;10:525-7.

30. Horne G, Ming-Lum C, Kirkpatrick AW, Parker RL. High-grade neuroendocrine carcinoma arising in a gastric duplication cyst: a case report with literature review. Int J Surg Pathol 2007;15:187-91.

31. Kuraoka K, Nakayama H, Kagawa T, Ichikawa T, Yasui W. Adenocarcinoma arising from a gastric duplication cyst with invasion to the stomach: a case report with literature review. J Clin Pathol 2004;57:428-31.

32. Rashid F, Aber A, Iftikhar SY. A review on gastric diverticulum. World J Emerg Surg 2012;7:1.

33. Marianne C, Ur Rehman M, Min Hoe C. A case report of large gastric diverticulum with literature review. Int J Surg Case Rep 2018;44:82-4.

34. Schneider NI, Plieschnegger W, Geppert M, et al. Pancreatic acinar cells—a normal finding at the gastroesophageal junction? Data from a prospective central European multicenter study. Virchows Arch 2013;463:643-50.

35. Johansson J, Hakansson HO, Mellblom L, et al. Prevalence of precancerous and other metaplasia in the distal oesophagus and gastro-oesophageal junction. Scand J Gastroenterol 2005;40:893-902.

36. Johansson J, Hakansson HO, Mellblom L, et al. Pancreatic acinar metaplasia in the distal oesophagus and the gastric cardia: prevalence, predictors and relation to gord. J Gastroenterol 2010;45:291-9.

37. Wang HH, Zeroogian JM, Spechler SJ, Goyal RK, Antonioli DA. Prevalence and significance of pancreatic acinar metaplasia at the gastroesophageal junction. Am J Surg Pathol 1996;20:1507-10.

38. Jhala NC, Montemor M, Jhala D, et al. Pancreatic acinar cell metaplasia in autoimmune gastritis. Arch Pathol Lab Med 2003;127:854-7.

39. Krishnamurthy S, Dayal Y. Pancreatic metaplasia in Barrett's esophagus. An immunohistochemical study. Am J Surg Pathol 1995;19:1172-80.

40. Yuan Z, Chen J, Zheng Q, Huang XY, Yang Z, Tang J. Heterotopic pancreas in the gastrointestinal tract. World J Gastroenterol 2009;15:3701-3.

41. Jun SY, Son D, Kim MJ, et al. Heterotopic pancreas of the gastrointestinal tract and associated precursor and cancerous lesions: systematic pathologic studies of 165 cases. Am J Surg Pathol 2017;41:833-48.

42. Frantzides CT, Carlson MA, Zografakis JG, Moore RE, Zeni T, Madan AK. Postoperative gastrointestinal complaints after laparoscopic nissen fundoplication. JSLS 2006;10:39-42.

43. Bityutskiy LP, Soykan I, McCallum RW. Viral gastroparesis: a subgroup of idiopathic gastroparesis—clinical characteristics and long-term outcomes. Am J Gastroenterol 1997;92:1501-4.

44. Jung HK, Choung RS, Locke GR 3rd, et al. The incidence, prevalence, and outcomes of patients with gastroparesis in Olmsted county, Minnesota, from 1996 to 2006. Gastroenterology 2009;136:1225-33.

45. Hyett B, Martinez FJ, Gill BM, et al. Delayed radionucleotide gastric emptying studies predict morbidity in diabetics with symptoms of gastroparesis. Gastroenterology 2009;137:445-52.

46. Choung RS, Locke GR 3rd, Schleck CD, Zinsmeister AR, Melton LJ 3rd, Talley NJ. Risk of gastroparesis in subjects with type 1 and 2 diabetes in the general population. Am J Gastroenterol 2012;107:82-8.

47. Liu N, Abell T. Gastroparesis updates on pathogenesis and management. Gut Liver 2017;11:579-89.

48. Camilleri M, Parkman HP, Shafi MA, Abell TL, Gerson L, American College of G. Clinical guideline: management of gastroparesis. Am J Gastroenterol 2013;108:18-37.

49. Abell TL, Camilleri M, Donohoe K, et al. Consensus recommendations for gastric emptying scintigraphy: a joint report of the American neurogastroenterology and motility society and the society of nuclear medicine. J Nucl Med Technol 2008;36:44-54.

50. Bashashati M, McCallum RW. Motility: is 'icc-opathy' present in gastroparesis-like syndrome? Nat Rev Gastroenterol Hepatol 2015;12:375-6.

51. Angeli TR, Cheng LK, Du P, et al. Loss of interstitial cells of cajal and patterns of gastric dysrhythmia in patients with chronic unexplained nausea and vomiting. Gastroenterology 2015;149:56-66.

52. Zarate N, Mearin F, Wang XY, Hewlett B, Huizinga JD, Malagelada JR. Severe idiopathic gastroparesis due to neuronal and interstitial cells of cajal degeneration: pathological findings and management. Gut 2003;52:966-70.

53. Stocker A, Abell TL, Rashed H, Kedar A, Boatright B, Chen J. Autonomic evaluation of patients with gastroparesis and neurostimulation: comparisons of direct/systemic and indirect/cardiac measures. Gastroenterology Res 2016;9:10-6.

54. Harberson J, Thomas RM, Harbison SP, Parkman HP. Gastric neuromuscular pathology in gastroparesis: analysis of full-thickness antral biopsies. Dig Dis Sci 2010;55:359-70.

55. Gyger G, Baron M. Systemic sclerosis: gastrointestinal disease and its management. Rheum Dis Clin North Am 2015;41:459-73.

56. Fraser RJ, Horowitz M, Maddox AF, Harding PE, Chatterton BE, Dent J. Hyperglycaemia slows gastric emptying in type 1 (insulin-dependent) diabetes mellitus. Diabetologia 1990;33:675-80.

57. Sturm A, Holtmann G, Goebell H, Gerken G. Prokinetics in patients with gastroparesis: a systematic analysis. Digestion 1999;60:422-7.

58. Erbas T, Varoglu E, Erbas B, Tastekin G, Akalin S. Comparison of metoclopramide and erythromycin in the treatment of diabetic gastroparesis. Diabetes Care 1993;16:1511-4.

59. Abell TL, Van Cutsem E, Abrahamsson H, et al. Gastric electrical stimulation in intractable symptomatic gastroparesis. Digestion 2002;66:204-12.

60. Parkman HP, Hasler WL, Fisher RS, American Gastroenterological A. American Gastroenterological Association medical position statement: diagnosis and treatment of gastroparesis. Gastroenterology 2004;127:1589-91.

61. Mihai C, Mihai B, Drug V, Cijevschi Prelipcean C. Gastric bezoars—diagnostic and therapeutic challenges. J Gastrointestin Liver Dis 2013;22:111.

62. Park SE, Ahn JY, Jung HY, et al. Clinical outcomes associated with treatment modalities for gastrointestinal bezoars. Gut Liver 2014;8:400-7.

63. Gaya J, Barranco L, Llompart A, Reyes J, Obrador A. Persimmon bezoars: a successful combined therapy. Gastrointest Endosc 2002;55:581-3.

64. Moriel EZ, Ayalon A, Eid A, Rachmilewitz D, Krausz MM, Durst AL. An unusually high incidence of gastrointestinal obstruction by persimmon bezoars in Israeli patients after ulcer surgery. Gastroenterology 1983;84:752-5.

65. Granot E, Fich A, Ayalon A, et al. An epidemic of persimmon bezoars in Israel. Isr J Med Sci 1984;20:167-9.

66. Altintoprak F, Degirmenci B, Dikicier E, et al. CT findings of patients with small bowel obstruction due to bezoar: a descriptive study. ScientificWorldJournal 2013;2013:298392.

67. Iwamuro M, Okada H, Matsueda K, et al. Review of the diagnosis and management of gastrointestinal bezoars. World J Gastrointest Endosc 2015;7:336-45.

68. Ghosheh B, Salameh JR. Laparoscopic approach to acute small bowel obstruction: review of 1061 cases. Surg Endosc 2007;21:1945-9.

69. Cifuentes Tebar J, Robles Campos R, Parrilla Paricio P, et al. Gastric surgery and bezoars. Dig Dis Sci 1992;37.1694-6.

70. Iwamuro M, Tanaka S, Shiode J, et al. Clinical characteristics and treatment outcomes of nineteen Japanese patients with gastrointestinal bezoars. Intern Med 2014;53:1099-105.

71. Lee BJ, Park JJ, Chun HJ, et al. How good is cola for dissolution of gastric phytobezoars? World J Gastroenterol 2009;15:2265-9.

72. Sharma D, Srivastava M, Babu R, Anand R, Rohtagi A, Thomas S. Laparoscopic treatment of gastric bezoar. JSLS 2010;14:263-7.

73. Zhang RL, Yang ZL, Fan BG. Huge gastric disopyrobezoar: a case report and review of literatures. World J Gastroenterol 2008;14:152-4.

74. Ladas SD, Kamberoglou D, Karamanolis G, Vlachogiannakos J, Zouboulis-Vafiadis I. Systematic review: coca-cola can effectively dissolve gastric phytobezoars as a first-line treatment. Aliment Pharmacol Ther 2013;37:169-73.

75. Krausz MM, Moriel EZ, Ayalon A, Pode D, Durst AL. Surgical aspects of gastrointestinal persimmon phytobezoar treatment. Am J Surg 1986;152:526-30.

76. Gorter RR, Kneepkens CM, Mattens EC, Aronson DC, Heij HA. Management of trichobezoar: case report and literature review. Pediatr Surg Int 2010;26:457-63.

77. Stack PE, Thomas E. Pharmacobezoar: an evolving new entity. Dig Dis 1995;13:356-64.

78. Frohna WJ. Metamucil bezoar: an unusual cause of small bowel obstruction. Am J Emerg Med 1992;10:393-5.

79. Stack PE, Patel NR, Young MF, Ferslew KE, Thomas E. Pharmacobezoars—the irony of the antidote: first case report of nifedipine xl bezoar. J Clin Gastroenterol 1994;19:264-5.

80. Heinz-Erian P, Gassner I, Klein-Franke A, et al. Gastric lactobezoar - a rare disorder? Orphanet J Rare Dis 2012;7:3.

81. Dwivedi AJ, Chahin F, Agrawal S, Patel J, Khalid M, Lakra Y. Gastric phytobezoar: treatment using meat tenderizer. Dig Dis Sci 2001;46:1013-5.

82. Iwamuro M, Kawai Y, Shiraha H, Takaki A, Okada H, Yamamoto K. In vitro analysis of gastric phytobezoar dissolubility by coca-cola, coca-cola zero, cellulase, and papain. J Clin Gastroenterol 2014;48:190-1.

83. Javed A, Agarwal AK. A modified minimally invasive technique for the surgical management of large trichobezoars. J Minim Access Surg 2013;9:42-4.

84. Sarin SK, Sreenivas DV, Lahoti D, Saraya A. Factors influencing development of portal hypertensive gastropathy in patients with portal hypertension. Gastroenterology 1992;102:994-9.

85. Merli M, Nicolini G, Angeloni S, Gentili F, Attili AF, Riggio O. The natural history of portal hypertensive gastropathy in patients with liver cirrhosis and mild portal hypertension. Am J Gastroenterol 2004;99:1959-65.

86. Kim MY, Choi H, Baik SK, et al. Portal hypertensive gastropathy: correlation with portal hypertension and prognosis in cirrhosis. Dig Dis Sci 2010;55:3561-7.

87. Ohta M, Hashizume M, Higashi H, et al. Portal and gastric mucosal hemodynamics in cirrhotic patients with portal-hypertensive gastropathy. Hepatology 1994;20:1432-6.

88. Villanueva C, Colomo A, Bosch A, et al. Transfusion strategies for acute upper gastrointestinal bleeding. N Engl J Med 2013;368:11-21.

89. Perez-Ayuso RM, Pique JM, Bosch J, et al. Propranolol in prevention of recurrent bleeding from severe portal hypertensive gastropathy in cirrhosis. Lancet 1991;337:1431-4.

90. Zhou Y, Qiao L, Wu J, Hu H, Xu C. Comparison of the efficacy of octreotide, vasopressin, and omeprazole in the control of acute bleeding in patients with portal hypertensive gastropathy: a controlled study. J Gastroenterol Hepatol 2002;17:973-9.

91. Herrera S, Bordas JM, Llach J, et al. The beneficial effects of argon plasma coagulation in the management of different types of gastric vascular ectasia lesions in patients admitted for gi hemorrhage. Gastrointest Endosc 2008;68:440-6.

92. Watson M, Hally RJ, McCue PA, Varga J, Jimenez SA. Gastric antral vascular ectasia (watermelon stomach) in patients with systemic sclerosis. Arthritis Rheum 1996;39:341-6.

93. Acosta RD, Wong RK. Differential diagnosis of upper gastrointestinal bleeding proximal to the ligament of trietz. Gastrointest Endosc Clin N Am 2011;21:555-66.

94. Dulai GS, Jensen DM, Kovacs TO, Gralnek IM, Jutabha R. Endoscopic treatment outcomes in watermelon stomach patients with and without portal hypertension. Endoscopy 2004;36:68-72.

95. Han S, Chaudhary N, Wassef W. Portal hypertensive gastropathy and gastric antral vascular ectasia. Curr Opin Gastroenterol 2015;31:506-12.

96. Gostout CJ, Viggiano TR, Ahlquist DA, Wang KK, Larson MV, Balm R. The clinical and endoscopic spectrum of the watermelon stomach. J Clin Gastroenterol 1992;15:256-63.

97. Jabbari M, Cherry R, Lough JO, Daly DS, Kinnear DG, Goresky CA. Gastric antral vascular ectasia: the watermelon stomach. Gastroenterology 1984;87:1165-70.

98. Charneau J, Petit R, Cales P, Dauver A, Boyer J. Antral motility in patients with cirrhosis with or without gastric antral vascular ectasia. Gut 1995;37:488-92.

99. Brijbassie A, Osaimi AA, Powell SM. Hormonal effects on nodular gave. Gastroenterology Res 2013;6:77-80.

100. Quintero E, Pique JM, Bombi JA, Bordas JM, Sentis J, Elena M, et al. Gastric mucosal vascular ectasias causing bleeding in cirrhosis. A distinct entity associated with hypergastrinemia and low serum levels of pepsinogen I. Gastroenterology 1987;93:1054-61.

101. Spahr L, Villeneuve JP, Dufresne MP, et al. Gastric antral vascular ectasia in cirrhotic patients: absence of relation with portal hypertension. Gut 1999;44:739-42.

102. Roman S, Saurin JC, Dumortier J, Perreira A, Bernard G, Ponchon T. Tolerance and efficacy of argon plasma coagulation for controlling bleeding in patients with typical and atypical manifestations of watermelon stomach. Endoscopy 2003;35:1024-8.

103. Probst A, Scheubel R, Wienbeck M. Treatment of watermelon stomach (GAVE syndrome) by means of endoscopic argon plasma coagulation (APC): long-term outcome. Z Gastroenterol 2001;39:447-52.

104. Mathou NG, Lovat LB, Thorpe SM, Bown SG. Nd:Yag laser induces long-term remission in transfusion-dependent patients with watermelon stomach. Lasers Med Sci 2004;18:213-8.

105. Marrone GC, Silen W. Pathogenesis, diagnosis and treatment of acute gastric mucosal lesions. Clin Gastroenterol 1984;13:635-50.

106. Panarelli NC. Drug-induced injury in the gastrointestinal tract. Semin Diagn Pathol 2014;31:165-75.

107. Ananthakrishnan N, Parthasarathy G, Kate V. Acute corrosive injuries of the stomach: a single unit experience of thirty years. ISRN Gastroenterol 2011;2011:914013.

108. Genta RM. Differential diagnosis of reactive gastropathy. Semin Diagn Pathol 2005;22:273-83.

109. Mo C, Sun G, Lu ML, et al. Proton pump inhibitors in prevention of low-dose aspirin-associated upper gastrointestinal injuries. World J Gastroenterol 2015;21:5382-92.

110. Matsumoto S, Wakatsuki K, Migita K, et al. Predictive factors for delayed gastric emptying after distal gastrectomy with roux-en-y reconstruction. Am Surg 2018;84:1086-90.

111. Yang D, He L, Tong WH, Jia ZF, Su TR, Wang Q. Randomized controlled trial of uncut roux-en-y vs billroth II reconstruction after distal gastrectomy for gastric cancer: which technique is better for avoiding biliary reflux and gastritis? World J Gastroenterol 2017;23:6350-6.

112. Greywoode G, Szuts A, Wang LM, Sgromo B, Chetty R. Iatrogenic deep epithelial misplacement ("gastritis cystica profunda") in a gastric foveolar-type adenoma after endoscopic manipulation: a diagnostic pitfall. Am J Surg Pathol 2011;35:1419-21.

113. Bouquot M, Dokmak S, Barbier L, Cros J, Levy P, Sauvanet A. Gastric stump carcinoma as a long-term complication of pancreaticoduodenectomy: report of two cases and review of the English literature. BMC Gastroenterol 2017;17:117.

114. Gorospe M, Fadare O. Gastric mucosal calcinosis: clinicopathologic considerations. Adv Anat Pathol 2007;14:224-8.

115. Nayak HK, Mohindra S, Iqbal S, Saraswat VA, Agarwal V, Pande G. Gastric mucosal calcinosis mimicking malignancy. Am J Gastroenterol 2016;111:1380.

116. Hamada J, Tamai K, Ono W, Saotome K. Uremic tumoral calcinosis in hemodialysis patients: clinicopathological findings and identification of calcific deposits. J Rheumatol 2006;33:119-26.

117. Movilli E, Feliciani A, Camerini C, et al. A high calcium-phosphate product is associated with high c-reactive protein concentrations in hemodialysis patients. Nephron Clin Pract 2005;101:c161-7.

118. Greenson JK, Trinidad SB, Pfeil SA, et al. Gastric mucosal calcinosis. Calcified aluminum phosphate deposits secondary to aluminum-containing antacids or sucralfate therapy in organ transplant patients. Am J Surg Pathol 1993;17:45-50.

119. Li K, Xu Y. Citrate metabolism in blood transfusions and its relationship due to metabolic alkalosis and respiratory acidosis. Int J Clin Exp Med 2015;8:6578-84.

120. Nishikawa Y, Sakurai T, Miyamoto S. Multiple white plaques in the body of the stomach in a patient undergoing hemodialysis. Gastroenterology 2016;151:e18-9.

121. Matsukuma K, Gui D, Olson KA, Tejaswi S, Clayton EF, Thai A. Osmoprep-associated gastritis: a histopathologic mimic of iron pill gastritis and mucosal calcinosis. Am J Surg Pathol 2016;40:1550-6.

122. Abraham SC, Yardley JH, Wu TT. Erosive injury to the upper gastrointestinal tract in patients receiving iron medication: an underrecognized entity. Am J Surg Pathol 1999;23:1241-7.

123. Haig A, Driman DK. Iron-induced mucosal injury to the upper gastrointestinal tract. Histopathology 2006;48:808-12.

124. Marginean EC, Bennick M, Cyczk J, Robert ME, Jain D. Gastric siderosis: patterns and significance. Am J Surg Pathol 2006;30:514-20.

125. Conte D, Velio P, Brunelli L, et al. Stainable iron in gastric and duodenal mucosa of primary hemochromatosis patients and alcoholics. Am J Gastroenterol 1987;82:237-40.

126. Haratake J, Yasunaga C, Ootani A, Shimajiri S, Matsuyama A, Hisaoka M. Peculiar histiocytic lesions with massive lanthanum deposition in dialysis patients treated with lanthanum carbonate. Am J Surg Pathol 2015;39:767-71.

127. Hoda RS, Sanyal S, Abraham JL, et al. Lanthanum deposition from oral lanthanum carbonate in the upper gastrointestinal tract. Histopathology 2017;70:1072-8.

128. Hashash JG, Proksell S, Kuan SF, Behari J. Iron pill-induced gastritis. ACG Case Rep J 2013;1:13-5.

129. Affolter K, Samowitz W, Boynton K, Kelly ED. Doxycycline-induced gastrointestinal injury. Hum Pathol 2017;66:212-5.

130. Xiao SY, Zhao L, Hart J, Semrad CE. Gastric mucosal necrosis with vascular degeneration induced by doxycycline. Am J Surg Pathol 2013;37:259-63.

131. Lee SJ, Flowers ME. Recognizing and managing chronic graft-versus-host disease. Hematology Am Soc Hematol Educ Program 2008:134-41.

132. Naymagon S, Naymagon L, Wong SY, et al. Acute graft-versus-host disease of the gut: considerations for the gastroenterologist. Nat Rev Gastroenterol Hepatol 2017;14:711-26.

133. Harris AC, Young R, Devine S, et al. International, multicenter standardization of acute graft-versus-host disease clinical data collection: a report from the Mount Sinai Acute GVHD International Consortium. Biol Blood Marrow Transplant 2016;22:4-10.

134. Weisdorf DJ, Snover DC, Haake R, et al. Acute upper gastrointestinal graft-versus-host disease: clinical significance and response to immunosuppressive therapy. Blood 1990;76:624-9.

135. Unanue ER, Allen PM. The basis for the immunoregulatory role of macrophages and other accessory cells. Science 1987;236:551-7.

136. Laster SM, Wood JG, Gooding LR. Tumor necrosis factor can induce both apoptic and necrotic forms of cell lysis. J Immunol 1988;141:2629-34.

137. Shono Y, Docampo MD, Peled JU, Perobelli SM, Jenq RR. Intestinal microbiota-related effects on graft-versus-host disease. Int J Hematol 2015;101:428-37.

138. Yeh SP, Liao YM, Hsu CH, et al. Gastric bleeding due to graft-vs-host disease: discrepancy between endoscopic and histologic assessment. Am J Clin Pathol 2004;122:919-25.

139. Cruz-Correa M, Poonawala A, Abraham SC, et al. Endoscopic findings predict the histologic diagnosis in gastrointestinal graft-versus-host disease. Endoscopy 2002;34:808-13.

140. Washington K, Jagasia M. Pathology of graft-versus-host disease in the gastrointestinal tract. Hum Pathol 2009;40:909-17.

141. Myerson D, Steinbach G, Gooley TA, Shulman HM. Graft-versus-host disease of the gut: a histologic activity grading system and validation. Biol Blood Marrow Transplant 2017;23:1573-9.

142. Lerner KG, Kao GF, Storb R, Buckner CD, Clift RA, Thomas ED. Histopathology of graft-vs.-host reaction (GvHR) in human recipients of marrow from HL-A-matched sibling donors. Transplant Proc 1974;6:367-71.

143. Shulman HM, Cardona DM, Greenson JK, et al. NIH consensus development project on criteria for clinical trials in chronic graft-versus-host disease: II. The 2014 pathology working group report. Biol Blood Marrow Transplant 2015;21:589-603.

144. Crowell KR, Patel RA, Fluchel M, Lowichik A, Bryson S, Pohl JF. Endoscopy in the diagnosis of intestinal graft-versus-host disease: is lower endoscopy with biopsy as effective in diagnosis as upper endoscopy combined with lower endoscopy? Pediatr Blood Cancer 2013;60:1798-800.

145. Weidner AS, Panarelli NC, Rennert H, Jessurun J, Yantiss RK. Immunohistochemistry improves the detection of adenovirus in gastrointestinal biopsy specimens from hematopoietic stem cell transplant recipients. Am J Clin Pathol 2016;146:627-31.

146. Reggiani Bonetti L, Losi L, Di Gregorio C, et al. Cytomegalovirus infection of the upper gastrointestinal tract: a clinical and pathological study of 30 cases. Scand J Gastroenterol 2011;46:1228-35.

147. Mills AM, Guo FP, Copland AP, Pai RK, Pinsky BA. A comparison of CMV detection in gastrointestinal mucosal biopsies using immunohistochemistry and PCR performed on formalin-fixed, paraffin-embedded tissue. Am J Surg Pathol 2013;37:995-1000.

148. Nguyen T, Park JY, Scudiere JR, Montgomery E. Mycophenolic acid (cellcept and myofortic) induced injury of the upper GI tract. Am J Surg Pathol 2009;33:1355-63.

149. Star KV, Ho VT, Wang HH, Odze RD. Histologic features in colon biopsies can discriminate mycophenolate from GVHD-induced colitis. Am J Surg Pathol 2013;37:1319-28.

150. Ruutu T, Gratwohl A, Niederwieser D, et al. The EBMT-ELN working group recommendations on the prophylaxis and treatment of GvHD: a change-control analysis. Bone Marrow Transplant 2017;52:357-62.

151. Schwartz JM, Wolford JL, Thornquist MD, et al. Severe gastrointestinal bleeding after hematopoietic cell transplantation, 1987-1997: incidence, causes, and outcome. Am J Gastroenterol 2001;96:385-93.

152. Harb AH, Abou Fadel C, Sharara AI. Radiation enteritis. Curr Gastroenterol Rep 2014;16:383.

153. Kavanagh BD, Pan CC, Dawson LA, et al. Radiation dose-volume effects in the stomach and small bowel. Int J Radiat Oncol Biol Phys 2010;76(Suppl):S101-7.

154. Coia LR, Myerson RJ, Tepper JE. Late effects of radiation therapy on the gastrointestinal tract. Int J Radiat Oncol Biol Phys 1995;31:1213-36.

155. Tatsis V, Peponi E, Papadopoulos G, Tsekeris P, Fatouros M, Glantzounis G. Subtotal gastrectomy for diffused hemorrhagic gastritis induced by radiation, following liver resection for hilar cholangiocarcinoma. A case report. Int J Surg Case Rep 2016;18:30-2.

156. Yantiss RK. Eosinophils in the GI tract: how many is too many and what do they mean? Mod Pathol 2015;28(Suppl 1):S7-21.

157. Zhang L, Xie XY, Wang Y, Wang YH, Chen Y, Ren ZG. Treatment of radiation-induced hemorrhagic gastritis with prednisolone: a case report. World J Gastroenterol 2012;18:7402-4.

158. Townsend A, Price T, Karapetis C. Selective internal radiation therapy for liver metastases from colorectal cancer. Cochrane Database Syst Rev 2009:cd007045.

159. King J, Quinn R, Glenn DM, et al. Radioembolization with selective internal radiation microspheres for neuroendocrine liver metastases. Cancer 2008;113:921-9.

160. Reardon KA, McIntosh AF, Shilling AT, et al. Treatment of primary liver tumors with yttrium-90 microspheres (therasphere) in high risk patients: analysis of survival and toxicities. Technol Cancer Res Treat 2009;8:71-7.

161. Murthy R, Brown DB, Salem R, et al. Gastrointestinal complications associated with hepatic arterial yttrium-90 microsphere therapy. J Vasc Interv Radiol 2007;18:553-61.

162. Salem R, Lewandowski RJ, Sato KT, et al. Technical aspects of radioembolization with 90y microspheres. Tech Vasc Interv Radiol 2007;10:12-29.

163. Song SY, Chung JW, Lim HG, Park JH. Nonhepatic arteries originating from the hepatic arteries: angiographic analysis in 250 patients. J Vasc Interv Radiol 2006;17:461-9.

164. Riaz A, Lewandowski RJ, Kulik LM, et al. Complications following radioembolization with yttrium-90 microspheres: a comprehensive literature review. J Vasc Interv Radiol 2009;20:1121-30.

165. Sjoquist KM, Goldstein D, Bester L. A serious complication of selected internal radiation therapy: case report and literature review. Oncologist 2010;15:830-5.

166. Sangro B, Martínez-Urbistondo D, Bester L, et al. Prevention and treatment of complications of selective internal radiation therapy: expert guidance and systematic review. Hepatology 2017;66:969-82.

167. Moss SF. The clinical evidence linking helicobacter pylori to gastric cancer. Cell Mol Gastroenterol Hepatol 2017;3:183-91.

168. Nguyen T, Ramsey D, Graham D, et al. The prevalence of helicobacter pylori remains high in African American and Hispanic veterans. Helicobacter 2015;20:305-15.

169. Eusebi LH, Zagari RM, Bazzoli F. Epidemiology of helicobacter pylori infection. Helicobacter 2014;19(Suppl 1):1-5.

170. de Martel C, Parsonnet J. Helicobacter pylori infection and gender: a meta-analysis of population-based prevalence surveys. Dig Dis Sci 2006;51:2292-301.

171. Chey WD, Leontiadis GI, Howden CW, Moss SF. ACG clinical guideline: treatment of helicobacter pylori infection. Am J Gastroenterol 2017;112:212-39.

172. Singhal AV, Sepulveda AR. Helicobacter heilmannii gastritis: a case study with review of literature. Am J Surg Pathol 2005;29:1537-9.

173. Wroblewski LE, Peek RM, Jr., Wilson KT. Helicobacter pylori and gastric cancer: factors that modulate disease risk. Clin Microbiol Rev 2010;23:713-39.

174. Lopes AI, Vale FF, Oleastro M. Helicobacter pylori infection - recent developments in diagnosis. World J Gastroenterol 2014;20:9299-313.

175. Dixon MF, Genta RM, Yardley JH, Correa P. Classification and grading of gastritis. The updated Sydney system. International workshop on the histopathology of gastritis, Houston 1994. Am J Surg Pathol 1996;20:1161-81.

176. Sarem M, Corti R. [Role of helicobacter pylori coccoid forms in infection and recrudescence]. Gastroenterol Hepatol 2016;39:28-35. [Spanish]

177. Panarelli NC, Yantiss RK. The importance of biopsy sampling practices in the pathologic evaluation of gastrointestinal disorders. Curr Opin Gastroenterol 2016;32:374-81.

178. Wu TT, Hamilton SR. Lymphocytic gastritis: association with etiology and topology. Am J Surg Pathol 1999;23:153-8.

179. Zagari RM, Rabitti S, Greenwood DC, Eusebi LH, Vestito A, Bazzoli F. Systematic review with meta-analysis: diagnostic performance of the combination of pepsinogen, gastrin-17 and anti-helicobacter pylori antibodies serum assays for the diagnosis of atrophic gastritis. Aliment Pharmacol Ther 2017;46:657-67.

180. Wang YK, Kuo FC, Liu CJ, et al. Diagnosis of helicobacter pylori infection: current options and developments. World J Gastroenterol 2015;21:11221-35.

181. Batts KP, Ketover S, Kakar S, et al. Appropriate use of special stains for identifying helicobacter pylori: recommendations from the Rodger C. Haggitt Gastrointestinal Pathology Society. Am J Surg Pathol 2013;37:e12-22.

182. Wang XI, Zhang S, Abreo F, Thomas J. The role of routine immunohistochemistry for helicobacter pylori in gastric biopsy. Ann Diagn Pathol 2010;14:256-9.

183. Panarelli NC, Ross DS, Bernheim OE, et al. Utility of ancillary stains for helicobacter pylori in near-normal gastric biopsies. Hum Pathol 2015;46:397-403.

184. Hu Q, Zhang Y, Zhang X, Fu K. Gastric mucosa-associated lymphoid tissue lymphoma and helicobacter pylori infection: a review of current diagnosis and management. Biomark Res 2016;4:15.

185. Chen ZM, Shah R, Zuckerman GR, Wang HL. Epstein-Barr virus gastritis: an underrecognized form of severe gastritis simulating gastric lymphoma. Am J Surg Pathol 2007;31:1446-51.

186. Takeuchi K, Yokoyama M, Ishizawa S, et al. Lymphomatoid gastropathy: a distinct clinicopathologic entity of self-limited pseudomalignant NK-cell proliferation. Blood 2010;116:5631-7.

187. Mansoor A, Pittaluga S, Beck PL, Wilson WH, Ferry JA, Jaffe ES. NK-cell enteropathy: a benign NK-cell lymphoproliferative disease mimicking intestinal lymphoma: clinicopathologic features and follow-up in a unique case series. Blood 2011;117:1447-52.

188. Takata K, Noujima-Harada M, Miyata-Takata T, et al. Clinicopathologic analysis of 6 lymphomatoid gastropathy cases: expanding the disease spectrum to cd4-cd8+ cases. Am J Surg Pathol 2015;39:1259-66.

189. Park JY, Cornish TC, Lam-Himlin D, Shi C, Montgomery E. Gastric lesions in patients with autoimmune metaplastic atrophic gastritis (AMAG) in a tertiary care setting. Am J Surg Pathol 2010;34:1591-8.

190. Betterle C, Zanchetta R. Update on autoimmune polyendocrine syndromes (APS). Acta Biomed 2003;74:9-33.

191. Massironi S, Cavalcoli F, Rossi RE, et al. Chronic autoimmune atrophic gastritis associated with primary hyperparathyroidism: a transversal prospective study. Eur J Endocrinol 2013;168:755-61.

192. Coati I, Fassan M, Farinati F, Graham DY, Genta RM, Rugge M. Autoimmune gastritis: pathologist's viewpoint. World J Gastroenterol 2015; 21:12179-89.

193. Torbenson M, Abraham SC, Boitnott J, Yardley JH, Wu TT. Autoimmune gastritis: distinct histological and immunohistochemical findings before complete loss of oxyntic glands. Mod Pathol 2002;15:102-9.

194. Rusak E, Chobot A, Krzywicka A, Wenzlau J. Anti-parietal cell antibodies - diagnostic significance. Adv Med Sci 2016;61:175-9.

195. Bergman MP, D'Elios MM. Cytotoxic T cells in H. Pylori-related gastric autoimmunity and gastric lymphoma. J Biomed Biotechnol 2010;2010:104918.

196. Pittman ME, Voltaggio L, Bhaijee F, Robertson SA, Montgomery EA. Autoimmune metaplastic atrophic gastritis: recognizing precursor lesions for appropriate patient evaluation. Am J Surg Pathol 2015;39:1611-20.

197. Cockburn AN, Morgan CJ, Genta RM. Neuroendocrine proliferations of the stomach: a pragmatic approach for the perplexed pathologist. Adv Anat Pathol 2013;20:148-57.

198. Vannella L, Lahner E, Annibale B. Risk for gastric neoplasias in patients with chronic atrophic gastritis: a critical reappraisal. World J Gastroenterol 2012;18:1279-85.

199. Borch K, Ahren B, Ahlman H, Falkmer S, Granerus G, Grimelius L. Gastric carcinoids: biologic behavior and prognosis after differentiated treatment in relation to type. Ann Surg 2005;242:64-73.

200. Lagorce-Pages C, Fabiani B, Bouvier R, Scoazec JY, Durand L, Flejou JF. Collagenous gastritis: a report of six cases. Am J Surg Pathol 2001;25:1174-9.

201. Ma C, Park JY, Montgomery EA, et al. A comparative clinicopathologic study of collagenous gastritis in children and adults: the same disorder with associated immune-mediated diseases. Am J Surg Pathol 2015;39:802-12.

202. Kamimura K, Kobayashi M, Sato Y, Aoyagi Y, Terai S. Collagenous gastritis: review. World J Gastrointest Endosc 2015;7:265-73.

203. Arnason T, Brown IS, Goldsmith JD, et al. Collagenous gastritis: a morphologic and immunohistochemical study of 40 patients. Mod Pathol 2015;28:533-44.

204. Brain O, Rajaguru C, Warren B, Booth J, Travis S. Collagenous gastritis: reports and systematic review. Eur J Gastroenterol Hepatol 2009;21:1419-24.

205. Leung ST, Chandan VS, Murray JA, Wu TT. Collagenous gastritis: histopathologic features and association with other gastrointestinal diseases. Am J Surg Pathol 2009;33:788-98.

206. Winslow JL, Trainer TD, Colletti RB. Collagenous gastritis: a long-term follow-up with the development of endocrine cell hyperplasia, intestinal metaplasia, and epithelial changes indeterminate for dysplasia. Am J Clin Pathol 2001;116:753-8.

207. Nielsen OH, Riis LB, Danese S, Bojesen RD, Soendergaard C. Proximal collagenous gastroenteritides: clinical management. A systematic review. Ann Med 2014;46:311-7.

208. Choi EY, McKenna BJ. Olmesartan-associated enteropathy: a review of clinical and histologic findings. Arch Pathol Lab Med 2015;139:1242-7.

209. Dixon MF, Wyatt JI, Burke DA, Rathbone BJ. Lymphocytic gastritis—relationship to campylobacter pylori infection. J Pathol 1988;154:125-32.

210. Jaskiewicz K, Price SK, Zak J, Louwrens HD. Lymphocytic gastritis in nonulcer dyspepsia. Dig Dis Sci 1991;36:1079-83.

211. De Giacomo C, Gianatti A, Negrini R, et al. Lymphocytic gastritis: a positive relationship with celiac disease. J Pediatr 1994;124:57-62.

212. Wolber R, Owen D, DelBuono L, Appelman H, Freeman H. Lymphocytic gastritis in patients with celiac sprue or spruelike intestinal disease. Gastroenterology 1990;98:310-5.

213. Perardi S, Todros L, Musso A, David E, Repici A, Rizzetto M. Lymphocytic gastritis and protein-losing gastropathy. Dig Liver Dis 2000;32:422-5.

214. Haot J, Berger F, Andre C, Moulinier B, Mainguet P, Lambert R. Lymphocytic gastritis versus varioliform gastritis. A historical series revisited. J Pathol 1989;158:19-22.

215. Haot J, Jouret A, Willette M, Gossuin A, Mainguet P. Lymphocytic gastritis—prospective study of its relationship with varioliform gastritis. Gut 1990;31:282-5.

216. Cui I, Chen Z, Panarelli N, et al. Patterns of lymphocytic gastritis may reflect the underlying etiology. Mod Pathol 2016;29(Suppl 2):167A.

217. Polydorides AD. Pathology and differential diagnosis of chronic, noninfectious gastritis. Semin Diagn Pathol 2014;31:114-23.

218. Choi WT, Lauwers GY. Patterns of gastric injury: beyond helicobacter pylori. Surg Pathol Clin 2017;10:801-22.

219. Kahkouee S, Samadi K, Alai A, Abedini A, Rezaiian L. Serum ace level in sarcoidosis patients with typical and atypical HRCT manifestation. Pol J Radiol 2016;81:458-61.

220. Pulimood AB, Amarapurkar DN, Ghoshal U, et al. Differentiation of Crohn's disease from intestinal tuberculosis in India in 2010. World J Gastroenterol 2011;17:433-43.

221. Telisinghe L, Amofa-Sekyi M, Maluzi K, et al. The sensitivity of the QuantiFERON®-TB gold plus assay in Zambian adults with active tuberculosis. Int J Tuberc Lung Dis 2017;21:690-6.

222. Kaneki T, Koizumi T, Yamamoto H, et al. Gastric sarcoidosis—a single polypoid appearance in the involvement. Hepatogastroenterology 2001;48:1209-10.

223. Arabi NA, Musaad AM, Ahmed EE, Ibnouf MM, Abdelaziz MS. Primary gastric tuberculosis presenting as gastric outlet obstruction: a case report and review of the literature. J Med Case Rep 2015;9:265.

224. Ushiku T, Moran CJ, Lauwers GY. Focally enhanced gastritis in newly diagnosed pediatric inflammatory bowel disease. Am J Surg Pathol 2013;37:1882-8.

225. Ye Z, Lin Y, Cao Q, He Y, Xue L. Granulomas as the most useful histopathological feature in distinguishing between Crohn's disease and intestinal tuberculosis in endoscopic biopsy specimens. Medicine (Baltimore) 2015;94:e2157.

226. Miller AI, Smith B, Rogers AI. Phlegmonous gastritis. Gastroenterology 1975;68:231-8.

227. Stein LB, Greenberg RE, Ilardi CF, Kurtz L, Bank S. Acute necrotizing gastritis in a patient with peptic ulcer disease. Am J Gastroenterol 1989;84:1552-4.

228. Schultz MJ, van der Hulst RW, Tytgat GN. Acute phlegmonous gastritis. Gastrointest Endosc 1996;44:80-3.

229. Tierney LM Jr, Gooding G, Bottles K, Montgomery CK, Fitzgerald FT. Phlegmonous gastritis and hemophilus influenzae peritonitis in a patient with alcoholic liver disease. Dig Dis Sci 1987;32:97-101.

230. Kim GY, Ward J, Henessey B, et al. Phlegmonous gastritis: case report and review. Gastrointest Endosc 2005;61:168-74.

231. Lee BS, Kim SM, Seong JK, et al. Phlegmonous gastritis after endoscopic mucosal resection. Endoscopy 2005;37:490-3.

232. Choi SJ, Kim HJ, Kim JS, Bak YT, Kim JS. Radiation recall gastritis secondary to combination of gemcitabine and erlotinib in pancreatic cancer and response to PPI–a case report. BMC Cancer 2016;16:588.

233. Huang CT, Liao WY. Emphysematous gastritis: a deadly infectious disease. Scand J Infect Dis 2009;41:317-9.

234. Jung JH, Choi HJ, Yoo J, Kang SJ, Lee KY. Emphysematous gastritis associated with invasive gastric mucormycosis: a case report. J Korean Med Sci 2007;22:923-7.

235. Cherney CL, Chutuape A, Fikrig MK. Fatal invasive gastric mucormycosis occurring with emphysematous gastritis: case report and literature review. Am J Gastroenterol 1999;94:252-6.

236. Al Rasheed MR, Senseng CG. Sarcina ventriculi: review of the literature. Arch Pathol Lab Med 2016;140:1441-5.

237. Sopha SC, Manejwala A, Boutros CN. Sarcina, a new threat in the bariatric era. Hum Pathol 2015;46:1405-7.

238. Lam-Himlin D, Tsiatis AC, Montgomery E, et al. Sarcina organisms in the gastrointestinal tract: a clinicopathologic and molecular study. Am J Surg Pathol 2011;35:1700-5.

239. Dib JR, Liebl W, Wagenknecht M, Farias ME, Meinhardt F. Extrachromosomal genetic elements in micrococcus. Appl Microbiol Biotechnol 2013;97:63-75.

240. Coffey RJ Jr, Tanksley J. Pierre Menetrier and his disease. Trans Am Clin Climatol Assoc 2012;123:126-33.

241. Coffey RJ, Washington MK, Corless CL, Heinrich MC. Menetrier disease and gastrointestinal stromal tumors: hyperproliferative disorders of the stomach. J Clin Invest 2007;117:70-80.

242. Beneck D. Hypertrophic gastropathy in a newborn: a case report and review of the literature. Pediatr Pathol 1994;14:213-21.

243. Singh B, Coffey RJ. From wavy hair to naked proteins: the role of transforming growth factor alpha in health and disease. Semin Cell Dev Biol 2014;28:12-21.

244. Wang X, Huong SM, Chiu ML, Raab-Traub N, Huang ES. Epidermal growth factor receptor is a cellular receptor for human cytomegalovirus. Nature 2003;424:456-61.

245. Cardenas A, Kelly C. Menetrier disease. Gut 2004;53:330, 8.

246. Gonzalez RS, Adsay V, Graham RP, et al. Massive gastric juvenile-type polyposis: a clinicopathological analysis of 22 cases. Histopathology 2017;70:918-28.

247. Burdick JS, Chung E, Tanner G, et al. Treatment of Menetrier's disease with a monoclonal antibody against the epidermal growth factor receptor. N Engl J Med 2000;343:1697-701.

248. Mendelson AH, Donowitz M. Catching the zebra: clinical pearls and pitfalls for the successful diagnosis of Zollinger-Ellison syndrome. Dig Dis Sci 2017;62:2258-65.

249. Kulke MH, Anthony LB, Bushnell DL, et al. NANETS treatment guidelines: well-differentiated neuroendocrine tumors of the stomach and pancreas. Pancreas 2010;39:735-52.

250. Johnbeck CB, Knigge U, Kjaer A. Pet tracers for somatostatin receptor imaging of neuroendocrine tumors: current status and review of the literature. Future Oncol 2014;10:2259-77.

251. Thakker RV, Newey PJ, Walls GV, et al. Clinical practice guidelines for multiple endocrine neoplasia type 1 (MEN1). J Clin Endocrinol Metab 2012;97:2990-3011.

252. Berna MJ, Hoffmann KM, Long SH, Serrano J, Gibril F, Jensen RT. Serum gastrin in Zollinger-Ellison syndrome: II. Prospective study of gastrin provocative testing in 293 patients from the National Institutes of Health and comparison with 537 cases from the literature. Evaluation of diagnostic criteria, proposal of new criteria, and correlations with clinical and tumoral features. Medicine (Baltimore) 2006;85:331-64.

253. Jain RN, Samuelson LC. Differentiation of the gastric mucosa. II. Role of gastrin in gastric epithelial cell proliferation and maturation. Am J Physiol Gastrointest Liver Physiol 2006;291:G762-5.

254. Peghini PL, Annibale B, Azzoni C, et al. Effect of chronic hypergastrinemia on human enterochromaffin-like cells: insights from patients with sporadic gastrinomas. Gastroenterology 2002;123:68-85.

255. Roy PK, Venzon DJ, Shojamanesh H, et al. Zollinger-Ellison syndrome. Clinical presentation in 261 patients. Medicine (Baltimore) 2000;79:379-411.

256. Krampitz GW, Norton JA. Current management of the Zollinger-Ellison syndrome. Adv Surg 2013;47:59-79.

257. Krampitz GW, Norton JA, Poultsides GA, Visser BC, Sun L, Jensen RT. Lymph nodes and survival in pancreatic neuroendocrine tumors. Arch Surg 2012;147:820-7.

258. La Rosa S, Inzani F, Vanoli A, et al. Histologic characterization and improved prognostic evaluation of 209 gastric neuroendocrine neoplasms. Hum Pathol 2011;42:1373-84.

259. Bassullu N, Turkmen I, Uraz S, et al. Xanthomatous hyperplastic polyps of the stomach: clinicopathologic study of 5 patients with polypoid gastric lesions showing combined features of gastric xanthelasma and hyperplastic polyp. Ann Diagn Pathol 2013;17:72-4.

260. Diaz Del Arco C, Alvarez Sanchez A, Fernandez Acenero MJ. Non-gastric gastrointestinal xanthomas: case series and literature review. J Gastrointestin Liver Dis 2016;25:389-94.

261. Arnold CA, Frankel WL, Guo L, et al. Crystal-storing histiocytosis in the stomach: a clue to subtle hematolymphoid malignancies. Am J Surg Pathol 2018;42:1317-24.

262. Stolte M. Clinical consequences of the endoscopic diagnosis of gastric polyps. Endoscopy 1995;27:32-7.

263. Cooper JE, Roberts-Thomson IC. Gastrointestinal: fundic gland polyps. J Gastroenterol Hepatol 1999;14:395.

264. Kumar KR, Iqbal R, Coss E, Park C, Cryer B, Genta RM. Helicobacter gastritis induces changes in the oxyntic mucosa indistinguishable from the effects of proton pump inhibitors. Hum Pathol 2013;44:2706-10.

265. Vieth M, Stolte M. Fundic gland polyps are not induced by proton pump inhibitor therapy. Am J Clin Pathol 2001;116:716-20.

266. Levy MD, Bhattacharya B. Sporadic fundic gland polyps with low-grade dysplasia: a large case series evaluating pathologic and immunohistochemical findings and clinical behavior. Am J Clin Pathol 2015;144:592-600.

267. de Boer WB, Ee H, Kumarasinghe MP. Neoplastic lesions of gastric adenocarcinoma and proximal polyposis syndrome (GAPPS) are gastric phenotype. Am J Surg Pathol 2018;42:1-8.

268. Torbenson M, Lee JH, Cruz-Correa M, et al. Sporadic fundic gland polyposis: a clinical, histological, and molecular analysis. Mod Pathol 2002;15:718-23.

269. Abraham SC, Nobukawa B, Giardiello FM, Hamilton SR, Wu TT. Sporadic fundic gland polyps: common gastric polyps arising through activating mutations in the beta-catenin gene. Am J Pathol 2001;158:1005-10.

270. Abraham SC, Nobukawa B, Giardiello FM, Hamilton SR, Wu TT. Fundic gland polyps in familial adenomatous polyposis: neoplasms with frequent somatic adenomatous polyposis coli gene alterations. Am J Pathol 2000;157:747-54.

271. Li J, Woods SL, Healey S, et al. Point mutations in exon 1b of APC reveal gastric adenocarcinoma and proximal polyposis of the stomach as a familial adenomatous polyposis variant. Am J Hum Genet 2016;98:830-42.

272. Bianchi LK, Burke CA, Bennett AE, Lopez R, Hasson H, Church JM. Fundic gland polyp dysplasia is common in familial adenomatous polyposis. Clin Gastroenterol Hepatol 2008;6:180-5.

273. Wood LD, Salaria SN, Cruise MW, Giardiello FM, Montgomery EA. Upper GI tract lesions in familial adenomatous polyposis (FAP): enrichment of pyloric gland adenomas and other gastric and duodenal neoplasms. Am J Surg Pathol 2014;38:389-93.

274. Lloyd IE, Kohlmann WK, Gligorich K, et al. A clinicopathologic evaluation of incidental fundic gland polyps with dysplasia: implications for clinical management. Am J Gastroenterol 2017;112:1094-102.

275. Carmack SW, Genta RM, Graham DY, Lauwers GY. Management of gastric polyps: a pathology-based guide for gastroenterologists. Nat Rev Gastroenterol Hepatol 2009;6:331-41.

276. Brosens LA, Keller JJ, Offerhaus GJ, Goggins M, Giardiello FM. Prevention and management of duodenal polyps in familial adenomatous polyposis. Gut 2005;54:1034-43.

277. Beer A, Streubel B, Asari R, Dejaco C, Oberhuber G. Gastric adenocarcinoma and proximal polyposis of the stomach (GAPPS) - a rare recently described gastric polyposis syndrome - report of a case. Z Gastroenterol 2017;55:1131-4.

278. Gonzalez-Obeso E, Fujita H, Deshpande V, et al. Gastric hyperplastic polyps: a heterogeneous clinicopathologic group including a distinct subset best categorized as mucosal prolapse polyp. Am J Surg Pathol 2011;35:670-7.

279. Lauwers GY, Wahl SJ, Melamed J, Rojas-Corona RR. p53 expression in precancerous gastric lesions: an immunohistochemical study of PAb 1801 monoclonal antibody on adenomatous and hyperplastic gastric polyps. Am J Gastroenterol 1993;88:1916-9.

280. Nogueira AM, Carneiro F, Seruca R, et al. Microsatellite instability in hyperplastic and adenomatous polyps of the stomach. Cancer 1999;86:1649-56.

281. Arnason T, Lauwers GY. Extruded highly proliferative benign mucous neck cells: a peculiar histologic mimic of poorly cohesive gastric carcinoma. Int J Surg Pathol 2014;22:623-8.

282. Rahman MA, Karam SM. Gastric parietal cell vacuolation mimicking gastric carcinoma. Histopathology 2013;63:735-7.

283. Wang K, Weinrach D, Lal A, et al. Signet-ring cell change versus signet-ring cell carcinoma: a comparative analysis. Am J Surg Pathol 2003;27:1429-33.

284. Boncher J, Bronner M, Goldblum JR, Liu X. Reticulin staining clarifies florid benign signet ring cell change with mitotic activity in a penetrating gastric ulcer. Am J Surg Pathol 2011;35:762-6.

DISEASES OF THE SMALL INTESTINE AND COLORECTUM

CONGENITAL ABNORMALITIES

Atresias and Stenoses

Definition. *Atresia* is the complete obliteration of the bowel lumen. *Stenosis* is segmental luminal narrowing.

Clinical Features. Intestinal atresias and stenoses affect approximately 1 in every 5,000 live births and are most common in the duodenum (1,2). Between 20 and 40 percent of duodenal atresias and stenoses develop in patients with Down syndrome; duodenal atresia is the most common gastrointestinal anomaly to occur in this population (3). Atresias also occur in combination with cardiovascular malformations, skeletal and limb deformities, VATER (vertebrate, anus, trachea, esophagus, renal) syndrome, and renal dysplasia (4–6). Multiple jejunoileal atresias and stenoses are common in patients with cystic fibrosis, biliary atresia, and immunodeficiencies (7). Colonic atresias occur in patients with Hirschsprung disease; rectal atresia is associated with sirenomelia (8,9).

Intestinal atresias are usually suspected at the time of fetal ultrasound owing to detection of polyhydramnios and bowel dilatation proximal to the atretic segment. Approximately 50 percent of cases are associated with elevated maternal serum alpha-fetoprotein (AFP) levels. Atresias and stenoses produce abdominal distention and vomiting shortly after birth; some patients develop meconium peritonitis. Duodenal atresias produce a characteristic "double bubble" sign on abdominal imaging, reflecting air in the stomach and duodenum proximal to the atresia (10). Lesions of the distal small bowel and colon are associated with distended loops of air-filled bowel proximal to the atresia.

Pathogenesis. Familial atresias are due to germline *TTC7A* mutations and are inherited in an autosomal recessive fashion (11). Atresias and stenoses also occur in combination with 17q12 deletions (4–6). Isolated cases likely result from *in utero* ischemia due to vascular accidents, intussusceptions, or intrapartum asphyxia.

Gross Findings. Atresias produce complete occlusion of the lumen, whereas stenoses appear as segmental narrowing or diaphragm-like strictures. Atretic segments can be completely separate from the distal bowel or connected by a fibrous cord. The proximal bowel is usually dilated (fig. 4-1A). Dull serosal discoloration is accompanied by hemorrhage, ulcers, and edema.

Microscopic Findings. Atretic and stenotic segments feature mural fibrosis and mucosal denudation. Calcified meconium may be accompanied by mixed inflammation (fig. 4-1B). The proximal bowel often displays ischemic mucosal injury with edema and ulcers.

Treatment and Prognosis. Initial treatment consists intravenous rehydration and nasogastric tube placement to remove gastroduodenal contents. Atresias require surgical resection, which is associated with an excellent prognosis. The mortality rate is less than 5 percent; complications are more common among patients with other congenital anomalies (12).

Duplication Cysts

Definitions. *Duplication cyst* is a tubular or cystic structure containing all layers of the intestinal wall and contiguous with the small bowel or colon. Synonyms include *enteric duplication cyst* and *enterogenous cyst*.

Clinical Features. Duplications occur throughout the gastrointestinal tract: they are most common in the ileum (60 percent) followed by the foregut (30 percent) and colorectum (10 percent). Multiple duplications occur in 10 to 20 percent of affected patients. The prevalence is 0.0002 percent in the general population; boys are more often affected.

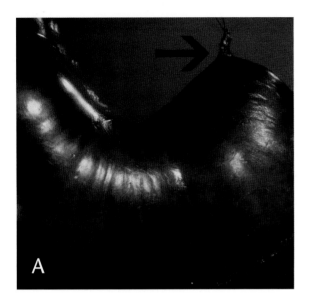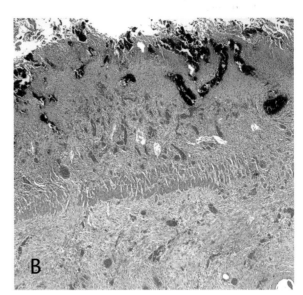

Figure 4-1

JEJUNAL ATRESIA

The jejunum proximal to the atresia (arrow) is distended and discolored secondary to ischemia (A). Atretic segments display replacement of the muscularis propria by fibrosis, granulation tissue, and calcifications (B).

Symptomatic lesions usually present within the first 2 years of life and cause bowel obstruction secondary to direct compression, intussusception, or volvulus (13). Duodenal duplications can compress the biliary tree, resulting in jaundice or pancreatitis (14). Erosion of the cyst lining manifests with chronic blood loss and iron deficiency anemia.

Pathogenesis. Most duplications result from aberrant recanalization of the gut lumen during the second to third months of embryogenesis. Less commonly, they develop following incomplete separation of the primitive gut from the notochord. Intrauterine ischemia may play a pathogenic role in some cases.

Gross Findings. Enterocolic duplications are cystic intramural lesions that frequently communicate with the lumen (fig. 4-2). They contain all layers of the bowel wall. The mucosa may be normal, although it is often denuded.

Microscopic Findings. As stated, duplication cysts contain all layers of the bowel wall (fig. 4-3A). They are lined by cuboidal to columnar enteric epithelium with variable inflammation (fig. 4-3B). Small intestinal duplications feature variable villous architectural abnormalities. Ciliated epithelial cells and gastric heterotopias may be present (fig. 4-3C,D).

Treatment and Prognosis. Enterocolic duplication cysts are frequently resected due to the risk of developing neoplasia (15,16). Symptomatic lesions compressing the biliary tree can be managed by creating a transduodenal window between the duodenum and the duplication.

Congenital Diverticula and Remnants of the Vitelline Duct

Definition. A *diverticulum* is a mural outpouching containing all layers of the intestinal wall. *Vitelline duct remnants* are diverticula, cysts, or fibrous cords representing incompletely involuted vitelline (omphalomesenteric) ducts. Synonyms include *true diverticulum* for congenital diverticulum and *Meckel diverticulum* and *umbilical fistula* for vitelline duct remnant.

Clinical Features. Almost all congenital diverticula of the distal small intestine are Meckel diverticula. They occur in 2 percent of the population and show a predilection for males. Only 2 percent produce symptoms, usually in the form of abdominal pain or gastrointestinal bleeding (5). Abdominal pain results from inversion of the diverticulum, which forms the lead point of an intussusception. Meckel diverticula containing exuberant gastric heterotopias can develop peptic ulcers and are an important consideration

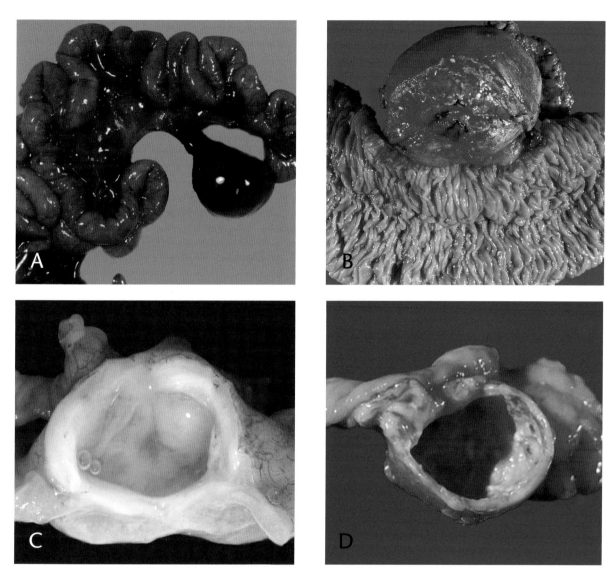

Figure 4-2

INTESTINAL DUPLICATION CYSTS

A large duplication cyst is continuous with the small intestine (A). (Courtesy of Dr. D. Beneck, New York, NY.) Another cystic duplication is intimately associated with the small intestinal wall (B). Cross sections demonstrate continuity of the cyst wall with the muscularis propria of the small bowel (C). Colonic duplication produces a large cyst in the muscularis propria (D).

in young patients with abdominal pain and intestinal bleeding.

Other congenital diverticula develop throughout the length of the intestine. Most are asymptomatic. Large lesions compress adjacent structures, producing vague abdominal symptoms. Diverticula with ulcers are detected due to iron deficiency anemia or bleeding.

Pathogenesis. Meckel diverticula occur when the vitelline duct is incompletely obliterated

during embryogenesis (17). Other diverticula probably result from incomplete recanalization of the gut during embryogenesis, similar to duplications.

Gross Findings. Meckel diverticula are located within 2 meters of the ileocecal valve. They appear as blind-ended pouches, cysts, or variably fibrotic cords, and may be attached to the abdominal wall (fig. 4-4A). Those with acid-related perforation feature fibrin plaques and erythema on the serosa, particularly at the

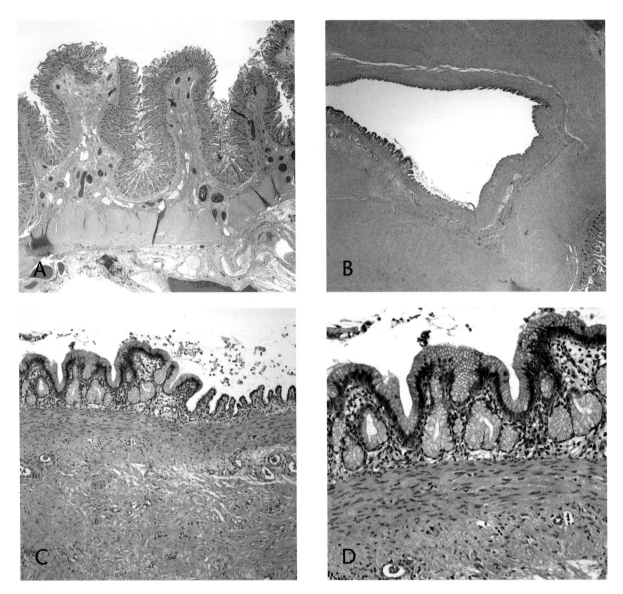

Figure 4-3

INTESTINAL DUPLICATION CYSTS

This cyst is lined by nearly normal small intestinal mucosa supported by thick, fibrotic submucosa (A). Another enteric duplication is present in the muscularis propria of the small bowel (B). The attenuated mucosa (C) is surfaced by gastric-type epithelium (D).

base of the diverticulum (fig. 4-4B). Those that drain to the skin surface cause local irritation.

Microscopic Findings. Meckel diverticula contain all layers of the intestinal wall (fig. 4-5A). Persistent vitelline arteries are often identified in the submucosa and more than half of cases harbor ectopic gastric or pancreatic tissue (fig. 4-5B). The former secrete acid that causes ulcers at the junction between gastric

and enteric mucosa. Ulcers overlying large caliber arteries can lead to severe gastrointestinal bleeding (fig. 4-5C,D). Omphalomesenteric duct remnants that extend to the skin surface form an umbilical polyp that may contain a fibrous cord, inflamed sinus tract, or gastroenteric epithelium (fig. 4-6).

Congenital diverticula contain all layers of the intestinal wall and feature variable mucosal

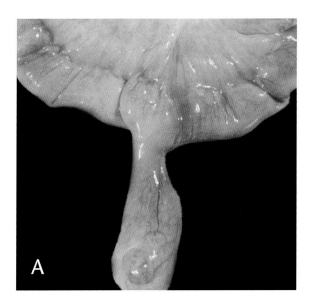 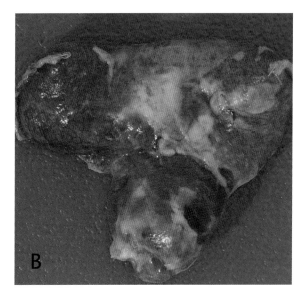

Figure 4-4

MECKEL DIVERTICULA

A long, blind-ended diverticulum is present on the antimesenteric aspect of the small bowel (A). Diverticula that contain gastric mucosa develop peptic ulcers accompanied by fibrin plaques at the junction between the diverticulum and the small intestine (B).

inflammation and architectural distortion. Occasional cases show segmental hyperplasia of interstitial cells of Cajal that replaces the muscularis propria and predisposes to perforation (fig. 4-7) (18,19).

Treatment and Prognosis. Symptomatic diverticula are generally resected. Management of asymptomatic diverticula is somewhat controversial. Congenital diverticula are prone to inflammation and can occasionally give rise to neoplasms (20).

Heterotopias

Heterotopias are structurally normal elements in an abnormal location. Synonyms include *ectopic tissue* and *choristoma*.

Gastric Heterotopia. Congenital rests of gastric mucosa occur throughout the small bowel and colon, as well as in congenital diverticula and cysts, particularly Meckel diverticula (17). Most are located in the duodenal bulb where they are endoscopically inapparent or form velvety, occasionally confluent plaques (fig. 4-8) (21). Small polyps and microscopic foci are asymptomatic, whereas larger ones are more likely to cause bleeding, obstruction, intussusception, or malabsorption. Rectal heterotopias appear as small polyps and plaques. Pain, itching, or bleeding result from mucosal irritation due to acid-related injury (22,23).

Mucosal heterotopias feature lobules of tightly packed oxyntic glands surfaced by foveolar epithelium (fig. 4-9). Large, pedunculated polyps subjected to luminal trauma contain variably dilated oxyntic glands separated by arborizing smooth muscle cell bundles that emanate from the muscularis propria, as well as submucosal fibrosis (fig. 4-10). Lesions in the proximal duodenum can be colonized by *Helicobacter pylori* when patients also have *H. pylori*-related chronic gastritis (24). Large ileal heterotopias frequently show features of ischemic injury due to intussusception (fig. 4-11).

Treatment of asymptomatic heterotopias is unnecessary but large lesions that bleed or obstruct the lumen are generally removed. Adenocarcinomas can rarely develop in heterotopic mucosa (25).

Pancreatic Heterotopia. Enterocolic pancreatic heterotopias occur most commonly in the proximal duodenum, followed in frequency by congenital cysts and diverticula. They may be confined to the mucosa, in which case they produce no symptoms, or involve the deeper wall. Mural lesions can cause symptoms related to inflammation or intussusception. They show a predilection for the periampullary region and

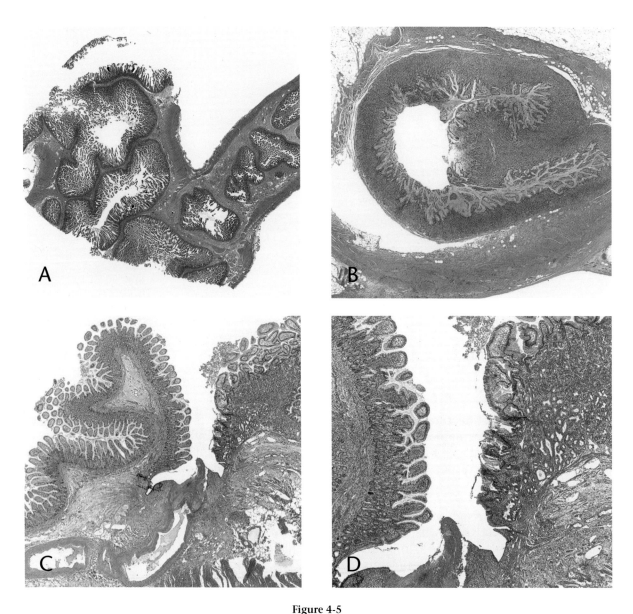

Figure 4-5

MECKEL DIVERTICULA

The diverticulum is continuous with the small bowel lumen and contains all the layers of the intestinal wall (A). Another diverticulum contains confluent sheets of oxyntic glands (B). Large gastric heterotopias (right) cause peptic ulcers at the base of the diverticulum (C) that can erode into large caliber submucosal arteries and cause hemorrhage (D).

minor papilla where they are prone to chronic pancreatitis, particularly among adult males with a history of alcohol use. Affected patients usually have a normal pancreas, raising the possibility that variant ductal anatomy near the papilla predisposes them to a localized form of alcohol-induced pancreatitis (26).

Pancreatic heterotopias represent remnants that separate from the embryonic pancreas during fore-gut rotation. Those confined to the mucosa and superficial submucosa consist of acini arranged in lobules. Acini contain polarized cells with amphophilic or basophilic granular cytoplasm and basal nuclei (fig. 4-12). Pancreatic islets are seen in one third of cases; lesions composed entirely of endocrine cells are uncommon.

Mural heterotopias can simulate the normal pancreas, but usually display some degree of

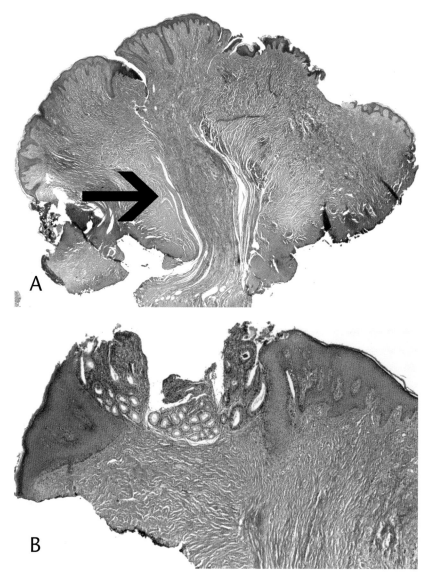

Figure 4-6

OMPHALOMESENTERIC DUCT REMNANT

Incomplete involution of the omphalomesenteric duct forms a cellular fibrous cord (arrow) and an umbilical polyp (A). Foci of residual gastroenteric mucosa can be present on the skin surface (B).

parenchymal atrophy and chronic pancreatitis. Severe pancreatitis with acinar atrophy leads to variably dilated ductal elements enmeshed in fibromuscular stroma that may create a polypoid mass (fig. 4-13). Such lesions have been termed *myoepithelial hamartoma, adenomyoma, cystic dystrophy of heterotopic pancreas, groove pancreatitis,* and *paraduodenal pancreatitis* (fig. 4-14). The latter designation is preferable because it most closely describes the pathogenesis of this lesion (26,27).

Large heterotopias commonly feature low-grade pancreatic intraepithelial neoplasia, but malignant transformation is rare (28). Virtually every type of neoplasm that can develop in the

pancreas has been reported to occur in large mural pancreatic heterotopias (28–30).

DISORDERS OF INFANCY AND EARLY CHILDHOOD

Microvillus Inclusion Disease

Definition. *Microvillus inclusion disease* is a heritable malabsorptive disorder resulting from failed development of the small intestinal brush border. Synonyms include *Davidson disease, congenital microvillus atrophy,* and *familial enteropathy.*

Clinical Features. Patients present with intractable diarrhea and an inability to absorb

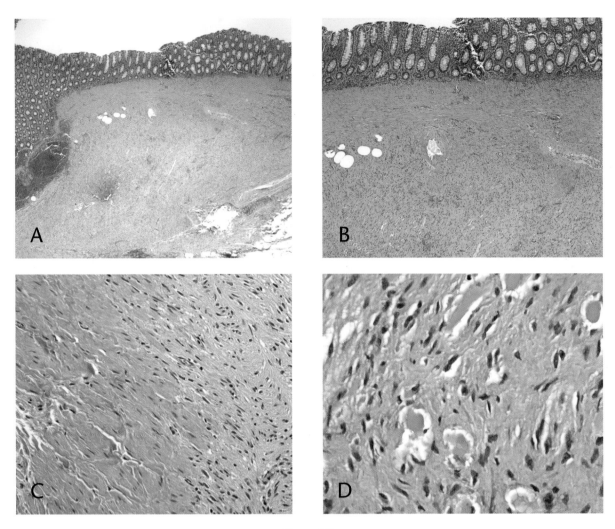

Figure 4-7

CONGENITAL DIVERTICULUM OF THE COLON

Congenital enteric diverticula contain all layers of the bowel wall (A) and may feature hyperplasia of interstitial cells of Cajal that replace the muscularis propria (B). Hyperplastic foci (right) of interstitial cells of Cajal closely resemble the cells of gastrointestinal stromal tumors (C), including skeinoid fibers (D).

Figure 4-8

GASTRIC HETEROTOPIA

Gastric heterotopias are most common in the proximal duodenum where they form polyps and plaques.

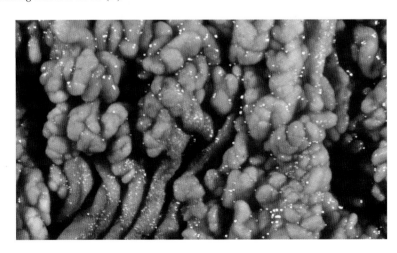

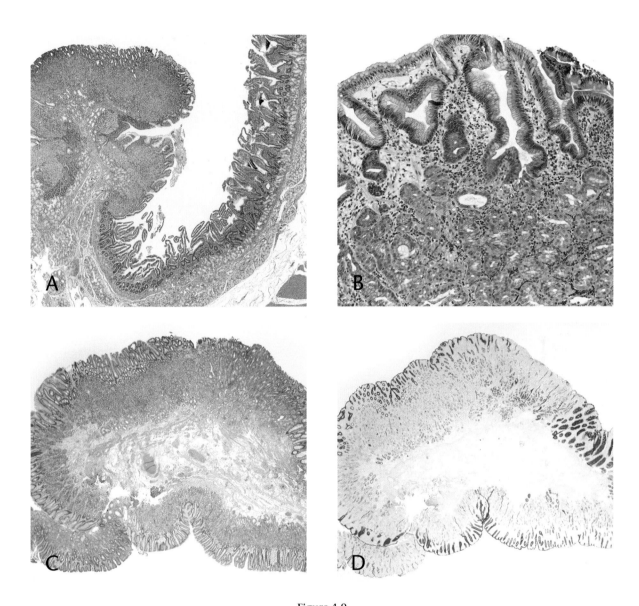

Figure 4-9

GASTRIC HETEROTOPIAS

Mucosa-based rests have a polypoid appearance (A) and are surfaced by foveolar epithelium (B). Rectal lesions also contain oxyntic glands and may be large (C). Alcian blue/periodic acid–Schiff with diastase (PAS-D) stains distinguish the neutral mucin-containing foveolar lining cells from acid mucin-rich colonocytes (D). (Courtesy of Dr. E. Montgomery, Baltimore, MD.)

nutrients within the first few days of life. These symptoms are accompanied by electrolyte imbalances, metabolic acidosis, and dehydration.

Pathogenesis. Microvillus inclusion disease displays an autosomal recessive pattern of inheritance and results from defects in *MYO5B*. The product of this gene facilitates trafficking of apical transporters that, when dysregulated, lead to malabsorption (31). Occasional cases have been linked to alterations affecting *STXBP2* and *STX3*,

both of which produce proteins involved in transport across the enterocyte membrane (32).

Gross and Microscopic Findings. Endoscopic examination may be normal or reveal loss of villi. Duodenal samples feature slightly blunted villi with crypt hyperplasia and minimal, if any, lamina propria inflammation. Intraepithelial lymphocytosis is lacking. Epithelial cells at the villous tips show mild nuclear irregularities but the most striking finding is patchy or diffuse loss

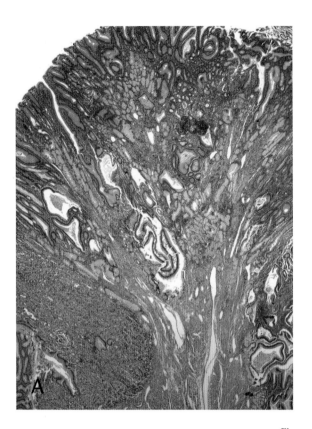
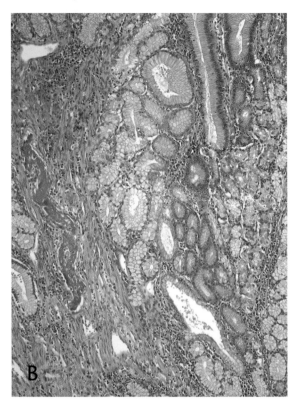

Figure 4-10

GASTRIC HETEROTOPIA

Large gastric heterotopias are subject to luminal trauma and may develop superimposed inflammatory changes. Bundles of smooth muscle cells emanate from the muscularis mucosae (A) and fibrin thrombi in submucosal vessels (B).

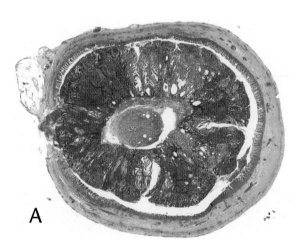
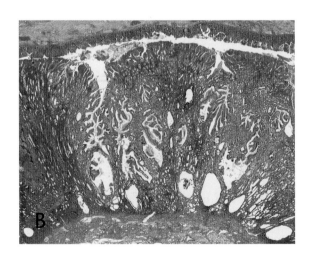

Figure 4-11

GASTRIC HETEROTOPIA

A large gastric heterotopia forms the lead point of an intussusception (A). Erosions and mucosal hemorrhage obscure ectopic gastric glands (B).

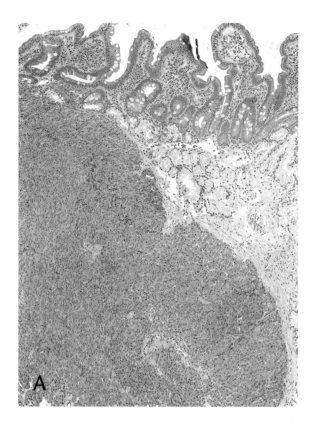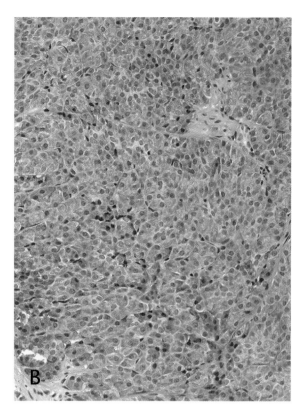

Figure 4-12

PANCREATIC HETEROTOPIA

Lobules of heterotopic pancreatic tissue are frequently encountered in the duodenal mucosa and submucosa (A). They contain tightly packed acini consisting of polarized cells with granular eosinophilic or basophilic cytoplasm (B).

of the villous brush border with small vacuoles in the superficial cytoplasm (fig. 4-15).

Immunostains for CD10, polyclonal carcinoembryonic antigen (CEA), and villin demonstrate patchy loss of the brush border with staining of microvillus components within cytoplasmic vacuoles (fig. 4-16A) (33,34). Fragmented microvilli are periodic acid–Schiff (PAS) positive, diastase resistant, and visible with electron microscopy (fig. 4-16B) (35).

Treatment and Prognosis. Left untreated, microvillus inclusion disease is generally fatal. Patients require parenteral nutrition or small intestinal transplantation. Those receiving parenteral nutrition are at risk for hepatic complications and infections.

Congenital Tufting Enteropathy

Definition. *Congenital tufting enteropathy* is a heritable malabsorptive disorder resulting from

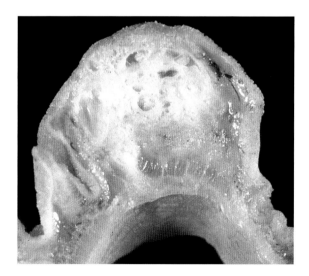

Figure 4-13

PANCREATIC HETEROTOPIA

Large ectopic rests undergo progressive fibrosis and atrophy of acinar elements accompanied by cystic dilation of pancreatic ductules and smooth muscle hyperplasia.

183

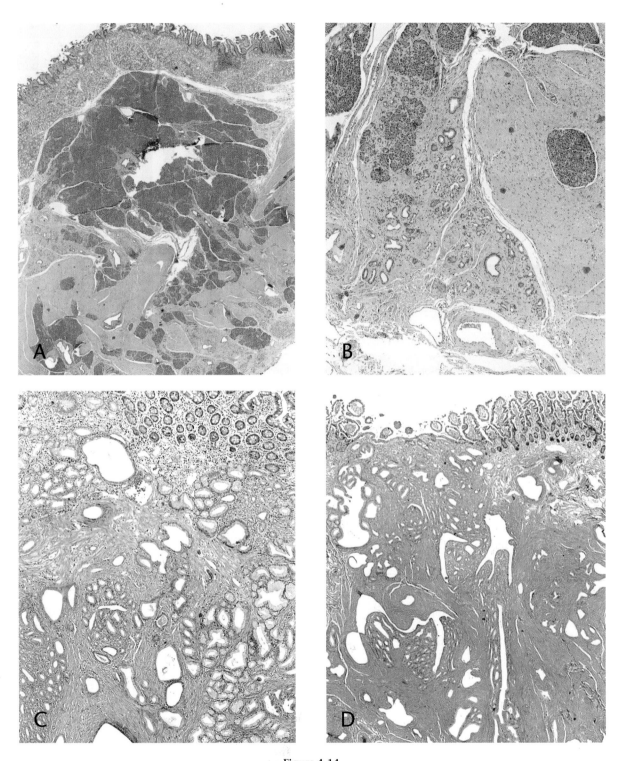

Figure 4-14

PANCREATIC HETEROTOPIA

Ectopic pancreatic tissue in the wall near the ampulla is associated with thick bundles of smooth muscle cells (A) and scattered ductules (B). Atrophy of acini leads to a proliferation of dilated ductules in fibromuscular stroma (C) that can become quite large and simulate a neoplasm (D).

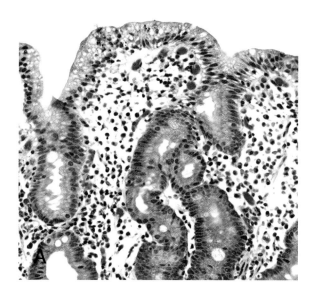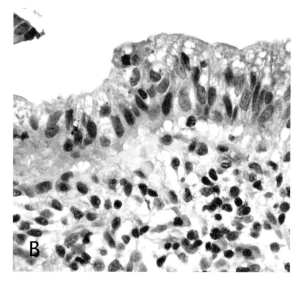

Figure 4-15

MICROVILLUS INCLUSION DISEASE

Villous blunting is associated with crypt hyperplasia, normal cellularity of the lamina propria, and vacuolated surface enterocytes (A). Nuclei in the superficial epithelium are slightly disorganized and accompanied by cellular debris, as well as cytoplasmic vacuoles in the apical cytoplasm (B). (Courtesy of Dr. J. Goldsmith, Boston, MA.)

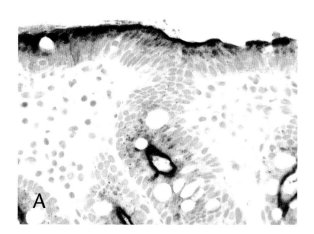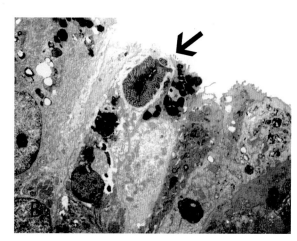

Figure 4-16

MICROVILLUS INCLUSION DISEASE

An immunostain for CD10 stains the brush border with accumulation of CD10-positive microvilli in the cytoplasm (A). (Courtesy of Dr. J. Goldsmith, Boston, MA.) Ultrastructural analysis demonstrates microvilli (arrow) in apical cytoplasmic vacuoles (B). (Courtesy of Dr. J. Hart, Chicago, IL.)

defective enterocytes. Synonyms include *intestinal epithelial dysplasia* and *congenital enteropathy*.

Clinical Features. Congenital tufting enteropathy is a rare disorder with a prevalence of 1 per 50,000 to 100,000 births, although it is more common in groups with higher rates of consanguinity

(36). Affected patients present a few months after birth with severe intractable diarrhea, electrolyte imbalances, and dehydration (37). Chronic intestinal insufficiency leads to failure to thrive. Although some patients have isolated diarrheal symptoms, others have a syndromic form of

185

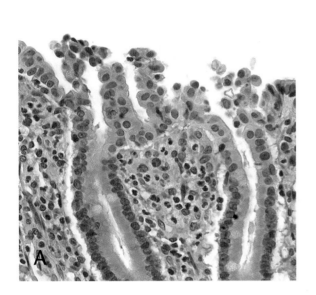
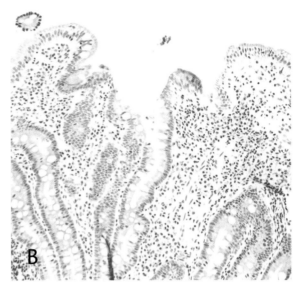

Figure 4-17

CONGENITAL TUFTING ENTEROPATHY

Surface epithelial cells show cytoplasmic depletion. They are dyshesive, forming tufted cell clusters at the surface (A). An immunostain demonstrates complete loss of membranous EPCAM staining (B). (Courtesy of Dr. J. Goldsmith, Boston, MA.)

disease manifested by keratitis, dysmorphic features, and skeletal dysplasia. Prenatal testing may be offered to families with an affected member, but is not widely used as a screening tool due to the infrequent nature of the disorder.

Pathogenesis. Congenital tufting enteropathy is inherited in an autosomal recessive manner. Nearly 75 percent of affected patients have *EPCAM* mutations that lead to abnormal enterocyte differentiation (38,39). Slightly more than 20 percent of patients have *SPINT2* mutations, which encodes HAI-2, a serine protease inhibitor that normally inhibits prostasin and other proteases on the cell membrane (40). Mutations in *EPCAM* are associated with diarrheal symptoms alone, whereas *SPINT2* mutations underlie the syndromic form of disease (41).

Gross Findings. Endoscopic examination may be completely normal or demonstrate mucosal atrophy with villous flattening.

Microscopic Findings. Duodenal samples feature villous blunting associated with crypt hyperplasia and increased mitotic activity (fig. 4-17A). Enterocytes are crowded and disorganized; buds or tufts of epithelial cells are scattered along the surface (fig. 4-17B). The lamina propria contains normal numbers of inflammatory cells or shows slightly increased cellularity.

Immunohistochemical stains demonstrate complete loss of EPCAM staining in the surface epithelia of patients with germline *EPCAM* mutations (42). Abnormal EPCAM loss and epithelial tufts can also be seen in gastric and colonic mucosae (fig. 4-18) (43).

Treatment and Prognosis. Oral and enteric feedings worsen diarrheal symptoms and, as a result, most patients require parenteral nutrition. Unfortunately, long-term parenteral nutrition can cause hepatic fibrosis and may not be sufficient to maintain nutritional status. Small intestinal transplantation is often considered in affected patients.

Abetalipoproteinemia

Definition. *Abetalipoproteinemia* is an enteropathy characterized by decreased absorption of fats and fat-soluble vitamins. Synonyms include *Bassen-Kornzweig syndrome, low-density lipoprotein deficiency*, and *microsomal triglyceride transfer protein deficiency*.

Clinical Features. Patients typically present in infancy with steatorrhea, malabsorption, vomiting, and failure to thrive. The diagnosis is suspected based on lipid profile results. Affected patients have absent or extremely diminished levels of chylomicrons, very low-density

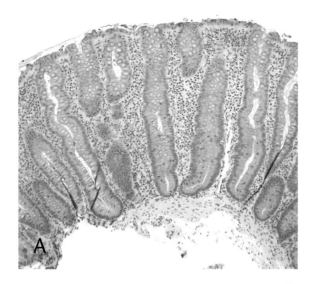 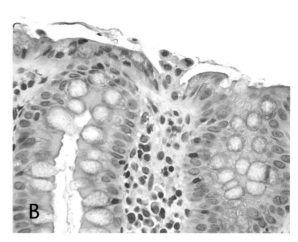

Figure 4-18

CONGENITAL TUFTING ENTEROPATHY

The disorder can cause abnormalities in the colon (A). Small tufts of disorganized epithelial cells are present at the surface (B). (Courtesy of Dr. J. Goldsmith, Boston, MA.)

lipoprotein (VLDL), low-density lipoprotein (LDL), cholesterol, triglycerides, and apolipoprotein (44). Hematologic manifestations include acanthocytosis, anemia, and reticulocytosis; red blood cell abnormalities can lead to hemolysis and hyperbilirubinemia. Increased international normalized ratio (INR) reflects malabsorption of fat-soluble vitamins.

Pathogenesis. Abetalipoproteinemia is inherited in an autosomal recessive fashion and results from alterations in *MTTP*, which encodes microsomal triglyceride transfer protein. This protein plays an important role in very low-density lipoprotein synthesis and transport of apoprotein B from intestinal absorptive cells. Loss of function results in the virtual absence of apolipoprotein-containing lipoproteins in the blood (45).

Gross Findings. Lipid accumulation imparts yellow discoloration to the mucosa, although examination may be normal in some cases.

Microscopic Findings. The villous architecture is preserved or only mildly altered. Surface enterocytes contain apical fat vacuoles (fig. 4-19). Fine lipid vacuoles may also be present above the basement membrane.

Treatment and Prognosis. Treatment consists of a low-fat diet with oral supplementation of essential fatty acids and fat-soluble vitamins (A, D, E, and K). Untreated individuals may develop retinitis pigmentosa, vision loss, decreased deep tendon reflexes, loss of vibratory sense and proprioception, and muscle weakness. Ataxia can develop in young adulthood.

Enteroendocrine Cell Dysgenesis

Definition. *Enteroendocrine cell dysgenesis* is a congenital enteropathy associated with absence of intestinal endocrine cells. It is also termed *enteric anendocrinosis*.

Clinical Features. Infants present with intractable diarrhea and decreased absorption of all nutrients. Water absorption is normal. Similar to other congenital enteropathies, symptoms worsen with oral feedings.

Pathogenesis. Affected patients have germline *NEUROG3* mutations resulting in arrested development of endocrine cells in the small bowel and colon.

Gross and Microscopic Findings. The endoscopic examination is essentially normal. Small bowel samples feature normal villous architecture without increased lamina propria cellularity. Goblet cells and Paneth cells are present in normal numbers, but endocrine cells are markedly decreased or absent (fig. 4-20). Chromogranin immunostains reveal decreased numbers of positive cells, often with faint staining. Similar findings are present in

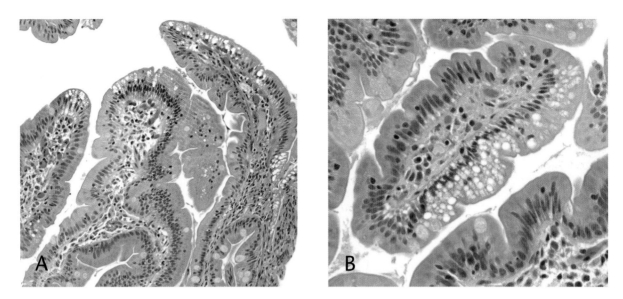

Figure 4-19

ABETALIPOPROTEINEMIA

The villous architecture is essentially normal, as is lamina propria cellularity (A). Clustered epithelial cells contain numerous small lipid vacuoles in their cytoplasm (B).

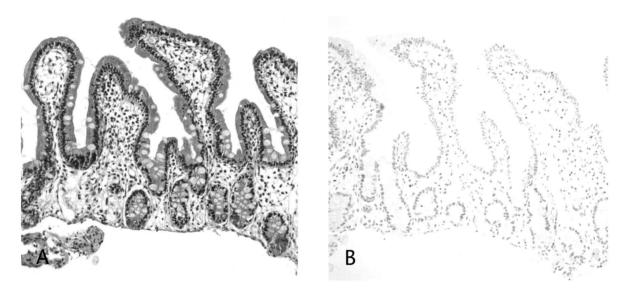

Figure 4-20

ENTEROENDOCRINE CELL DYSGENESIS

The proximal small bowel displays nearly normal villous architecture and lamina propria cellularity. Enterocytes, Paneth cells, and goblet cells are present in normal numbers (A) but chromogranin immunostains demonstrate an absence of endocrine cells (B). (Courtesy of Dr. G. Cortina, Los Angeles, CA.)

the colon, although gastric endocrine cells are generally present in normal numbers (46). Pathologic features that distinguish this entity from other childhood enteropathies are detailed in Table 4-1.

Treatment and Prognosis. Most patients require parenteral nutrition, which can cause hepatic fibrosis over time. Patients with hepatic complications and those with intestinal failure may undergo small intestinal transplantation.

Table 4-1

DISTINGUISHING FEATURES OF PAUCI-INFLAMMATORY CONGENITAL ENTEROPATHIES

Disorder	Epithelial Cell Abnormalities	Ancillary Stain Results	Underlying Defect
Microvillus inclusion disease	Loss of brush border Vacuoles in enterocytes	Vacuoles stain for PAS-D[a], villin, and CD10; cytoplasmic vacuoles contain microvilli	*MYO5B* mutations *STXBP2* and *STX3* changes
Congenital tufting enteropathy	Disorganized enterocytes with tufts of epithelium	Complete loss of EPCAM immuno-staining	*EPCAM* mutations
Abetalipoproteinemia	Numerous lipid vacuoles in enterocyte cytoplasm	Lipid accumulation can be confirmed with oil red O or Sudan black stains	*MTPP* mutations
Enteroendocrine cell dysgenesis	Decreased or absent endocrine cells	Decreased/absent chromogranin-positive cells in crypts	*NEUROG3* mutations

[a]PAS-D = periodic acid–Schiff with diastase.

Intestinal Aganglionosis

Definition. *Intestinal aganglionosis* is the absence of ganglion cells in myenteric and submucosal plexuses. Synonyms include *Hirschsprung disease* and *congenital megacolon.*

Clinical Features. Intestinal aganglionosis affects approximately 1 in 5,000 newborns (47). It is more common in patients with other congenital disorders and affects nearly 1 percent of children with trisomy 21 (3,9). Risk is also higher among siblings of affected children. Neonates present with delayed passage of meconium (after 48 hours) or explosive diarrhea upon digital rectal examination. Babies are more likely to develop signs and symptoms of intestinal obstruction or perforation compared with older patients. Children and adults present with a long history of abdominal distention and severe constipation that is not alleviated with medications (48). Additional symptoms include nausea and vomiting, unexplained fever, and failure to thrive. Imaging reveals an abrupt transition between the dilated colon proximal to the aganglionic segment and an absence of bowel gas in the affected distal region.

Pathogenesis. Intestinal aganglionosis results from disrupted neural crest cell development and migration. Its pathogenesis is linked to defects in a number of genes that regulate neural crest cell proliferation, differentiation, and survival, including *RET, GDNF, SOX10, SHH, PHOX2b, ZFHX1B, ET3, GFRα1, NRT,* and *EDNRB* (49). These alterations, however, are detected in only 50 percent of cases, suggesting that other mechanisms play substantial roles in the development of the disorder (50).

Gross Findings. Intestinal aganglionosis affects the bowel in a retrograde fashion: the distal rectum is always involved and the process variably extends into more proximal regions. Most patients have short segment aganglionosis limited to the distal colorectum. Some have aganglionosis affecting the entire colon or distal small bowel, and rare patients lack ganglion cells throughout the entire small bowel and colon. Resection specimens display narrowing in the region of aganglionosis with dilatation of the proximal bowel (fig. 4-21).

Microscopic Findings. Sections obtained from the aganglionic segment demonstrate a complete absence of ganglion cells in the myenteric and submucosal plexuses, often accompanied by neuronal hypertrophy (fig. 4-22). Detection of ganglion cells can be difficult, as they tend to be smaller and less conspicuous in samples from young children. The extreme distal end of the rectum is normally aganglionic; failure to detect ganglion cells in samples from within a centimeter of the anorectal transitional area should be considered inconclusive rather than evidence of aganglionosis (51).

Acetylcholinesterase stains performed on frozen tissue sections highlight abnormal cholinergic fibers in the muscularis mucosae and colonic lamina propria, although these stains are not widely available. Calretinin immunohistochemical stains are much easier to interpret and can be performed on formalin-fixed paraffin-embedded tissue. Calretinin normally stains ganglion cells and their associated neurites in the lamina propria and submucosa (52). Thus, the absence of calretinin-positive ganglion cells and nerve twigs is essentially diagnostic of intestinal aganglionosis in the appropriate setting (fig. 4-23) (53,54).

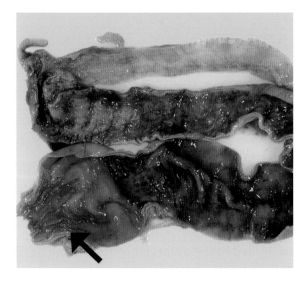

Figure 4-21

COLONIC AGANGLIONOSIS

The colon is markedly dilated (arrow) proximal to the aganglionic segment. (Courtesy of Dr. D. Beneck, New York, NY.)

Treatment and Prognosis. Intestinal aganglionosis requires surgical resection. A pull-through colectomy entails removal of the affected segment and anastomosis of the healthy bowel to the anus. Alternatively, patients undergo surgical resection of the bowel with creation of a temporary or permanent ostomy.

The prognosis following surgery is generally excellent. Some patients develop post-surgical anal stenosis, diarrhea or constipation, and anal leakage. Others develop intestinal aganglionosis-associated enterocolitis, either before or after surgery. This complication is a major cause of morbidity and mortality, and is characterized by megacolon with ulcers, mural necrosis, fever, abdominal distention, diarrhea, and sepsis. Treatment requires antibiotic therapy, bowel rest with hydration, and colonic irrigation (55).

Cystic Fibrosis

Definition. *Cystic fibrosis* is a systemic disorder characterized by thick, tenacious secretions of the respiratory tract and gastrointestinal tract.

Clinical Features. Cystic fibrosis is most common among individuals of Northern European descent and affects approximately 1 in 3,000 persons. The diagnosis is often suspected when newborn infants fail to pass meconium due to obstruction by thick mucoid secretions; meconium ileus occurs in approximately 20 percent of affected patients (56). Approximately 10 percent of affected

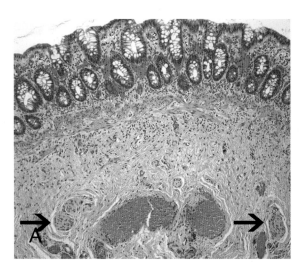

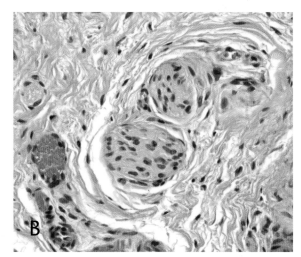

Figure 4-22

COLONIC AGANGLIONOSIS

An aganglionic segment contains hypertrophic nerves (arrows) in the submucosa (A) unaccompanied by ganglion cells (B).

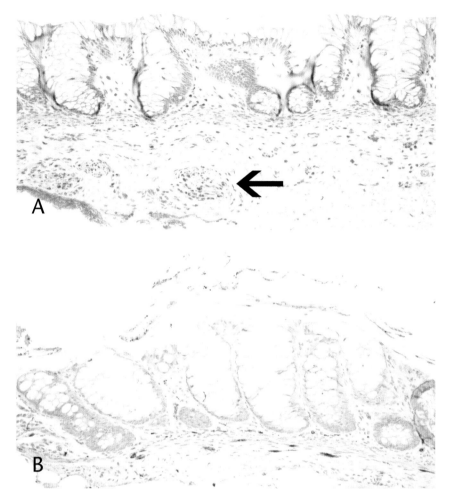

Figure 4-23

COLONIC AGANGLIONOSIS

A calretinin immunostain demonstrates hypertrophic submucosal nerves (arrow). There is no staining of submucosal ganglion cells or nerve twigs in the lamina propria (A). In contrast, the normal colon contains calretinin-positive ganglion cells in the submucosa and scattered neurites in the mucosa (B).

children develop rectal prolapse as a result of straining, with hard stools, malnutrition, and cough-induced increased intra-abdominal pressure (57). Thick secretions impede absorption, resulting in failure to thrive. Respiratory symptoms are more apparent in slightly older children, and pancreatic insufficiency often develops by adulthood. Newborn screening for elevated trypsinogen levels can direct further evaluation with sweat tests and genetic assessment.

Pathogenesis. Cystic fibrosis is an autosomal recessive heritable disorder that results from biallelic inactivation of *CFTR*. This gene encodes the cystic fibrosis transmembrane conductance regulator protein, which is a chloride ion channel.

Gross Findings. Bowel obstruction is caused by thick mucoid secretions that occlude the lumen and cause variable distention and necrosis.

Microscopic Findings. The bowel contains copious amounts of thick layered eosinophilic mu-

coid material (fig. 4-24). The mucosa is frequently normal or shows variably severe ischemic changes, depending on the interval between the onset of obstructive symptoms and surgical resection.

Treatment and Prognosis. Newborns with intestinal obstruction frequently require surgical resection, whereas adults are treated symptomatically with preparatory agents and pancreatic enzyme replacement. Recurrent infections necessitate chronic antibiotic therapy. End-stage lung and liver disease may lead to solid organ transplantation. Recent research efforts aimed at gene, phage, and small molecule therapies have met with limited success (58).

Necrotizing Enterocolitis

Definition. *Necrotizing enterocolitis* is intestinal necrosis affecting newborns.

Clinical Features. Necrotizing enterocolitis typically presents within the first 2 weeks of

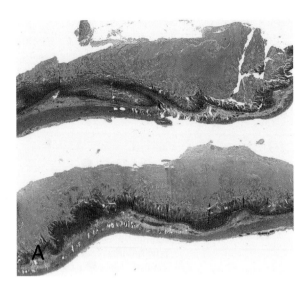
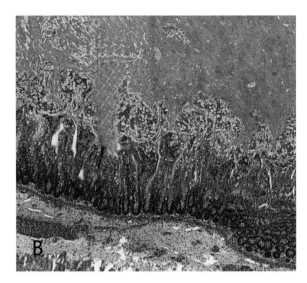

Figure 4-24

CYSTIC FIBROSIS

Thick, tenacious secretions cause luminal obstruction in cystic fibrosis patients (A). They consist of dense layers of eosinophilic mucus and are accompanied by mild inflammatory changes in the mucosa (B).

life. It is more common in premature babies, affecting 5 to 10 percent of infants weighing less than 1,500 grams (59). Risk is increased in formula-fed infants and those with congenital heart disease and or other comorbidities.

Symptoms include bloating, vomiting, bloody stools, and difficulty breathing. The disease may rapidly progress to perforation and peritonitis with systemic hypotension. Clinical signs include decreased bowel sounds and abdominal tenderness, radiographically evident visible pneumatosis intestinalis or portal venous air, and laboratory evidence of acidosis (60).

Pathogenesis. The mechanism by which necrotizing enterocolitis develops is not clear. Presumably, loss of mucosal integrity facilitates bacterial invasion of the intestinal wall. Sluggish blood flow through the region promotes infection and ischemic injury (61).

Gross Findings. Necrotizing enterocolitis causes abdominal distention, usually due to bowel dilatation. Affected intestinal segments show gray-green discoloration of the serosa with full-thickness necrosis (fig. 4-25).

Microscopic Findings. Surgical resection specimens display ischemic-type necrosis with mural necrosis. Older injuries feature calcifications, granulation tissue, and fibrosis of the muscularis propria.

Treatment and Prognosis. Premature infants are provided with small amounts of breast milk and probiotics while receiving intravenous nutrition in order to prevent necrotizing enterocolitis (62). Initial treatment of affected patients consists of bowel rest, decompression by nasogastric tube, intravenous fluids, and antibiotic therapy (63). Patients with progressive mural necrosis or perforation may be initially managed with peritoneal drainage or surgical resection of the affected bowel (59). Nearly 80 percent of infants with necrotizing enterocolitis survive. Complications include malabsorption, short gut syndrome, intestinal strictures, and developmental delays.

Inborn Errors of Metabolism

Definition. *Inborn errors of metabolism* are progressive neurodegenerative disorders due to abnormal accumulation of glycoproteins, lipids, and other cellular products.

Clinical Features. A variety of metabolic disorders are characterized by abnormal accumulation of glycoproteins and lipids, and have intestinal manifestations. Regardless of the underlying abnormality, presenting features are rarely limited to the gastrointestinal tract. Symptomatic patients frequently have developmental delays, hearing and visual impairment, and failure to thrive. Hepatosplenomegaly, coarse facial

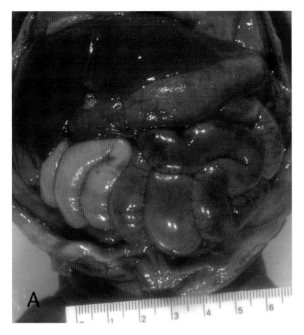 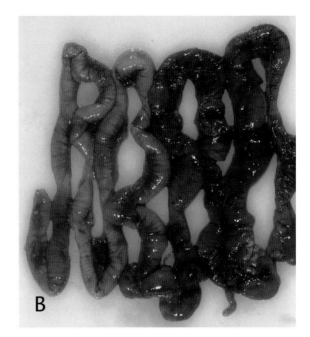

Figure 4-25

NECROTIZING ENTEROCOLITIS

A long segment of necrotic bowel is dusky green-gray and dilated (A). There is an abrupt transition between viable (left) and necrotic (right) areas in the mid small bowel (B). (Courtesy of Dr. D. Beneck, New York, NY.)

Table 4-2

INBORN ERRORS OF METABOLISM THAT FEATURE MACROPHAGE ACCUMULATION IN THE INTESTINAL MUCOSA

Disorder	Defective Protein	Accumulated Cell Product
Sialidosis	Neuraminidase	Sialyloligosaccharides
Wolman disease/cholesterol ester storage disease	Lysosomal acid lipase	Cholesterol and triglycerides
Fabry disease	Alpha-galactosidase A	Ceramide trihexosidase
Gangliosidoses	Hexosaminidase A	GM2 ganglioside
Niemann-Pick disease	Sphingomyelinase	Sphingomyelinase
Mucopolysaccharidoses (Hurler and Hunter syndrome)	Lysosomal enzymes that degrade mucopolysaccharides	Heparan sulfate and dermatan sulfate

features, skeletal abnormalities, and neurologic symptoms begin to develop within a year of birth.

Pathogenesis. Most inborn errors of metabolism are autosomal recessive disorders due to inherited genetic defects affecting a variety of enzymes. Accumulation of glycoproteins, lipids, and other molecules in macrophages, nerves, muscle, and other cell types leads to clinical symptoms (Table 4-2).

Microscopic Findings. Biopsy findings include expansion of the lamina propria by aggregates of foamy macrophages that show variable staining for PAS-D (fig. 4-26). Biopsy samples that include the submucosa and its nerve plexus may facilitate the diagnosis of the gangliosidoses. Ultimate classification of disease requires a combination of lysosomal enzyme activity assays and molecular tests.

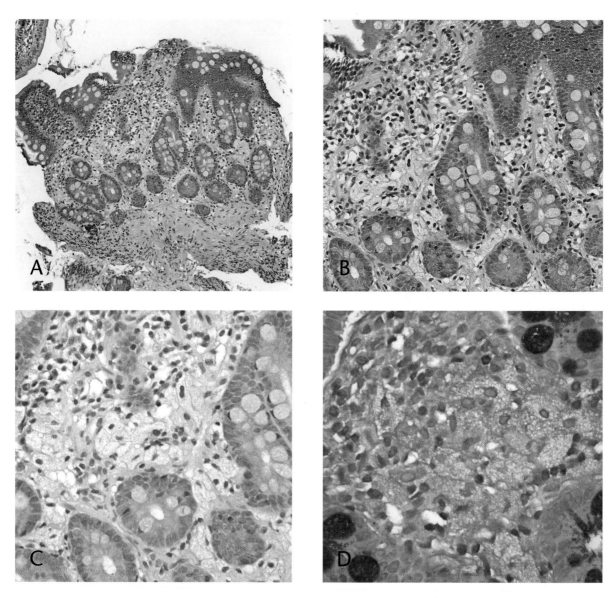

Figure 4-26

SIALIDOSIS

Inborn errors of metabolism affecting neuraminidase function lead to accumulation of sialyloligosaccharides in macrophages (A). Foamy macrophages are dispersed between the crypts throughout the colon, rather than confined to the superficial mucosa of the distal rectum, as is typical of muciphages (B). Aggregates of macrophages are unaccompanied by increased numbers of other inflammatory cell types (C) and show weak PAS-D staining (D).

Treatment and Prognosis. Treatment options are limited and mostly directed at supportive care. Efforts are made to maximize nutrition and seizure control.

Primary Intestinal Lymphangiectasia

Definition. *Primary intestinal lymphangiectasia* (also termed *Waldmaan disease*) is a progressive disorder resulting from congenital malformation of the lymphatic system.

Clinical Features. Primary intestinal lymphangiectasia is uncommon and fewer than 200 cases have been reported in the literature. The disease shows a slight female predilection. It presents in infancy with diarrhea, protein-losing enteropathy, lower extremity edema, chylous ascites, and failure to thrive (64). Some patients have autoimmune polyglandular disorder type 1, DiGeorge syndrome, thymic hypoplasia, Noonan syndrome, or nephrotic syndrome. Patients often have multiple serologic abnormalities, including hypoproteinemia, lymphopenia, decreased immunoglobulin, low numbers of circulating CD4-positive T-cells, deficiencies in fat-soluble vitamins, and hypocalcemia. Ascitic fluid is high in triglycerides with low levels of albumin. Imaging reveals thickened mucosal folds and distended small bowel loops (65).

Pathogenesis. Primary intestinal lymphangiectasia reflects a structural abnormality in the lymphatic system that leads to progressive dilatation and tortuosity of lymphatic channels and lymph stasis.

Gross Findings. Dilated lacteals are endoscopically apparent, producing white dots, nodules, or plaques that tend to be most pronounced on the crests of edematous mucosal folds (fig. 4-27). They frequently leak chylous fluid when sampled.

Microscopic Findings. Dilated endothelium-lined lymphatic channels permeate the mucosa and submucosa, resulting in variably bulbous villi. Lymphatic channels contain faintly eosinophilic proteinaceous material accompanied by foamy macrophages on a background of normal mucosa (fig. 4-28).

Differential Diagnosis. The differential diagnosis includes secondary, or acquired, intestinal lymphangiectasia, which results from chronic outflow obstruction. Most affected patients are asymptomatic adults with underlying disorders such as cardiac disease, prior liver transplantation, radiation therapy, Crohn disease, or retroperitoneal lymphadenopathy. Endoscopic and histologic changes are similar to those of primary intestinal lymphangiectasia but tend to be localized.

Treatment and Prognosis. Patients with primary intestinal lymphangiectasia usually require nutritional therapy with high protein diets and low levels of triglycerides. Parenteral nutrition may be of benefit in some patients. Somatostatin analogues may slow motility to enhance protein absorption, while diuretics and paracentesis can be used to minimize fluid overload (66). Patients are also at increased risk for infection due to hypogammaglobulinemia. Those

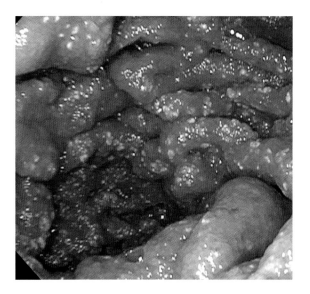

Figure 4-27

INTESTINAL LYMPHANGIECTASIA

Lymphangiectasias appear as small yellow flecks on the mucosal surface.

with concomitant pulmonary manifestations may develop chylothorax and respiratory failure.

Protein Allergy

Definition. Hypersensitivity to proteins in cow's milk, soy milk, or breast milk is termed *protein allergy.* Synonyms include *allergic proctocolitis* and *milk protein allergy.*

Clinical Features. Protein allergy is common, affecting 2 to 5 percent of formula-fed infants and approximately 0.5 percent of breast-fed infants. Most patients present within weeks to months after birth, although symptoms may manifest in children up to 2 years of age. Symptoms include diarrhea, rectal bleeding, and failure to thrive (67). Some patients have systemic manifestations with wheezing, coughing, and urticaria. Potential allergens can be tested with a skin prick test. Small amounts of protein are injected into the skin and the appearance of a rash or urticaria is used to identify specific sensitivities. Serologic abnormalities include peripheral eosinophilia with elevated serum IgE levels.

Pathogenesis. Protein allergy results from an IgE-mediated type 1 hypersensitivity reaction. Mast cells are stimulated to degranulate when bound to IgE, resulting in recruitment of eosinophils.

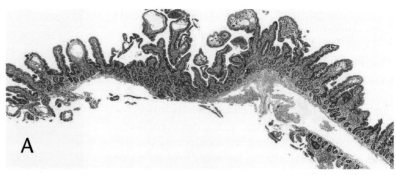

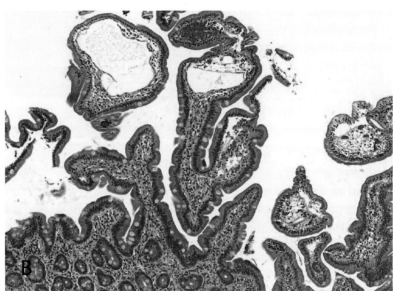

Figure 4-28

PRIMARY INTESTINAL LYMPHANGIECTASIA

Numerous large villi (A) are distended by dilated lymphatic channels (B).

Gross Findings. Most infants undergo examination of the rectosigmoid colon alone, although more diffuse inflammatory changes are likely present. The mucosa displays a decreased vascular pattern with edema, nodularity, erythema, friability, erosions, and occasional ulcers.

Microscopic Findings. Biopsy samples display increased mucosal eosinophils, often in excess of 60 per high-power field, accompanied by neutrophilic or eosinophil-rich crypt abscesses and cryptitis. Eosinophils tend to be dispersed, rather than aggregated, in the lamina propria (fig. 4-29). The infiltrate is often patchy and, thus, multiple tissue samples may be required to establish a diagnosis (68).

Treatment and Prognosis. Treatment consists of dietary modification. Formula-fed babies may be offered hydrolyzed, casein-based formula, soy, or an elemental diet. Breastfeeding mothers with symptomatic babies may try modifying their own diets. Mild symptoms can be managed with antihistamines, whereas anaphylaxis can be treated with epinephrine injection.

VASCULAR ABNORMALITIES AND ISCHEMIC ENTEROCOLITIS

Caliber-Persistent Artery

Definition. *Caliber-persistent artery* is an abnormally large caliber artery in the submucosa. Synonyms include *Dieulafoy lesion*, *exulceratio simplex*, *submucosal arterial malformation*, and *cirsoid aneurysm*.

Clinical Features. Caliber-persistent arteries account for less than 5 percent of all episodes of nonvariceal upper gastrointestinal tract bleeding in adult patients (69). They show a predilection to affect older men with chronic renal insufficiency, chronic liver disease, cardiovascular disease, alcohol use, and other comorbidities (70,71). Chronic nonsteroidal anti-inflammatory drug (NSAID) use and anticoagulant therapy

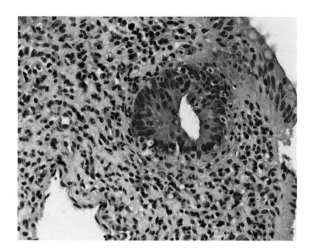

Figure 4-29

MILK PROTEIN ALLERGY

Neutrophilic cryptitis is accompanied by eosinophil-rich inflammation in the lamina propria.

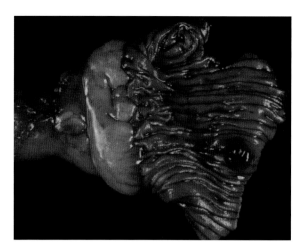

Figure 4-30

CALIBER-PERSISTENT ARTERY OF SMALL BOWEL

The lesion is a sharply circumscribed hemorrhagic nodule with a central nipple-like protrusion.

increase bleeding risk. Patients usually present with acute onset hematemesis or melena (72).

Pathogenesis. Large, pulsatile arteries in the submucosa irritate the mucosa, leading to erosions and potential hemorrhage. Occasional lesions bleed when primary inflammatory disorders, such as *H. pylori* infection, cause ulcers.

Gross Findings. Caliber-persistent arteries are most common in the stomach, particularly in the lesser curvature within 6 cm of the gastroesophageal junction, but they can occur anywhere in the gastrointestinal tract (70). They appear as violaceous submucosal polyps with adherent clot surrounded by erythema or erosions (fig. 4-30). They may show pulsatile flow during episodes of active bleeding.

Microscopic Findings. Caliber-persistent arteries are large with a diameter of 1 to 5 mm. Intimal hyperplasia and fibrinoid necrosis of the arterial wall are present at the bleeding site, but aneurysmal dilatation is lacking (fig. 4-31).

Treatment and Prognosis. Endoscopic therapy consists of sclerotherapy, electrocautery, argon plasma coagulation, band ligation, or hemoclip placement. Angiography can be used to identify and embolize the bleeding vessel. Surgical intervention with suture ligation is also effective; resection is reserved for patients who do not respond to other methods (73). Resolution of symptoms follows adequate therapy.

Telangiectasia

Definition. *Telangiectasia* is an acquired vascular proliferation composed of dilated capillaries and venules.

Clinical Features. Isolated telangiectasias are generally asymptomatic. Multiple lesions occur in patients with calcinosis, Raynaud phenomenon, esophageal dysmotility, sclerodactyly, and telangiectasia (CREST) syndrome, as well as in dialysis-dependent individuals who have end-stage renal disease. Patients with hereditary hemorrhagic telangiectasia develop telangiectasias and other vascular abnormalities of the gastrointestinal tract that cause substantial morbidity, as described below (74).

Pathogenesis. Telangiectasias presumably result from mural irregularities in small veins and venules. Loss of smooth muscle cells or the elastic lamina promotes vascular dilatation and blood pooling that lead to engorgement and red blood cell extravasation.

Gross Findings. Telangiectasias are flat, often stellate areas of vascular enhancement. They span only a few millimeters and do not entirely disappear upon compression owing to the presence of associated hemorrhage (fig. 4-32).

Microscopic Findings. Histologic sections reveal flat or slightly tufted mucosa containing aggregates of engorged capillaries and venules

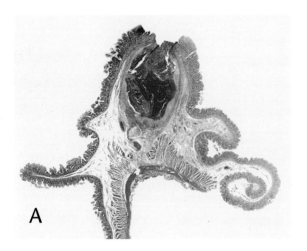
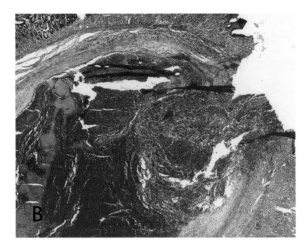

Figure 4-31

CALIBER-PERSISTENT ARTERY OF THE SMALL BOWEL

A massively enlarged artery is present in the submucosa and extends to the eroded mucosal surface (A). Mural fibrin deposits are present in the arterial wall at the bleeding site, but the artery does not show aneurysmal dilatation (B).

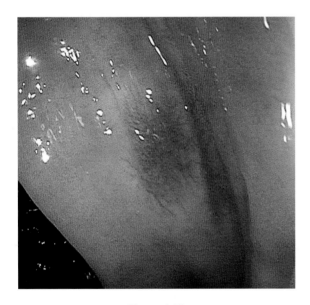
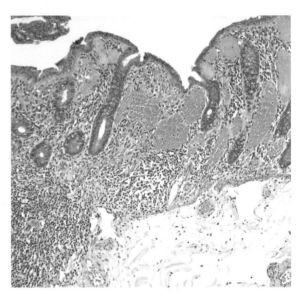

Figure 4-32

MUCOSAL TELANGIECTASIA

The lesion is small and flat. Tiny vessels emanate from the erythematous center.

Figure 4-33

MUCOSAL TELANGIECTASIA

The colonic mucosa is expanded and slightly raised due to the presence of numerous dilated, thin-walled vessels engorged with blood.

(fig. 4-33). Extravasated red blood cells are variably present in the lamina propria.

Differential Diagnosis. Telangiectasias resemble angiodysplasias and both types of lesions occur in the same patient populations, suggesting they are pathogenetically related. Distinguishing features of various benign vascular lesions are summarized in Table 4-3.

Treatment and Prognosis. Isolated telangiectasias require no treatment and patients have an excellent prognosis. Patients with multiple lesions are asymptomatic in many cases, although some individuals with numerous telangiectasias or additional vascular anomalies may require endoscopic ablation due to recurrent bleeding. The prognosis

Table 4-3

DISTINGUISHING FEATURES OF NON-NEOPLASTIC VASCULAR LESIONS OF THE SMALL INTESTINE AND COLON

	Telangiectasia	Angiodysplasia	Arteriovenous Malformation	Venous Malformation
Epidemiology	Acquired Present at any age	Acquired Increase with age	Congenital Present at any age	Congenital Grow with age
Associated disorders	HHT[a] Scleroderma	HHT Hemodialysis	HHT	Blue rubber bleb nevus syndrome
Endoscopic appearance	Small, erythematous Flat or slightly raised	Flat or slightly raised Delicate vessels	Large, multinodular Purple or red	Smooth, dome-shaped Blue or purple
Pathologic features	Superficial clusters of dilated capillaries and venules	Tortuous and thick submucosal veins Dilated mucosal vessels	Aggregates of thick-walled veins and and arteries	Aggregates of dilated veins in submucosa with extensive hemorrhage

[a]HHT = Hereditary hemorrhagic telangiectasia.

for patients with multifocal telangiectasias is determined by the nature of any associated conditions.

Angiodysplasia

Definition. *Angiodysplasia* is an acquired vascular lesion composed of small and medium-sized submucosal veins and venules.

Clinical Features. Angiodysplasia is the most common vascular anomaly of the gastrointestinal tract. It is a frequent cause of bleeding in elderly patients and those with dialysis-dependent renal failure (75,76). Most affected patients are over 60 years of age. Lesions may be associated with chronic or intermittent blood loss, although life-threatening acute hemorrhage occurs in 10 to 15 percent of patients (77). Bleeding risk is increased in patients with coagulation disorders.

Pathogenesis. Age-related laxity of connective tissues contributes to the development of angiodysplasia. Presumably, diminished support of vascular structures, combined with intermittent venous outflow obstruction during peristalsis, leads to elevated mural venous pressures (75). As a result, submucosal veins become progressively dilated and transmit increased pressure to mucosal venules and capillaries. The latter subsequently dilate, leading to incompetence of pre-capillary sphincters.

Gross Findings. Lesions are flat or slightly elevated and bright red (fig. 4-34). They usually occur in the colon and show a predilection for the right colon where wall tensions are greatest. Imaging techniques that facilitate a diagnosis include selective angiography of mesenteric arteries, radio-

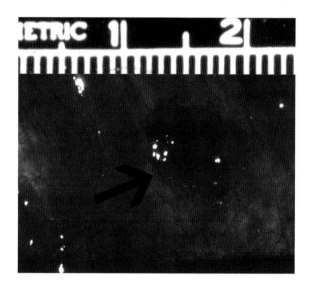

Figure 4-34

COLONIC ANGIODYSPLASIA

Angiodysplasias are round, slightly raised, erythematous lesions that span a few millimeters (arrow).

nuclide scanning, and helical CT angiography, as well as colonoscopy and capsule endoscopy.

Microscopic Findings. It is almost impossible to recognize angiodysplasias in endoscopically obtained biopsy material because most abnormal vessels are located in the submucosa where they are not amenable to sampling. Recognizing lesions in resection specimens can also be challenging; ectatic vessels are compressed following formalin fixation. Angiodysplasias are composed of disorganized aggregates of dilated, tortuous veins in the submucosa accompanied

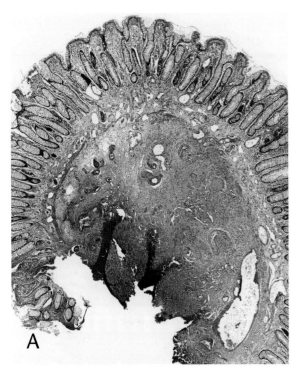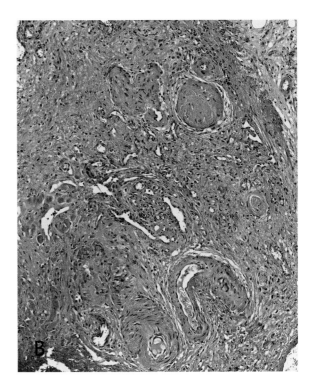

Figure 4-35

COLONIC ANGIODYSPLASIA

Large, irregularly shaped vessels are present in the submucosa and are accompanied by ectatic vascular spaces in the lamina propria (A). Aggregates of thick-walled veins and arteries display organizing thrombi and recanalization (B).

by variably dilated capillaries and venules that expand the mucosa (fig. 4-35).

Differential Diagnosis. The dilated mucosal vessels overlying angiodysplasias are indistinguishable from mucosal telangiectasias, although the former tend to be larger and contain disorganized vascular aggregates in the submucosa.

Treatment and Prognosis. Endoscopic treatment with argon plasma coagulation is usually effective. Alternatively, angiographic identification of actively bleeding lesions can be followed by highly selective embolization. Surgical resection is reserved for select patients with multiple lesions or uncontrolled bleeding. Pharmacologic treatment with thalidomide, somatostatin analogues, and other agents has gained popularity in some settings (78–80).

Arteriovenous Malformation

Definition. *Arteriovenous malformation* is a congenital anomaly featuring direct communications between arteries and veins.

Clinical Features. Arteriovenous malformations manifest at any age. Most patients present with acute or recurrent hemorrhage from the lower gastrointestinal tract. Some lesions are detected during evaluation of iron deficiency anemia. Individuals with multiple or large malformations may present with high-output cardiac failure due to arteriovenous shunting, or symptoms of portal hypertension that reflect direct communication between the portal venous system and arterial circulation. Individuals with heart failure who are managed with continuous-flow left ventricular assist devices are at increased bleeding risk (81). Multiple arteriovenous malformations occur in patients with hereditary hemorrhagic telangiectasia as well as in individuals who have juvenile polyposis syndrome due to *SMAD4* mutations (82).

Gross Findings. Arteriovenous malformations are red, dusky nodules or plaques that blanch with pressure and rapidly refill. Imaging reveals ill-defined segmental thickening due to

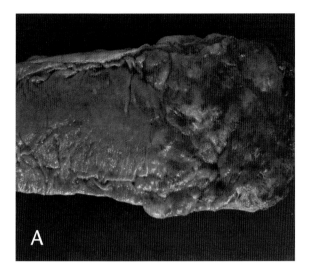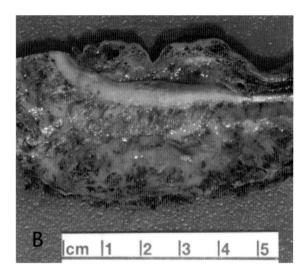

Figure 4-36

ARTERIOVENOUS MALFORMATION

A large arteriovenous malformation expands the rectal mucosa, imparting a blue, mottled appearance (A). The spongy mass expands the submucosa and extends through the muscularis propria into perirectal fat (B).

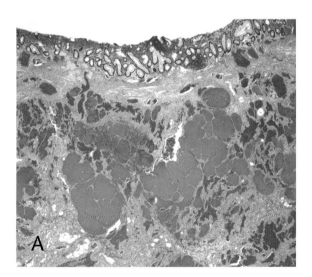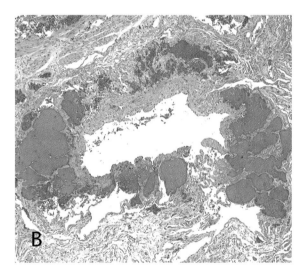

Figure 4-37

ARTERIOVENOUS MALFORMATION

Engorged vascular spaces and thick-walled veins expand the colonic submucosa and extend into the muscularis propria (A). A large, irregularly shaped vein is surrounded by numerous thin-walled vascular channels (B).

variably sized cystic spaces that permeate the bowel wall (fig. 4-36).

Microscopic Findings. Arteriovenous malformations consist of congeries of tortuous, variably dilated arteries and veins with thick muscular walls (fig. 4-37). Elastin stains distinguish arterialized veins from arteries.

Treatment and Prognosis. Angiographic guidance of embolization is the treatment of choice for arteriovenous malformations that are small and solitary. Large or multifocal lesions often require surgical resection (83). Once definitively treated, the prognosis is excellent.

Table 4-4

DIAGNOSTIC CRITERIA FOR HEREDITARY HEMORRHAGIC TELANGIECTASIA

Criteria Evaluated	Clinical Diagnosis of Disease
Clinical Manifestations	Definite Disease
1. Mucocutaneous telangiectasias	Findings from >3 categories
Lips	Possible Disease
Tongue	Findings from >2 categories
Nose	Unlikely Disease
Fingers	Findings from only 1 category
2. Recurrent epistaxis	Absence of any diagnostic criteria
3. Visceral arteriovenous malformations	
Lung	
Gastrointestinal tract	
Liver	
Brain	
Spine	
Family History	
4. Affected 1st degree relative	

Data from Shovlin CL, Guttmacher AE, Buscarini E, et al. Diagnostic criteria for hereditary hemorrhagic telangiectasia (Rendu-Osler-Weber syndrome). Am J Med Genet 2000;91:66-7.

Hereditary Hemorrhagic Telangiectasia

Definition. *Hereditary hemorrhagic telangiectasia* is an autosomal dominant disorder characterized by telangiectasias, angiodysplasias, and arteriovenous malformations of multiple organ systems. It is also known as *Osler-Weber-Rendu syndrome*.

Clinical Features. Hereditary hemorrhagic telangiectasia features mucosal and cutaneous telangiectasias, gastrointestinal angiodysplasias, pulmonary and visceral arteriovenous malformations, and vascular abnormalities of the central nervous system. The disease has a prevalence of approximately 1 per 10,000 individuals and affects men and women at similar rates (84). Nearly 10 percent of patients are diagnosed in infancy due to intracranial hemorrhage; most other affected individuals develop symptoms in childhood or early adulthood.

Common manifestations include epistaxis, hemoptysis, and gastrointestinal bleeding. Approximately 75 percent of patients have radiographically evident hepatic arteriovenous malformations of the liver, but most of these are clinically asymptomatic. Diagnostic criteria consist of a combination of clinical features and family history (Table 4-4) (85).

Pathogenesis. Hereditary hemorrhagic telangiectasia results from germline *HHT1* (*ENG*) or *HHT2* (*ALK1/ACVRL1*) mutations, which encode endoglin or activin receptor-like kinase (ALK1), respectively (86). Patients with juvenile polyposis syndrome due to *SMAD4* mutations also have hereditary hemorrhagic telangiectasia (82). Protein products from all three genes are involved in TGF-α-mediated cell signaling, which promotes blood vessel integrity and regulates vascular remodeling (87,88).

Gross and Microscopic Findings. Telangiectasias, angiodysplasias, and arteriovenous malformations that develop in association with hereditary hemorrhagic telangiectasia are indistinguishable from sporadic lesions (fig. 4-38).

Treatment and Prognosis. Approximately 90 percent of patients with hereditary hemorrhagic telangiectasia have a normal life expectancy; the remainder die of hemorrhage or related complications. Bleeding intracranial and pulmonary lesions can have catastrophic effects and thus, patients with hereditary hemorrhagic telangiectasia are routinely screened for cerebral and pulmonary arteriovenous malformations (89).

Gastrointestinal lesions are managed to attain symptomatic relief and control bleeding. Iron supplementation and blood transfusions counter chronic blood loss, especially after heavy bleeding episodes. Hormonal regulation with estrogens and estrogen receptor modulators can decrease bleeding; they also increase endoglin and ALK1 mRNA transcripts, partially compensating for haploinsufficiency (90). Superficial

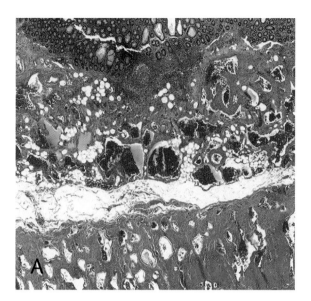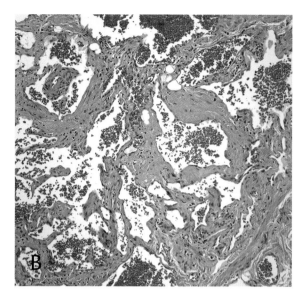

Figure 4-38

HEREDITARY HEMORRHAGIC TELANGIECTASIA

An arteriovenous malformation features innumerable vascular channels that permeate the full thickness of the colonic wall (A). Vessels vary in size and shape, and many contain interrupted mural aggregates of smooth muscle cells (B).

telangiectasias and angiodysplasias are managed endoscopically with argon plasma coagulation or ablation, whereas arteriovenous malformations require embolization or resection. The life expectancy and treatment of patients with underlying *SMAD4* mutations are influenced by manifestations of juvenile polyposis syndrome.

Blue Rubber Bleb Nevus Syndrome

Definition. *Blue rubber bleb nevus syndrome* is a congenital disorder featuring mucocutaneous venous malformations.

Clinical Features. Blue rubber bleb nevus syndrome is a rare disorder characterized by multiple venous malformations of the skin and gastrointestinal tract, particularly the small intestine. Lesions are present at birth but may not be conspicuous at that time; most patients are diagnosed within the first year of life.

Cutaneous lesions are firm, rubbery, blue or purple nodules that are most numerous on the upper trunk and arms, although they can also occur on palms and soles. Blebs blanch with pressure and slowly refill upon release. Patients with numerous gastrointestinal lesions develop chronic iron deficiency anemia by adulthood. Intussusception of polypoid mucosal lesions can account for recurrent abdominal pain in some patients.

Pathogenesis. Most available data suggest that blue rubber bleb syndrome is a non-hereditary disorder of unclear etiology. Rare reports describe an autosomal dominant mode of inheritance (91).

Gross Findings. Sharply circumscribed nodules are centered in the submucosa, with a normal mucosal surface (fig. 4-39). Traumatized lesions show erosions and oozing (92).

Microscopic Findings. Vascular lesions consist of dilated, thin-walled veins that may contain thrombi or phleboliths (fig. 4-40). The overlying mucosa is usually normal, although erosions, granulation tissue, and hemorrhage may be present. Mucosal inflammatory changes presumably reflect intussusception or luminal trauma.

Treatment and Prognosis. Patients with blue rubber bleb nevus syndrome are conservatively managed with iron supplementation or blood transfusions to correct anemia (83). Multiple large lesions may require sclerotherapy, laser coagulation, or even surgical resection. Octreotide, alpha-interferon and other pharmacologic agents that effectively treat other types of vascular lesions have limited value in the management of blue rubber bleb nevi; some data suggest that sirolimus can reduce nodule size (93,94). Blue rubber bleb nevus syndrome is unassociated with increased cancer risk.

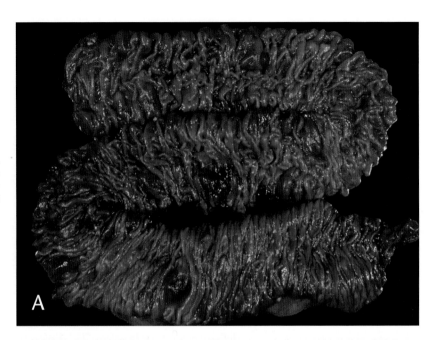

Figure 4-39

BLUE RUBBER BLEB NEVUS SYNDROME

This small bowel resection specimen contains numerous polypoid vascular tumors (A). Blue-black lesions are centered in the submucosa (B). (Courtesy of Drs. R. Gonzalez, Boston, MA and D. Agostini-Vulaj, Rochester, NY.)

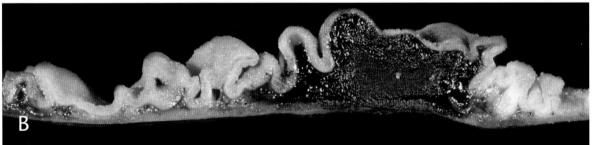

Portal Hypertensive Enterocolopathy

Definition. *Portal hypertensive enterocolopathy* is defined by the presence of mucosal ectasias and intestinal varices resulting from portal hypertension.

Clinical Features. Portal hypertensive enterocolopathy represents an important cause of chronic blood loss among cirrhotic patients. Nearly 66 percent of patients with established cirrhosis have portal hypertensive enterocolopathy, particularly those with higher hepatic venous pressure gradients (95). Most patients with this finding also have gastroesophageal varices, whereas the converse is not true: less than one-third of cirrhotic patients with gastroesophageal varices have portal hypertensive enterocolopathy (96).

Pathogenesis. Elevated portal venous pressures usually result from increased resistance to flow in the setting of cirrhosis. Portal vein thrombosis, nodular regeneration of hepatic parenchyma, and other disorders less frequently lead to elevated portal venous pressures that are transmitted to mucosal capillaries and venules throughout the gastrointestinal tract.

Gross Findings. Portal hypertensive enterocolopathy imparts a mottled, congested appearance to the mucosa with bulbous, edematous villi in the proximal small bowel (95,97). Lesions of the colon appear as irregular erythematous patches, reflecting vascular ectasias in the mucosa (fig. 4-41).

Microscopic Findings. Elevated portal venous pressures are transmitted to mucosal capillaries and venules, resulting in vascular ectasias (fig. 4-42). Dilated vascular spaces may be accompanied by extravasated red blood cells and lamina propria fibrosis, but also occur on a background of normal, or nearly normal, mucosa.

Treatment and Prognosis. Iron supplementation and endoscopic ablation of bleeding sites

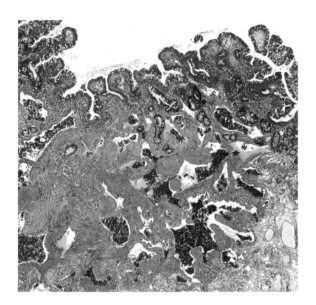

Figure 4-40

BLUE RUBBER BLEB NEVUS SYNDROME

A large submucosal lesion consists of irregular aggregates of ectatic veins accompanied by sclerosis. (Courtesy of Drs. R. Gonzalez, Boston, MA and D. Agostini-Vulaj, Rochester, NY.)

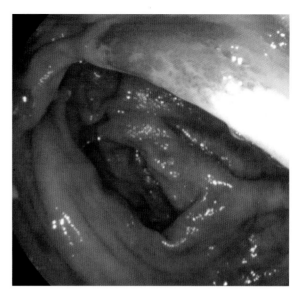

Figure 4-41

PORTAL HYPERTENSIVE COLOPATHY

Scattered erythematous patches are present in the proximal colon.

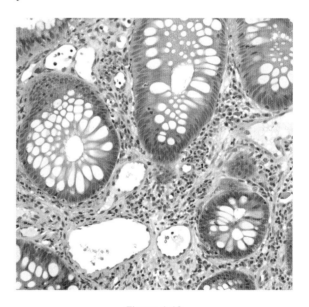

Figure 4-42

PORTAL HYPERTENSIVE COLOPATHY

Prominent ectatic capillaries are dispersed in the lamina propria, which shows patchy fibrosis.

temporarily manage gastrointestinal bleeding. Pharmacologic agents that may be of benefit include non-selective beta-blockers, long-acting octreotide-containing compounds, and hemostatic powder (98,99). Definitive treatment requires reversal of liver disease or transplantation.

Ischemic Enterocolitis

Definition. *Ischemic enterocolitis* is enterocolic injury and necrosis secondary to hypoperfusion.

Clinical Features. Ischemic enterocolitis is a common condition, particularly among elderly patients. Vascular occlusion by atheroma, thrombus, or embolus accounts for approximately 50 percent of cases (100,101). The remainder reflect decreased splanchnic blood flow resulting from left ventricular failure, aortic insufficiency, cardiogenic shock, septic physiology, increased blood viscosity, vasculitis, and certain medications. Cytomegalovirus (CMV) and *Clostridium difficile* both elicit an ischemic-type pattern of injury with extensive ulcers and mural necrosis, as discussed below (102,103).

Ischemic enterocolitis is more common in patients with peripheral vascular disease, diabetes mellitus, amyloidosis, and chronic renal insufficiency requiring hemodialysis (104). Most patients present with crampy abdominal pain and tenderness, accompanied by hematochezia. Symptom severity tends to correlate with the extent of intestinal injury, although some elderly patients have surprisingly mild symptoms

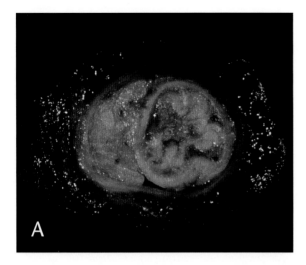
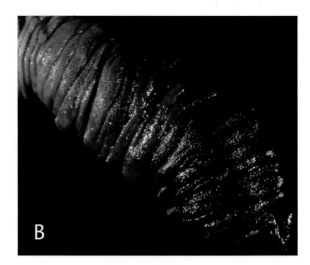

Figure 4-43

INTESTINAL INTUSSUSCEPTION

Cross section through the intussusception demonstrates a telescoped segment of small bowel within the distal bowel (A). The proximal tip of the intussusceptum is ischemic (B).

despite severe enterocolitis. Classic radiographic features include bowel dilatation, mural thickening, and mucosal nodularity reflecting hemorrhage and edema (i.e., "thumb-printing").

Pathogenesis. Diminished blood flow through the mucosa leads to the accumulation of toxic metabolites as well as the depletion of proteins, carbohydrates, lipids, water, electrolytes, and vitamins. Transient ischemia may cause reversible cell damage, whereas persistent hypoperfusion irreversibly alters epithelial cell structure and metabolism. These changes result in epithelial cell death and decreased mucosal integrity, thereby increasing susceptibility to bacterial translocation (105). Local activation of the complement cascade causes endothelial cell damage, edema, and recruitment of inflammatory cells (106).

Arterial Occlusion. Complete arterial occlusion usually reflects rupture of atheromatous plaques, which are most pronounced at the root of the superior mesenteric artery (101,107,108). Ruptured complicated plaques of the superior mesenteric artery shower distal arteries with emboli. Alternatively, intracardiac thrombi that develop in the setting of atrial fibrillation and myocardial infarction may embolize the superior mesenteric artery and its branches (101,109). Volvulus, intussusception, and strangulated hernias all cause complete arterial occlusion

as well (fig. 4-43). Other etiologies are far less frequent. Endovascular treatment of aortic aneurysms can result in iatrogenic segmental ischemic enterocolitis; hydrophilic polymers that coat endovascular surgical devices may be sheared during the procedure and embolize downstream arteries (fig. 4-44). Intermittent compression of the celiac artery by the median arcuate ligament can cause occlusive ischemic enteritis in patients with anomalous anatomy of the celiac plexus (110). Cocaine promotes vasoconstriction and thrombotic occlusion of mesenteric arteries and short branches from the vasa recta (111).

Venous Occlusion. Venous outflow obstruction accounts for nearly 15 percent of ischemic enterocolitis cases (112). Extrinsic compression by incarcerated hernias, lymphadenopathy, adhesions, and thrombosis are the most common causes. Hypercoagulable states due to protein C or S deficiencies, abdominal malignancy, and some medications increase the risk of thrombus formation. Of these, estrogens are most studied; these agents are prothrombotic and accelerate platelet aggregation, particularly at high doses (113–115). Venous thrombi originating in smaller veins can propagate to affect larger vessels, and portal vein thrombi may extend into mesenteric veins. Risk of venous thrombosis is increased by smoking, hypertension, diabetes mellitus, and obesity.

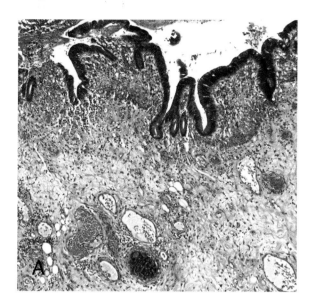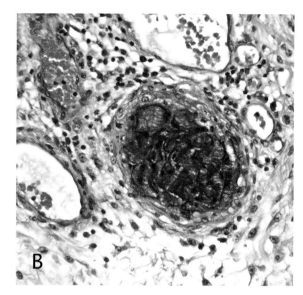

Figure 4-44

IATROGENIC POLYMER EMBOLIZATION OF SMALL BOWEL

Lubricating polymers on endovascular surgical devices can be dislodged during aortic instrumentation, resulting in small bowel embolization (A). Basophilic embolic material is associated with fibrin (B). (Courtesy of Dr. C. A. Arnold, Aurora, CO.)

Nonocclusive Ischemia. Nonocclusive ischemic enterocolitis is a common complication in patients who require high-dose vasopressor therapy, as well as those with disseminated intravascular coagulation, severe dehydration, hemoconcentration, and other disorders that increase blood viscosity (116–118). Extreme physical activity and profound hypotension due to any cause can reduce splanchnic blood flow, thereby promoting nonocclusive ischemic enterocolitis. Several pharmacological agents, including NSAIDs, cocaine, and oral contraceptives, can substantially decrease splanchnic blood flow and produce ischemic injury (119,120).

Gross Findings. The endoscopic features of mild ischemic enteritis include patchy erythema or pale edematous mucosa, petechial hemorrhages, and erosions (fig. 4-45A). Severe enterocolitis is characterized by dusky or purple discoloration of the mucosa with longitudinal ulcers and adherent fibrin (fig. 4-45B). Profound ischemia results in expansion of the mucosa and submucosa by edema and hemorrhage that can simulate the endoscopic appearance of malignancy, especially in the right colon (fig. 4-46) (121).

Non-occlusive and occlusive forms of ischemic enterocolitis produce similar features in resection specimens, although the latter tend to cause segmental, rather than patchy injury. Venous outflow obstruction usually results in marked mural thickening owing to vascular congestion and hemorrhage (fig. 4-47). Nonocclusive ischemia results in patchy edema, erythema, and ulcers overlying a normal muscularis propria, whereas more extensive injury results in attenuation of the bowel wall with gray-green or black discoloration (fig. 4-48).

Microscopic Findings. *Acute Ischemic Enterocolitis.* Histologic abnormalities are most pronounced in the superficial mucosa of the anti-mesenteric aspect of the gut where oxygen and nutrient levels are lowest. Changes of ischemic enteritis are first evident in the villi, which show nearly normal architecture with sloughed epithelial cells and mucus in the lumen (fig. 4-49A). Progressive injury results in variable villous shortening, cytoplasmic depletion of epithelial cells, enlarged nuclei, and prominent nucleoli. Epithelial cell necrosis and detachment of the villous surface epithelium are followed by crypt cell apoptosis and lamina propria hemorrhage (fig. 4-49B). More severe injury results in extensive mucosal necrosis, hemorrhage and edema of the submucosa, and scattered necrotic smooth muscle cells in the muscularis propria (122).

207

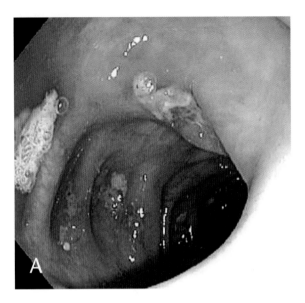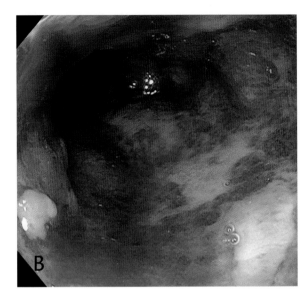

Figure 4-45

ISCHEMIC COLITIS

Early ischemia results in a loss of the vascular pattern, edema, and patchy erosions (A). More severe injury produces mucosal congestion and distorted folds; fibrinous exudates overlie ulcers (B).

Ischemic colitis produces epithelial cell changes similar to those seen in the small bowel: small regenerative crypts have a withered appearance with large, smooth nuclei and increased mitotic activity (fig. 4-50). The lamina propria contains congested capillaries and venules accompanied by extravasated fibrin, imparting a hyalinized, eosinophilic appearance. Fibrinous exudates containing necrotic epithelial cells may be present in cases that show extensive ulceration (fig. 4-50D). Fibrin thrombi are commonly detected near ulcers and are generally considered pathogenic only when detected in mucosae surfaced by intact epithelium. However, the presence of multiple fibrin thrombi can be a clue to a specific diagnosis, such as thrombotic thrombocytopenic purpura, which may require plasmapheresis or other therapy (fig. 4-51) (123). Ischemic enterocolitis is pauci-inflammatory: neutrophilic inflammation is generally mild or absent except in areas of erosion or ulceration.

Prolonged ischemia results in injury to deeper layers of the bowel wall. Scattered smooth muscle cells in the muscularis propria display pyknotic or absent nuclei and hypereosinophilic cytoplasm. Lysis of smooth muscle cells is accompanied by mural edema and an influx of inflammatory cells as well as translocation of luminal bacteria. Infection can involve mesenteric tissues, producing striking inflammatory changes in extramural vessels (fig. 4-52). Inflammatory changes in mesenteric vessels should not be considered evidence of vasculitis if confined to regions of extensive mural necrosis.

Acute mucosal ischemia can heal completely. The granulation tissue is gradually replaced by lamina propria surfaced by attenuated epithelium, which is remodeled to restore the normal architecture of the enteric and colonic mucosae. Ischemic injury to the submucosa or muscularis propria does not resolve with complete restoration of normal components. Granulation tissue in these areas is largely replaced by fibrosis, resulting in strictures or fistulae.

Chronic Ischemic Entertocolitis. Recurrent or sustained hypoperfusion of the small bowel or colon can lead to chronic ischemic enterocolitis. Injury usually involves the submucosa or muscularis propria. Affected patients may develop strictures that cause post-prandial pain, weight loss, or intestinal obstruction (124). Recurrent volvulus, internal hernias, prior radiation therapy, severe atherosclerotic disease, and vasculitis are risk factors for chronic ischemic injury (125).

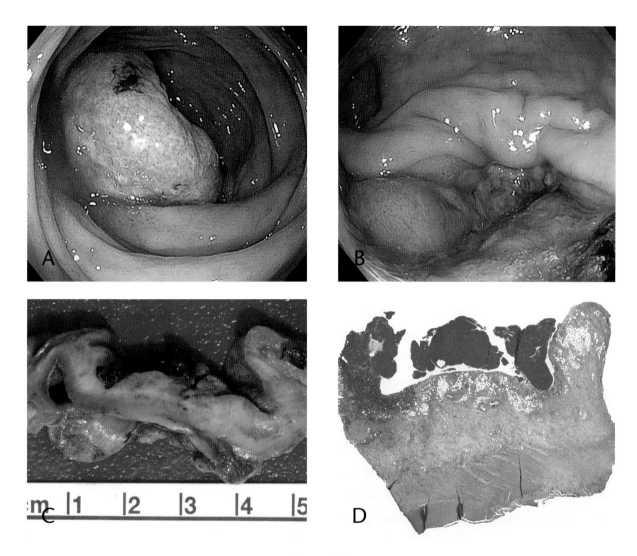

Figure 4-46

ISCHEMIC COLITIS SIMULATING A NEOPLASM

Localized ischemia simulates a polypoid (A) or partially obstructing mass (B). The corresponding resection specimen contains a large polypoid area in the right colon (C) resulting from ulcer-related inflammation, edema, and expansion of the submucosa (D).

Ischemic strictures are concentric and may be multifocal (126). They usually contain atrophic mucosa with architectural distortion, Paneth and pyloric metaplasia, and mural fibrosis (fig. 4-53). Chronic ulcers are sharply circumscribed and usually located on the antimesenteric aspect of the bowel. Hemosiderin-laden macrophages are inconspicuous (127).

Differential Diagnosis. Acute ischemic enterocolitis is pauci-inflammatory and, thus, readily distinguished from most types of infectious enterocolitis and idiopathic inflammatory

bowel disease. Some findings, such as cholesterol emboli, thrombi, amyloidosis, and various types of vasculitis, may show features to suggest a more specific diagnosis, especially in resection specimens (fig. 4-54).

Treatment and Prognosis. Treatment of transient ischemic enterocolitis is usually supportive, whereas mural necrosis requires surgical resection. Prognosis is dependent on the extent of disease and associated comorbidities. Perforation due to necrosis is associated with high mortality rates.

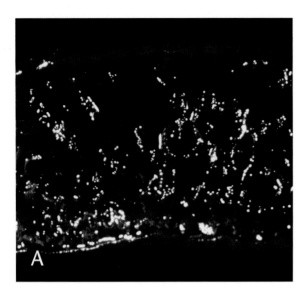 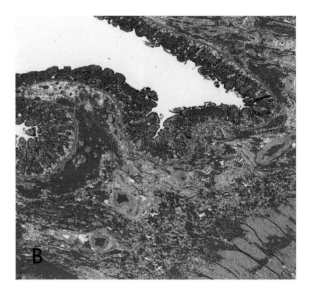

Figure 4-47

ISCHEMIC ENTERITIS

Mesenteric thrombosis results in venous outflow obstruction, vascular engorgement, edema, and mural hemorrhage (A), with relative preservation of the mucosa (B).

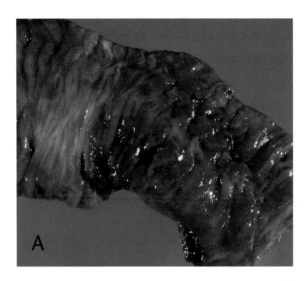 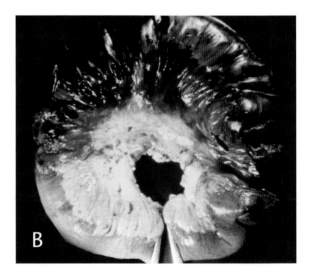

Figure 4-48

ISCHEMIC ENTERITIS

Mucosal edema obscures the normal folds; erythema and erosions are present (A). Occlusive ischemic injury produces segmental bowel infarction. There is an abrupt transition between necrotic, dilated small bowel and the adjacent uninvolved intestine (B).

Polyarteritis Nodosa

Polyarteritis nodosa is a necrotizing vasculitis of medium-sized arteries. Polyarteritis nodosa tends to affect middle-aged adults, with a predilection for men. Although its etiology is not precisely known, polyarteritis nodosa is clearly associated with immune-mediated disorders as well as both hepatitis B and hepatitis C virus infections (128,129). Nearly half of affected patients have gastrointestinal manifestations with abdominal pain, diarrhea, hematochezia, or even

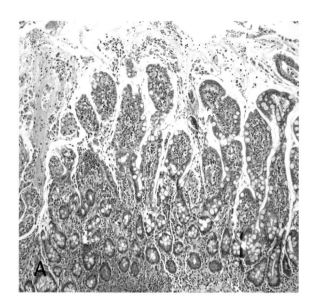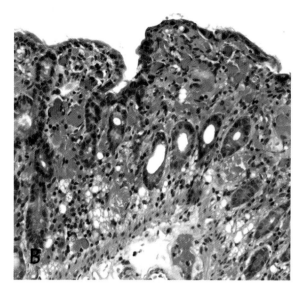

Figure 4-49

ISCHEMIC ENTERITIS

Early ischemic enteritis manifests in the villous tips; surface epithelial cells are mucin-depleted and necrotic cells are sloughed in the lumen (A). Progressive injury results in mucosal and submucosal hemorrhage, villous flattening, and cytoplasmic depletion of enterocytes (B).

malabsorptive symptoms (130–132). Abdominal imaging with angiography reveals aneurysmal dilatations and stenoses along the mesenteric arteries, particularly small straight arteries.

Polyarteritis nodosa causes variably severe ischemic enterocolitis, often in a segmental distribution. Mucosal friability and sharply demarcated ulcers are most pronounced on the antimesenteric aspect. Deeply penetrating ulcers, hemorrhagic infarcts, and perforation occur in some cases (133).

Variably severe acute ischemic injury is accompanied by fibrinoid necrosis with thrombus formation (fig. 4-55) (134). Chronic changes include strictures accompanied by crypt distortion and cellular metaplasia, as well as intimal hyperplasia of mural and mesenteric arteries (fig. 4-55D). Elastin stains demonstrate destruction of the internal elastic lamina within arteries.

Antineutrophil Cytoplasmic Antibody-Associated Vasculitis

Definition. This type of necrotizing vasculitis affects small to medium-sized vessels and is associated with antineutrophil cytoplasmic antibodies (ANCA).

Clinical Features. There are three distinct variants of ANCA-associated small vessel vasculitis, each characterized by their clinical features and associated human leukocyte antigen (HLA) polymorphisms. *Granulomatosis with polyangiitis* (*Wegener granulomatosis with polyangiitis*) is linked to HLA-DP1, whereas *microscopic polyangiitis* is associated with HLA-DQ, and *eosinophilic granulomatosis with polyangiitis* (*Churg-Strauss syndrome*) occurs in patients with the HLA-DRB4 haplotype. Most patients suffering from granulomatosis with polyangiitis and microscopic polyangiitis lack gastrointestinal manifestations of disease, whereas 30 to 60 percent of those who have eosinophilic granulomatosis with polyangiitis frequently develop intestinal involvement (135,136).

Eosinophilic granulomatosis with polyangiitis shows a predilection for middle-aged adults. Patients typically have a several-year history of allergic rhinitis, nasal polyposis, and asthma, and may also have involvement of the skin, heart, nervous system, and kidneys (137).

Pathogenesis. All of the ANCA-associated vasculitides are associated with polymorphic variants encoding proteinase 3, the antigenic target of ANCA, or alpha-1-antitrypsin, an

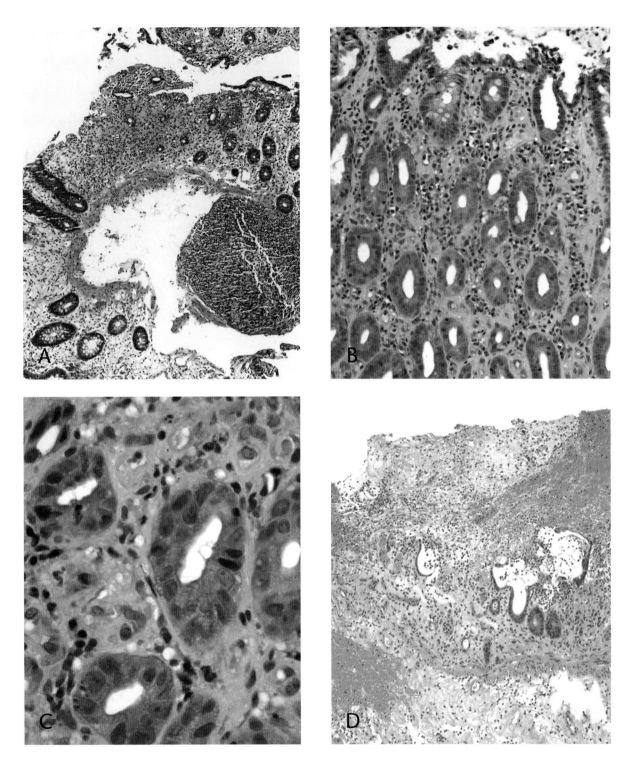

Figure 4-50

ISCHEMIC COLITIS

Ischemia causes mucosal injury with crypt loss accompanied by lamina propria eosinophilia (A). Regenerative microcrypts are lined by mucin-depleted colonocytes (B). These "withered" crypts display increased mitotic activity (C). Severe injury causes sloughing of necrotic colonocytes with adherent blood and fibrin, simulating pseudomembranes (D).

ANCA inhibitor (138). Disease likely develops as a result of the interplay between these genetic factors and environmental stimuli, such as exposure to allergens or drugs. Most (50 to 75 percent) patients who develop eosinophilic granulomatosis with polyangiitis have elevated serum ANCA (anti-MPO) or cANCA levels accompanied by peripheral blood eosinophilia (greater than 1,500/mL) (139).

Gross Findings. Ischemic-type changes with segmental erythema, edema, and ulcers occur throughout the tubular gut.

Microscopic Findings. Ischemic enterocolitis is accompanied by inflammatory changes in small arteries, arterioles, capillaries, and venules (fig. 4-56). Necrotizing vasculitis features eosinophil-rich mural inflammation, nuclear debris, fibrin, and poorly formed granulomas (140).

Differential Diagnosis. Gastrointestinal involvement by eosinophilic granulomatosis with polyangiitis may simulate eosinophilic gastroenteritis owing to the presence of high numbers of eosinophils. However, the eosinophils associated with vasculitis tend to be more pronounced in the submucosa and ischemic-type injury predominates in the mucosa.

Treatment and Prognosis. Treatment of eosinophilic granulomatosis with polyangiitis requires immunosuppressive therapy.

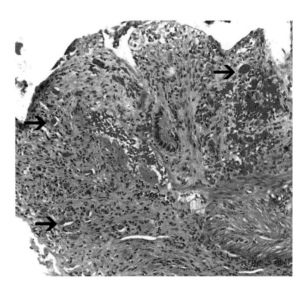

Figure 4-51

THROMBOTIC THROMBOCYTOPENIC PURPURA

Colonic biopsy samples display near-complete loss of the colonic epithelium with hyaline thrombi (arrows) and hemorrhage in the lamina propria (left).

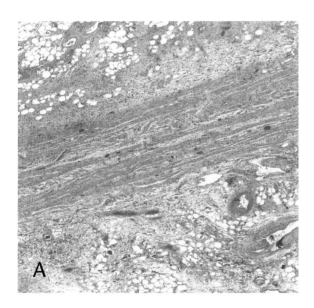
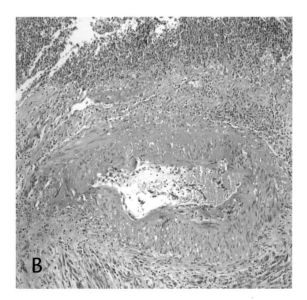

Figure 4-52

MURAL CHANGES OF ISCHEMIC INJURY

Progressive ischemic injury causes striking edema and necrosis of the bowel wall. The muscularis propria is attenuated and infiltrated by inflammatory cells; scattered necrotic smooth muscle cells are present (A). Vessels underlying ulcers can show luminal or mural fibrin deposits accompanied by neutrophils and necrotic cellular debris; these abnormalities should not be considered pathogenic unless they are detected beneath uninflamed, intact mucosa (B).

213

Corticosteroids and cyclophosphamide are considered first-line agents; rituximab and omalizumab are beneficial in some cases (141,142).

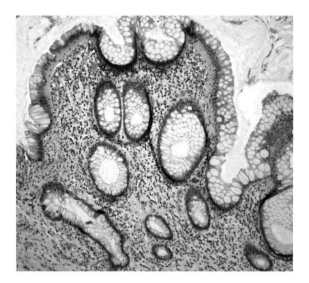

Figure 4-53

CHRONIC ISCHEMIC COLITIS

Persistent ischemia leads to mucosal abnormalities similar to those of quiescent inflammatory bowel disease. The lamina propria cellularity is mildly increased and crypts show architectural abnormalities.

IgA-Associated Vasculitis

Definition. *IgA-associated vasculitis* is a hypersensitivity and leukocytoclastic vasculitis characterized by IgA-predominant immune complex deposition. Synonyms include *Henoch–Schönlein purpura, anaphylactoid purpura,* and *purpura rheumatica.*

Clinical Features. IgA-associated vasculitis affects the skin, kidneys, joints, and gastrointestinal tract, particularly the small bowel (143–146). Most cases occur in children, often following an episode of streptococcal pharyngitis. Cases that develop in adults may be related to drug exposures (quinidine, ranitidine, clarithromycin) (147).

Gross Findings. Endoscopy reveals petechial hemorrhages, diffuse erythema with an edematous or mottled appearance, and irregular ulcers (fig. 4-57). Duodenal involvement may mimic peptic injury, although vasculitis shows a predilection for the distal duodenum and generally spares the bulb. Submucosal hemorrhages can produce polypoid protrusions that form the lead points for intussusceptions.

Microscopic Findings. Histologic findings present in biopsy samples simulate an inflammatory enteritis because they display mild ischemic-type changes accompanied by striking

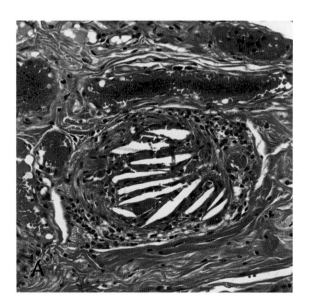
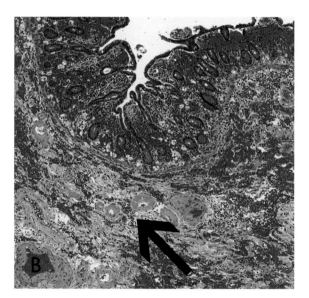

Figure 4-54

HISTOLOGICALLY EVIDENT CAUSES OF ISCHEMIC ENTEROCOLITIS

Cholesterol clefts are present in association with foreign body-type giant cells in an artery (A). A resection specimen obtained for indications of ischemic enteritis demonstrates extensive vascular amyloid deposits (arrow) associated with mucosal injury and hemorrhage (B).

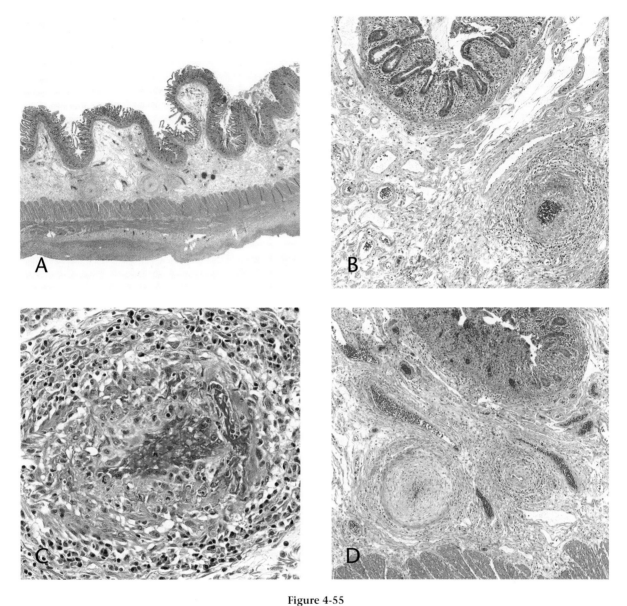

Figure 4-55

POLYARTERITIS NODOSA

This small bowel resection displays increased cellularity around thickened arteries in the submucosa (A). Submucosal arteries feature mural fibrinoid necrosis (B) with a cuff of inflammatory cells (C). Established vascular lesions show striking intimal hyperplasia with near-occlusion of arteries (D).

neutrophil-rich inflammation (fig. 4-58A). Lamina propria hemorrhage with fibrin deposits are seen in combination with sheets of neutrophils that spare the epithelium and are more pronounced in the deep mucosa (fig. 4-58B). Leukocytoclastic vasculitis affects arterioles, capillaries, and venules (fig. 4-58C). Fibrinoid necrosis and mixed inflammation in vascular walls are accompanied by karyorrhectic debris, often with fibrin thrombi (fig. 4-58D) (148). Vascular IgA and complement (C3) deposits are typically present in untreated patients.

Treatment and Prognosis. Most patients respond well to corticosteroid therapy. Accurate diagnosis and prompt treatment are associated with an excellent prognosis.

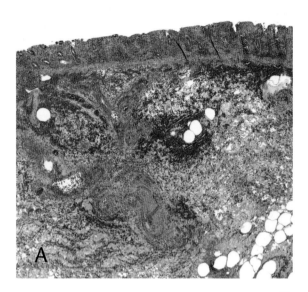
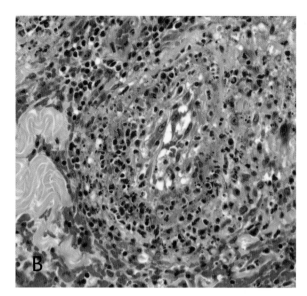

Figure 4-56

EOSINOPHILIC GRANULOMATOSIS WITH POLYANGIITIS

Mucosal ischemia is accompanied by vasculitis affecting submucosal vessels (A). Small arteries display fibrinoid necrosis and mural inflammation accompanied by eosinophil-rich perivascular inflammation (B).

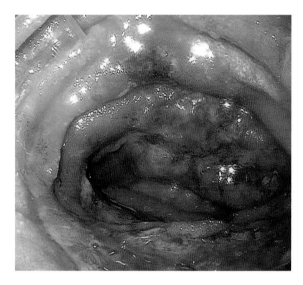

Figure 4-57

IgA-ASSOCIATED VASCULITIS

IgA-associated vasculitis shows a predilection for the proximal small bowel where it causes segmental ischemic injury, mottled mucosa, and erosions.

Behçet Disease

Definition. *Behçet disease* is an immune-mediated systemic vasculitis affecting small and medium-sized veins.

Clinical Features. Behçet disease is a chronic, relapsing condition affecting multiple mucocutaneous sites. The disease is more common in Japan than Western countries and is associated with HLA-B51 (149). Most affected patients are young adults, particularly women. Clinical findings include ulcers of the oral mucosa and genitalia, ocular inflammation, and gastrointestinal bleeding (Table 4-5) (150).

Gross Findings. Approximately 25 percent of patients have gastrointestinal ulcers, particularly in the distal ileum and right colon. The ulcers are large, sharply demarcated, and unassociated with inflammatory changes in the intervening mucosa (fig. 4-59A) (151).

Microscopic Findings. Behçet disease-related ulcers develop over Peyer patches and extend into the submucosa or deeper bowel wall (152,153). Dense mononuclear cell-rich inflammation is present around small- and medium-caliber veins deep to ulcers and distant from areas of injury (fig. 4-59B,C). Veins and venules display perivascular mononuclear cell-rich inflammation, intimal thickening, and occasional thrombosis (fig. 4-59D). Loose macrophage aggregates may be present, but well-formed granulomas are lacking.

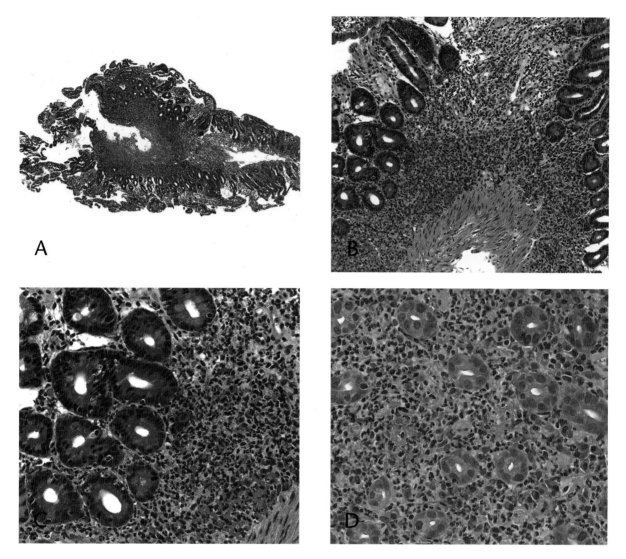

Figure 4-58

IgA-ASSOCIATED VASCULITIS

Striking neutrophil-rich inflammation simulates acute enteritis (A). The infiltrate tends to be most pronounced in the deep mucosa (B) and mostly spares the crypts (C). Superficial aggregates of neutrophils and fibrin deposits surround injured capillaries and venules (D).

Treatment and Prognosis. Treatment consists of immunosuppression, particularly with infliximab and related biologic agents. Relapsing symptoms are common.

Enterocolic Lymphocytic Phlebitis

Definition. *Enterocolic lymphocytic phlebitis* is a lymphocytic venulitis limited to the gastrointestinal tract. The term is synonymous with mesenteric veno-occlusive disease.

Clinical Features. Enterocolic lymphocytic phlebitis is more common in adults than children and affects men more frequently than women. Patients present with intermittent ischemic symptoms such as recurrent abdominal pain, nausea, and bloody diarrhea. The disorder is confined to the gastrointestinal tract and usually affects a single organ (154).

Enterocolic lymphocytic phlebitis probably represents an immune-mediated vasculitis; it has

Table 4-5

INTERNATIONAL CLINICAL CRITERIA FOR BEHÇET DISEASE[a]

Sign or Sympton	Points Assigned (≥4 Required for Diagnosis)
Recurrent oral ulcers	2
Genital ulcers	2
Uveitis	2
Retinal vasculitis	2
Erythema nodosum, pseudofolliculitis, papulopustular lesions, acneiform nodules in adults untreated with corticosteroid therapy	1
Neurologic manifestations	1
Vascular manifestations	1
Positive pathergy test read by a physician within 24-48 hours of testing	1 (optional extra point if testing performed)

[a]Data from International Team for the revision of the international criteria for Behçet's disease (ITR-ICBD). The international criteria for Behçet's disease (ICBD): a collaborative study of 27 countries on the sensitivity and specificity of the new criteria. J Eur Acad Dermatol Venereol 2014;28:338-47.

been described in association with lymphocytic enterocolitis and some medications (155). Involvement of mesenteric veins is frequent and, thus, most patients have disease affecting the small bowel, colon, or appendix (156).

Gross Findings. Ulcers and ischemic mucosal injury are accompanied by prominent mural veins and hemorrhagic infarction.

Microscopic Findings. Dense lymphocyte-rich infiltrates are present in and around veins and venules of the viscera and mesentery. They may be associated with mural fibrin deposits, neutrophils, and karyorrhectic debris (fig. 4-60) (157). Most of the infiltrating lymphocytes are CD3/CD8-positive T-cells accompanied by smaller populations of B-cells. Loose aggregates of macrophages may be seen in some cases, but well-formed granulomas are lacking. Myointimal hyperplasia and venous thrombosis are often striking.

Treatment and Prognosis. Surgical resection of the affected organ is generally curative (158).

Idiopathic Myointimal Hyperplasia of Mesenteric Veins

Definition. *Idiopathic myointimal hyperplasia of mesenteric veins* is a type of ischemic colitis resulting from progressive occlusion of mesenteric and mural veins.

Clinical Features. Idiopathic myointimal hyperplasia of mesenteric veins is an under-recognized type of chronic ischemic colitis that

occurs almost exclusively in middle-aged, previously healthy men (159). Patients present with intermittent abdominal pain accompanied by progressively severe bloody diarrhea.

Pathogenesis. The mechanism by which this disorder develops is unknown. Consistent involvement of the sigmoid colon raises the possibility that intermittent volvulus leads to tension on mesenteric veins, myointimal hyperplasia, and ischemic colitis due to venous outflow obstruction. Morphologic similarities between mesenteric vein changes and saphenous vein grafts in coronary artery bypass patients have led some authors to postulate a role for arteriovenous shunting.

Gross Findings. The disease almost always affects the left colon and upper rectum, causing strictures accompanied by ulcerated, friable mucosa (fig. 4-61) (160). Resection specimens feature segmental strictures surrounded by indurated and enlarged epiploica (fig. 4-62).

Microscopic Findings. Biopsy samples show pauci-inflammatory ischemic colitis with small, withered crypts and hyalinized lamina propria (fig. 4-63A). Thick-walled capillaries lined by prominent endothelial cells, often with subendothelial fibrin deposits, represent a consistent feature (159,161). Fibrin thrombi are often present within venules, which also contain brightly eosinophilic fibrin deposits in their walls (fig. 4-63B). These vascular changes likely reflect chronically increased venous pressure.

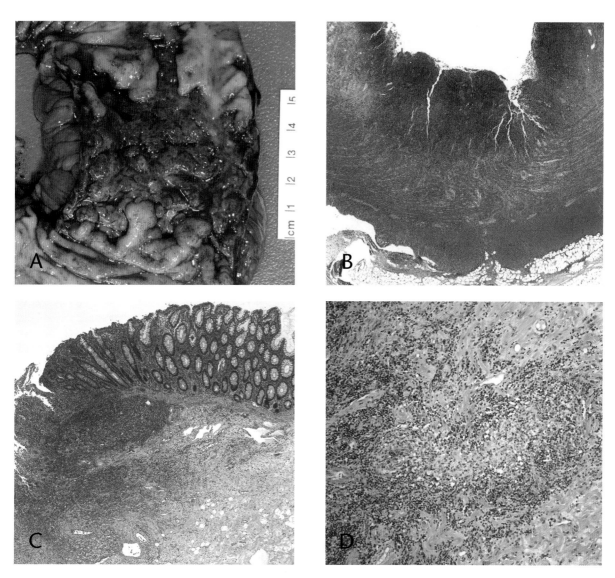

Figure 4-59

BEHÇET DISEASE

Large, irregular ulcers are separated by normal intervening mucosa (A). The histologic features are not specific; superficial mononuclear cell-rich granulation tissue is present at the ulcer base but mural lymphoid aggregates typical of Crohn disease are lacking (B). An abrupt transition to nearly normal mucosa is characteristic (C). Lymphocyte-rich phlebitis may be accompanied by loose aggregates of macrophages (D).

Myointimal hyperplasia occurs in veins of the submucosa and deeper bowel wall, as well as the mesentery (fig. 4-63C,D). Intimal hyperplasia and proliferation of smooth muscle cells is unaccompanied by inflammation (fig. 4-63E,F). The arteries are entirely spared (162).

Treatment and Prognosis. Surgical resection of the affected colonic segment is curative. For this reason, distinction from other types of ischemic colitis and inflammatory bowel disease is critically important. Most forms of ischemic enterocolitis are managed expectantly with supportive care, and inflammatory bowel disease is treated with various types of immunosuppressive agents including corticosteroids. Some data suggest that the use of corticosteroid therapy promotes bowel perforation in patients with idiopathic myointimal hyperplasia of mesenteric veins (159).

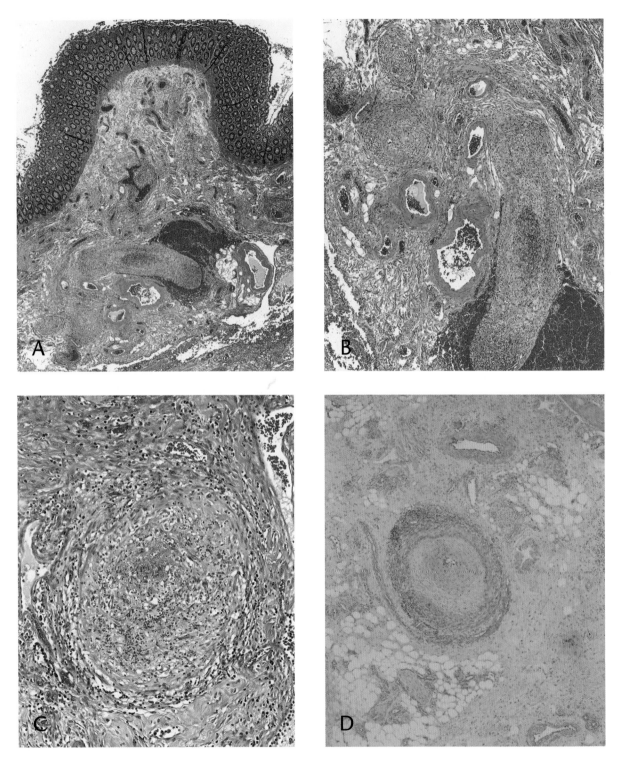

Figure 4-60

ENTEROCOLIC LYMPHOCYTIC PHLEBITIS

Ischemic colitis is associated with lymphoid inflammation around mural veins (A) and venous thrombi (B). Inflammatory cells infiltrate the vein wall and obliterate the lumen while entirely sparing arteries (C). Burnt-out lesions feature myointimal hyperplasia and occlusion associated with chronic inflammation (D).

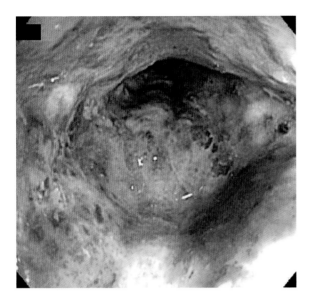

Figure 4-61

**IDIOPATHIC MYOINTIMAL
HYPERPLASIA OF MESENTERIC VEINS**

Sigmoidoscopy reveals ischemic-type mucosal changes with ulcers and dusky discoloration.

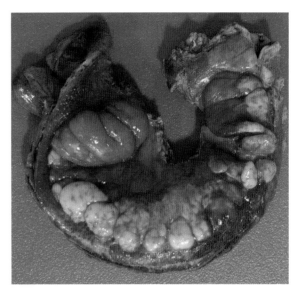

Figure 4-62

**IDIOPATHIC MYOINTIMAL
HYPERPLASIA OF MESENTERIC VEINS**

The disease causes segmental ischemic colitis characterized by luminal narrowing and prominent, indurated epiploica.

Other Types of Vasculitis and Vasculopathy

Thromboangiitis Obliterans (Buerger Disease). Thromboangiitis obliterans most commonly affects men with a long history of cigarette smoking. The disease features pauci-inflammatory obliteration of small to medium-sized arteries, and may affect veins and nerves (163). Most patients have peripheral disease affecting the limbs, but some with involvement of superior mesenteric artery branches present with chronic ischemic enterocolitis (164). Occlusion of arteries and arterioles results from organizing thrombi accompanied by endothelial proliferation and medial fibrosis; the internal elastic lamina is preserved.

Mesenteric Phlebosclerosis. Mesenteric phlebosclerosis is an infrequent cause of chronic ischemic enterocolitis that shows a predilection for Asian patients. This disorder was once considered an idiopathic disease, but emerging data suggest a relationship to herbal medications that contain gardenia fruit (i.e., sanshishi) (165).

Patients present with the insidious onset of abdominal pain and progressive diarrhea. The diagnosis is based on a combination of radiographic and endoscopic abnormalities. Imaging reveals linear calcifications of mesenteric veins. Endoscopic features include mottled and edematous mucosa with prominent blue-black submucosal vessels and shallow ulcers.

Biopsy samples and resection specimens display ischemic-type mucosal changes with striking mural fibrosis that may be pronounced enough to cause stenosis and obstructive symptoms (fig. 4-64A,B). Veins are thickened and sclerotic (fig. 4-64C,D) (166). Surgical resection of the affected bowel is curative.

Malignant Atrophic Papulosis (Köhlmeier–Degos Syndrome). Malignant atrophic papulosis is a rare arteriopathy affecting cutaneous vessels, often in combination with gastrointestinal involvement. It affects men and women equally and can occur at any age. The small bowel is the most common site of extracutaneous involvement.

Patients with gastrointestinal involvement present with recurrent abdominal pain and hematochezia. Early endoscopic findings are mild and non-specific, but more severe disease is associated with multifocal ulcers that can perforate (167).

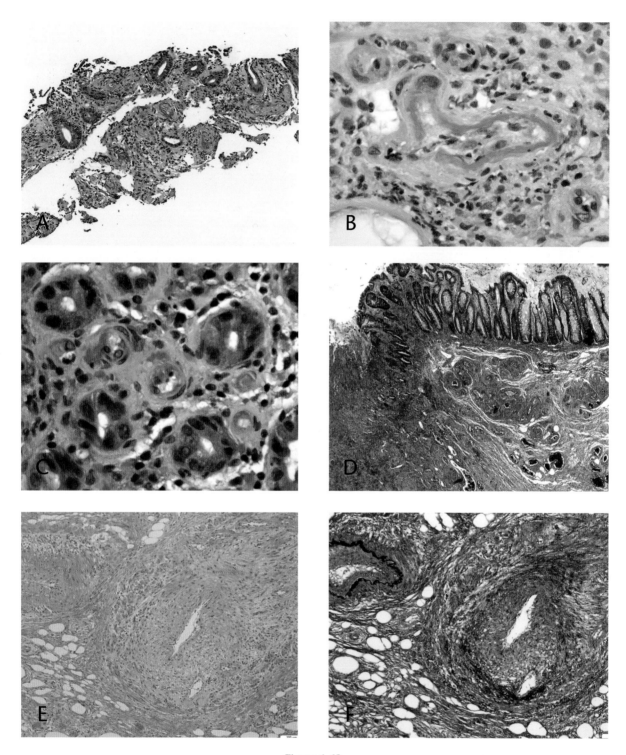

Figure 4-63

IDIOPATHIC MYOINTIMAL HYPERPLASIA OF MESENTERIC VEINS

Biopsy samples feature ischemic colitis (A) with brightly eosinophilic deposits in lamina propria vessels (B). Thick-walled mucosal capillaries show subendothelial fibrin and red cells due to increased venous pressure (C). Submucosal vessels display similar vascular hyalinization and organizing thrombi (D). Myointimal hyperplasia affects mesenteric veins and completely spares the arteries (E). Elastin stains confirm the absence of an internal elastic lamina in the affected vessels; adjacent arteries (upper left) are unaffected (F).

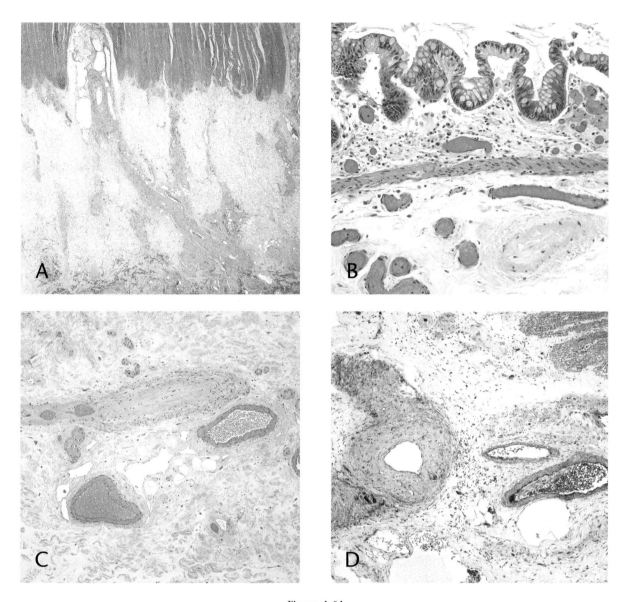

Figure 4-64

MESENTERIC PHLEBOSCLEROSIS

The bowel wall is expanded and contains thickened veins (A), which may be present in the submucosa (B). Fibrous thickening of the vascular wall is accompanied by minimal inflammation (C). Arterial sparing is accentuated by a trichrome stain (D). (Courtesy of Dr. E. Montgomery, Baltimore, MD.)

Microscopic perforation sites appear as numerous fibrin plaques on the serosa and are essentially pathognomonic of the disease (168). Histologic features include sclerosis of small and medium-sized arteries with prominent endothelial cells and increased cellularity of the intima (fig. 4-65). Vascular changes are unaccompanied by mural inflammation, although a mild infiltrate may be seen when superimposed arterial thrombi are present. Nearly all patients with gastrointestinal involvement die of their disease (169).

MEDICATION-RELATED ENTEROCOLOPATHIES AND ENTEROCOLITIDES

Antibiotic Agents

Symptomatic gastrointestinal toxicity is uncommon in patients receiving antibiotic

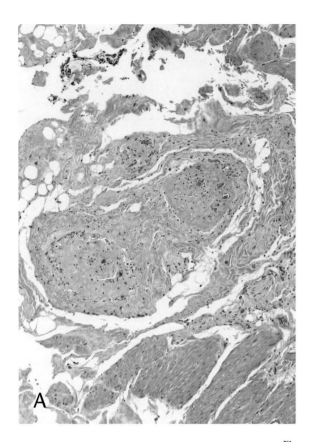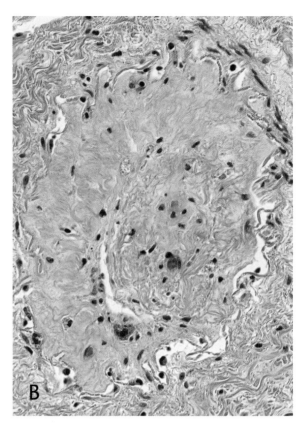

Figure 4-65

MALIGNANT ATROPHIC PAPULOSIS

Chronic intestinal injury is accompanied by pauci-inflammatory obliteration of arteries (A). Fragments of the elastic lamina are visible in an occluded artery (B).

therapy. Antimicrobial agents that alter intestinal flora, however, can cause diarrheal symptoms and facilitate the development of infectious colitis due to *Clostridium difficile* or *Klebsiella oxytoca* (170,171). Some patients receiving penicillin or related agents develop an immune complex-mediated hypersensitivity vasculitis with gastrointestinal, cutaneous, and/or renal manifestations (172). Biopsy samples in these cases display the typical features of leukocytoclastic vasculitis with basal neutrophil-rich inflammation in the mucosa, perivascular karyorrhectic debris, fibrinoid necrosis, and microthrombi, as described in the previous section.

Bisphosphonates

Alendronate and related aminobisphosphonates selectively inhibit osteoclast-mediated bone resorption and are used in the management of osteoporosis, Paget disease, and malignancy-related hypercalcemia. These medications are directly caustic to mucosal surfaces, presumably due to elaboration of free radicals during oxidation of amino acid side chains (173). As discussed in Chapter 2, these agents are best known for their propensity to cause severe pill esophagitis, although they can also cause duodenal erosions and ulcers (174,175).

Iron Deposition and Related Injury

Oral ferrous sulfate is commonly used to treat iron deficiency anemia. It is corrosive to mucosal surfaces due to the elaboration of reactive oxygen species upon hydrolysis, particularly in an acidic environment (176). Gastric injury is most common ("iron pill gastritis") and can be detected in nearly 1 percent of all gastric biopsy samples (177). Duodenal injury is infrequent; erosions and ulcers are rarely seen in affected patients (178,179).

Similar to gastroesophageal injury, iron-related duodenal erosions feature coarse, yellow-brown crystalline material in the superficial lamina propria. This finding should be distinguished from the accumulation of fine, granular hemosiderin in epithelial cells, which reflects systemic iron overload due to hemolysis or hemochromatosis, as discussed in Chapter 3 (180,181).

Pseudomelanosis intestinalis is an incidental finding in patients receiving oral iron supplements, those with systemic iron overload, and individuals treated with anti-hypertensive agents that contain benzene rings metabolized to melanin-like pigment, such as hydralazine and thiazides (182,183). Endoscopic findings include spotty brown-to-black pigmentation of the duodenal mucosa without associated inflammation (fig. 4-66) (184). Pigment-laden macrophages are seen in the lamina propria of the villous tips (fig. 4-67) (185). Pigment related to anti-hypertensive drugs is finely granular, black, and may show weak staining with Prussian blue histochemical stains.

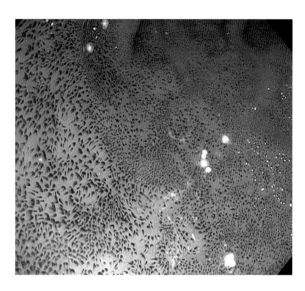

Figure 4-66

PSEUDOMELANOSIS DUODENII

Spotty brown discoloration of the duodenal mucosa can reflect ferritin deposits or accumulation of melanin-like pigment resulting from drug metabolism.

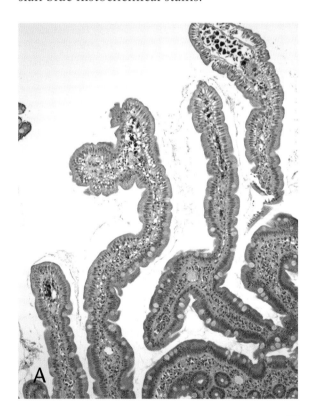

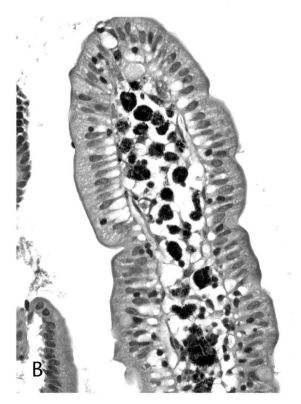

Figure 4-67

PSEUDOMELANOSIS DUODENII

The villous architecture is generally normal (A). Brown-black pigment is unassociated with mucosal inflammation (B).

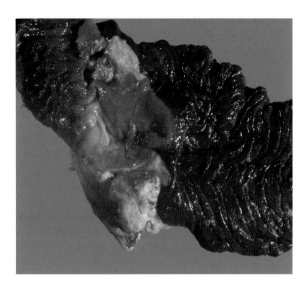

Figure 4-68

MELANOSIS COLI

The colonic mucosa (right) shows brown discoloration compared with the normal-appearing ileum.

Melanosis Coli

The relationship between phenolphthalein-containing stimulant laxatives and melanosis coli is well recognized but phenolphthalein-related melanosis is infrequent in the modern era; most phenolphthalein-containing agents were voluntarily withdrawn from the market in the late 1990s due to concerns regarding their carcinogenic properties (186). However, similar colonic findings occur following ingestion of senna-containing compounds and other plant glycosides. Mucosal pigmentation is usually an incidental finding during colonoscopy. Most patients complain of chronic constipation, although a minority may have diarrheal symptoms (i.e., factitious diarrhea).

Stimulant laxatives cause epithelial cell injury and apoptosis, resulting in the accumulation of cellular debris in macrophages of the colonic lamina propria. Although the nature of the pigment is not entirely clear, it likely represents a combination of lipofuscin and ceroid from degenerated epithelial cells as well as a melanin-like substance derived from anthracoid medications (187). Large aggregates of pigment-laden macrophages produce yellow-brown or dark mucosal pigmentation that tends to be more prominent in the proximal

colon (fig. 4-68). Lymphoid aggregates and adenomas are relatively spared, reflecting fewer lamina propria macrophages in these areas compared with the background mucosa (fig. 4-69). Macrophages are dispersed throughout the lamina propria and contain chunky, dark brown pigment (fig. 4-69D). The pigment stains strongly with PAS-D, as would be expected of ceroid or lipofuscin, but is negative with Fontana-Masson and Prussian blue stains. Other inflammatory cells are present in normal numbers. Increased surface epithelial cell apoptosis may be present but crypt cell injury is lacking.

Preparatory Effects

Oral sodium phosphate and magnesium citrate create a hyperosmolar luminal environment, whereas polyethylene glycol lavage solutions are more osmotically balanced. Senna, bisacodyl, and sodium picosulfate are stimulant laxatives. All of these bowel preparatory agents can cause colonic mucosal injury.

Endoscopic findings include patchy erythema and occasional aphthous erosions. Cytoplasmic depletion and degeneration of surface epithelial cells is accompanied by scattered apoptotic debris and mucosal edema (fig. 4-70A). Neutrophilic cryptitis and superficial scattered neutrophils are variably present (fig. 4-70B) (188). Alterations tend to be more severe in patients receiving large volume polyethylene glycol and sodium phosphate-based regimens compared with recently available oral sulfate solutions. Mucosal injury and ulcers can also result from local irritation induced by cleansing agents present on colonoscopes (189).

Nonsteroidal Anti-Inflammatory Drugs

Clinical Features. NSAIDs are highly effective in the treatment of arthritis, musculoskeletal pain, and fever, and are widely prescribed for their anti-thrombotic effects. Unfortunately, NSAIDs commonly cause gastrointestinal injury; more than 70 percent of chronic users develop gastrointestinal inflammation and nearly 25 percent have ulcers, mostly in the proximal small bowel (190). The inflammatory effects of NSAIDs are amplified when used in combination with anticoagulants, corticosteroids, alcohol, and tobacco, especially in elderly patients (191). Gastrointestinal signs and

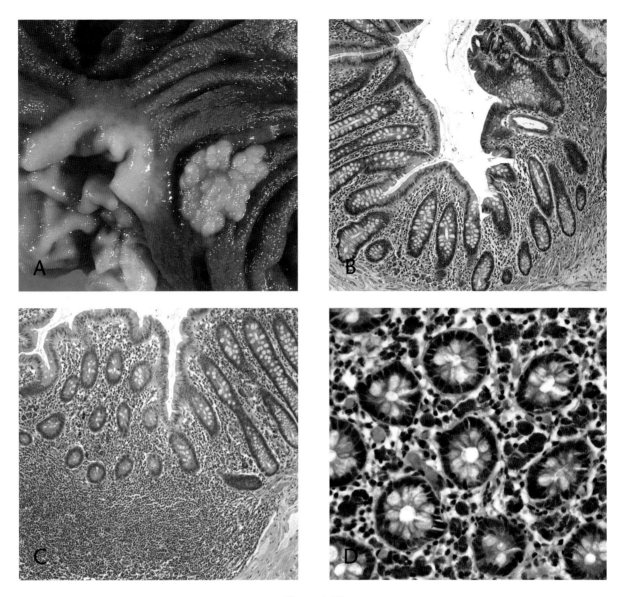

Figure 4-69

MELANOSIS COLI

Melanosis coli is less pronounced in adenomas (A), reflecting fewer pigmented macrophages in the lamina propria of an adenoma (right) compared with non-lesional mucosa (B). Pigmented macrophages are also less numerous in lymphoid aggregates (C). The macrophages contain coarse brown material and are evenly dispersed between colonic crypts (D).

symptoms of NSAID-related injury include iron deficiency anemia, bleeding, and abdominal pain, although many patients are asymptomatic.

Pathogenesis. NSAIDs cause gastrointestinal injury through the inhibition of the cyclooxygenase (COX) pathway, resulting in decreased prostaglandin synthesis and compromised mucosal integrity (192). Non-selective inhibitors of both COX-1 and COX-2 tend to cause more severe gastrointestinal injury than COX-2 inhibitors (193,194).

Gross Findings. Ulcers and erosions are more pronounced on the crests of mucosal folds and on the anti-mesenteric aspect of the bowel. Patchy edema and erythema are common in the background mucosa. Circumferential diaphragms appear as one or more circumferential membranes that narrow the orifice to only 3 to 4

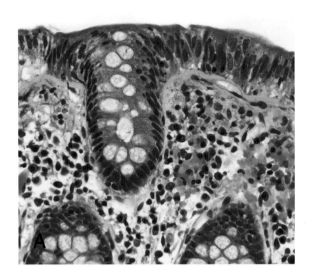
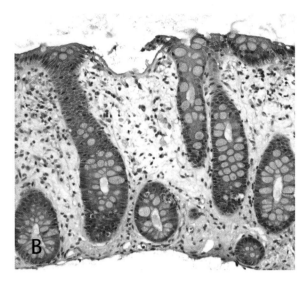

Figure 4-70

BOWEL PREPARATORY EFFECT

Preparatory agents irritate the colonic mucosa, resulting in reparative changes in the surface epithelium with apoptotic debris (A) and mucosal edema accompanied by patchy neutrophilic cryptitis (B).

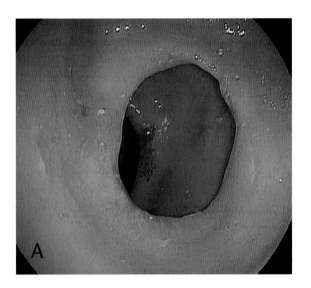
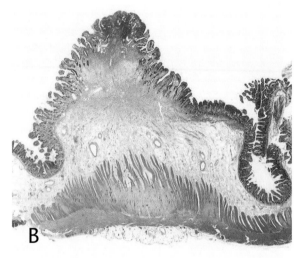

Figure 4-71

NONSTEROIDAL ANTI-INFLAMMATORY DRUG (NSAID)-RELATED DIAPHRAGM DISEASE

A smooth diaphragm narrows the lumen (A), mostly reflecting submucosal fibrosis (B). (A: courtesy of Dr. E. Montgomery, Baltimore, MD.)

mm (fig. 4-71A). Diaphragms consist of collagen fibers that are perpendicularly oriented to the muscularis propria (fig. 4-71B) (195–199). Heavy NSAID users can develop strictures, presumably resulting from intermittent ischemia induced by drug-related alterations in local perfusion (fig. 4-72).

Microscopic Findings. Proximal duodenal findings include plasma cell-rich lamina propria inflammation with neutrophils, patchy intraepithelial lymphocytosis, and mild villous blunting (fig. 4-73A). Acute ileal injury causes patchy areas of neutrophilic inflammation accompanied by mucosal edema, cytoplasmic depletion

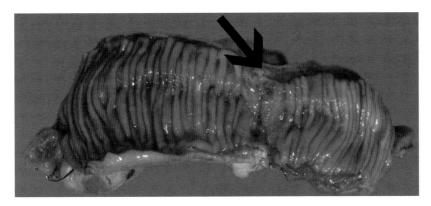

Figure 4-72

NSAID-RELATED STRICTURE

Chronic NSAID users may develop strictures (arrow) that reflect marked submucosal fibrosis.

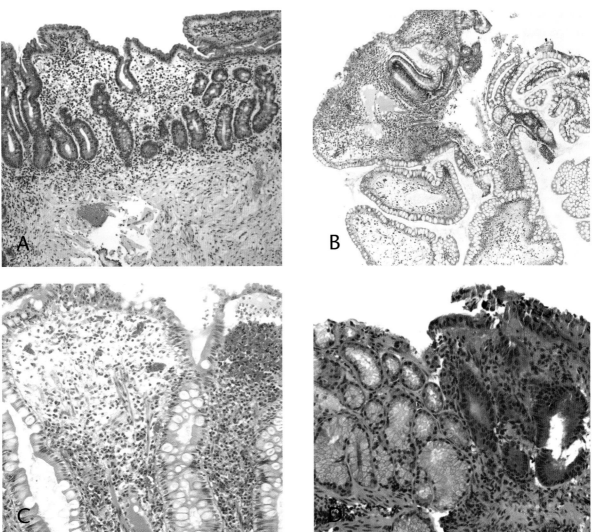

Figure 4-73

NSAID-RELATED ENTERITIS

Duodenal samples display partial villous shortening and crypt hyperplasia associated with intraepithelial lymphocytosis and plasma cell-rich inflammation in the lamina propria (A). Ileal villi are edematous (B) and show patchy inflammation with superficial neutrophils (C). Longstanding NSAID use can lead to chronic ileitis and pyloric metaplasia (D).

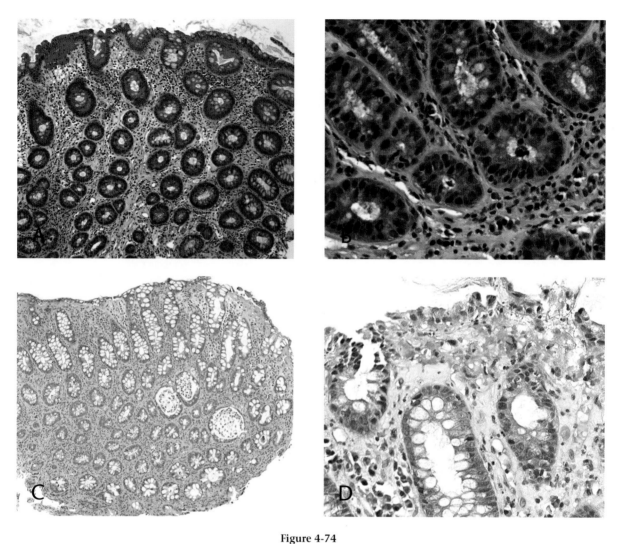

Figure 4-74

NSAID-RELATED COLITIS

Mucin-depleted regenerative crypts (A) are accompanied by lamina propria inflammation rich in eosinophils (B). Collagenous colitis can result from NSAID-related injury, and may show neutrophilic inflammation (C) with superficial hemorrhage (D).

of surface and crypt epithelium, intraepithelial neutrophilic clusters, and crypt abscesses (fig. 4-73B,C). Pyloric metaplasia, villous blunting, and patchy chronic active inflammation can occur in chronic NSAID users (fig. 4-73D) (200). Although distinction from Crohn disease may not be possible based on biopsy evaluation alone, correlation with clinical and endoscopic findings allows correct classification of most cases. Patients with minimal symptoms and few endoscopic abnormalities are far more likely to have NSAID-related injury than Crohn disease, regardless of the presence of pyloric metaplasia in biopsy material (201).

NSAIDs elicit an acute pattern of colitis. The lamina propria contains inflammatory cells and edema, with or without hemorrhage. Neutrophils are present in the lamina propria and crypt epithelium; crypt abscesses may be seen. Macrophages, eosinophils, and plasma cells are often numerous, especially when the injury persists more than a couple of weeks. Small, regenerative crypts show increased mitotic activity and apoptotic debris (fig. 4-74A,B). Erosions, ischemic-type features, and changes simulating lymphocytic or collagenous colitis also occur (fig. 4-74C,D). Distinction from microscopic colitis is based on clinical and histologic features: 1) patients with NSAID-related injury tend to present with a shorter duration of gastrointestinal symptoms and bleeding, rather than chronic watery diarrhea; 2) NSAID-related injury usually produces endoscopically apparent enterocolitis or erosions that are lacking in most patients with lymphocytic or collagenous colitis; and 3) intraepithelial lymphocytosis and collagen deposition due to NSAIDs tend to be patchy and less well-developed than typically seen in lymphocytic and collagenous colitis (202).

Ion Exchange Resins and Sequestrants

Sodium Polystyrene Sulfonate. Resins and sequestrants are nonabsorbable compounds that facilitate excretion of ions through ion-exchange mechanisms. Only one of these, sodium polystyrene sulfonate (i.e., kayexalate), has been implicated as an unequivocal cause of gastrointestinal injury. This cation exchange resin can be administered orally or as an enema to treat the hyperkalemia of chronic renal failure. It was once delivered in a pre-mixed sorbitol suspension that caused severe gastrointestinal injury through the osmotic effects of luminal sorbitol (fig. 4-75) (203). Patients with decreased bowel transit time were at increased risk of injury due to prolonged mucosal contact with sorbitol (204–206). Common presenting symptoms included severe abdominal pain, gastrointestinal hemorrhage, or peritonitis shortly after administration of the drug. This agent is now delivered in powder form or water-based solutions and, thus, the incidence of kayexalate-induced gastrointestinal injury has drastically decreased over time.

Similar to all ion exchange resins and sequestrants, sodium polystyrene sulfonate can adhere to a variety of tissue surfaces, including ulcers; detection of crystals in biopsy material confirms that the patient received the drug but does not imply causality. Thus, pathologists should not implicate kayexalate as the cause of an ulcer, unless they confirm that the drug was administered in a sorbitol carrier. Crystals are rhomboidal or triangular, with jagged edges and an internal mosaic pattern that resembles fish scales or stacks of bricks (fig. 4-76) (205). They are refractile and deeply basophilic in routine

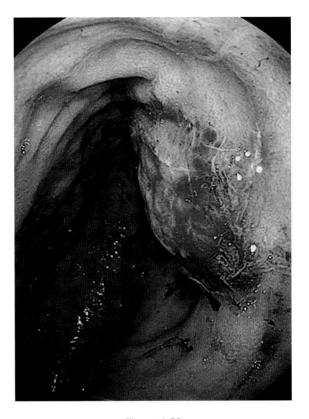

Figure 4-75

KAYEXALATE-INDUCED GASTROINTESTINAL INJURY

Large indurated ulcers are accompanied by striking mucosal edema.

sections but stain black with acid-fast and magenta with PAS-D stains (207).

Sevelamer. Sevelamer is an anion exchange resin used to treat hyperphosphatemia in uremic patients. The crystals are similar in size and shape to those of sodium polystyrene sulfonate and also have an internal mosaic structure. However, the broad, curved internal ridges are slightly larger than those seen in sodium polystyrene sulfonate and the crystals have a two-toned appearance (207). They contain central bright pink linear accentuations on a yellow background or are rusty brown with yellow discoloration at the periphery (fig. 4-77). Sevelamer crystals are magenta-colored in acid-fast stains and do not polarize. They also adhere to a variety of tissues including ulcers, adenomas, and normal tissues. Despite early reports, there are no compelling data to suggest that sevelamer causes gastrointestinal injury. Like kayexalate, it should not

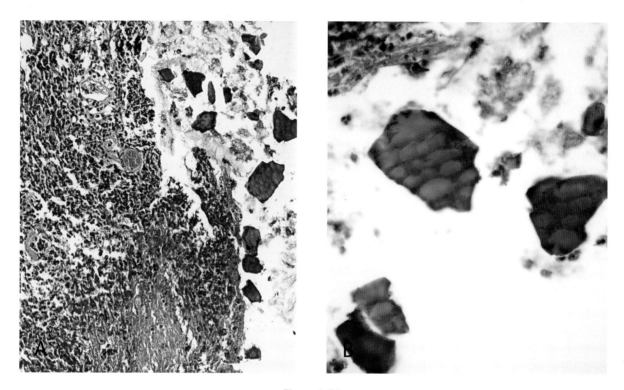

Figure 4-76

KAYEXALATE-INDUCED MUCOSAL NECROSIS

Inflamed granulation tissue and necrotic debris are associated with kayexalate crystals (A). Crystals are basophilic and irregularly shaped, with internal structures reminiscent of fish scales or stacked bricks (B).

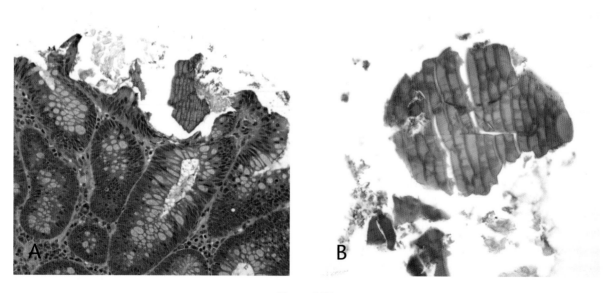

Figure 4-77

SEVELAMER CRYSTALS

Crystals are adherent to a colonic adenoma (A). They resemble sodium polystyrene sulfonate, although they are usually pink or rusty brown with peripheral yellow discoloration (B).

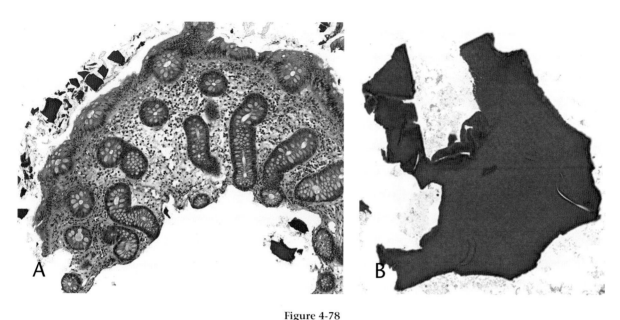

Figure 4-78

BILE SALT SEQUESTRANTS

Cholestyramine and other bile salt sequestrants are similar in size and shape to kayexalate crystals (A), but are brightly eosinophilic without internal structures (B).

be considered pathogenic even when found in association with ulcers (208).

Bile Acid Sequestrants. Cholestyramine, colesevelam, colestipol, and related agents are frequently used in the management of patients with hyperlipidemia and cholestatic liver disease. Resin fragments are rhomboidal or triangular, similar in size and shape to kayexalate crystals. However, they lack an internal mosaic structure and are not basophilic. Rather, they appear dark brown, magenta, orange, bright red, or purple in hematoxylin and eosin (H&E)-stained tissue sections depending on the tissue thickness and staining conditions (fig. 4-78). They are dull yellow with acid-fast stains (209). Bile acid sequestrants do not cause mucosal injury and need not be commented upon when detected in biopsy samples (207).

Olmesartan and Related Compounds

Clinical Features. Sartans are angiotensin II receptor antagonists that function as powerful antihypertensive agents. Olmesartan and related drugs cause severe enterocolitis in approximately 1 percent of patients taking them (210,211). Symptomatic patients are usually in their seventh to eighth decades of life and present with profound malabsorptive diarrhea and weight loss. More than 50 percent require hospitalization for severe illness. The interval between initiation of treatment and onset of symptoms is highly variable, and may be months to years (212).

Pathogenesis. The mechanism of sartan-induced mucosal injury is unclear. Some investigators have hypothesized roles for HLA-DQ haplotypes and immune dysregulation, whereas others suggest that sartans inhibit transforming growth factor (TGF)-α leading to an aberrant cellular immune response in the intestinal mucosa (213–215). Olmesartan seems to elicit inflammatory cell infiltrates and overexpression of cytokines, similar to those seen in celiac disease; *in vitro* studies suggest it disrupts the tight junction protein, ZO-1 (216). Patients may have autoantibodies typical of celiac disease but do not respond to gluten withdrawal.

Gross Findings. Endoscopic findings in patients with sartan-related gastrointestinal injury are variable. Some patients have an entirely normal examination, whereas others have mucosal atrophy or scalloped duodenal folds (fig. 4-79). Erythema and/or ulcers are often identified during upper and lower endoscopic examinations (211,212,217).

Microscopic Findings. Histologic abnormalities occur throughout the gastrointestinal tract.

Gastric changes include chronic active gastritis with variable intraepithelial lymphocytosis and apoptotic debris in deep glands (fig. 4-80). Duodenal samples display variable villous shortening with mononuclear cell-rich inflammation and intraepithelial lymphocytosis (fig. 4-81A,B)

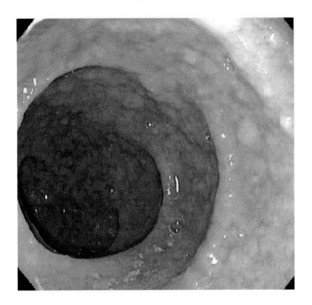

Figure 4-79

OLMESARTAN-INDUCED DUODENAL INJURY

The duodenal mucosa is flat and pale with scalloped folds.

(217,218). Crypt cell apoptosis and neutrophilic inflammation tend to be more prominent than seen in celiac disease (fig. 4-81C). Loss of Paneth cells, goblet cells, and endocrine cells can simulates the features of autoimmune enteropathy in some cases (fig. 4-81D). Ileal and colonic changes include mildly increased intraepithelial lymphocytosis, and plasma cell-rich chronic active inflammation that mimics inflammatory bowel disease (fig. 4-82) (219).

Nearly one-third of patients with sartan-related enteropathy have subepithelial collagen deposits, which are most common in the proximal small bowel (fig. 4-80) (220). The combination of chronic mucosal inflammation, neutrophilic aggregates, apoptosis, and subepithelial collagen deposits should prompt consideration of a sartan-related injury, especially in an older patient. Drug withdrawal is associated with complete resolution of clinical symptoms, although it can take several months for histologic abnormalities to completely resolve (211,212).

Medications that Affect the Cell Cycle

Clinical Features. Colchicine and paclitaxel are alkaloid preparations that exert cytotoxic effects by inducing mitotic arrest during metaphase. Both agents can cause cytologic

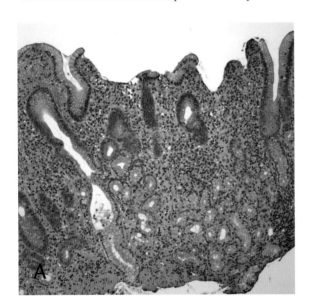
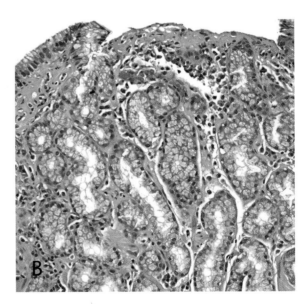

Figure 4-80

OLMESARTAN-INDUCED GASTRITIS

The antral mucosa is expanded by dense plasma cell-rich inflammation (A). Subepithelial collagen deposits are present in association with chronic inflammation (B).

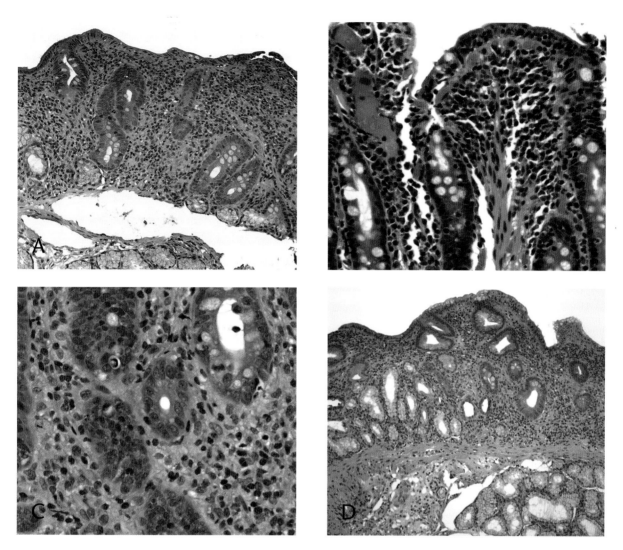

Figure 4-81

OLMESARTAN-INDUCED DUODENITIS

Complete villous shortening and crypt hyperplasia are accompanied by dense chronic inflammation (A). The surface epithelium is attenuated and infiltrated by lymphocytes (B). Crypts contain scattered apoptotic epithelial cells and neutrophils (C). Goblet cells are diminished and Paneth cells are absent (D).

changes in the proliferative mucosa of the gastrointestinal tract. Paclitaxel is an antineoplastic agent that binds microtubules of the mitotic spindle (221). It is used to treat carcinomas of the breast, esophagus, and lung, and causes non-neoplastic epithelial cell injury, particularly in the small bowel and colon. Colchicine prevents tubulin protein polymerization and mitotic spindle formation. It is used to treat gout, Mediterranean fever, pleuritis, and pericarditis.

Microscopic Findings. Paclitaxel effect is associated with numerous ring mitotic forms and increased numbers of normal-appearing mitotic figures in the crypt epithelium (fig. 4-83) (222). Small bowel biopsy samples show variable villous abnormalities, but the amount of associated inflammation is minimal unless erosions or ulcers are present. Colchicine toxicity elicits similar histologic features, although arrested mitotic figures tend to be more numerous and drug-related injury is more pronounced in the stomach and small bowel but not the colon (fig. 4-84).

Treatment and Prognosis. Gastrointestinal manifestations of treatment are expected in

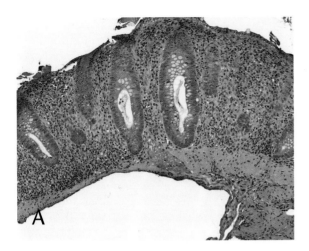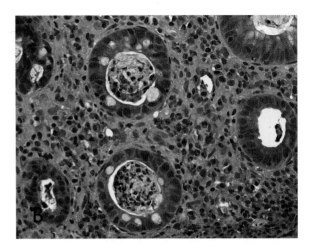

Figure 4-82

OLMESARTAN-INDUCED COLITIS

Dense plasma cell-rich inflammation expands the colonic lamina propria (A) and is accompanied by neutrophilic cryptitis (B), simulating the features of idiopathic inflammatory bowel disease.

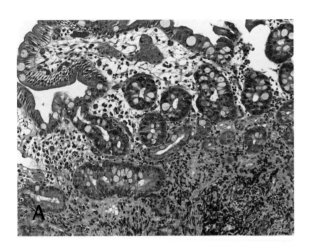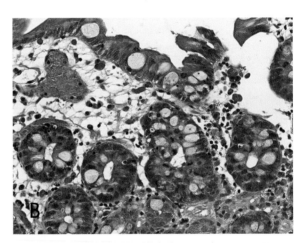

Figure 4-83

PACLITAXEL EFFECT

Paclitaxel causes inflammatory changes in the intestinal mucosa (A). Numerous typical and ring mitotic figures are present in the crypts (B).

patients receiving paclitaxel and do not imply toxic effects of this agent; they are related to the interval between drug administration and the biopsy procedure. However, histologic changes associated with colchicine generally reflect higher than therapeutic levels; their detection warrants immediate communication with the treating physician because toxicity can cause severe gastrointestinal injury and neurologic symptoms. Of note, any proliferative lesion (e.g., adenoma or carcinoma) can contain ring mitotic figures at therapeutic

levels of colchicine. These findings do not imply toxicity when confined to such lesions. Paclitaxel and colchicine related changes may be confused with dysplasia in some cases (223).

Mycophenolate-Induced Gastrointestinal Injury

Clinical Features. Mycophenolate is an anti-proliferative agent used to maintain immunosuppression in solid organ and bone marrow transplant recipients. There are two

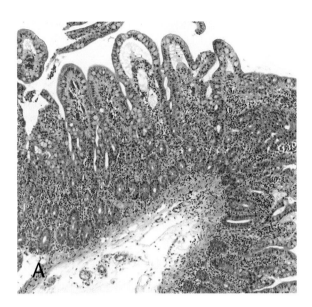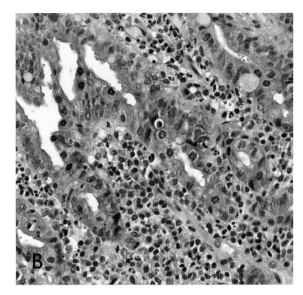

Figure 4-84

COLCHICINE TOXICITY

Colchicine induces variably severe villous abnormalities with crypt hyperplasia and increased lamina propria inflammation (A). Crypts contain cuboidal epithelial cells with ring mitotic figures (B).

available formulations: mycophenolate mofetil is absorbed in the stomach and mycophenolate sodium is absorbed in the small intestine. Gastrointestinal manifestations of drug injury occur in nearly half of patients receiving mycophenolate and can develop at any point during the course of therapy (224). Patients present with diarrhea, nausea and vomiting, abdominal pain, malabsorption, and gastrointestinal bleeding. The likelihood of gastrointestinal symptoms increases in patients receiving high doses and those with impaired renal function.

Pathogenesis. Mycophenolate is a pro-drug that is converted to metabolically active mycophenolic acid. The latter non-competitively inhibits inosine 5'-monophosphate dehydrogenase in the *de novo* pathway of purine synthesis, which is important to B- and T-cell proliferation. Intestinal epithelial cells utilize the same metabolic pathway, making them particularly susceptible to drug-related injury (224,225). Lymphocyte depletion potentiates injury by rendering the mucosa susceptible to infection (226,227).

Gross Findings. The endoscopic features of drug-induced injury are variable. Patients may develop erythema, erosions, or ulcers anywhere in the gastrointestinal tract.

Microscopic Findings. Mycophenolate-related injury features apoptotic epithelial cells in the deep crypt or gland region with atrophy and dropout, as well as patchy lamina propria infiltrates composed of neutrophils and eosinophils (fig. 4-85A). Destroyed crypts and glands are slightly dilated and lined by attenuated epithelial cells; they contain luminal apoptotic cellular debris and neutrophils (fig. 4-85B,C) (228). Injury tends to be most pronounced in the small bowel and colon.

Differential Diagnosis. The most problematic differential diagnoses include graft-versus-host disease (GVHD) and viral infection. Endocrine cell nests are more prominent in GVHD than in drug-related injury, whereas mycophenolate induces a greater degree of mucosal eosinophilia and apoptotic luminal debris in crypts and deep glands (fig. 4-85D). In fact, the combination of more than 15 lamina propria eosinophils per high-power field, luminal aggregates of apoptotic debris in crypts, and an absence of endocrine cell aggregates is more than 90 percent specific for a diagnosis of mycophenolate-related injury in patients at risk for GVHD (229). Adenovirus, varicella, and cytomegalovirus can cause epithelial cell apoptosis in the deep mucosa, simulating the effects of mycophenolate. These viruses produce characteristic viral inclusions and can

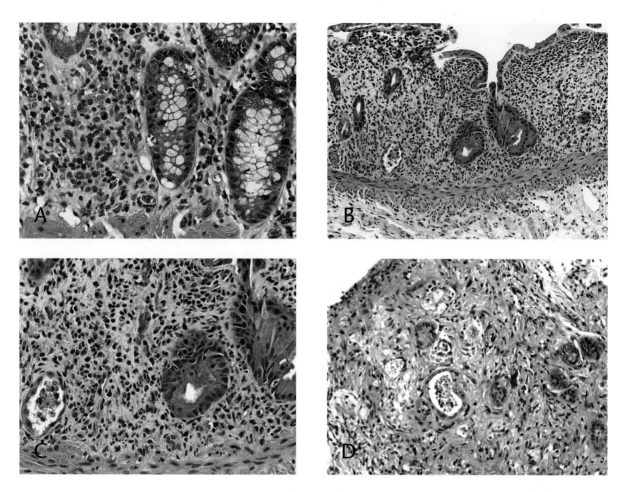

Figure 4-85

MYCOPHENOLATE-RELATED COLITIS

Apoptotic crypt debris and eosinophil-rich mucosal inflammation are common (A). Severe injury results in crypt loss; regenerative crypts are lined by cuboidal epithelium (B). Dilated crypts lined by attenuated epithelium and containing cellular debris are characteristic (C). Mycophenolate causes diffuse crypt injury and does not spare endocrine cells (D).

be detected using immunohistochemical stains, as described subsequently.

Chronic mycophenolate-related injury can simulate the features of idiopathic inflammatory bowel disease (fig. 4-86): up to 82 percent of patients who chronically receive mycophenolate have crypt architectural abnormalities in their colonic biopsy samples (230). The incidence of chronic active colitis indistinguishable from idiopathic inflammatory bowel disease is also increased in this patient population compared with the general population, possibly reflecting the chronic immunomodulatory effects of mycophenolate (231). It is unwise to render a new diagnosis of idiopathic inflammatory bowel disease in an immunosuppressed patient unless other etiologies, including immunomodulatory agents, have been excluded.

Immune Checkpoint Inhibitors

Clinical Features. Immune checkpoint inhibitors are highly effective against several tumor types. This class of drugs includes cytotoxic T-lymphocyte antigen-4 (CTLA-4) inhibitors (e.g., ipilimumab, tremelimumab), programmed cell death protein-1 (PD-1) inhibitors (e.g., nivolumab, pembrolizumab, avelumab), and programmed cell death protein ligand-1 (PD-L1) inhibitors (e.g., atezolizumab). Anti-CTLA-4 antibodies are mostly used in the treatment of melanoma and renal cell carcinoma, whereas anti-PD-1 and anti-PD-L1 medications are approved therapies

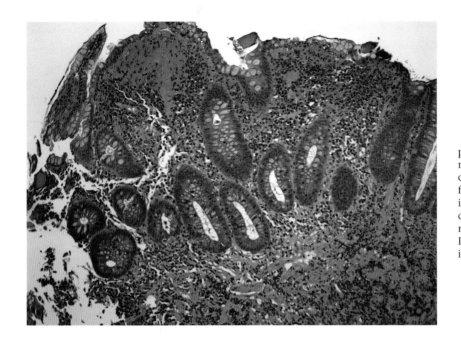

Figure 4-86

POST-TRANSPLANT CHRONIC COLITIS

Some solid organ transplant patients who are maintained with mycophenolate develop a form of chronic colitis indistinguishable from that seen in patients with idiopathic inflammatory bowel disease. Plasma cell-rich inflammation, basal plasmacytosis, and Paneth cell metaplasia are present in the distal colon.

for several solid tumor types of the gastrointestinal tract and other sites. Checkpoint inhibitors can increase immune-mediated destruction of tumor cells and produce dramatic clinical responses in some patients (232,233).

Checkpoint inhibitors also cause immune dysregulation in the gastrointestinal tract, which can lead to severe gastrointestinal symptoms including diarrhea, abdominal pain, and bleeding. Symptoms usually begin within a few months of the initial dose and even sooner when multiple agents are used in combination. Endoscopically evident mucosal erythema, friability, and ulcers are often present. Although rare, severe injury can result in colonic perforation (234,235). Inflammatory changes tend to be most pronounced in the colon, particularly the rectosigmoid region. Cessation of therapy is usually an effective treatment strategy, although patients with severe symptoms may also require systemic corticosteroids or infliximab.

Pathogenesis. Checkpoint inhibitors stimulate the immune system by blocking the co-inhibitory receptors present on T-cells that impede an antitumor inflammatory reaction. Physiologic activation of T-cells requires simultaneous interactions at two binding sites on antigen presenting cells. First, antigens must bind T-cell receptors presented by major histocompatibility complex molecules. Second, CD80 or B7 ligands on anti-

gen presenting cells must bind CD28 receptors on T-cells. A T-cell surface glycoprotein, CTLA-4, binds CD80 and B7, thereby competitively inhibiting CD28-mediated T-cell activation. Antibodies to CTLA-4 essentially enhance T-cell–mediated immunity by preventing inactivation of CD28-mediated signaling. On the other hand, PD-1 is a T-cell receptor that binds to PD-L1 or PD-L2 on antigen presenting cells and inhibits T-cell activation. Antibodies to these molecules suppress this inhibitory pathway and, thus, stimulate an anti-tumor immune response.

Microscopic Findings. All of the checkpoint inhibitors cause similar types of gastrointestinal mucosal injury, although CTLA-1 inhibitors cause more severe and widespread injury than PD-1 and PD-L1 inhibitors. Mucositis is characterized by variably severe neutrophilic inflammation and prominent epithelial cell apoptosis in the deep mucosa (fig. 4-87). Intraepithelial lymphocytosis is often present in the crypts (fig. 4-88) (236–238). Small bowel injury usually manifests with variable villous architectural abnormalities. Colonic changes can be accompanied by mononuclear cell-rich inflammation in the lamina propria, pseudopolyps, and crypt distortion that simulate the features of idiopathic inflammatory bowel disease, especially when patients are maintained on these agents for long periods of time (fig. 4-89) (239,240). Some

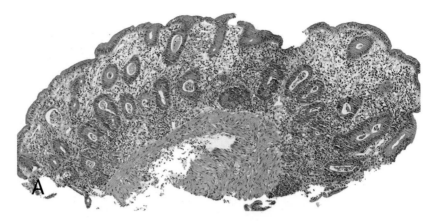

Figure 4-87

PEMBROLIZUMAB-ASSOCIATED COLITIS

The lamina propria contains a patchy mononuclear cell-rich inflammatory infiltrate associated with cryptitis and crypt abscesses (A). Dilated crypts contain necrotic cellular debris (B).

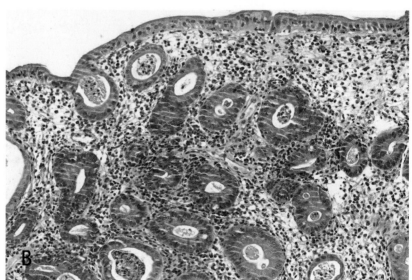

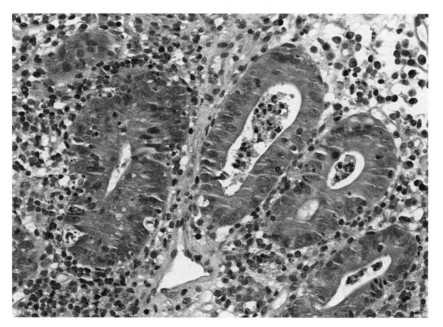

Figure 4-88

PEMBROLIZUMAB-ASSOCIATED COLITIS

Numerous inraepithelial lymphocytes and luminal neutrophils are accompanied by apoptotic crypt cells.

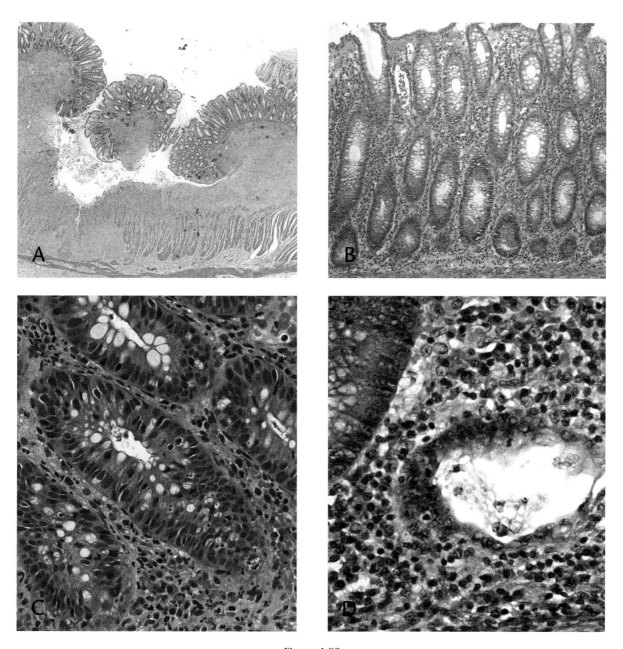

Figure 4-89

IPILIMUMAB-ASSOCIATED COLITIS

Severe colonic injury can result in ulcers and pseudopolyp development (A). Chronic colitis develops in some patients, featuring plasma cell-rich mucosal inflammation (B), neutrophilic cryptitis (C), and apoptotic luminal debris (D).

patients receiving ipilimumab develop deep fissuring ulcers and colonic perforation (234).

Idelalisib

Idelalisib inhibits the PI3Kδ isoform, which is involved in membrane receptor-mediated B-cell signaling. This agent was recently approved for treatment of several types of low-grade B-cell malignancies. It can cause gastrointestinal toxicity in a significant proportion of treated patients, especially when used in combination with other chemotherapeutic agents. Severe, debilitating diarrhea is the most important side effect.

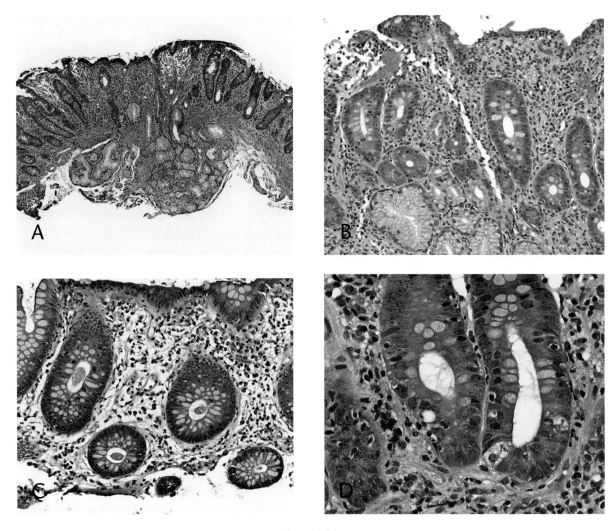

Figure 4-90

IDELALISIB-ASSOCIATED ENTEROCOLITIS

Similar to other targeted therapies, idelalisib can cause severe villous abnormalities (A) with intraepithelial lymphocytosis, cryptitis, and epithelial cell apoptosis (B). Colonic injury features intraepithelial lymphocytosis (C) with crypt cell apoptosis (D).

Histologic features of gastrointestinal toxicity include variable villous blunting, intraepithelial lymphocytosis, neutrophilic cryptitis, and epithelial cell apoptosis (fig. 4-90). Intraepithelial lymphocytes are CD3/CD8-positive T-cells and tend to be more numerous in the crypts than surface epithelium (148,241).

Other Chemotherapeutic Agents

Chemotherapeutic agents that promote cellular necrosis can injure the gastrointestinal epithelium, resulting in loss of mucosal integrity, increased permeability, and translocation of organisms from the lumen (242). The risk of gastrointestinal morbidity is highest in young children, elderly patients, and those with poor nutritional status or neutropenia (243).

Chemotherapy-induced injury to the esophagus typically causes odynophagia or dysphagia due to erosions, ulcers or desquamation, as described in Chapter 2. Injury to the remaining gastrointestinal tract produces nausea and vomiting, failure to thrive, abdominal pain, and diarrhea, which may be bloody. Endoscopic findings include erythema, erosions, and ulcers that are usually patchy. Severe toxicity with extensive ulcers

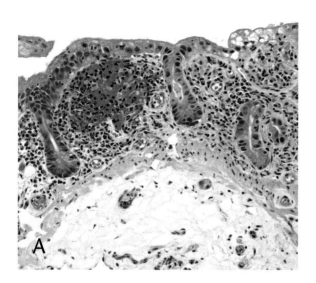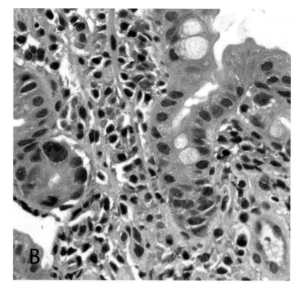

Figure 4-91

5-FLUOROURACIL-INDUCED DUODENITIS

Villous blunting is accompanied by striking cytologic atypia, cytoplasmic depletion, and nucleomegaly (A). Atypical nuclei have smooth borders and are accompanied by clearly benign cells (B).

or perforation is rare, and when present, raises the possibility of an underlying predisposing metabolic defect. For example, *DPYD* mutations that prolong the serum half-life of 5-fluorouracil are identified in approximately 20 percent of patients who develop severe gastrointestinal toxicity due to this agent (244,245).

Chemotherapeutic agents that injure the gastrointestinal epithelium feature scattered crypts and glands lined by attenuated epithelial cells; the latter show irregular nuclear spacing and acidophilic cytoplasm. Necrotic epithelial cells and neutrophils are often present in the lumen. Small bowel samples may demonstrate villous blunting associated with marked cytologic abnormalities, hyperchromatic nuclei, and prominent nucleoli, as well as numerous apoptotic bodies in the deep crypts (fig. 4-91). These features occasionally simulate dysplasia, although crypts are not crowded. Ample cytoplasm, smudgy chromatin, and minimal mitotic activity are clues to a non-neoplastic interpretation, especially in the appropriate clinical setting.

Medications that Cause Ischemic Injury

Some medications cause ischemic injury to the gastrointestinal tract through direct vasoconstrictive actions or by modulating bioactive molecules that regulate splanchnic blood flow (Table 4-6) (119,120). Cocaine, NSAIDs, and oral contraceptives are the best documented drugs that cause gastrointestinal injury through an ischemic mechanism. The histologic changes caused by these agents are similar to those of other types of intestinal ischemia, although NSAIDs are also associated with other inflammatory patterns, as previously described.

Cocaine causes ischemic enteritis through two primary mechanisms: vasoconstriction and thrombotic occlusion of arteries, particularly short branch arteries from the vasa recta. Most patients with cocaine-induced ischemic enterocolitis develop symptoms within 3 days of drug ingestion (246). Extensive regional infarction and bowel perforation can occur in patients with vasospasm or thrombosis of larger arteries (111).

The pro-thrombotic effects of oral contraceptive drugs are well known, although low-dose agents are associated with a much lower risk of thrombosis (49). Risk factors for thrombosis include smoking, hypertension, diabetes mellitus, obesity, and underlying genetic abnormalities that promote coagulation, such as protein C or S deficiencies. Estrogens accelerate platelet aggregation and are prothrombotic (114). Mesenteric vein thromboses are most common, although

243

Table 4-6

MEDICATIONS THAT CAUSE ISCHEMIC ENTEROCOLITIS

Hormonal Agents	**Antineoplastic Agents**
Oral contraceptive agents	Vinorelbine
Danazol	Paclitaxel and related compounds
Flutamide	**Diuretic Agents**
Estrogen	Furosemide
Anti-Inflammatory Agents	Ethacrynic acid
Interferon	**Laxatives and Resins**
Azathioprine	Magnesium citrate
Anti-tumor necrosis factor (TNF)	Bisacodyl
Nonsteroidal anti-inflammatory drugs (NSAIDs)	Kayexalate in sorbitol carrier
Cardiovascular Medications	**Illicit Drugs**
Calcium channel blockers	Cocaine
Vasopressins	Amphetamines
Digitalis	**Miscellaneous Drugs**
Psychotropic Medications	Serotonin agonists and antagonists
Anti-epileptics	Decongestants
Oxybutynin	Ergot alkaloids
Tricyclic antidepressants	Simvastatin and related agents
Phenothiazine and related agents	Opiates

some patients develop progressive occlusion of arteries (115). Discontinuation of therapy usually results in reversal of these changes.

OTHER THERAPY-RELATED ENTEROCOLOPATHIES AND ENTEROCOLITIDES

Graft-versus-Host Disease

Definition. *Graft-versus-host disease* (GVHD) is an immune-mediated tissue injury resulting from donor T-cells following stem cell transplantation.

Clinical Features. GVHD is a major cause of mortality in bone marrow transplant patients. It is classified based on the interval of time between transplantation and onset of symptoms: acute GVHD occurs less than 100 days after transplant, whereas chronic GVHD occurs more than 100 days after transplant (247). Acute GVHD develops in up to 50 percent of allogeneic transplant recipients, as well as in 5 to 6 percent of autologous bone marrow transplant recipients, particularly those with underlying multiple myeloma (248). Rare cases follow blood transfusion or solid organ transplantation.

Gastrointestinal symptoms include nausea, vomiting, and diarrhea, and many patients have a cutaneous maculopapular rash. Patients with liver involvement have abnormal liver function tests with a cholestatic pattern of injury. Chronic GVHD is associated with sclerotic cutaneous lesions and cholestatic liver disease, reflecting loss of bile ducts.

Pathogenesis. Donor T-lymphocytes recognize allo-antigens on recipient epithelial cells, resulting in elaboration of cytokines and B-cell activation (247).

Gross Findings. GVHD causes diffuse mucosal injury throughout the gastrointestinal tract. Mild GVHD may produce minimal changes, with loss of the normal vascular pattern or erythema. Edema, nodularity, erosions, and ulcers are only seen in patients with severe disease (fig. 4-92) (249,250). Mucosal atrophy develops in patients with chronic GVHD.

Microscopic Findings. Acute GVHD causes a similar pattern of injury throughout the gastrointestinal tract: single cell necrosis in the proliferative compartment is accompanied by a pauci-inflammatory mucosal infiltrate (fig. 4-93A) (251). Crypts and deep mucosal glands are cystically dilated and lined by attenuated epithelial cells (fig. 4-93B). Crypts contain abundant apoptotic debris and cytoplasmic

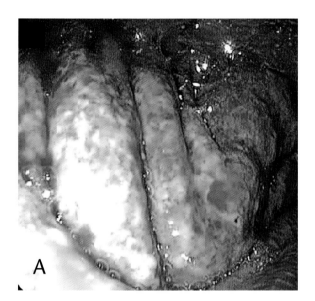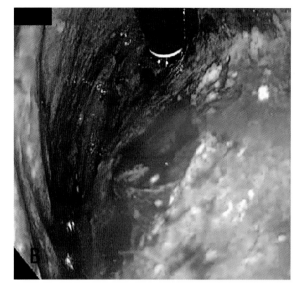

Figure 4-92

GRAFT-VERSUS-HOST DISEASE

Severe injury features marked edema and a mottled mucosal surface (A) with ulcers and exudates (B).

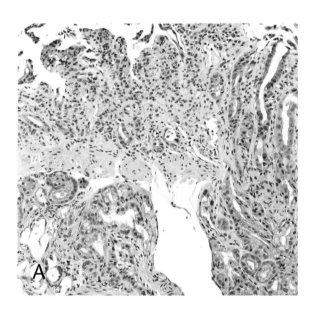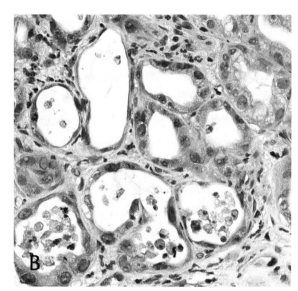

Figure 4-93

GRAFT-VERSUS-HOST DISEASE

The duodenal villi are flattened. Crypts contain insured epithelium and drop-out is evident (A). Dilated Brunner glands are lined by attenuated epithelial cells with necrotic cellular debris (B).

vacuoles filled with karyorrhectic material (fig. 4-94) (252). Crypt loss is accompanied by villous blunting in the small bowel and ulcers or erosions in severe cases (fig. 4-95). Endocrine cells are relatively preserved (fig. 4-96) (253). Histo-

logic grading schemes are based on the extent of epithelial cell damage (Table 4-7) (254,255). Chronic GVHD displays crypt architectural distortion, patchy loss of crypts and glands, and fibrosis of the lamina propria, but crypt cell

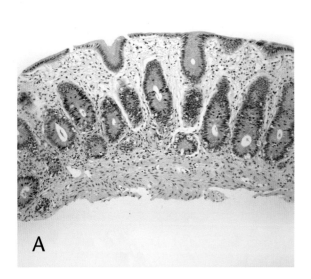
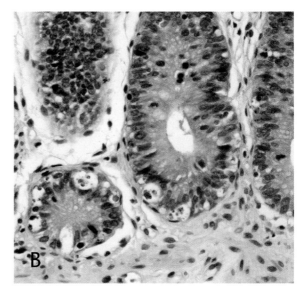

Figure 4-94

GRAFT-VERSUS-HOST DISEASE

The colonic crypt architecture is preserved and the lamina propria is uninflamed, yet crypts contain abundant necrotic cellular debris (A). Exploding crypt cells consist of abundant apoptotic debris in vacuoles (B).

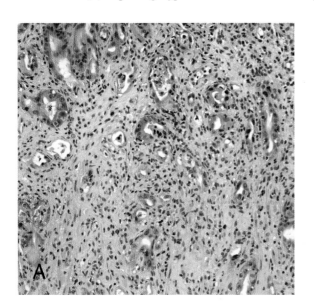
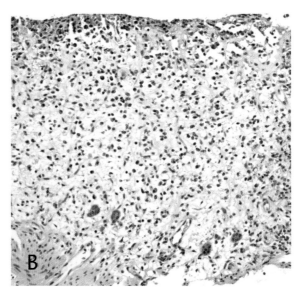

Figure 4-95

GRAFT-VERSUS-HOST DISEASE

Severe GVHD results in multifocal crypt destruction (A) that may progress to complete crypt loss (B).

apoptosis is not a prominent feature in most cases (256).

Differential Diagnosis. Several medications and infections can cause features that resemble mild GVHD. Mycophenolate, proton pump inhibitors, oral sodium bowel preparations, and NSAIDs can all increase epithelial cell apoptosis. Infections with CMV and adenovirus characteristically elicit cellular disarray and spotty necrosis; they should be excluded when assessing biopsy

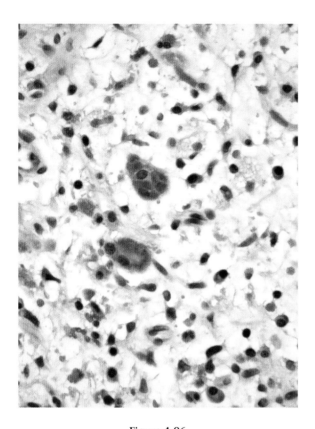

Figure 4-96

GRAFT-VERSUS-HOST DISEASE

Endocrine cells are spared in cases of severe GVHD and often appear as residual nests.

Table 4-7

GRADING SCHEME FOR GASTROINTESTINAL GRAFT-VERSUS-HOST DISEASE[a]

GVHD Grade	Histology
1	Scattered apoptotic epithelial cells, >6/10 contiguous crypts
2	Entire crypt contains apoptotic debris ("exploding crypts")
3	Crypt dropout
4	Totally denuded mucosa

[a]Data from Lerner KG, Kao GF, Storb R, Buckner CD, Clift RA, Thomas ED. Histopathology of graft-vs.-host reaction (GvHR) in human recipients of marrow from HL-A-matched sibling donors. Transplant Proc 1974;6:367-71.

samples from patients with suspected GVHD. Samples obtained within 20 days after conditioning chemotherapy frequently feature cellular changes indistinguishable from those of GVHD, and thus, a definite diagnosis of GVHD cannot be made in the immediate transplant period (257).

Treatment and Prognosis. Immunosuppression is the mainstay of therapy for patients with GVHD. Various combinations of corticosteroid therapy, mycophenolate mofetil, tacrolimus, and other agents can be effective, although mortality rates range from 10 to 15 percent. Some data suggest that severe injury is less likely to respond to therapy (258).

Cord Colitis Syndrome

Definition. Antibiotic responsive culture-negative diarrheal symptoms in patients receiving transplanted stem cells have been called *cord colitis syndrome*.

Clinical Features. "Cord colitis syndrome" is probably an infectious disorder that follows stem cell transplantation, rather than a *bona fide* entity (259–261). It usually develops following umbilical cord transplant but can occur after peripheral blood stem cell or bone marrow transplant (260). Patients typically present with abdominal pain and severe, protracted diarrhea.

Pathogenesis. Cord colitis syndrome likely represents a pattern of mucosal injury resulting from a variety of pathogens that are difficult to detect using routine methods. *Bradyrhizobium enterica* and other infectious agents have been identified in patients with this condition (262,263).

Microscopic Findings. Affected patients have a non-specific pattern of inflammation. Some have patchy active colitis with variable numbers of mononuclear cells in the lamina propria (fig. 4-97). Apoptotic debris is usually present in colonic crypts. Loose granulomatous inflammation is often seen in the superficial lamina propria and may represent prior epithelial injury.

Treatment and Prognosis. Treatment consists of antibacterial therapy. Patients respond well to fluoroquinolones and metronidazole. Relapses following cessation of therapy are common, and patients may require prolonged antibiotic therapy (259).

Neutropenic Enterocolitis

Definition. *Neutropenic enterocolitis* is intestinal necrosis developing in neutropenic patients. *Typhlitis* is a synonym.

247

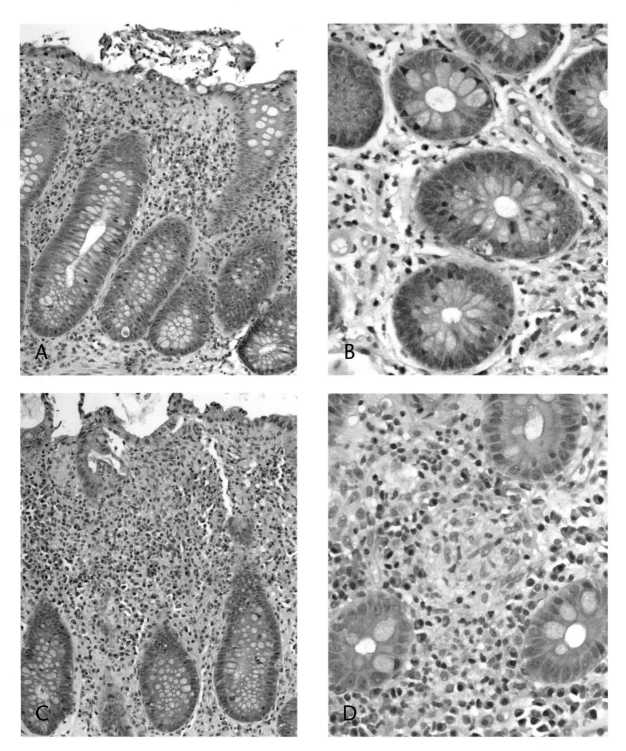

Figure 4-97

CORD COLITIS SYNDROME

Patchy active colitis is present on a background of mild plasma cell-rich inflammation in the lamina propria (A) and scattered apoptotic crypt epithelial cells (B). Poorly formed granulomatous inflammation may reflect crypt destruction or prior surface injury (C), but some cases contain well-formed epithelioid granulomas (D).

Clinical Features. Neutropenic enterocolitis is a serious complication of chemotherapy, most frequently developing in patients treated for hematologic malignancies. It shows a predilection for the terminal ileum and ascending colon, producing rapidly progressive abdominal pain and distention (264,265). Imaging reveals dilated loops of bowel with mural thickening or perforation.

Pathogenesis. The combined effects of cytotoxic drug-induced cellular damage and immunosuppression diminish the mucosal barrier, allowing *Klebsiella pneumonia*, *Escherichia coli*, *Enterobacter* sp., *Staphylococcus aureus*, *Streptococcus viridans*, *Clostridium difficile*, *Candida* sp., and other organisms to invade the intestinal wall (264). *Clostridium septicum* occasionally causes neutropenic enterocolitis and necrotizing fasciitis in patients with gastrointestinal malignancies (266).

Gross Findings. Thick yellow-brown exudates coat the mucosal surface, reflecting confluent ulcers (fig. 4-98). The bowel wall is often thickened owing to marked submucosal edema and hemorrhage.

Microscopic Findings. Striking mural edema and extensive necrosis are accompanied by hemorrhage. Neutrophils may be present in small numbers, but the extent of the host response is disproportionately mild compared with the severity of injury (fig. 4-99). Gram and Gomori methenamine silver (GMS) stains frequently highlight invasive organisms (fig. 4-100).

Treatment and Prognosis. Supportive care with antibiotic therapy, bowel rest, and fluid resuscitation can lead to reversal of mild to moderate injury. Mural necrosis and intestinal perforation are life-threatening and require surgical resection.

Radiation Enterocolitis

Definition. Enterocolic injury secondary to therapeutic ionizing radiation is termed *radiation enterocolitis*.

Clinical Features. Acute radiation enterocolitis develops hours to weeks after therapy, whereas chronic radiation-induced injury manifests months to years after cessation of treatment. Acute radiation injury causes symptoms in 25 to 50 percent of patients receiving treatment. The rectum is most commonly affected, although disease can occur in any intestinal segment

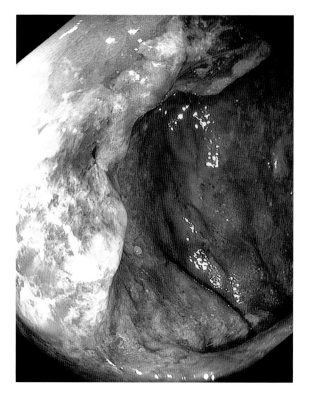

Figure 4-98

NEUTROPENIC ENTEROCOLITIS

Viable edematous mucosa is adjacent to an area of extensive necrosis surfaced by a shaggy exudate.

in the field of radiation. Patients present with tenesmus, urgency, and mucoid discharge.

Chronic radiation-induced enterocolitis is less common, affecting 5 to 15 percent of patients. Symptoms include nausea, vomiting, constipation, and lower gastrointestinal bleeding. Imaging reveals mural thickening and angulated bowel loops secondary to adhesions.

Pathogenesis. Ionizing radiation is directly toxic to proliferative epithelial cells. Chronic injury leads to progressive obliteration of arteries, resulting in ischemic enteritis and strictures.

Gross Findings. Acute injury produces striking mucosal edema, erythema, and loss of the normal vascular pattern (fig. 4-101). Erosions and ulcers are present in severe cases. Chronic radiation-induced enterocolitis results in patchy erythema on a background of mucosal atrophy, loss of mucosal folds, strictures, fistulae, and chronic ulcers associated with mucosal friability (fig. 4-102).

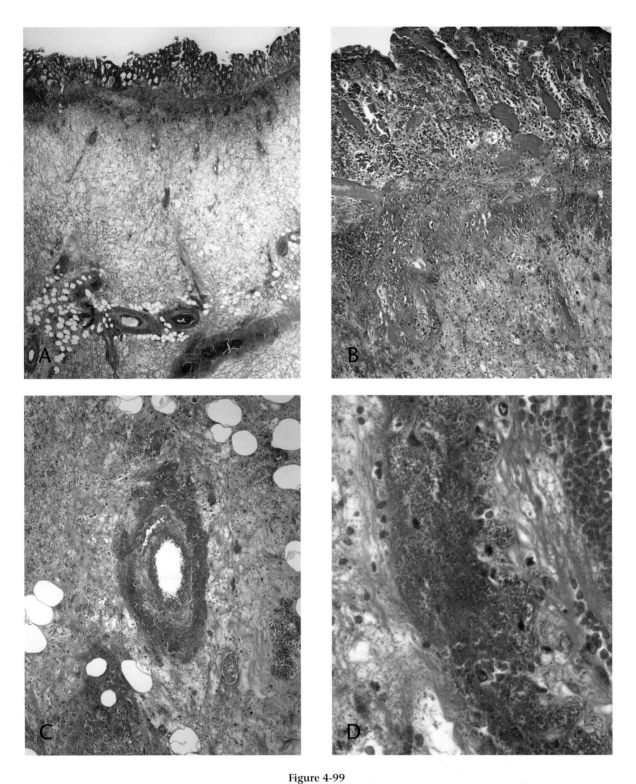

Figure 4-99

NEUTROPENIC ENTEROCOLITIS

Marked submucosal edema (A) is accompanied by mucosal necrosis and hemorrhage (B). Clouds of bacteria are present in the mucosa and submucosa, and surround blood vessels (C). Bacteria consist of mixed filamentous forms, rods, and cocci (D).

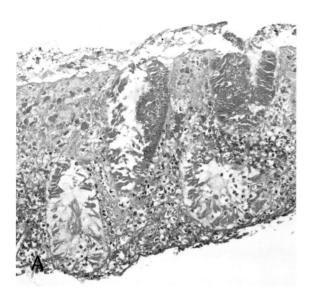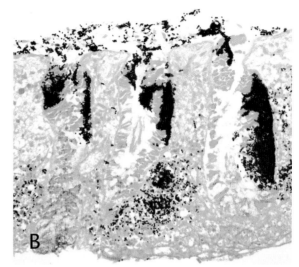

Figure 4-100

NEUTROPENIC ENTEROCOLITIS

The diagnosis is suspected when biopsy samples feature extensive mucosal necrosis and invasive organisms without a neutrophilic tissue reaction (A). A Gomori methenamine silver (GMS) stain demonstrates numerous yeast forms in the tissue and crypt lumens (B).

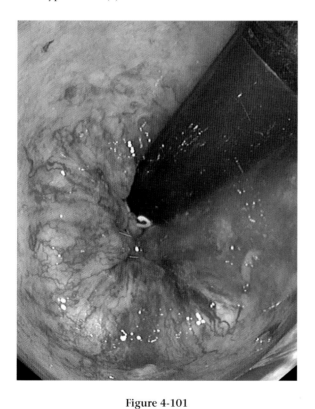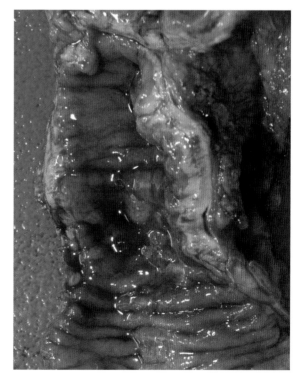

Figure 4-101

RADIATION PROCTITIS

The mucosa is erythematous, with prominent vessels and ectasias.

Figure 4-102

RADIATION-INDUCED ENTERITIS

Edematous mucosal folds overlie a segmental stricture.

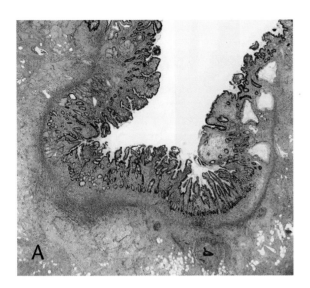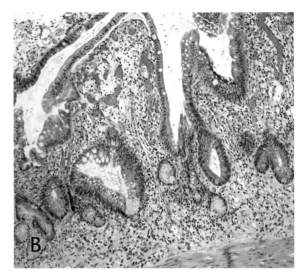

Figure 4-103

RADIATION-INDUCED ENTERITIS

Submucosal fibrosis and elastosis underlie villous architectural distortion and pseudopyloric metaplasia (A). Proliferating vessels and fibrosis are present in the mucosa, which also shows cellular evidence of chronic injury (B).

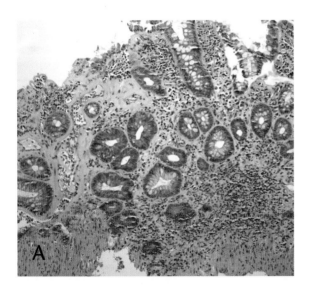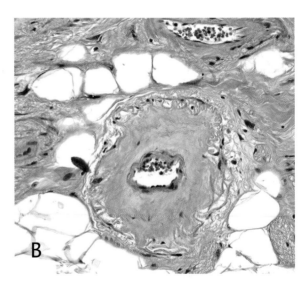

Figure 4-104

RADIATION-INDUCED COLITIS

Mucosal ectasias are associated with hyalinized collagen in the lamina propria (A). There is fibrous obliteration of the intima of submucosal arteries (B).

Microscopic Findings. Acute radiation enterocolitis displays dilated crypts lined by attenuated epithelial cells with dense eosinophilic cytoplasm and atypical nuclei. Crypt loss and regeneration are accompanied by increased numbers of apoptotic epithelial cells (267).

Chronic changes include submucosal fibrosis, mucosal architectural disarray, and pyloric metaplasia associated with minimal lamina propria inflammation (fig. 4-103). Telangiectatic mucosal capillaries are surrounded by hyalinized fibrosis (fig. 4-104A). Arteries display mural hyalinization, intimal hyperplasia, and foamy macrophages (fig. 4-104B).

Treatment and Prognosis. Acute radiation enterocolitis is treated with supportive care. Most symptoms spontaneously resolve within days to weeks, whereas histologic alterations heal within weeks to months. Chronic radiation-related injury is managed with argon plasma coagulation or other methods for bleeding control, including thalidomide treatment (80). Approximately one-third of patients require surgical resection of strictures or fistulae. Patients are at increased risk for cancer development at sites of radiation.

INFECTIONS OF THE SMALL BOWEL AND COLON

Acute Infectious Enterocolitis, Inflammatory Pattern

Definition. *Acute infectious enterocolitis* with an inflammatory pattern (*acute self-limited enterocolitis*) is the result of enterocolic injury caused by a variety of pathogens.

Clinical Features. Infectious enterocolitis results from a variety of organisms that spread through contaminated food and water sources or contact with secretions. Common pathogens in contaminated dairy, meat, and fish products include *Campylobacter, Salmonella*, several *Escherichia coli* strains, and Norwalk virus. *Shigella, Yersinia*, Coxsackie virus, rotavirus, enterovirus, and adenovirus are transmitted through secretions (268).

Symptoms include generalized abdominal distress, nausea, vomiting, pain, and bloody or nonbloody diarrhea. Most patients do not undergo colonoscopy and mucosal biopsy analysis unless they present with atypical clinical findings, prolonged symptoms, or severe disease due to immunocompromise. Patients with acute infectious enterocolitis are diagnosed based on a combination of clinical symptoms, laboratory findings, and stool studies.

Pathogenesis. Organisms that adhere to enterocytes generally cause high-volume malabsorptive or secretory diarrhea without inducing substantial changes to the mucosal architecture. Those that infiltrate the mucosa elicit an inflammatory infiltrate that elaborates cytokines, resulting in crypt destruction.

Gross Findings. Endoscopic changes are variable: non-invasive organisms are associated with normal findings or mild erythema, whereas enteroinvasive pathogens cause mucosal granularity, erosions, and ulcers that may produce inflammatory masses in some cases (fig. 4-105A). *Campylobacter*, and *Salmonella* show a predilection for the proximal colon.

Microscopic Findings. Cases of acute infectious enterocolitis may feature prominent inflammatory changes, ischemic injury, or a combination of both. *Campylobacter* and enteroinvasive strains of *E. coli* are the most common bacterial causes of acute infectious colitis with an inflammatory pattern. Two enteroinvasive, non-typhoid *Salmonella enterica* serovars, *enteritidis* and *typhimurium*, cause acute infectious enterocolitis, as well as septicemia in some cases (268).

All of these pathogens produce similar histologic abnormalities. Mucosal edema is accompanied by neutrophils dispersed in the lamina propria and crypt epithelium; crypt abscesses and destruction are commonly present (fig. 4-105). Regenerative crypts contain immature, mucin-depleted epithelial cells with increased mitotic activity (269). Neutrophils gradually disappear over the course of a few weeks and are replaced by a patchy or diffuse inflammatory infiltrate that contains plasma cells (fig. 4-106) (270). In contrast to chronic colitis, however, plasma cells are accompanied by similar numbers of macrophages and eosinophils, and the inflammatory infiltrate does not expand the full thickness of the mucosa. Microbiologic cultures and stool polymerase chain reaction (PCR) assays are required to establish a specific diagnosis.

Treatment and Prognosis. Most cases of acute infectious enterocolitis are self-limited and spontaneously resolve within a few weeks of symptom onset. Treatment during this time consists of supportive care for diarrheal symptoms. The overall prognosis is excellent. Debilitated patients, however, may develop colonic perforation or other complications that lead to severe morbidity or even death.

Acute Infectious Colitis, Ischemic/Hemorrhagic Pattern

Definition. *Acute infectious colitis, ischemic/hemorrhagic pattern* is toxin-mediated infectious colitis resulting in damage to mucosal microvasculature.

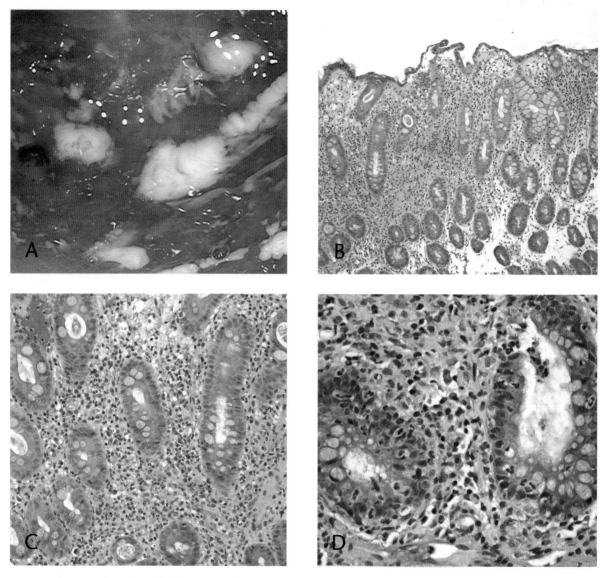

Figure 4-105

ACUTE INFECTIOUS COLITIS

Yellow-white fibrin plaques are present on a background of edematous mucosa (A). Biopsy samples from these areas reveal normal mucosal architecture, although crypts show regenerative features with cytoplasmic depletion (B). The lamina propria contains a patchy infiltrate composed of neutrophils, eosinophils, and other cell types (C), as well as foci of neutrophilic cryptitis (D).

Clinical Features. Toxin-secreting bacteria spread through contaminated food and water sources (268). Patients present with nausea, vomiting, pain, and bloody diarrhea that may be accompanied by tenesmus. Most are diagnosed based on a combination of clinical symptoms, laboratory findings, and stool studies, rather than endoscopy and biopsy analysis.

Pathogenesis. Bacteria secrete shiga toxin or verotoxin that directly damages endothelial cells, resulting in thrombosis and altered blood flow through the mucosal microvasculature.

Gross Findings. Hemorrhagic colitis is usually a segmental process with a predilection for the right colon. Occasional patients have more diffuse inflammatory changes. Features

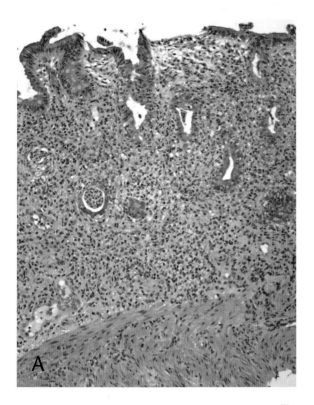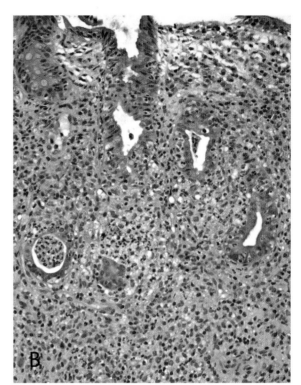

Figure 4-106

ACUTE INFECTIOUS COLITIS MIMICKING CHRONIC COLITIS

Neutrophil-rich infiltrates are replaced by plasma cells within a few weeks of symptom onset (A). Unlike cases of chronic colitis, plasma cells are accompanied by similar numbers of macrophages and other cell types (B).

include erythema, mucosal granularity, ulcers, and edema.

Microscopic Findings. The histologic features are similar to those of ischemic colitis due to vascular compromise, as previously described. Withered, regenerative crypts are accompanied by fibrin in the lamina propria (fig. 4-107). Fibrin thrombi may be present in some cases, but this finding is not specific. Gram-negative rods may be detected at the epithelial surface.

Treatment and Prognosis. Symptoms resolve spontaneously with supportive care in most cases. Antibiotic therapy is generally avoided because it can precipitate hemolytic uremia syndrome in patients infected by organisms that elaborate verotoxin or shiga toxin (271).

Bacterial Causes of Ischemic Hemorrhagic Colitis. *Shigellosis.* Shigella species are highly virulent organisms that represent a leading bacterial cause of diarrheal symptoms. More than 100 million individuals are infected worldwide, and the disease is responsible for

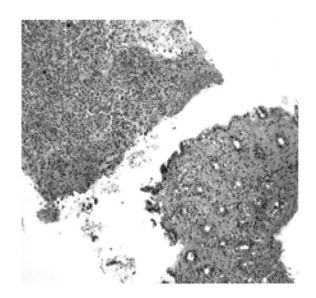

Figure 4-107

HEMORRHAGIC COLITIS SECONDARY TO *E. COLI O157:H7*

Ischemic colitis is accompanied by fibrinopurulent exudates and mucosal hemorrhage.

several hundred thousand deaths each year. Infection is more common in areas with poor sanitation, contaminated food and water sources, and crowded living conditions. Organisms are classified in three serogroups (serogroup A: *S. dysenteriae,* serogroup B: *S. flexneri,* and serogroup C: *S. boydii*), and one serotype (*S. sonnei*). The first three serogroups are more prevalent in developing countries, whereas *S. sonnei* accounts for most cases in the United States. The latter result from travel exposures or spread within daycare centers and institutionalized patients. *Shigella* invade the mucosa through the basolateral aspects of M cells dispersed in the intestinal epithelium (272). *S. flexneri* strains produce enterotoxin-1 (ShET1) and enterotoxin-2 (ShET2), which promote intestinal secretion (273). *S. dysentery* elaborates shiga toxin, causing microvascular injury in the mucosa similar to verotoxin.

Enterohemorrhagic E. Coli O157:H7. Enterohemorrhagic *E. coli* O157:H7 is a verotoxin-secreting organism that causes hemorrhagic colitis. It accounts for more than 70,000 clinically significant infections, 3,000 hospitalizations, and 500 deaths in the United States each year (274,275). Bacteria can infect any part of the colon, but tend to colonize the right colon, causing high-volume diarrhea (275). Approximately 10 percent of patients develop hemolytic uremia syndrome and thrombocytopenic purpura, which can be life-threatening (275,276).

Klebsiella Oxytoca. Klebsiella oxytoca is a Gram-negative rod originally believed to be a non-pathogenic commensal organism. It has since been recognized as an important cause of antibiotic-associated hemorrhagic colitis. The bacterium produces β-lactamase, allowing it to persist in the colons of patients treated with penicillin and similar agents (171). Affected patients develop crampy abdominal pain, bloody diarrhea, and a segmental colitis that resolves shortly after discontinuation of antibiotic therapy (171). Unlike other pathogens that elicit an ischemic and hemorrhagic pattern of injury, *K. oxytoca* generally causes hemorrhage without an ischemic component.

Pseudomembranous Colitis

Definition. *Pseudomembranous colitis* is acute or recurrent colitis characterized by adherent plaques of fibrin and cellular debris.

Clinical Features. Pseudomembranous colitis usually results from *Clostridium difficile* infection, although similar endoscopic findings can be seen in patients infected with *E. coli* 0157 and shiga toxin-producing organisms, acute ischemic or radiation injury, and medications that cause ischemic enterocolitis (277). Its incidence has increased from 4.5 per 1,000 in 2001 to 8.2 per 1,000 in 2010, and the proportion of severe cases has also increased (278,279). *C. difficile* infection is usually hospital-acquired. Risk factors include recent antibiotic use, advanced age, acid suppressive therapy, exposure to infected individuals, and comorbid conditions (278). Some patients are asymptomatic carriers, although most present with persistent watery diarrhea, bloating, and abdominal pain.

Radiographic findings include focal or diffuse mural thickening with pericolic fat stranding, prominent haustral folds, and proximal colon dilatation, especially among patients with evolving toxic megacolon (280,281). Enzyme-linked immunoassays are available for both toxins and are widely used in clinical practice (280). The gold standard for diagnosis requires either the cytotoxin neutralizing assay or toxigenic culture, although both tests require several days for interpretation (277). Other assays detect bacterial DNA or glutamate dehydrogenase, an enzyme produced by *C. difficile*.

Pathogenesis. *C. difficile* was recently renamed *Clostridiodes difficile*. This Gram-positive, anaerobic bacterium elaborates two toxins, TcdA and TcdB. These molecules inactivate a subgroup of GTPases, resulting in epithelial cell necrosis. The bacterium produces other virulence factors that facilitate binding to colonocytes and inhibit growth of other microbes.

Gross Findings. Endoscopy reveals yellow-white plaques on a background of edematous mucosa with variable granularity and ulcers (fig. 4-108). Patients with *C. difficile* infection may lack pseudomembranes but have erosions or granular mucosa at endoscopy and diagnostic changes in biopsy samples (280). Patients with toxic megacolon may require surgical resection, in which case the colon is dilated and edematous with numerous pseudomembranes (fig. 4-109).

Microscopic Findings. Biopsy findings are variable. Classic cases feature mushroom-shaped pseudomembranes composed of parallel arrays of necrotic epithelium and neutrophils enmeshed in mucine-rich exudates with fibrin. Underlying crypts are dilated with attenuated epithelium, but the adjacent epithelium is normal (fig. 4-110). Disrupted crypts slough their epithelial lining cells into the lumen; goblet cells may simulate signet ring cells when detached from the basement membranes (fig. 4-111). The lamina propria and submucosa are frequently edematous with minimal inflammation early in the course of disease.

Progressive mural edema compromises blood flow, resulting in superimposed ischemic-type changes and extensive ulcers with hemorrhage and intravascular fibrin thrombi. In fact, distinguishing *C. difficile*-related pseudomembranous colitis from ischemic colitis with exudates can be challenging. Clues to the diagnosis of noninfectious ischemic colitis include localized plaques and edema, abundant fibrin in the lamina propria with small regenerative crypts, and minimal inflammation (fig. 4-112) (282).

C. difficile-induced pseudomembranous colitis is a well-described complication of established inflammatory bowel disease, especially in hospitalized patients. In this situation, pseudomembranes and necrotic crypts in areas uninvolved by chronic colitis may suggest a superimposed infection (283). Many ulcerative colitis patients with *C. difficile* infection have

mucosal biopsy samples that feature acute colitis but lack pseudomembranes.

Treatment and Prognosis. Patients with pseudomembranous colitis are at risk for toxic megacolon, which is associated with increased mortality risk. Surgical resection is often necessary

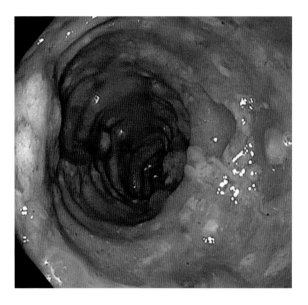

Figure 4-108

***CLOSTRIDIUM DIFFICILE* INFECTION**

Confluent yellow-white plaques coat the colon. The background mucosa is edematous and erythematous.

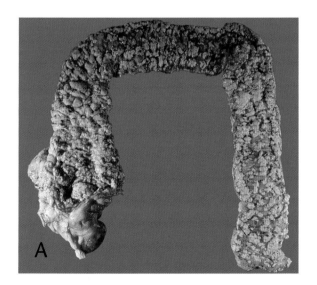

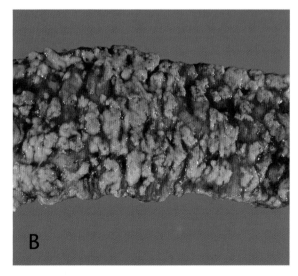

Figure 4-109

***CLOSTRIDIUM DIFFICILE* INFECTION**

The entire colon is surfaced by variably sized brown-yellow plaques (A) that coalesce in several areas (B).

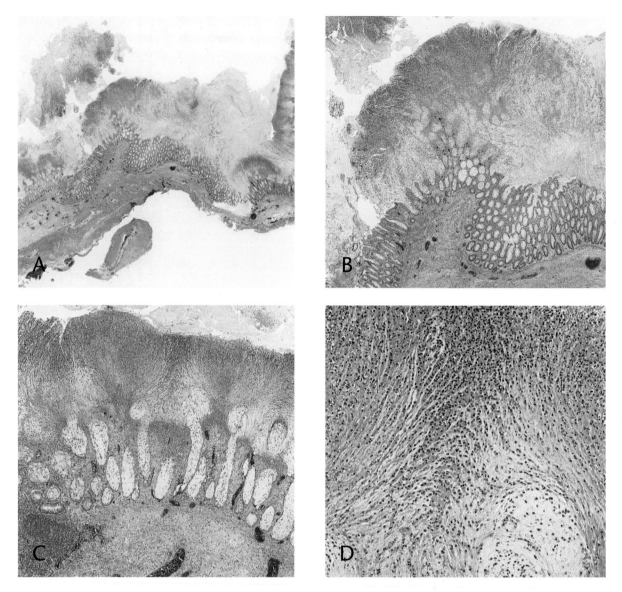

Figure 4-110

CLOSTRIDIUM DIFFICILE **INFECTION**

Pseudomembranes erupt from dilated crypts flanked by essentially normal mucosa (A). Mushroom-shaped exudates (B) and confluent pseudomembranes overlying areas of crypt destruction coat the surface (C). Pseudomembranes consist of linear arrays of necrotic epithelium and neutrophils embedded in fibrin and mucus (D).

in this situation, in which case symptoms dramatically improve following colectomy (284).

Other Bacterial Enterocolitis

Salmonella Typhi. *Salmonella enterica typhi* is a facultative Gram-negative rod that causes typhoid fever. The organism is transmitted through contaminated food and water, affecting 21 million people worldwide and causing 200,000

deaths per year (285). Initial infection is followed by spread of bacteria to macrophages in the liver and spleen, resulting in chronic infection with intermittent bacteremia. Fever and malaise develop a few weeks after infection, reflecting bacteremia. These symptoms are followed by nausea, vomiting, abdominal pain, and diarrhea. Sloughed epithelium admixed with blood results in gray-green discoloration of stool.

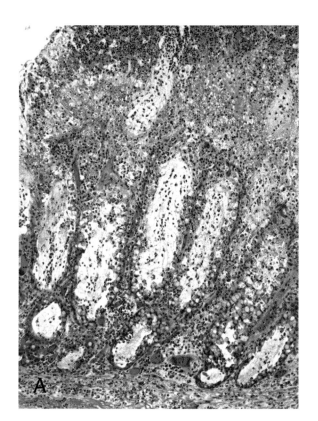 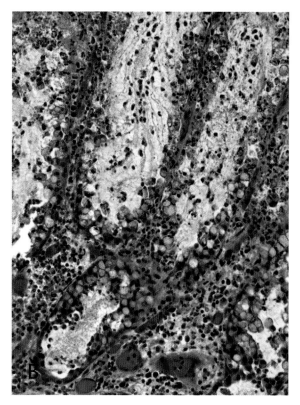

Figure 4-111

CLOSTRIDIUM DIFFICILE INFECTION

Necrotic epithelial cells are enmeshed in mucus from erupting crypts (A). Detached goblet cells superficially resemble signet ring cells; these "pseudosignet ring cells" are confined to areas of crypt rupture and lack cytologic atypia (B).

Endoscopic examination reveals mucosal edema in the proximal colon and ileum, as well as raised nodules corresponding to hyperplastic Peyer patches. Large Peyer patches can ulcerate and heal with fibrosis or progress to larger discoid or linear ulcers. Neutrophilic cryptitis and erosions are accompanied by mononuclear cell-rich inflammatory infiltrates that expand the lamina propria (fig. 4-113). Plasma cells may be prominent. Enlarged Peyer patches contain prominent germinal centers with tingible body macrophages. These structures are ultimately overrun by activated mononuclear cells and macrophages that harbor bacteria and show erythrophagocytosis (286). Well-formed granulomas are generally lacking.

Yersinia Enterocolitica* and *Y. Pseudotuberculosis. *Yersinia* is a Gram-negative coccobacillus transmitted through contaminated food and water (287). *Yersinia enterocolitica* and *Yersinia pseudotuberculosis* cause human enteric infections, and show a predilection for the ileo-colic region and appendix (288). The organisms enter Peyer patches through M cells, similar to *Salmonella*. They multiply in lymphoid follicles, then drain to regional lymph nodes, producing mesenteric lymphadenitis, ileocolitis, and appendicitis singly or in combination.

Infection elicits lymphoid hyperplasia associated with aphthous and linear ulcers. Biopsy findings include acute enterocolitis accompanied by lymphoid hyperplasia and occasional granulomas that may contain suppurative inflammation (fig. 4-114) (289). Although both species may elicit granulomas, suppurative granulomas are more frequently associated with *Yersinia pseudotuberculosis* (288,290). Fissures and transmural inflammation may also be present, simulating features of Crohn disease.

Intestinal Spirochetosis. Spirochetosis is a non-invasive infection caused by several types of Gram-negative spirochetes, including *Brachyspira aalborgi* and *Brachyspira pilosicoli*. Colonic

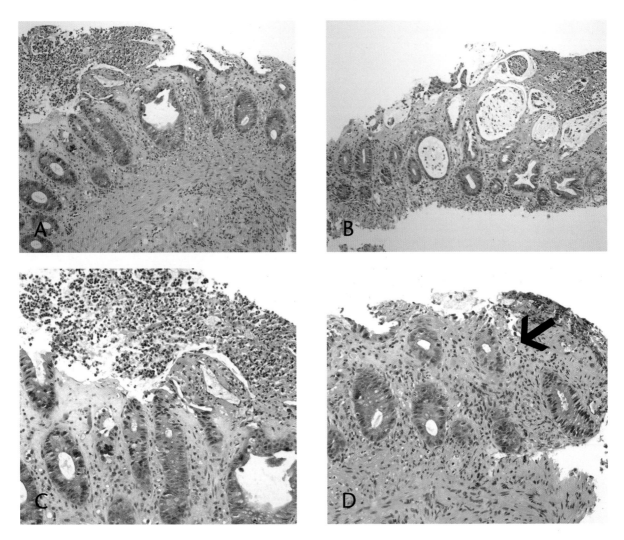

Figure 4-112

ISCHEMIC COLITIS WITH PSEUDOMEMBRANES

Ischemic injury can result in epithelial necrosis, denudation, and exudates that resemble pseudomembranes (A), particularly in the setting of mucosal prolapse (B). Sloughed debris, however, often contains round aggregates of necrotic cells, rather than linear cellular arrays (C). The adjacent mucosa shows ischemic-type changes with eosinophilic lamina propria, occasional fibrin thrombi (arrow), and regenerative microcrypts (D).

spirochetosis can affect both humans and animals, typically by fecal-oral transmission. The disorder was originally described in patients with human immunodeficiency virus (HIV)/acquired immunodeficiency syndrome (AIDS), although it may also occur in asymptomatic immunocompetent patients as well as those with diverticular disease or inflammatory bowel disease; infection in pediatric patients is common.

The prevalence of intestinal spirochetosis ranges up to approximately 15 percent in developed countries and is higher in developing countries,

particularly among homosexual men and patients with HIV infection (291). Infection may be asymptomatic, leading some investigators to believe the organisms are commensal rather than pathogenic. Immunocompromised patients, children, and critically ill individuals are more likely to have watery, nonbloody diarrhea, cramps, and occasional rectal bleeding (292). Symptoms generally resolve with antibiotic therapy.

Endoscopic examination is usually normal and biopsy samples lack substantial inflammation. The organisms appear as a fuzzy,

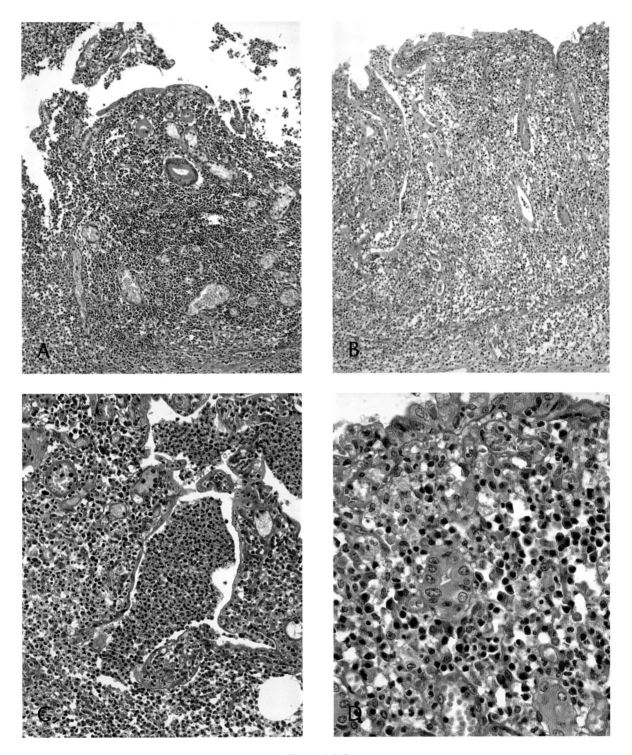

Figure 4-113

SALMONELLA TYPHI **ENTEROCOLITIS**

Early inflammatory changes occur overlying Peyer patches, which show aphthous ulcers (A). Mononuclear cell-rich infiltrates expand the mucosa and plasma cells are present in the deep crypt region (B). Crypt abscesses and architectural distortion simulate features of idiopathic inflammatory bowel disease (C). Germinal centers are overrun by sheets of activated lymphocytes and macrophages, some of which contain cellular fragments (D).

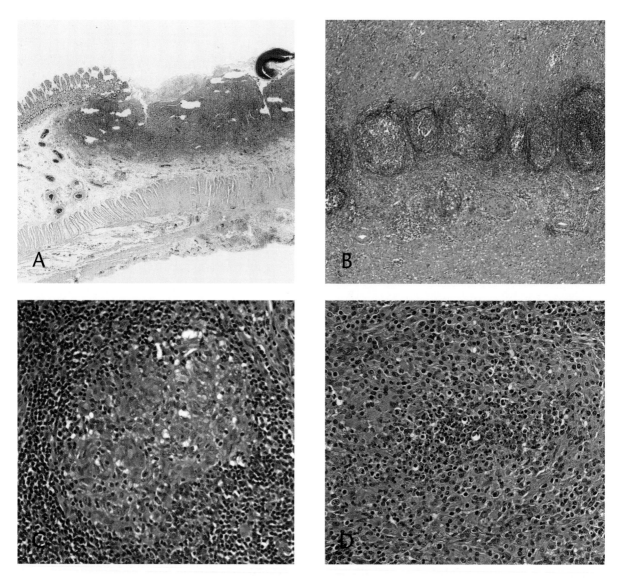

Figure 4-114

YERSINIA-ASSOCIATED ENTEROCOLITIS

Yersinia enterocolitica elicits an inflammatory pattern that simulates Crohn disease. Aphthous ulcers occur over hyperplastic Peyer patches (A) and mural lymphoid aggregates are common (B). Non-necrotic epithelioid granulomas are characteristic (C). *Yersinia pseudotuberculosis* is more commonly associated with suppurative granulomas (D).

basophilic fringe at the luminal aspect of the surface epithelium and may be patchy (fig. 4-115). Spirochetes have a corkscrew appearance and stain with silver impregnation stains (e.g., Warthin-Starry, Dieterle, Steiner), as well as commercially available spirochete immunostains (fig. 4-116).

Tropheryma Whippelii. Whipple disease is a chronic systemic inflammatory condition caused by *Tropheryma whipplei* (293). This Gram-positive rod accumulates in macrophages of patients with abnormal macrophage activation. Although no consistent immunologic abnormality has been identified, some cases are associated with HLA-B27 (294). The disease is more common in older white males who present with symptoms related to multiorgan involvement. Generalized lymphadenopathy, arthralgias, neurologic abnormalities, and diarrhea are common presenting symptoms (295).

Abnormal laboratory findings include increased erythrocyte sedimentation rate, fatty stools, anemia, and hypoproteinemia (296). Treatment consists of long-term antibiotic therapy with agents that cross the blood-brain barrier. Macrophages laden with organism fragments can be detected months to years after successful treatment.

Endoscopy typically reveals thickened folds and bulbous villi with white or yellow plaques. The villous architecture is somewhat effaced by macrophage-rich infiltrates that expand the lamina propria, often in combination with lymphangiectasia (fig. 4-117A). Macrophages contain foamy, faintly eosinophilic cytoplasm and small vacuoles (fig. 4-117B). These vacuoles contain partially degraded organisms, which are chunky and intensely PAS positive, but diastase resistant (fig. 4-117C). Well-formed granulomas are rarely encountered in the mucosa but may be observed in regional lymph nodes and liver. Neutrophils are variably present. Surface enterocytes may be vacuolated or show cytoplasmic depletion, but intraepithelial inflammation is lacking. Confirmatory immunohistochemical stains are available, although PCR-based assays are more widely used (fig. 4-117D) (297).

Mycobacterium Tuberculosis. Primary intestinal tuberculosis usually results from hematogenous spread of *Mycobacterium tuberculosis* from a pulmonary focus or primary infection; ingestion of unpasteurized milk can lead to zoonotic infection with *M. bovis* (298). *Mycobacterium tuberculosis* shows a predilection for Peyer patches of the ileocecal region.

Presenting symptoms include abdominal pain, fever, and night sweats, although some patients have a right lower quadrant mass and matted mesenteric lymphadenopathy that simulate malignancy. Strictures, fistulae, and adenopathy are radiographically apparent (299).

Endoscopic features include indurated mucosal folds, ulcers, and pseudopolyps that simulate Crohn disease (fig. 4-118). Localized disease can cause strictures (fig. 4-119). Chronic active ileocolitis features mononuclear cell-rich

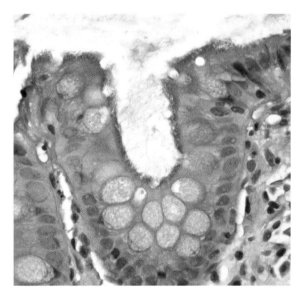

Figure 4-115

INTESTINAL SPIROCHETOSIS

A fuzzy, slightly blue fringe of bacteria is present at the luminal surface.

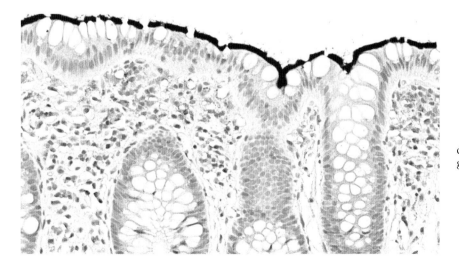

Figure 4-116

INTESTINAL SPIROCHETOSIS

A spirochete immunostain demonstrates innumerable organisms clinging to colonocytes.

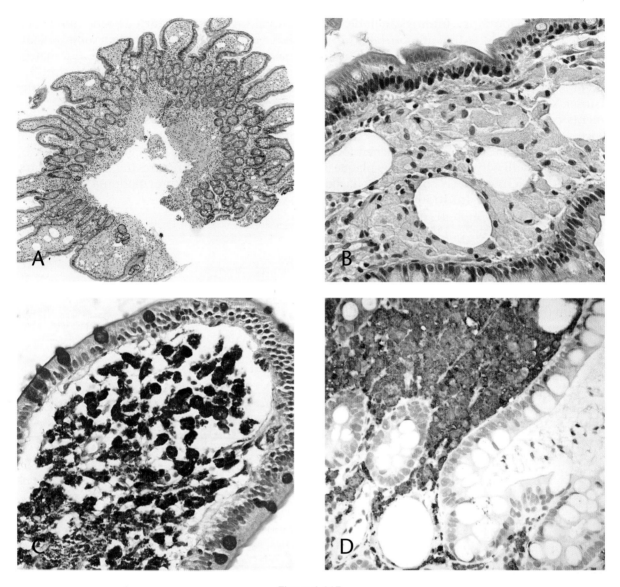

Figure 4-117

WHIPPLE DISEASE

Enlarged, bulbous villi contain a macrophage-rich infiltrate, dilated lacteals, and free lipid (A), unaccompanied by epithelial cell injury or inflammation (B). A PAS-D stain demonstrates chunky bacterial fragments within macrophages (C). An immunostain directed against bacterial antigens stains macrophages in the lamina propria (D).

inflammation and epithelioid granulomas arranged singly or in aggregates. Resection specimens generally contain confluent necrotic granulomas, but mucosal samples may only contain non-necrotic granulomas, further mimicking Crohn disease (fig. 4-120) (300).

Organism detection has historically required histochemical stains, such as Ziehl-Neelsen and Fite stains, although they have low sensitivity for organism detection, especially when bacilli are scarce. Commercially available immunohistochemical stains and PCR-based assays are more sensitive (301). Culture is the gold standard for establishing a diagnosis but requires several weeks to grow.

The differential diagnosis includes *Mycobacterium avium intracellulare* complex (MAI) and yersiniosis. The former are long, slender rods that tend to be more numerous than *M. tuberculosis*, although both pathogens can be present in high

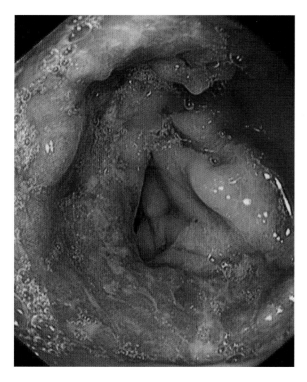

Figure 4-118

MYCOBACTERIUM TUBERCULOSIS **ENTEROCOLITIS**

The lumen is narrowed by a thick, indurated inflammatory mass that effaces the mucosal folds. (Courtesy of Dr. B. Odum, St. Louis, MO.)

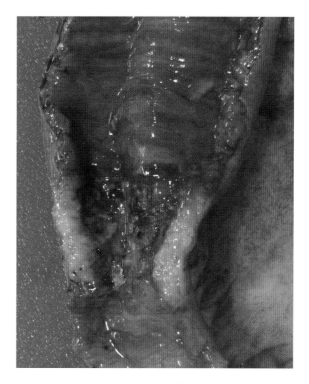

Figure 4-119

MYCOBACTERIUM TUBERCULOSIS **ENTERITIS**

A jejunal stricture is associated with ulcers and flattened mucosal folds.

numbers in severely immunocompromised individuals. The granulomas of yersiniosis tend to be epithelioid and non-necrotic. When present, necrosis is more often suppurative than coagulative. Distinguishing intestinal tuberculosis from Crohn disease can be challenging, especially in biopsy material. Infectious granulomas are often larger, more numerous, and show central necrosis compared with those of Crohn disease (299). Patients with Crohn disease who are treated with TNF-α inhibitors are at risk for reactivation of latent *M. tuberculosis* infection (302).

Mycobacterium Avium Intracellulare. Atypical mycobacteria are ubiquitous in soil and water, and can be found in animal reservoirs, dairy products, and most foods. Atypical mycobacteria are classified into four groups based on a combination of factors: pigment production, growth rate, and colony characteristics. *Mycobacterium avium intracellulare* (MAI) complex is the most common non-tuberculous organism to cause gastrointestinal illness. It may occur in

immunocompetent or immunocompromised patients. Immunocompetent patients mount a brisk inflammatory response to infection with epithelioid, variably necrotic granulomas, and scant organisms, whereas immunocompromised patients have a heavy infectious burden. Immunodeficient patients are at risk for disseminated disease and require multidrug antibiotic therapy.

Atypical mycobacteria show a predilection for the small bowel and colon, where they may cause thickened folds and yellow-white flecks that reflect macrophage-rich inflammatory infiltrates (fig. 4-121). Tissue samples feature sheets of macrophages that expand the lamina propria, but do not form epithelioid granulomas. Macrophages contain faintly eosinophilic or pale blue fibrillary cytoplasm resembling sheaves of wheat.

Mycobacteria are acid fast, stain with PAS-D, and may also be GMS positive when rapidly dividing (fig. 4-122) (256). The slender organisms are distinct from the chunky diastase-resistant

265

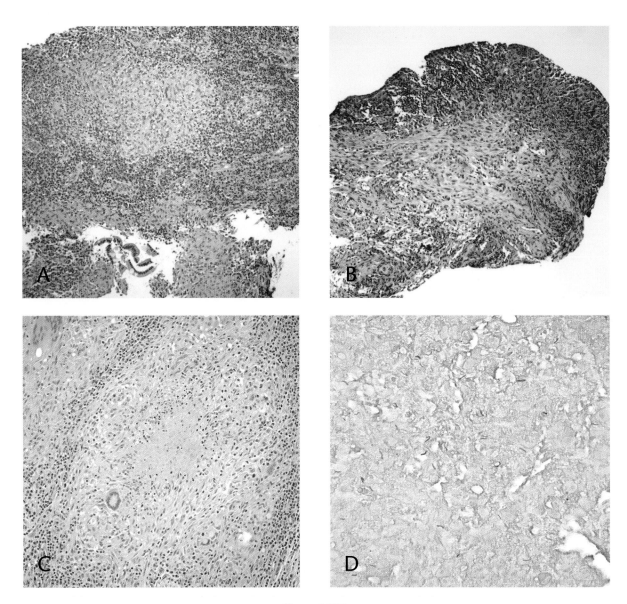

Figure 4-120

MYCOBACTERIUM TUBERCULOSIS ENTEROCOLITIS

Infection elicits a mononuclear cell-rich inflammatory response with granulomas that simulate the features of Crohn disease (A). Clues to a diagnosis of mycobacterial infection include mucosal fibrosis (B) and confluent, necrotic granulomas (C), both of which are unusual for Crohn disease. Organisms appear as short red rods with acid-fast stains (D).

material seen in macrophages of patients infected with *Tropheryma whipplei* (295). Infected macrophages may assume a spindled appearance in lymph nodes, spleen, and viscera, that simulates a spindle cell neoplasm (303).

Viral Enterocolitis

Human Immunodeficiency Virus (HIV) Enterocolopathy. Patients infected with HIV can develop unexplained diarrheal symptoms with minimal endoscopic and histologic abnormalities (304). Some patients with HIV and gastrointestinal symptoms suffer from the combined effects of HIV on enterocytes and altered mucosal immunity, whereas others are infected by non-HIV viral pathogens. Rotavirus, adenovirus, astrovirus, cytomegalovirus, and picobirnavirus have all been detected in

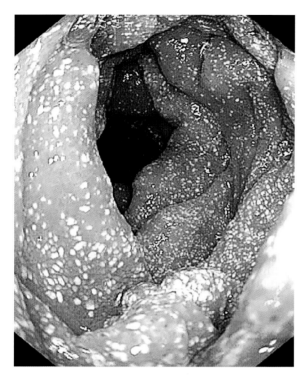

Figure 4-121

MYCOBACTERIUM AVIUM INTRACELLULARE
COMPLEX-ASSOCIATED DUODENITIS

The duodenal mucosal folds are thick with tiny white-yellow flecks.

stool specimens from HIV-positive patients with diarrhea (304).

The histologic abnormalities of HIV enterocolopathy are not specific. Small bowel biopsy samples show mild villous blunting, crypt hyperplasia, and intraepithelial apoptotic debris with patchy lymphocytosis (256,305). The incidence of HIV/AIDS enteropathy has decreased with the widespread use of highly active antiretroviral therapy (HAART) and improved methods for detecting other infectious agents (306).

Cytomegalovirus. Cytomegalovirus (CMV) is an important pathogen in immunosuppressed patients and can occasionally cause disease in immunocompetent hosts. It is a member of the Herpesviridae family that, similar to other herpesviruses, can cause new infection or reactivation of latent disease in the gastrointestinal tract.

Gastrointestinal manifestations include nausea and vomiting, abdominal pain, and watery or bloody diarrhea. Endothelial cell infection leads to thrombosis and mucosal ischemia, resulting in erythema, friability, and ulcers throughout the gastrointestinal tract; severe injury can result in segmental ischemic enterocolitis and perforation (fig. 4-123) (307). CMV-associated inflammatory reactions can be exuberant and simulate malignancy (308).

The amount of inflammation elicited by CMV infection depends on the immune status of the patient. Stem cell transplant patients often mount a minimal inflammatory response despite high numbers of viral inclusions, whereas viral inclusions in the setting of idiopathic inflammatory bowel disease tend to be scarce and are accompanied by plasma cell-rich inflammatory infiltrates (fig. 4-124). The virus infects endothelial cells, causing endothelial injury and thrombosis, which produce an acute ischemic-type injury with ulcers, fibrin thrombi, plump endothelial cells, and variable numbers of neutrophils around blood vessels (fig. 4-124D). The organism also infects glandular epithelium, particularly neutral mucin-containing Brunner glands in the duodenum, and may elicit epithelial cell apoptosis that simulates GVHD or a medication injury in specific clinical situations (fig. 4-125A). Fibroblasts can be infected, particularly in patients with high numbers of viral inclusions; ulcers and macrophage-rich inflammatory infiltrates are frequently present (fig. 4-125B). Amphophilic nuclear inclusions are surrounded by zones of rarified chromatin, whereas cytoplasmic inclusions are granular and brightly eosinophilic (fig. 4-125C).

Viral cytopathic changes are usually apparent in routinely stained histologic sections, although prophylactic ganciclovir therapy alters the morphologic features of virally infected cells (fig. 4-125D). Immunohistochemical stains can facilitate a diagnosis in this setting or when exuberant inflammation obscures infected cells; they should probably be used when a clinical suspicion for CMV infection exists (301,309–312). Antiviral treatment results in symptomatic improvement in most patients, even if only rare infected cells are detected (313). Molecular methods for detecting viral DNA in paraffin-embedded tissue are highly sensitive, but they are not widely used in current practice (314). Treatment consists of antiviral therapy with ganciclovir, valganciclovir, or related agents (315).

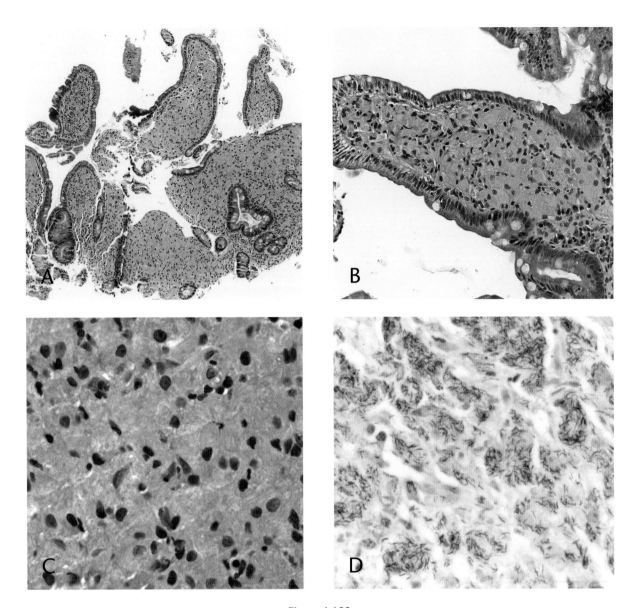

Figure 4-122

MYCOBACTERIUM AVIUM INTRACELLULARE **COMPLEX-ASSOCIATED DUODENITIS**

Villi are distended by a diffuse macrophage-rich infiltrate without prominent lacteals (A). Sheets of macrophages have slightly basophilic cytoplasm (B) with a fibrillar quality (C). An acid-fast stain demonstrates numerous delicate rods (D).

Adenovirus. Acute adenovirus infection causes self-limited enterocolitis in immuno-competent patients, but immunosuppressed patients can develop severe enterocolitis, nephritis, hepatitis, pneumonia, or life-threatening encephalitis (316). Endoscopic changes range from normal mucosa to granularity and friability with ulcers (fig. 4-126). The virus may elicit only mild histologic changes consisting of variable villous blunting, slightly tufted surface epithelium, and nuclear disarray with scattered apoptotic cellular debris (fig. 4-127). More severe changes include crypt injury with drop-out, erosions, and abundant nuclear debris that simulate GVHD (fig. 4-128).

Infected epithelial cells are often arranged in clusters and contain angulated or crescentic nuclei with smudgy, amphophilic inclusions (fig. 4-128C) (317). Routine use of adenovirus immunohisto-chemistry can facilitate their detection, especially when immunosuppressed patients present with unexplained gastrointestinal symptoms (311). Immunopositive cells are often clustered in the surface and crypts; occasional positive cells may be seen in the lamina propria when extensive crypt destruction is present (fig. 4-128D).

Immunocompetent patients require no further therapy. Bone marrow transplant patients may be treated with cidofovir during the immediate post-transplant period of severe immunocompromise (318).

Fungal Enterocolitis

Basidiobolomycosis. *Basidiobolus ranarum* is a member of the class Zygomycetes. It usually causes skin and soft tissue infections in individuals from tropical areas of Africa, South America, and Asia, but is an emerging pathogen in the United States. Unlike other fungi that tend to cause disease in the setting of immunocompromise, *Basidiobolus ranarum* infects immunocompetent individuals. Disease is most common in arid regions of the Southwest, particularly Arizona, where it likely results from exposure to contaminated soil, animal feces, and decaying plants. The organism shows a predilection for the gastrointestinal tract, especially the colon, and elicits an exuberant inflammatory reaction that simulates Crohn disease or a mass. Presenting symptoms include abdominal pain, fever, and weight loss, often accompanied by peripheral eosinophilia (319).

Basidiobolomycosis causes gastrointestinal disease characterized by marked wall thickening and granulomatous inflammation accompanied by intense tissue eosinophilia (fig. 4-129A). Granulomas contain fungal forms associated with Charcot-Leyden crystals and Splendore-Hoeppli phenomenon (320). Hyphae are thin walled, with irregularly branches and a few septations. They are large (8 to 40 µm) and readily visible in routinely-stained sections, although they can also be seen with silver stains (fig. 4-129B).

Microsporidiosis. Microsporidia were previously considered to be parasites but are now classified as fungi. The most clinically relevant microsporidia are *Enterocytozoon bieneusi* and *Encephalitozoon intestinalis* (321). Infection by ingestion of contaminated food or water sources is most common, although person-to-person transmission also occurs. Immunocompromised

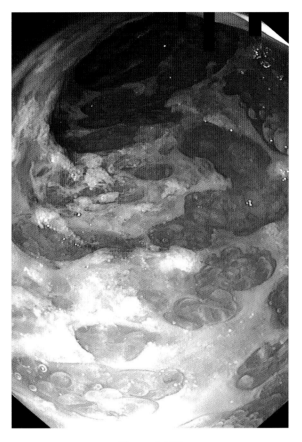

Figure 4-123

CYTOMEGALOVIRUS (CMV)-ASSOCIATED ENTEROCOLITIS

The ileal mucosa is diffusely erythematous, with numerous confluent ulcers.

individuals are at highest risk for severe infection. Typical presenting symptoms include watery, protracted diarrhea and dehydration that may be life threatening. Most patients have a normal endoscopic examination.

Small bowel biopsy samples display normal, or nearly normal, villous architecture and lamina propria cellularity. Intraepithelial lymphocytes are mildly increased or present in normal numbers. Supranuclear parasitophorous vacuoles are accompanied by apoptotic debris in the surface epithelium. These vacuoles contain small (2 to 3 mm), basophilic spores or slightly larger plasmodia; vacuoles may be overlooked or interpreted to represent goblet cells, especially when present in small numbers (fig. 4-130A). Organisms can also be detected in mucosal macrophages. Microsporidia are highlighted

269

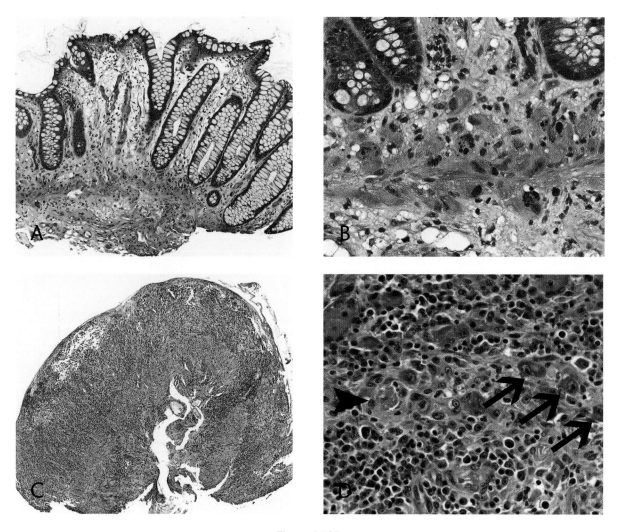

Figure 4-124

CYTOMEGALOVIRUS-ASSOCIATED COLITIS

Minimal inflammation is present in biopsy samples from a bone marrow transplant patient with diarrheal symptoms and normal endoscopic findings (A), although numerous CMV inclusions are present throughout the sample (B). In contrast, biopsy samples from corticosteroid-dependent patients with idiopathic inflammatory bowel disease feature erosions and plasma cell-rich inflammation (C). Fibrin thrombi (arrowhead) are associated with numerous CMV inclusions (arrows) in endothelial cells (D).

with modified trichrome or tissue Gram stains (fig. 4-130B). Stool studies and PCR-based assays facilitate a diagnosis (256).

Candidiasis. The gastrointestinal tract is a major reservoir of *Candida albicans, C. tropicalis,* and *C. (torulopsis) glabrata.* Most infections are limited to the esophagus; invasive enterocolic infections occur in the setting of neutropenic enterocolitis and in severely debilitated patients with altered mucosal immunity (322,323). Invasive fungi are associated with irregular,

confluent ulcers (fig. 4-131A). Organisms are most numerous at the luminal surface. Invasive organisms are associated with hemorrhage and necrosis but a brisk inflammatory reaction is often lacking due to decreased host immunity (fig. 4-131B).

Aspergillosis. *Aspergillus* sp. are ubiquitous in the environment. *Aspergillus fumigatus* is most commonly isolated from the gastrointestinal tract, followed by *A. flavus, A. terreus,* and *A. niger* (324). Aspergillosis is extremely

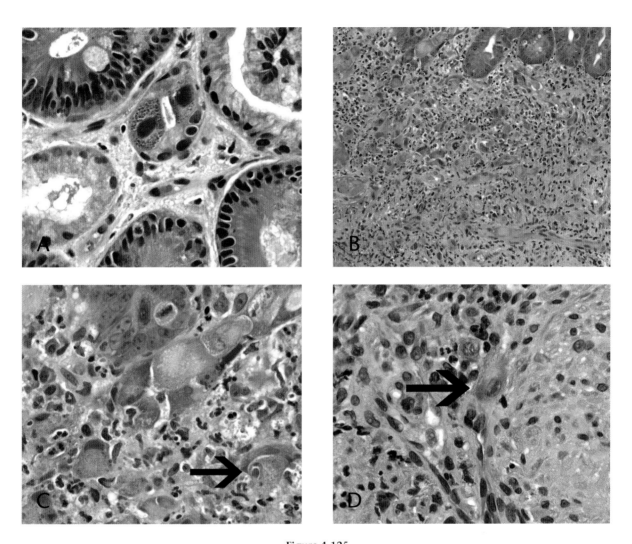

Figure 4-125

CYTOMEGALOVIRUS-ASSOCIATED ENTEROCOLITIS

The virus infects endothelial cells, fibroblasts, and glandular epithelial cells, particularly neutral mucin-containing Brunner glands (A). Similar to other herpesviruses, CMV elicits a macrophage-rich inflammatory reaction (B). Infected cells are large, with intranuclear inclusions surrounded by a pale halo of rarified chromatin (arrow), smaller, brightly eosinophilic cytoplasmic inclusions are also identified (C). Infected cells tend to be smaller, with less conspicuous inclusions (arrow) when detected in samples from patients receiving prophylactic antiviral agents (D).

uncommon among immunocompetent individuals but tends to develop in patients with prolonged neutropenia who inhale spores that subsequently spread hematogenously to the intestinal tract (325).

Aspergillus sp. are angioinvasive fungi, frequently causing thrombosis with mural infarction (fig. 4-132). Septate hyphae have parallel walls and branch at 45° angles. Intestinal infection is associated with a mortality rate of over 50 percent (325).

Mucormycosis. Mucormycosis occurs in bone marrow transplant patients and those with hematologic malignancies, as well as individuals who are immunocompromised for other reasons, including diabetes mellitus. Most gastrointestinal cases are limited to the stomach; intestinal involvement occurs in only 2 to 10 percent of patients and is associated with a mortality rate of nearly 50 percent (326). Invasive fungi cause an ischemic enterocolitis with extensive angioinvasion, similar to that of

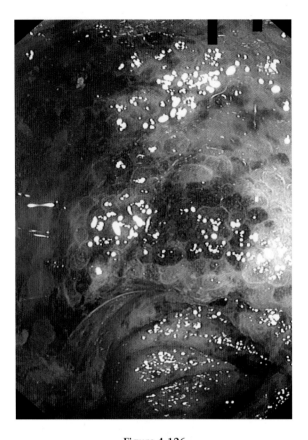

Figure 4-126

ADENOVIRUS-ASSOCIATED ENTEROCOLITIS

An area of eroded, friable mucosa with contact bleeding is present in the proximal colon of this stem cell transplant patient who presented with diarrhea and abdominal pain.

aspergillosis. *Mucor* feature pauci-septate, irregularly branched hyphae with a ribbon-like appearance and central clearing (fig. 4-133) (303).

Histoplasmosis. *Histoplasma capsulatum* is found in bird droppings and is endemic to the Mississippi and Ohio River valleys, Mexico, and regions of Central and South America (327). It exists in a filamentous form in the environment, and as a yeast in humans. Although limited disease occurs in immunocompetent individuals, dissemination can develop in immunocompromised individuals, particularly those with HIV/AIDS (328).

Endoscopic examination reveals thickened, distorted mucosa and ulcers (fig. 4-134A). Villi are expanded by a macrophage-rich infiltrate containing yeast but well-formed granulomas are generally lacking (fig. 4-134B). Ovoid yeast measure 2 to 4 μm and show narrow-based budding surrounded by a halo of rarified cyto-plasm within macrophages (fig. 4-134C). Silver stains highlight the intracellular organisms (fig. 4-134D).

***Talaromyces Marneffei* (Formerly *Penicillium Marneffei*).** This is a dimorphic fungus endemic to China and Southeast Asia that causes severe, often fatal, disease in patients with HIV/AIDS (329). Endoscopic abnormalities, including erosions, ulcers, and inflammatory masses, can mimic malignancy (330). The ovoid yeasts are 2 to 5 μm and closely simulate *Histoplasma capsulatum*, although some organisms are larger with curved ends (331).

Cryptococcus Neoformans. This organism causes extensive tissue necrosis and can affect any part of the gastrointestinal tract (332). The yeast are ovoid and span 4 to 7 μm. Some strains have a mucopolysaccharide capsule that is clear and colorless in routinely stained sections, but magenta with mucicarmine histochemical stains (333). Capsule-deficient strains are mucicarmine-negative, although encapsulated and capsule-deficient organisms are highlighted by GMS and PAS-D stains (334).

Protozoal Infections

Giardiasis. *Giardia lamblia* causes self-limited enteritis in otherwise healthy individuals, but immunocompromised individuals are at risk for recurrent or prolonged infection. Patients with HIV/AIDS, selective IgA deficiency, and common variable immunodeficiency are at highest risk because they often have impaired mucosal immunity (335). Giardiasis is frequently spread through contaminated water and food sources, although fecal-oral transmission occurs in institutions and daycare centers.

The organism usually infects the proximal small bowel where it completes its lifecycle; infection is rarely detected in the ileum (336). Trophozoites elicit minimal, if any, inflammatory changes in the mucosa and are easily overlooked (337,338). They are crescentic or pear-shaped and often have a "falling leaves" appearance when detected at the luminal surface or in intervillous spaces (fig. 4-135A). Organisms are flagellated, with two nuclei and a central karyosome. Their morphologic features are best appreciated in cytology preparations obtained from the formalin fixative of duodenal biopsies (fig. 4-135B) (339).

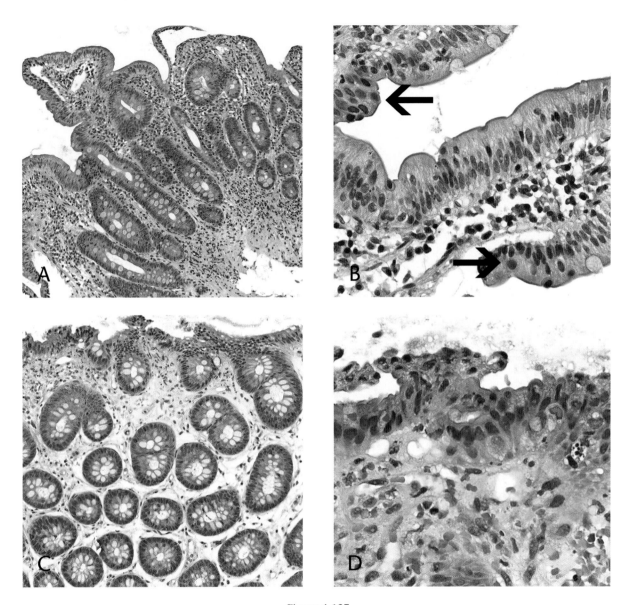

Figure 4-127

ADENOVIRUS-ASSOCIATED ENTEROCOLITIS

Duodenal samples from a child with severe combined immunodeficiency display mild villous architectural abnormalities, crypt hyperplasia, and slightly increased lamina propria cellularity (A). Apoptotic debris, loss of cell polarity, and scattered intranuclear viral inclusions (arrows) are evident in the surface epithelium (B). Colonic samples from a bone marrow transplant patient feature tufts of disorganized epithelial cells at the surface (C) that contain apoptotic cellular debris and numerous infected nuclei with smudgy inclusions (D).

Cyclosporiasis. *Cyclospora cayetanensis* is a protozoan transmitted through contaminated water sources and leafy vegetables. Cases in the United States have been linked to contaminated basil, raspberries, and other imported foods. Infected patients develop loose stools or watery diarrhea within 2 weeks of exposure; some also have fever, chills, myalgias, and fatigue (340). *C. cayetanensis* produces self-limited disease in immunocompetent individuals and protracted symptoms in immunodeficient patients. Chronic infection is associated with acalculous cholecystitis, Guillain-Barré syndrome, and arthritis. Trimethoprim-sulfamethoxazole is standard therapy (341,342).

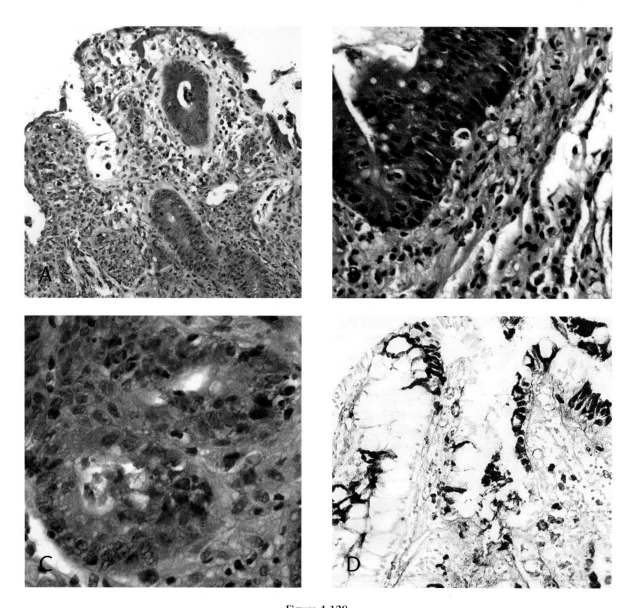

Figure 4-128

ADENOVIRUS-ASSOCIATED ENTEROCOLITIS

Duodenal samples feature crypt loss, erosions, and hemosiderin deposits in the lamina propria (A) accompanied by apoptotic crypt epithelial cells (B). Clustered glassy eosinophilic inclusions are present in crypt cell nuclei (C). Adenovirus immunostains demonstrate more numerous infected cells than are apparent in routinely stained sections (D).

C. cayetanensis is an obligate intracellular parasite that infects the proximal small bowel. Ingested sporulated oocysts contain two sporozoites that are released upon excystation within the gut. Sporozoites invade the intestinal epithelium and undergo at least two cycles of asexual reproduction within the cell, forming meronts that contain numerous merozoites. First generation meronts contain 8 to 12 mero-

zoites that undergo additional cycles of asexual reproduction. Second generation meronts each contain four merozoites that are released to penetrate other epithelial cells and subsequently form gametes. Gametes mature into female or male macrogamonts that undergo meiosis to form flagellated microgametes and are released to fertilize macrogamonts. The resulting zygote contains two sporocysts and becomes enveloped

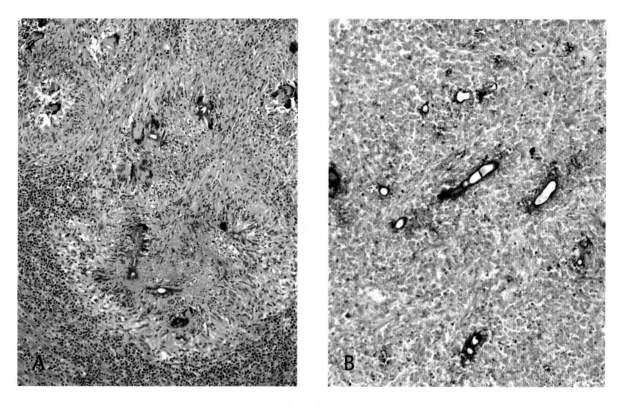

Figure 4-129

BASIDIOBOLOMYCOSIS

Fungal infection produces inflammatory masses composed of an exuberant granulomatous reaction to fungal forms. Eosinophilic Splendore-Hoeppli phenomenon accentuates hyphae within granulomas, which are associated with an eosinophil-rich infiltrate (A). A GMS stain demonstrates pauciseptate, thin-walled hyphae (B).

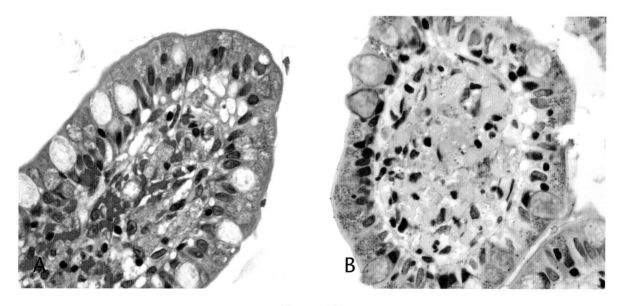

Figure 4-130

MICROSPORIDIOSIS

Supranuclear parasitophorous vacuoles contain slightly basophilic spores (A) that are enhanced with a tissue Gram stain (B).

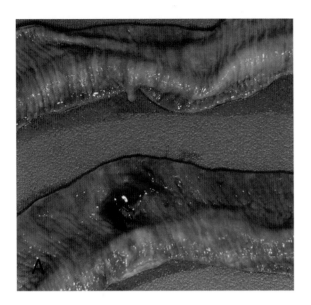
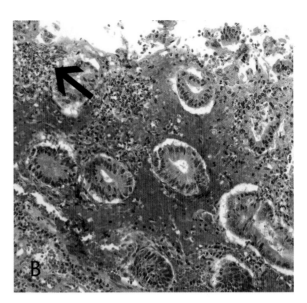

Figure 4-131

INTESTINAL CANDIDIASIS

A large, necrotic ulcer is surfaced by a gray-green pseudomembrane; smaller ulcers are also present (A). Invasive fungal forms (arrow) are associated with mucosal hemorrhage, superficial aggregates of neutrophils, and focal cryptitis (B).

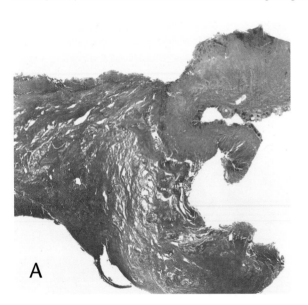
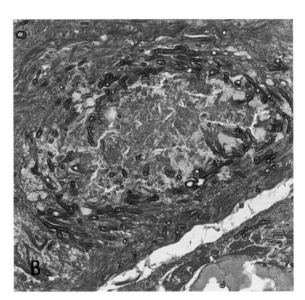

Figure 4-132

INTESTINAL ASPERGILLOSIS

The entire intestinal wall is necrotic and hemorrhagic (A). Numerous large caliber vessels feature invasive fungal forms (B).

in a resilient oocyst wall that is passed in the stool. Sporulation occurs in the environment and is complete within 1 to 2 weeks, although some evidence suggests that this stage of development may also occur within the human host (343,344).

Mucosal samples show variable villous abnormalities, crypt hyperplasia, and patchy inflammation. Organisms are apparent in routinely stained sections; they reside in parasitophorous vacuoles in the upper third of the enterocyte

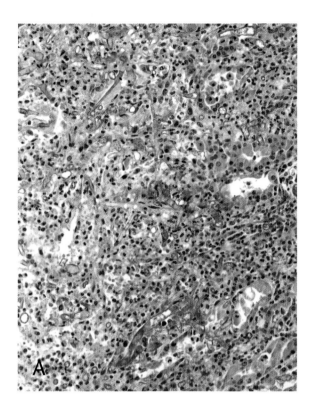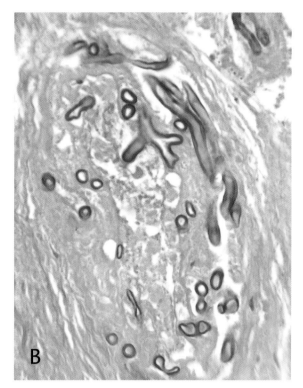

Figure 4-133

INVASIVE MUCORMYCOSIS

Scattered fungal forms are surrounded by neutrophil-rich inflammatory infiltrates (A). Broad, ribbon-like hyphae have thick walls and few septa which are better appreciated with a PAS-D stain (B).

cytoplasm (fig. 4-136). Various stages of the life cycle can be identified in histologic sections (343). Schizonts are round and 2 to 3 μm, whereas merozoites are 5 to 6 μm in length and banana-shaped. Infection is usually diagnosed with PCR-based DNA assays, stool evaluation, or intestinal aspirates from infected patients. Cysts are non-refractile with variable modified acid-fast staining and autofluorescence under ultraviolet illumination. *C. cayetanensis* is morphologically distinct from other coccidians and organisms in the differential diagnosis (Table 4-8).

Cryptosporidiosis. *Cryptosporidium parvum, C. hominis,* and *C. meleagridis* cause enteritis in humans. Children in daycare centers, institutionalized patients, travelers to developing countries, immigrants, and immunocompromised individuals are at highest risk for infection. Transmission usually occurs through contaminated food and water and person-to-person spread. The oocysts are chlorine and ozone resistant and, thus, outbreaks related to water-

parks and swimming pools occur intermittently during summer months (345). Symptoms include profuse watery diarrhea, abdominal cramps, malaise, nausea, and vomiting.

The diagnosis can be confirmed with acid-fast stains performed on stool and stool cultures. Immunocompetent patients generally do not require antibiotic therapy. Immunosuppressed individuals may require fluid resuscitation and antimotility agents. Antiparasitic agents, such as nitazoxanide, are variably effective. Symptoms usually improve in patients with HIV/AIDS who receive highly active antiretroviral therapy (HAART).

Cryptosporidia were previously classified as coccidians, although recent molecular data have led to their reclassification as gregarines, a subclass of *Conoidasida* closely related to coccidians (346). Infection elicits variable villous architectural abnormalities with patchy intraepithelial lymphocytosis (fig. 4-137). Surface epithelial cells may show disarray with loss of polarity and apoptotic debris. Neutrophilic cryptitis is

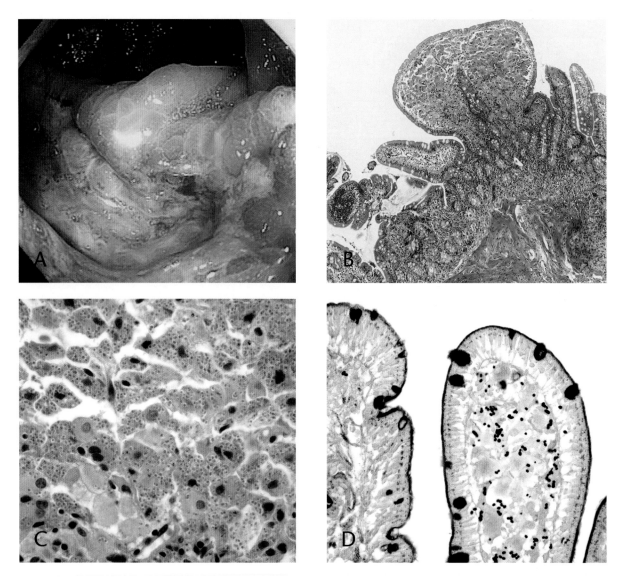

Figure 4-134

DUODENAL HISTOPLASMOSIS

Endoscopic abnormalities include thickened mucosal folds and bulbous villi (A) that reflect distension by sheets of macrophages expanding the lamina propria (B). (A: courtesy of Dr. B. Odum, St. Louis, MO.) Innumerable intracytoplasmic vacuoles contain yeast forms (C) that are highlighted with GMS histochemical stains (D).

occasionally present. Basophilic organisms are spherical and span 2 to 5 µm (303). They are located in cytoplasmic vacuoles at the apical surfaces of enterocytes but appear to be extracellular in tissue sections (256). They are apparent in routinely-stained sections and are highlighted by Gram stain. Although immunohistochemical stains are available, other organisms considered in the differential diagnosis are readily distinguished based on their morphologic features (Table 4-8).

Cystoisosporiasis. *Cystoisospora belli* is the largest coccidian, measuring up to 20 µm. It may infect immunocompetent or immunocompromised patients. Disease is usually self-limited among immunocompetent individuals but may lead to protracted watery diarrhea in immunosuppressed patients (347). The organism shows a predilection for the small bowel and rarely infects the colon. Infected patients often have peripheral eosinophilia. The diagnosis is

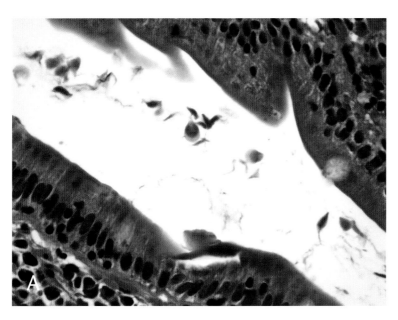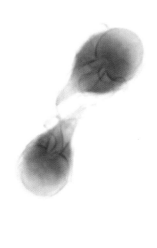

Figure 4-135

GIARDIASIS

Trophozoites reside in the intervillous space and have a crescentic or teardrop shape in routinely processed sections (A). Cytology specimens prepared from the formalin fixative of biopsy samples provide improved organism detail: flagella and nuclei are readily visible (B).

Table 4-8

DISTINGUISHING CHARACTERISTICS OF INTRACELLULAR ENTERIC PATHOGENS

Feature	*Microsporidia* sp.	*Cryptosporidia Parvum*	*Cyclospora Cayetanensis*	*Cystisospora Belli*
Location	Upper one third enterocyte	Apical vacuoles Appear extracellular	Superficial cytoplasm of enterocyte	Epithelial cells Macrophages
Size	2-3 μm spores 3-5 μm plasmodia	2-5 μm	2-3 μm schizonts 5-6 μm merozoites	15-20 μm
Morphology	Multiple round spores in single vacuole	Spherical sporozoites at luminal surface	Round schizonts Crescentic merozoites	Round sexual forms Elliptoid asexual forms
Stain characteristics	Modified trichrome, Giemsa, Gram, PAS/PAS-D[a], Silver	Giemsa Gram	Giemsa Acid fast	Giemsa Gram PAS/PAS-D

[a]PAS/PAS-D = periodic acid–Schiff (PAS) with diastase (PAS-D).

generally made based on stool studies, similar to other protozoal infections.

The endoscopic examination is generally normal. Biopsy findings include variable villous shortening with crypt hyperplasia and mild lamina propria inflammation. Enterocytes often show cytoplasmic depletion and disorganization in the superficial epithelium. Patchy intraepithelial lymphocytosis is frequently present (303). Organisms vary in size and shape,

reflecting a complex lifecycle. They are detected in parasitophorous vacuoles in the surface epithelium, either in a supranuclear or subnuclear location (fig. 4-138) (348). Giemsa, GMS, and PAS/PAS-D stains highlight the organisms, but they are usually unnecessary; organisms are readily evident in routinely stained sections.

Amebiasis. Several amebic species can infection humans, but *Entamoeba histolytica* is the best characterized organism responsible for clinically

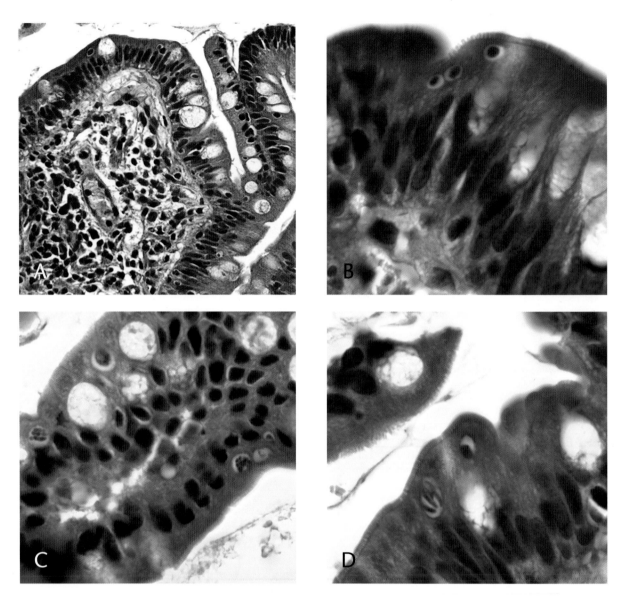

Figure 4-136

CYCLOSPORIASIS

The small intestinal epithelium contains slightly increased intraepithelial lymphocytes and several parasitophorous vacuoles (A). Sporozoites are located in the apical cytoplasm of surface absorptive cells (B). Parasitophorous vacuoles contain numerous meronts, which may develop into gametocytes and initiate sexual reproduction (C). Elongated merozoites are present in a parasitophorous vacuole (D).

significant gastrointestinal disease. *E. histolytica* infects 10 percent of the population globally and causes nearly 100,000 deaths each year (349). Water sources contaminated with cyst-containing feces account for most cases, although transmission also results from mucosal contact during sex and instrumentation with contaminated endoscopes and other equipment (350). Patients present with fever, abdominal pain, and bloody diarrhea with mucus. Leukocytosis is commonly present.

E. histolytica shows a predilection for the proximal colon where it causes discrete ulcers (fig. 4-139) (351). Ulcers are characteristically flask-shaped, featuring extensive tissue necrosis that reflects lysis of epithelial and inflammatory cells (fig. 4-140). Areas of necrosis contain finely

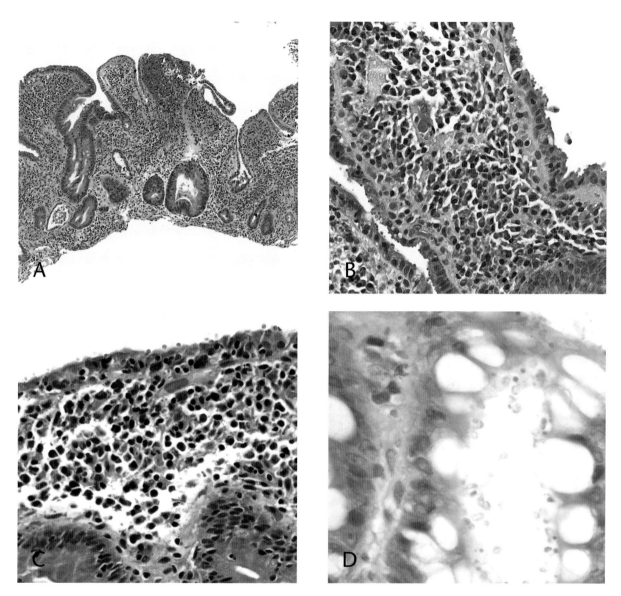

Figure 4-137

CRYPTOSPORIDIOSIS

The duodenal mucosa is mildly expanded by a mononuclear cell-rich inflammation and features partial villous blunting with crypt hyperplasia (A). Spherical organisms are lined up along the epithelial surface (B), eliciting intraepithelial lymphocytosis (C). Although they are usually basophilic, degenerated or poorly fixed organisms can appear pale with internal structures (D).

granular, eosinophilic material surrounded by neutrophils, lymphocytes, and macrophages (352–354). The immediately adjacent colonic mucosa shows mild inflammatory changes, but much of the intervening mucosa is normal. Trophozoites are located in intact mucosa adjacent to ulcers, at the advancing edges of ulcers, or in ulcer exudates. They contain pale, bubbly cytoplasm and central nuclei. They also contain

slightly eccentric karyosomes composed of condensed chromatin, which facilitates distinction from macrophages (fig. 4-140D). *E. histolytica* contain fragmented erythrocytes, whereas other species lack this finding.

Balantidiosis. *Balantidium coli* is a ciliated protozoan that normally resides in pigs; humans become infected through direct contact with pigs or their feces, as well as contaminated water

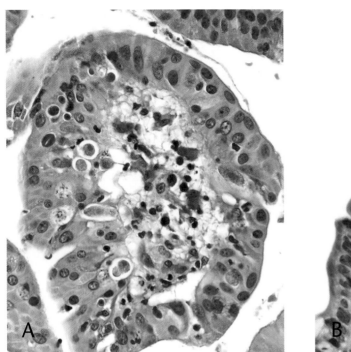
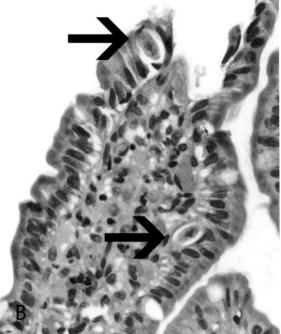

Figure 4-138

CYSTOISPORIASIS

Numerous round and elliptoid coccidians are present in supranuclear and subnuclear vacuoles. Epithelial cells display cytoplasmic depletion and disorganization; infiltrating inflammatory cells and cellular debris are present (A). (Courtesy of Dr. J. Greenson, Ann Arbor, MI.) Large parasitophorous vacuoles contain organisms (arrows) with prominent nuclei (B).

Figure 4-139

AMEBIASIS

Entamoeba histolytica cause discrete ulcers in the proximal colon accompanied by edema of the intervening mucosa. (Courtesy of Dr. K. Goto, Stockholm, Sweden.)

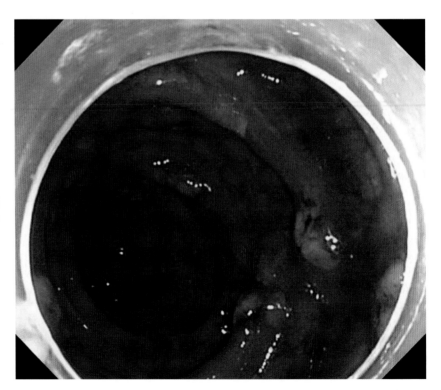

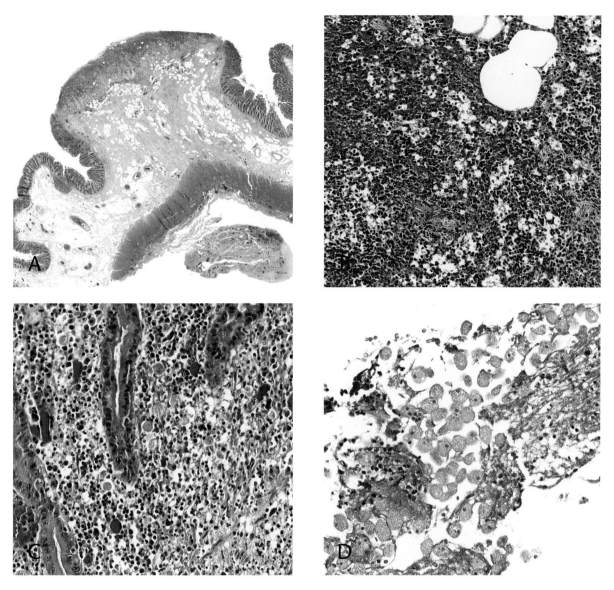

Figure 4-140

AMEBIASIS

Entamoeba histolytica induce sharply demarcated wedge-shaped ulcers (A) composed of necrotic, granular material (B). The adjacent mucosa shows mild inflammatory changes and invasive trophozoites (C). Organisms contain bubbly pale cytoplasm and karyosomes, as well as fragmented red blood cells (D).

sources. Disease is most common in Southeast Asia, the Western Pacific islands, and rural South America (355). Infection produces a variety of clinical symptoms ranging from generalized abdominal distress to bloody, mucus-containing diarrhea. Treatment includes antibiotic therapy with tetracycline or metronidazole.

The endoscopic features are similar to those associated with *E. histolytica* infection.

The organisms are large compared with other protozoans (356). They feature abundant frothy cytoplasm and prominent cell membranes as well as bean-shaped nuclei and cilia (fig. 4-141).

Helminthic Infections

Schistosomiasis. Schistosomes are trematodes, or blood flukes, that cause substantial morbidity worldwide. Approximately 10 percent of

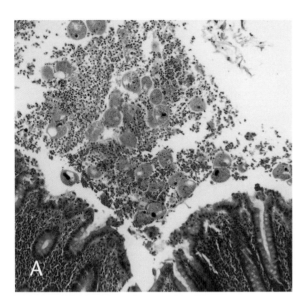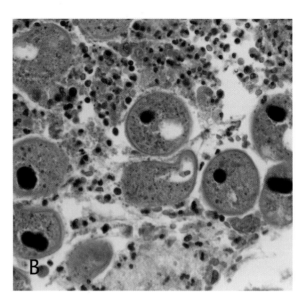

Figure 4-141

BALANTIDIOSIS

Balantidium coli are present in association with colitis and ulcer debris (A). The organisms are much larger than *E. histolytica*. They contain bean-shaped nuclei and a fringe of cilia; erythrophagocytosis may be present (B).

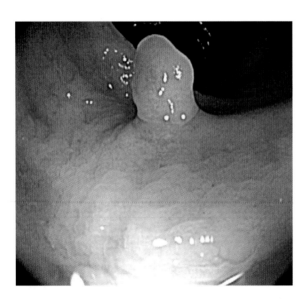

Figure 4-142

SCHISTOSOMIASIS

Inflammatory polyps are frequently present in patients with chronic schistosomiasis.

the global population is infected; endemic areas include parts of Africa, the Middle East, Central and South America, the Dominican Republic and Puerto Rico, China, Thailand, Indonesia, and the Philippines (357). The gastrointestinal tract is the target of *Schistosoma mansoni, S. japonicum, S. mekongi,* and *S. intercalatum,* but any species can affect this organ system. Snails represent intermediate hosts; human disease results from exposure to contaminated water. Flukes penetrate the skin and ultimately spread to the portal venous system where adults mate. Females shed eggs that embolize venules and capillaries in the small bowel and colon.

Most infected patients are asymptomatic, although some present with fever, myalgias and arthralgias, cough, and malaise shortly after infection. Bloody or non-bloody diarrhea, anemia, weight loss, and symptoms of bowel obstruction can develop in patients with chronic infections. The diagnosis is usually established following serologic studies or when ova are detected in stool or urine. Praziquantel is effective against all schistosomal species.

The endoscopic examination may be entirely normal, or display friability and granularity. Chronically infected patients often have endoscopically apparent pseudopolyps (fig. 4-142) that tend to be most pronounced in the rectosigmoid colon. Mucosal inflammation is directly attributable to ova: eggs lodged in vascular spaces are unaccompanied by inflammation (fig. 4-143A) but those that erode into the lamina propria

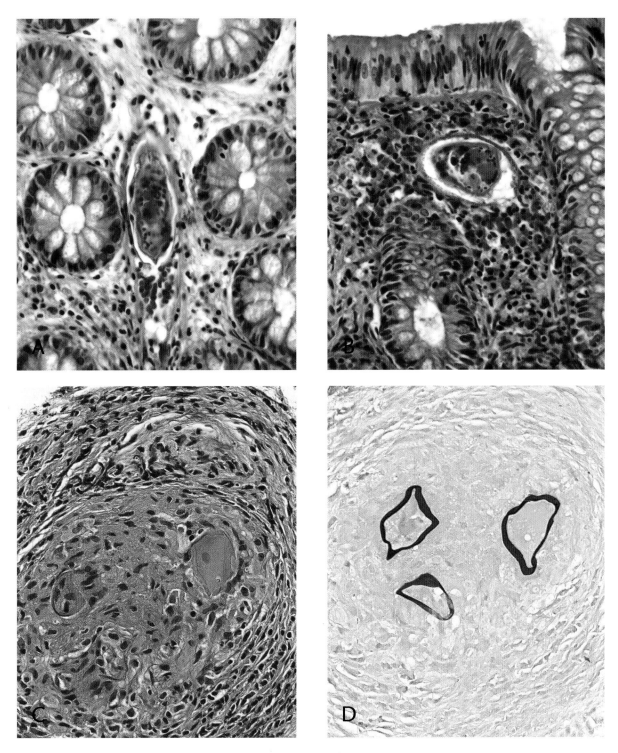

Figure 4-143

SCHISTOSOMIASIS

Ova embolize mucosal capillaries (A) and erode into the lamina propria, where they elicit an eosinophil-rich inflammatory response (B). Refractile egg fragments can be detected in epithelioid granulomas (C). They are bright red with acid-fast stains (D).

elicit an eosinophil-rich inflammatory infiltrate (fig. 4-143B) (358). Chronic infection leads to granuloma formation, fibrosis, and calcification of ova (fig. 4-143C). The shell and spine of the egg are variably acid fast and these qualities can facilitate morphologic speciation (fig. 4-143D). *S. mansoni*, *S. japonicum*, and *S. mekongi* have acid-fast shells and spines, whereas only the spine of *S. intercalatum* is acid fast.

Strongyloidiasis. *Strongyloides stercoralis* is a nematode that commonly causes gastrointestinal illness. It is endemic in tropical climates, the southeastern United States, and urban areas with large immigrant populations (359). Infection occurs primarily in adults with chronic illnesses, although up to 30 percent of infected patients are asymptomatic. Immunosuppression is an important risk factor for infection; patients at particular risk are those receiving corticosteroids, solid organ transplant recipients, and individuals with human T-lymphotropic virus (HTLV)-1 infection. The incidence of strongyloidiasis does not seem to be increased among patients with HIV/AIDS. Several cases have occurred in patients with common variable immunodeficiency, possibly reflecting impaired mucosal immunity (256).

Symptoms range from iron deficiency anemia and vague abdominal complaints to nausea, vomiting, diarrhea, and protein-losing enteropathy. Symptoms may be accompanied by mesenteric adenopathy, rash, urticaria, pruritis, and pulmonary symptoms. Leukocytosis and peripheral eosinophilia are commonly present. Documentation of active infection requires identification of larvae or eggs in stool or tissue. Immunoglobulins may reflect previously infection, so their detection does not necessarily imply active infection (360).

Infection occurs when filariform larvae in contaminated soil penetrate exposed skin. They make their way to the small bowel and mature in the lumen. Females lay eggs that hatch into rhabditiform larvae that can either be excreted into the environment to complete their lifecycle or differentiate into infectious filariform larvae in the gut. The latter situation leads to autoinfection and chronic infestation. Some immunosuppressed patients, especially those co-infected with HTLV-1 and those receiving corticosteroids, have periods of accelerated autoinfection with high parasite burdens (361). Disseminated disease can also develop in immunocompromised individuals. Many of these patients become bacteremic, presumably because worms carry enteric bacteria as they invade through the intestinal wall and migrate to other sites.

Endoscopic findings are non-specific. Mucosal edema and erythema are common. Patients with lymphatic obstruction by larvae may have duodenal lymphangiectasias. Ulcers, inflammatory masses, and pseudopolyps occur in some cases (362,363). Eggs, larvae, and adult worms can be found throughout the gastrointestinal tract, although worms show a predilection for the proximal small bowel (364). Adult worms are curved with pointed tails and long basophilic ova (fig. 4-144). Larvae range from 14 to 16 µm in length and have a thin cuticle that contains rows of small nuclei. Both adult worms and larvae reside in crypts where they do not elicit an inflammatory reaction. Only organisms that transgress the basement membrane elicit eosinophil-rich inflammation. Capillaria, parasites common to Southeast Asia and the Philippines, simulate the appearance of *S. stercoralis* in histologic sections, although they rarely invade the mucosa or cause enterocolitis.

Chronic *S. stercoralis* infection can produce mucosal injury that simulates the features of inflammatory bowel disease; the colon may contain skip lesions with a right-sided predominance or rectal sparing, as well as submucosal and mural inflammation. Crypt architectural abnormalities, atrophy, and villiform surface changes may be present, but they are unaccompanied by diffuse plasmacytosis in the mucosa. Intense lamina propria eosinophilia is often present and may raise concern for eosinophilic gastroenteritis. However, the latter generally lacks eosinophil microabscesses and clustered degranulating eosinophils in the lamina propria, both of which are often present in patients with chronic strongyloidiasis (fig. 4-144D). Misdiagnosing strongyloidiasis as idiopathic inflammatory bowel disease or eosinophilic gastroenteritis can be catastrophic. Immunosuppressive therapy may trigger hyperinfection, which has a 60 to 90 percent mortality rate (361).

Anisakiasis. *Anisakis simplex* is a nematode that parasitizes fish, marine invertebrates, and sea mammals. It causes human disease when contaminated raw or undercooked seafood is ingested (365). Larval forms penetrate the mucosa

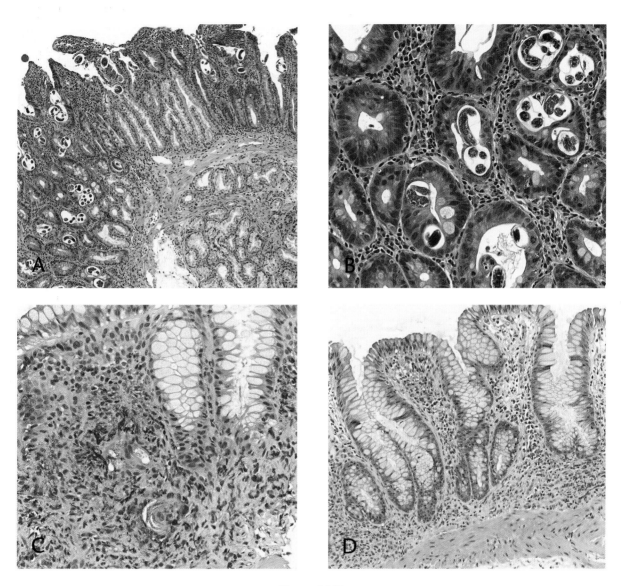

Figure 4-144

STRONGYLOIDIASIS

A corticosteroid-dependent renal transplant patient has many parasites in the duodenal crypts (A). Organisms are curved with pointed tails. Note the absence of eosinophilia in the lamina propria, despite the presence of numerous organisms (B). Worm fragments are embedded in eosinophilic abscesses and degranulated eosinophil debris in the lamina propria (C). Chronic infection can result in mucosal remodeling and crypt architectural distortion (D).

and burrow through the intestinal wall where they elicit an inflammatory reaction and produce symptoms of abdominal pain, bowel obstruction, and serositis (366). Disease in the distal small bowel mimics the clinical features of appendicitis and Crohn disease. Anisakiasis can also elicit a hypersensitivity reaction characterized by urticaria, angioedema, and anaphylaxis (367). It is an important consideration among young patients who

present with eosinophilic ascites. Infection is most common in the stomach but may occur anywhere in the gastrointestinal tract. Gastric ultrasonography is most useful in establishing a preoperative diagnosis; heterogeneously hypoechoic lesions containing tubular structures in the submucosa and deeper wall are characteristic (368). Humans are end-hosts, so infected patients do not require antihelminthic treatment.

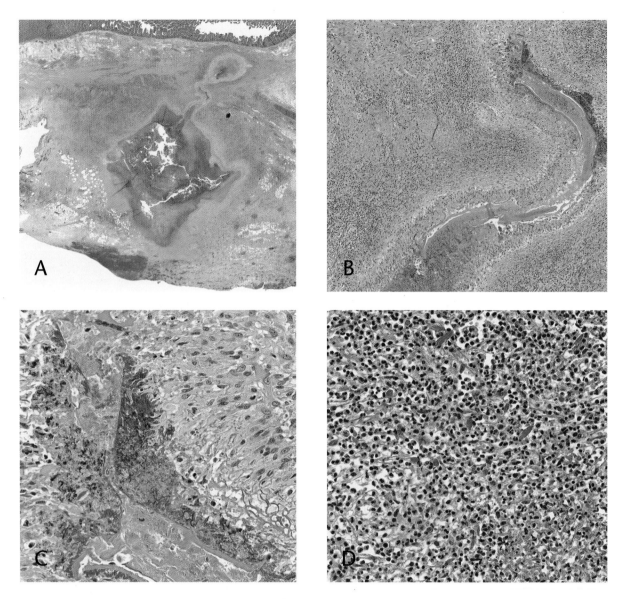

Figure 4-145

ANISAKIASIS

Parasites burrow into the bowel wall and die, eliciting a striking inflammatory reaction that extends to the serosal surface (A). The worm is surrounded by a palisaded granulomatous reaction and necrotic inflammatory cell debris (B). Foci of Splendore-Hoeppli phenomenon (C) are present in association with degranulating eosinophils and scattered Charcot-Leyden crystals (D).

Parasites elicit a granulomatous response intimately associated with an intense eosinophil-rich inflammatory reaction. The latter may be present distant from the site of infection, raising the possibility of mural or serosal eosinophilic gastroenteritis when incompletely sampled. Eosinophil-rich abscesses and Charcot-Leyden crystals are commonly encountered, especially in close proximity to the worms. Necrotic larvae are associated with Splendore-Hoeppli phenomenon (fig. 4-145) (369).

Other Helminthic Infections. A variety of hookworms, whipworms, flukes, tapeworms, and pinworms can infect the small and large intestines. These organisms generally do not invade the mucosa. Rather, they reside in the

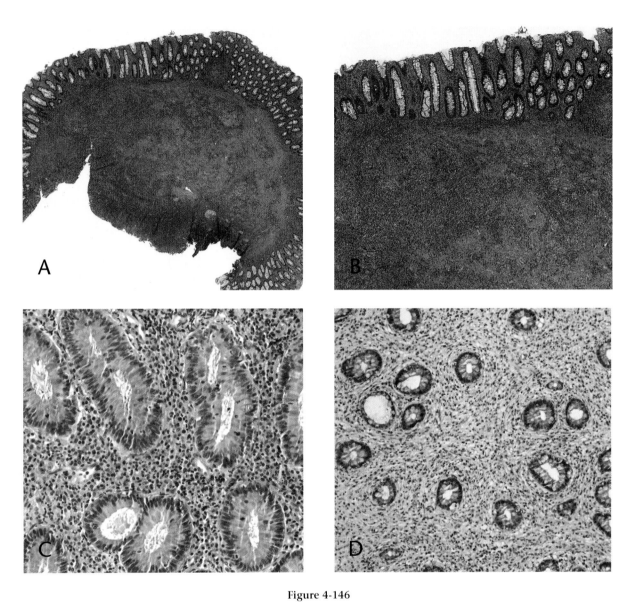

Figure 4-146

SYPHILITIC PROCTITIS

Syphilitic proctitis is characterized by lymphoplasmacytic inflammation in the lamina propria (A) that extends into the deep mucosa along vessels (B). Lymphoplasmacytic inflammation is associated with neutrophilic cryptitis, but crypt architectural distortion is minimal (C). Macrophage-rich infiltrates surround crypts and expand the lamina propria. This finding should raise concern for an infection, as this pattern is not typical of idiopathic inflammatory bowel disease (D).

lumen where they cause bleeding and malabsorption, resulting in abdominal pain, iron deficiency anemia, and diarrhea. Large aggregates of nematodes may obstruct the lumen. For the most part, classification of these pathogens requires stool examination for larvae, worms, or eggs, and serologic tests, rather than histologic assessment.

Proctitis Due to Sexually Transmitted Infections

These diseases are also discussed in Chapter 8.

Syphilis. Gastrointestinal syphilis is increasingly common, particularly in the anorectum. The causative organism, *Treponema pallidum,* is primarily transmitted through sexual contact. Homosexual men and patients with HIV/

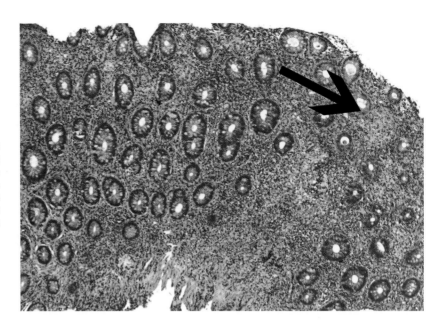

Figure 4-147

LYMPHOGRANULOMA VENEREUM

A distal rectal biopsy sample features a dense lymphohistiocytic infiltrate. Neutrophilic inflammation is minimal and crypt architectural distortion is lacking. Loose granulomatous inflammation is associated with crypt destruction (arrow).

AIDS are at highest risk of disease. Presenting symptoms related to proctitis include rectal pain exacerbated by defecation, tenesmus, and constipation, and mucoid or bloody stools accompanied by anal chancres and condylomata lata. The diagnosis often requires serologic tests, such as VDRL, RPR, and treponeme-specific antibodies (370). Penicillin therapy is the treatment of choice, although recurrent infection is common in individuals who practice high-risk sexual behavior (371).

Rectal disease can simulate idiopathic inflammatory bowel disease or a neoplasm when it produces an indurated mass or ulcer. Biopsy samples display chronic colitis with plasma cell-rich inflammation that may be present around vessels in the deep mucosa and superficial submucosa (372). Neutrophilic cryptitis, crypt abscesses, and crypt destruction are often present, but crypt architectural distortion is usually inconspicuous (fig. 4-146). Poorly formed granulomas and dispersed histiocytes are often present, and small vessels with prominent endothelial cells (i.e., proliferative endarteriolitis) may be noted. Diffuse macrophage-rich infiltrates and fibrosis of the lamina propria are important clues to the diagnosis; these findings are uncommon in patients with ulcerative colitis, especially early in the course of disease. Some cases of syphilitic proctitis manifest as an acute self-limited colitis without substantially increased plasma cells. The clinicopathologic features of syphilitic proctitis can mimic those of many other sexually transmitted proctocolitides, as described below (373). *Treponemes* are highlighted by silver impregnation, although widely available immunohistochemical stains show a much higher sensitivity.

Lymphogranuloma Venereum. Lymphogranuloma venereum results from infection with *Chlamydia trachomatis* serotypes L1, L2, and L3. Although it tends to cause anal disease, lymphogranuloma venereum can cause chronic proctitis. Affected patients present with mucoid or bloody discharge, anal pain, fever, tenesmus, and constipation. Inguinal lymphadenopathy is a common feature. Serologic testing is the gold standard for diagnosis. Treatment consists of antibiotic therapy with doxycycline or erythromycin (371).

Infected patients have active proctitis with ulcers, mucosal granularity, erythema, and friability (374). Chronic colitis features mild to moderate acute inflammation on a background of plasma cell-rich lamina propria inflammation. Loose aggregates of macrophages, lymphoid aggregates in the deep mucosa, neuronal hyperplasia, and fibrosis are often present; well-formed granulomas are occasionally encountered (fig. 4-147). Crypt architectural distortion, basal plasmacytosis, and Paneth cell metaplasia are less prominent than are typically seen in untreated chronic idiopathic inflammatory bowel disease (375). The inflammatory features are indistinguishable from those of syphilitic proctitis;

distinction requires spirochete immunohisto-chemistry and serologic evaluation (376).

Gonorrhea. *Neisseria gonorrhea* is a Gram-negative diplococcus that represents the second most commonly reported sexually transmitted infection (373). Proctitis results from anal receptive intercourse and occurs in women and men. It is common in patients with urogenital infection (377). The organism is an obligate human pathogen that expresses virulence factors to promote survival and replication. It can also attach to sperm, thereby facilitating transmission during intercourse. Infection is frequently asymptomatic (379). Symptomatic patients complain of mucoid stools, purulent discharge, anal bleeding, itching and irritation, rectal discomfort or fullness, and painful defecation. Development of a rash or arthritis may indicate disseminated infection (379). *Neisseria meningitidis* has been isolated from the anorectum but it not clear whether it represents colonization or an actual pathogen (378).

Organisms can be seen in slide preparations created from anal discharge (371). Although cultures can be used to establish a diagnosis and determine antibiotic susceptibility, the Centers for Disease Control and Prevention recently recommended nucleic acid amplification testing (NAAT) to identify extragenital gonorrhea because it shows superior sensitivity and specificity (373, 380). Screening of patients who engage in high-risk sexual practices is recommended (90). Treatment consists of antibiotic therapy with ceftriaxone or cefixime combined with empiric therapy for *Chlamydia,* given the high frequency of coinfection (371). Sexual partners should also be treated. Recurrence is common, so the threshold for retesting symptomatic patients should be low.

The mucosa may be endoscopically normal or show erythema and/or ulcers. Mucosal biopsy samples are often histologically normal. Some display mildly increased neutrophils and mononuclear cells, focal cryptitis, and crypt abscesses similar to other infections that cause an acute pattern of colitis. Bacteria colonize the mucosa and invade epithelial cells (381).

Herpes Simplex Virus. Herpes simplex virus (HSV) is transmitted through mucous membrane contact and affects immunocompetent and immunocompromised individuals. The esophagus and anorectum are the most common sites of gastrointestinal infection, as discussed in chapters 2 and 8. However, some patients develop herpetic proctitis, with or without concomitant anal disease. More proximal colitis is extremely rare and limited to immunocompromised patients. Affected individuals often have anorectal pain accompanied by fever, inguinal lymphadenopathy, mucopurulent discharge, and paresthesia. Both HSV1 and 2 can cause rectal disease, although the latter is far more common (382). Rectal swabs can be used to establish a diagnosis by viral culture or PCR for viral DNA (383,384). Treatment consists of acyclovir.

Clinically evident proctitis appears as shallow ulcers accompanied by erythema; intact vesicles of the rectal mucosa are uncommonly seen. Viral infection causes an acute self-limited colitis pattern of injury. Macrophage-rich inflammatory infiltrates are associated with abundant neutrophils and severe epithelial cell injury. Necrotic cellular debris is present in the colonic crypts, as well as the squamous epithelium of the transition zone (fig. 4-148). Acidophilic Cowdry A inclusions are surrounded by a rim of chromatin clearing, whereas Cowdry B inclusions are homogeneous and powdery blue; the former are more commonly encountered in rectal biopsy samples from infected patients. Immunohistochemical stains for HSV1 and HSV2 are commercially available (fig. 4-148D).

OTHER INFLAMMATORY CONDITIONS AND STRUCTURAL ABNORMALITIES

Peptic Duodenitis and Duodenal Ulcers

Definition. These conditions are the result of acid-related duodenal injury.

Clinical Features. *Peptic duodenitis* is a common disorder of the upper gastrointestinal tract, particularly in older adults.

Symptoms include dyspepsia and upper abdominal pain that may radiate to the back. Bleeding ulcers can cause iron deficiency anemia and melena. Abdominal pain may be exacerbated with meals. Duodenal ulcers account for approximately 40 percent of cases of acute-onset bleeding from the upper gastrointestinal tract.

Pathogenesis. *H. pylori* infection used to be a common cause of duodenitis because it promoted acid secretion and altered host defenses.

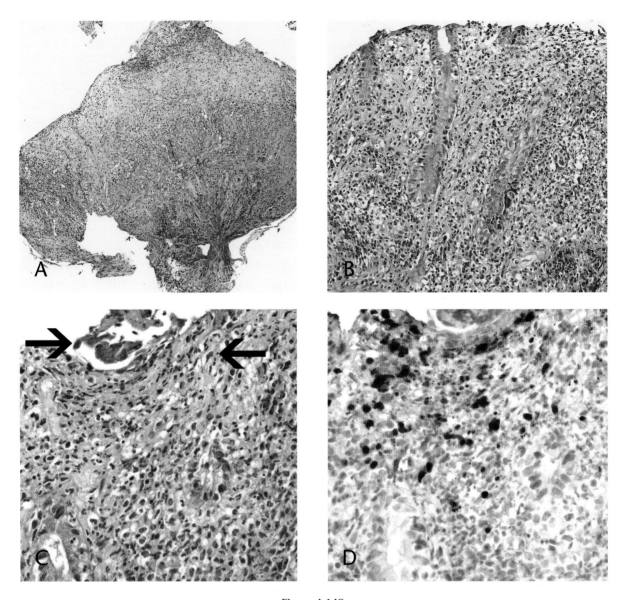

Figure 4-148

ANORECTAL HERPES SIMPLEX VIRUS INFECTION

Severe injury results in areas of complete denudation and edema (A). Intact mucosal fragments feature an acute colitis pattern of injury with extensive crypt destruction (B). Cryptitis is accompanied by mixed inflammation and numerous macrophages as well as a few viral inclusions (arrows) in the surface epithelium and destroyed crypts (C). Viral infection is confirmed with immunohistochemical stains (D).

Prior to widespread *H. pylori* eradication efforts, 90 percent of duodenal ulcers were attributed to infection with this pathogen. In the modern era, however, most cases result from acid-induced epithelial injury. Ulcer formation is facilitated by NSAIDs and other agents that promote injury to the mucosal barrier, such as smoking, chronic renal disease, and alcohol intake.

Gross Findings. Peptic duodenitis shows more severe changes in the proximal duodenum, particularly the duodenal bulb. Patchy or diffuse mucosal erythema is accompanied by petechial hemorrhages, erosions, or ulcers (385). The latter are round or ovoid with a clean base and usually span no more than a few centimeters (fig. 4-149). Multiple ulcers raise the possibility of hypergastrinemia due to an underlying gastrin-secreting endocrine tumor (Zollinger-Ellison syndrome).

Microscopic Findings. Acute peptic erosions or ulcers feature granulation tissue accompanied by marked epithelial cell injury. Surface cells show cytoplasmic depletion with nuclear enlargement. Regenerative crypts display increased mitotic activity. Goblet cells, Paneth cells, and endocrine cells may be inconspicuous in areas of severe injury (fig. 4-150A).

Chronic peptic duodenitis elicits a chronic inflammatory infiltrate with increased plasma cells in the lamina propria (fig. 4-150B) (386). Villi may be blunted, especially overlying Brunner glands. Foveolar metaplasia is frequently present in the surface epithelium (fig. 4-150C). Patchy intraepithelial lymphocytosis and clusters of neutrophils may be identified in symptomatic patients (fig. 4-150D) (387). Foci of foveolar metaplasia can be colonized by *H. pylori* when patients have *H. pylori* gastritis.

Differential Diagnosis. Peptic duodenitis can simulate the features of celiac disease, Crohn disease, and medication-related duodenitis. In contrast to celiac disease, peptic injury shows a predilection for the most proximal duodenum, with less severe changes in the second and third portions. Intraepithelial lymphocytosis tends to be less diffuse than that of celiac disease and neutrophils may be more prominent than expected. Crohn disease affects the small bowel in a segmental distribution and almost always occurs in combination with ileocolonic inflammation.

Treatment and Prognosis. Complications of peptic duodenitis are rare, although perforation can occur. Hemorrhage related to perforation may be life-threatening, with a mortality rate of 5 to 8 percent. Chronic and recurrent ulcers in the pyloric channel were once an important cause of gastric outlet obstruction but are less common in the modern era. Treatment of infection consists of eradication and *H. pylori* acid suppression with proton pump inhibitor therapy. Actively bleeding ulcers may be endoscopically treated with thermocoagulation, epinephrine injection, or other methods. Perforated ulcers and those associated with gastric outlet obstruction generally require surgical management (388).

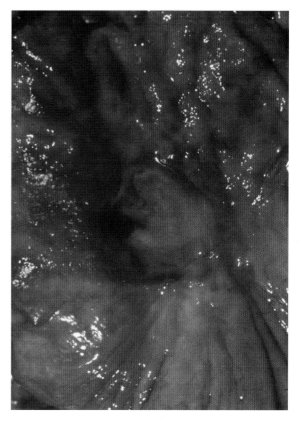

Figure 4-149

PEPTIC ULCER

This duodenal ulcer is round, with smooth borders and peripheral erythema. The background mucosa shows patchy inflammation and granularity.

Tropical Sprue

Definition. *Tropical sprue (postinfective tropical malabsorption)* is a malabsorptive disorder presumably related to an infectious etiology.

Clinical Features. Tropical sprue is endemic in equatorial regions around the globe, including India, Southeast Asia, West Africa, northern South America, and the Caribbean, where it likely accounts for up to 40 percent of malabsorption cases. The symptoms are classified as acute and chronic phases and differ among visitors to endemic areas and indigenous populations. Travelers have an insidious symptom onset with fevers, myalgias, and weakness, or acute diarrheal illness accompanied by abdominal pain, nausea, and flatulence. Malabsorptive diarrhea is uniformly present. Chronic manifestations of tropical sprue are more common in

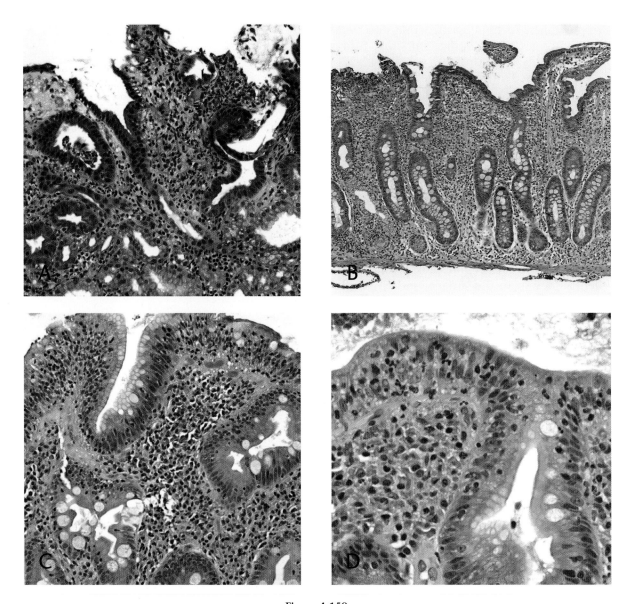

Figure 4-150

PEPTIC DUODENITIS

Superficial erosions are associated with marked epithelial regeneration and cytoplasmic depletion; neutrophils are present in the lamina propria and crypts (A). Chronic peptic injury elicits a plasma cell-rich infiltrate with crypt hyperplasia and variable villous shortening (B). Patchy lymphocytosis and foveolar metaplasia are present in the surface epithelium (C). Clusters of neutrophils are frequently identified in samples from the duodenal bulb (D).

indigenous populations. They include persistent diarrhea, abdominal pain, stomatitis, glossitis, and megaloblastic anemia secondary to folate and vitamin B12 deficiencies (389).

Pathogenesis. The etiology of tropical sprue is unknown. Aerobic bacterial overgrowth occurs in some patients and may be toxin-producing. Viral and parasitic etiologies have

been proposed, but no causal organism has been identified to date. Associations with the Aw-19 HLA haplotype suggest that innate immunity may play a role in disease pathogenesis.

Gross Findings. Endoscopic examination typically reveals essentially normal findings or only mild abnormalities such as scalloped folds and prominent mucosal vasculature.

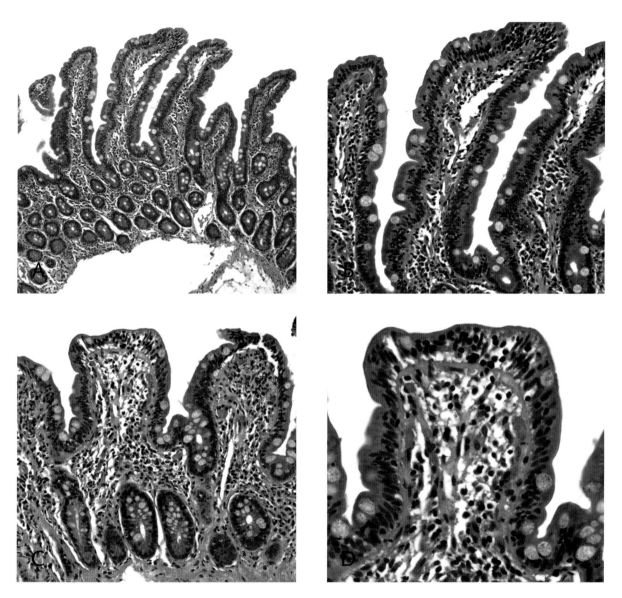

Figure 4-151

TROPICAL SPRUE

Villous abnormalities in the duodenum are less pronounced than those of celiac disease (A), although diffuse intraepithelial lymphocytosis is present (B). Broad, short villi in the ileum (C) show a similar degree of intraepithelial lymphocytosis (D).

Microscopic Findings. Tropical sprue can involve the entire small bowel and usually displays more severe mucosal alterations in the ileum than proximal duodenum. Changes include increased intraepithelial lymphocytes with variable villous blunting; completely flat villi are extremely uncommon and should prompt concern for another disorder (fig. 4-151). Tropical sprue also features more lamina propria eosinophils and fewer plasma cells than

are typically seen in celiac disease, especially if villous architectural abnormalities are present (389). Patients with vitamin B12 deficiency may have megaloblastic changes in enterocyte nuclei characterized by nuclear enlargement and decreased mitotic activity.

Treatment and Prognosis. Treatment consists of broad-spectrum antibiotic therapy, often combined with vitamin B12 and folate replacement.

Small Intestinal Bacterial Overgrowth

Definition. *Small intestinal bacterial overgrowth* is the result of increased bacterial numbers or alterations in the normal flora of in the small bowel.

Clinical Features. Small intestinal bacterial overgrowth is a common cause of chronic diarrhea in patients with impaired intestinal motility due to do a spectrum of disorders such as collagen vascular diseases, stricturing Crohn disease, cystic fibrosis, decreased mucosal immunity, prior small bowel surgery, or anatomic variations that result in blind pouches. Other risk factors include chronic pancreatitis, liver and kidney disease, celiac disease, and advanced age.

Patients typically complain of chronic diarrhea, weight loss, and bloating. Bacteria also deconjugate bile acids and compete for B12, resulting in fat malabsorption and vitamin deficiencies. The diagnosis is largely based on the presence of high numbers (10,000 or more) of colony-forming units (CFUs) per mL in duodenal aspirate cultures. It can also be established with hydrogen breath tests (390).

Pathogenesis. Bacterial florae are extremely important to the overall health and function of the gastrointestinal tract. The proximal small bowel normally contains very few bacteria owing to the sterilizing effects of acidic gastric juices. The motility of the luminal contents suppresses bacterial growth, such that nearly one-third of healthy individuals do not have detectable bacteria in cultures obtained from the jejunum (391). When present, proximal small bowel florae are similar to those of the oropharynx, largely consisting of aerobes and facultative anaerobes. Both aerobic and anaerobic bacteria are increasingly numerous in the distal small bowel. The colon contains the most bacteria, and a larger fraction of these is composed of anaerobes.

Direct injury to the brush border decreases disaccharidase activity, thereby increasing the luminal concentration of complex sugars. Bacterial metabolism of these substrates promotes their growth within the lumen, resulting in elaboration of lipopolysaccharides and other products that damage the mucosa and increase its permeability. These molecules stimulate the innate immune response, resulting in mucosal inflammation and cellular injury (392).

Microscopic Findings. Minimal, if any, histologic abnormalities are detected in approximately 50 percent of patients with clinically suspected bacterial overgrowth syndrome (393). Nearly one-fourth of cases show variable villous architectural abnormalities with decreased villous to crypt ratios (fig. 4-152A,B). Other less common changes include mixed mononuclear cell-rich inflammation in the lamina propria with occasional eosinophils and neutrophils. Surface epithelial cell injury may be disproportionately severe given the degree of intraepithelial lymphocytosis (fig. 4-152C). The histologic changes tend to be patchier and milder than those of celiac disease and show minimal crypt involvement (fig. 4-152D) (394).

Treatment and Prognosis. Antibiotic agents aimed at eradicating abnormal bacteria are the cornerstone of treatment. Patients with motility disorders may require multiple or sustained courses of antibiotic therapy. Fecal microbiota transplants have been used with variable success (395).

Secondary Intestinal Lymphangiectasia

Definition. *Secondary intestinal lymphangiectasia* is the acquired proliferation of lymphatic channels due to outflow obstruction.

Clinical Features. Secondary intestinal lymphangiectasia is often asymptomatic, although some patients with extensive disease present with protein-losing enteropathy and ascites. Diffuse lymphangiectasia is associated with underlying cardiac disease, prior liver transplantation, radiation therapy, Crohn disease, and retroperitoneal lymphadenopathy due to benign or malignant conditions (396). Patients with protein-losing enteropathy may also have decreased immunoglobulin and circulating lymphocytes, deficiencies in fat-soluble vitamins, and hypocalcemia. Ascitic fluid is rich in triglycerides with low levels of albumin. Localized lesions are usually asymptomatic.

Pathogenesis. Secondary intestinal lymphangiectasia reflects mechanical obstruction of lymph outflow.

Gross Findings. Dilated lacteals are endoscopically apparent, producing one or more white dots, nodules, or plaques (fig. 4-153). Lesions tend to be most pronounced on the crests of edematous mucosal folds and may leak chylous fluid when sampled.

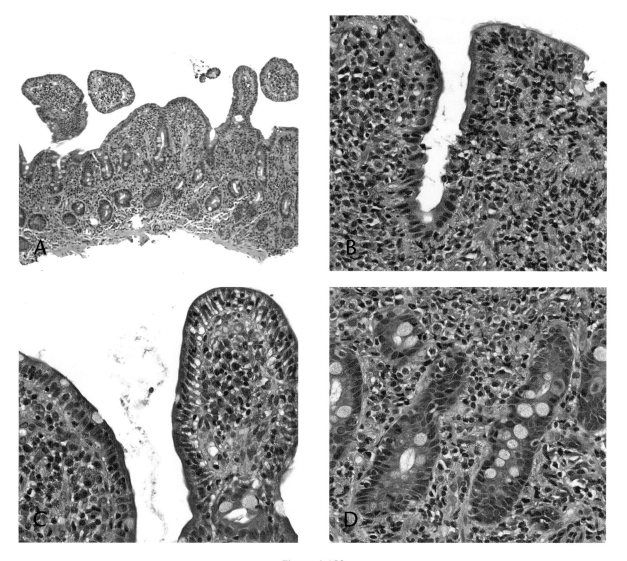

Figure 4-152

SMALL INTESTINAL BACTERIAL OVERGROWTH

Variable villous architectural abnormalities are accompanied by mononuclear cell-rich inflammation in the lamina propria (A) and patchy intraepithelial lymphocytosis (B). Distorted villi show a greater degree of epithelial cell injury than would be expected given the mild degree of lymphocytosis in this area (C). Crypts are essentially spared by an infiltrate rich in plasma cells and eosinophils (D).

Microscopic Findings. Dilated endothelium-lined lymphatic channels expand the villi. Lymphatic channels contain faintly eosinophilic proteinaceous material and foamy macrophages (fig. 4-154). The surrounding lamina propria is essentially normal.

Treatment and Prognosis. Secondary intestinal lymphangiectasia does not necessarily require therapy; treatment is aimed at alleviating the underlying disorder. Dietary modification with low-fat intake and medium-chain triglyceride supplementation is effective in some patients (396).

Small Intestinal Diverticulosis

Definition. *Small intestinal diverticulosis* is acquired herniation of mucosa and submucosa through muscularis propria. It is also termed *false diverticula*.

Clinical Features. Duodenal diverticula are detected in slightly more than 8 percent of the

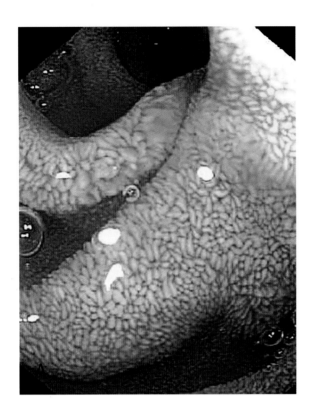
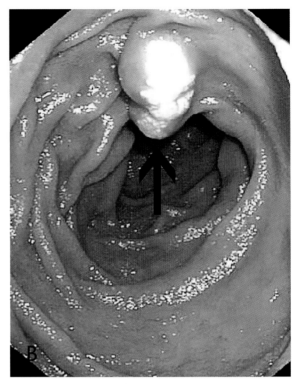

Figure 4-153

SECONDARY SMALL INTESTINAL LYMPHANGIECTASIA

Diffuse lymphangiectasia appears as multiple yellow-white flecks on the duodenal mucosa (A). Localized lymphangiectasia produces a sessile polyp with yellow discoloration (arrow) on a background of essentially normal mucosa (B).

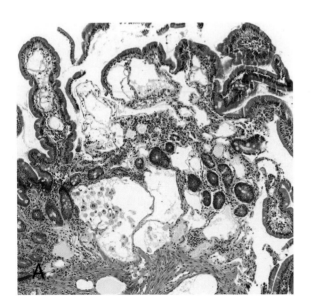
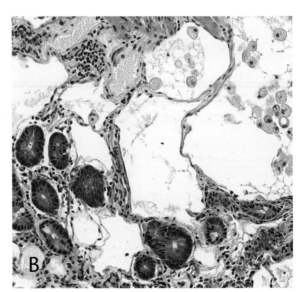

Figure 4-154

SECONDARY SMALL INTESTINAL LYMPHANGIECTASIA

Several villi are distended by dilated lymphatic channels (A) containing lymph and foamy macrophages (B).

population. Most are solitary lesions resulting from inflammatory conditions that weaken or destroy the duodenal wall, such as peptic ulcer disease and choledocholithiasis, although they also develop in patients with Marfan syndrome, Ehlers-Danlos syndrome, and other connective tissue diseases (397,398).

Jejunal and ileal diverticula are less common, affecting less than 5 and 0.5 percent of the population, respectively. They occur in the setting of collagen vascular disease, Fabry disease, visceral myopathies and neuropathies, neuronal inclusion disease, and other causes of intestinal dysmotility.

Small intestinal diverticulosis shows a predilection for adults older than 40 years of age. Most lesions are clinically silent (399). Some patients present with bleeding, diverticulitis, perforation, or fistulae (400). Multiple diverticula of the distal bowel can lead to bacterial overgrowth, producing malabsorptive symptoms.

Gross and Microscopic Findings. Diverticula appear as outpouchings on the mesenteric border (fig. 4-155). Most are smaller than 1 cm, although duodenal lesions can span several centimeters. The diverticular lining is usually ulcerated or shows villous blunting and inflammation.

Treatment and Prognosis. Symptomatic treatment includes dietary modification and antibiotic or probiotic therapy for bacterial overgrowth. Surgery is limited to patients with perforation, bleeding, and other complications (401).

Colonic Diverticulosis and Related Inflammatory Conditions

Definition. *Diverticulosis* is acquired herniation of mucosa and submucosa into or through the muscularis propria. *Diverticulitis* is variably severe diverticular and pericolic inflammation. *Diverticular disease-related colitis* is chronic colitis affecting diverticulosis and interdiverticular colon. Synonyms for diverticulosis are *false diverticula* or *pulsion diverticula*. Diverticular disease-related colitis is also termed *segmental colitis associated with diverticulosis*.

Clinical Features. Diverticulosis is a common problem in Western populations and increases in frequency with advanced age. Approximately 50 percent of patients older than 70 years of age and 70 percent of patients older than 85 years of age are affected. Risk is

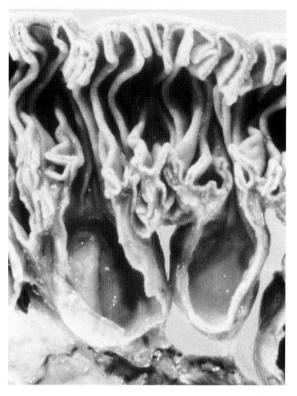

Figure 4-155

SMALL INTESTINAL DIVERTICULOSIS

Multiple large diverticula protrude through the muscularis propria.

increased among patients with progressive systemic sclerosis, Ehlers-Danlos syndrome, and other connective tissue disorders. Diverticulosis in Western populations shows a predilection for the descending and sigmoid colon, although it can involve the proximal colon or even affect the entire colon in some patients. Most patients are asymptomatic. Some complain of rectal bleeding or have iron deficiency anemia secondary to occult blood loss.

Up to 25 percent of patients with colonic diverticulosis coli develop diverticulitis. Diverticular inflammation is more common in patients with ulcerative colitis and Crohn disease; these individuals have a nearly 10-fold increased risk of diverticulitis (402–404). In addition, colonic diverticula are particularly prone to inflammation: more than 80 percent of patients with idiopathic inflammatory bowel disease and diverticulosis develop inflammation in areas affected by diverticulosis (405).

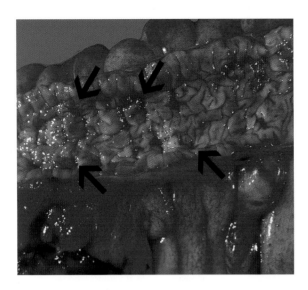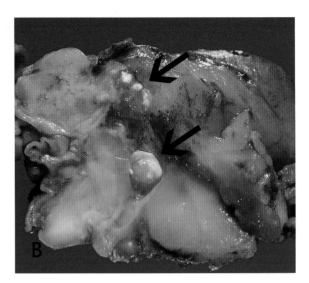

Figure 4-156

COLONIC DIVERTICULOSIS

The sigmoid colon is narrow with a thick wall. Several diverticular orifices (arrows) are visible on the mucosal surface (A). Mucus-filled diverticula (arrows) extend through the wall into pericolic fat (B).

Left-sided diverticulitis presents with hematochezia, left lower quadrant abdominal pain, episodic diarrhea, constipation, tenesmus, and symptomatic fistulae. Diverticulitis of the right colon simulates the clinical features of appendicitis. Imaging may demonstrate mesenteric fat stranding and mural thickening; extraluminal contrast or air can be seen in patients with perforated diverticulitis.

Approximately 5 percent of patients with diverticular disease develop diverticular disease-associated colitis (406). Most patients are older adults, and men are affected more often than women. These individuals often have distal colonic strictures and inflammation that cause diarrhea, constipation, tenesmus, and hematochezia. Some patients develop extraintestinal symptoms similar to those of idiopathic inflammatory bowel disease with arthralgias, cutaneous and ocular manifestations, and sacroiliitis (407–409). Imaging demonstrates a thickened sigmoid colon that may be accompanied by fistulae and fissures.

Pathogenesis. Diverticula result from chronically increased intraluminal pressures that promote herniation of mucosa and submucosa between the taenia coli where the vasa recta penetrate the muscularis propria. Luminal stasis or impacted feces cause localized mucosal irritation

and inflammation. Progressive injury results in peridiverticular abscesses and perforation.

The pathogenesis of diverticular disease-associated colitis is not clear, although it likely results from a combination of genetic, lifestyle, and environmental factors. Some patients have HLA-B27, raising the possibility that it reflects an abnormal host immune response in a patient with a genetic susceptibility to idiopathic inflammatory bowel disease (410). Emerging data suggest diverticulosis-associated inflammation results from persistent mucosal injury in the context of alterations in the fecal microbiome (411).

Gross Findings. Diverticula appear as wide-mouthed orifices on the mucosal surface. Left-sided diverticulitis is usually accompanied by luminal narrowing and mucosal edema, erythema, friability, or ulcers on the interdiverticular mucosa of the affected colonic segment (fig. 4-156). Polypoid prolapsing mucosal folds may surround diverticular orifices. Perforated diverticulitis is often accompanied by fat necrosis, hemorrhage, and abscesses in the pericolic fat (fig. 4-157). These changes organize over time and, thus, acute inflammatory changes may not be prominent when patients undergo resection weeks to months after an episode of diverticulitis. Diverticular disease-associated colitis features mucosal erythema, friability, and ulceration with fistulae and strictures similar to

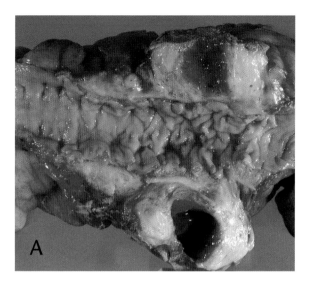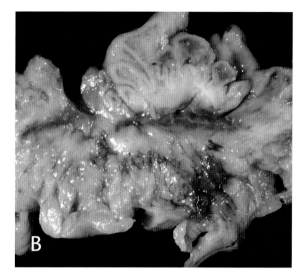

Figure 4-157

COLONIC DIVERTICULITIS

A large pericolic abscess corresponds to a perforated diverticulum. An indurated and inflamed fistulous tract extends into pericolic soft tissue (A). Polypoid, edematous mucosal folds overlie the hypertrophic muscularis propria and likely result from luminal trauma (B).

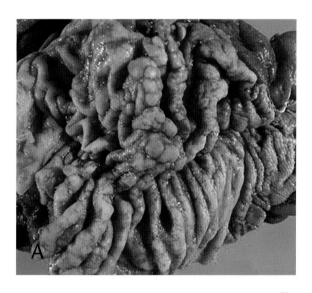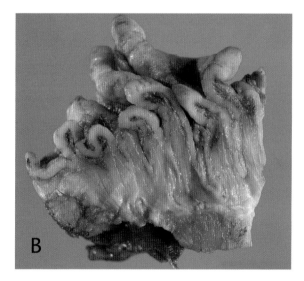

Figure 4-158

DIVERTICULAR DISEASE-ASSOCIATED COLITIS

Enlarged, indurated mucosal folds overlying a diverticulitis-related stricture simulate carcinoma (A). The interdiverticular mucosa displays prolapse-related polypoid projections associated with marked hypertrophy of the muscularis propria (B).

idiopathic inflammatory bowel disease. Some cases cause severe luminal narrowing and prominent mucosal folds that simulate the appearance of a malignancy (fig. 4-158). The rectum is uninvolved.

Microscopic Findings. Pulsion diverticula consist of mucosa and submucosa extending into, or through, the muscularis propria. Cases of diverticulitis display variable amounts of neutrophil-rich inflammation in the diverticular mucosa and peridiverticular soft tissue, frequently extending to the serosal surface or eroding into subserosal arteries (fig. 4-159). Cases of remote

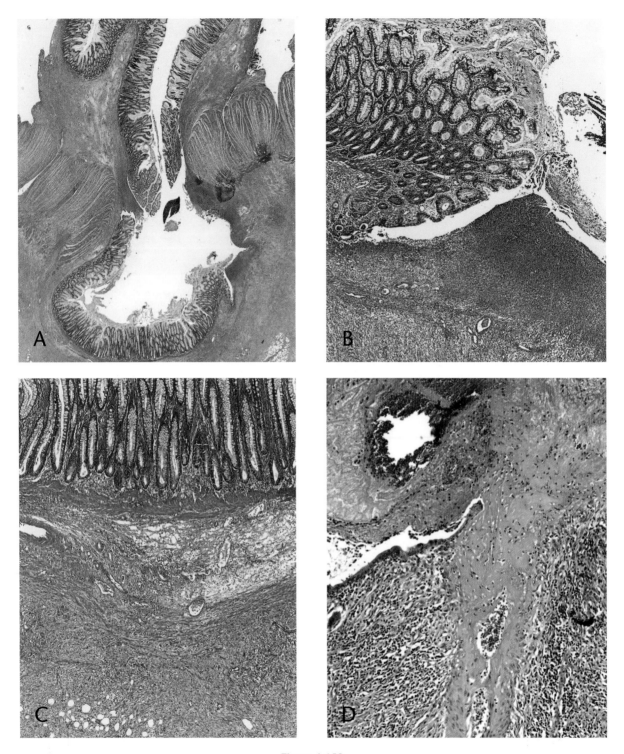

Figure 4-159

COLONIC DIVERTICULITIS

An inflamed diverticulum extends through the muscularis propria into subserosal fat (A). An ulcerated diverticulum is surrounded by edematous mucosa and inflammation (B). Inflammation and fibrosis obliterate the muscularis propria beneath the diverticulum; the mucosa, muscularis mucosae, and submucosa show minimal inflammatory changes (C). Inflamed and ulcerated diverticula can erode into submucosal arteries (D).

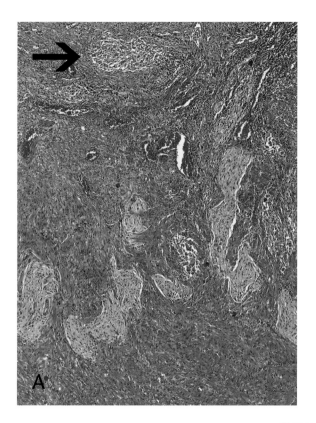 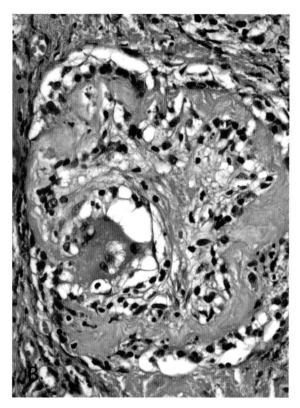

Figure 4-160

COLONIC DIVERTICULITIS

Remote diverticulitis features disorganization of the muscularis propria, with loose granulomatous inflammation (arrow) and neuronal hypertrophy (A). Pulse granulomas represent organizing inflammation surrounding fecal material (B).

diverticulitis feature hypertrophy of the muscularis propria with variable amounts of neuronal hyperplasia, chronic inflammation, and fibrosis, accompanied by loose granulomatous inflammation surrounding fecal material (fig. 4-160A). Hyalinized rings of fibrous tissue surrounded by acute and chronic inflammation (i.e., pulse granulomas) are often present at sites of prior perforation (fig. 4-160B).

All of the histologic features of ulcerative colitis and Crohn disease can be seen in patients with diverticular disease-associated colitis (283). Chronic active colitis with crypt architectural distortion, Paneth cell metaplasia, basal plasmacytosis, and transmural lymphoid aggregates accompany crypt abscesses, fissuring ulcers, and sinus tracts (fig. 4-161). Strictures, neuronal hyperplasia, and granulomas are frequently present, and some cases even show granulomatous vasculitis or granulomatous lymphadenitis (409). Most patients do not develop Crohn disease elsewhere in the gastrointestinal tract. In fact, patients with diverticulosis involved by chronic colitis usually have diverticulitis-associated chronic colitis rather than Crohn disease, especially if the inflammation is limited to the area of diverticula and the patient has no history of inflammatory bowel disease (283).

Treatment and Prognosis. Diverticulosis requires no therapy, although patients may consider lifestyle modification and increased fiber intake. Some patients develop hematochezia secondary to erosion of vessels at the base of the diverticulum; these individuals may undergo intravascular therapy for bleeding control or surgical resection in some cases. Uncomplicated diverticulitis is generally treated with a combination of high-fiber diet and antibiotic therapy. Resection is reserved for patients with persistent or recurrent symptoms: patients are initially managed with antibiotic therapy followed by surgical resection after the inflammation mostly

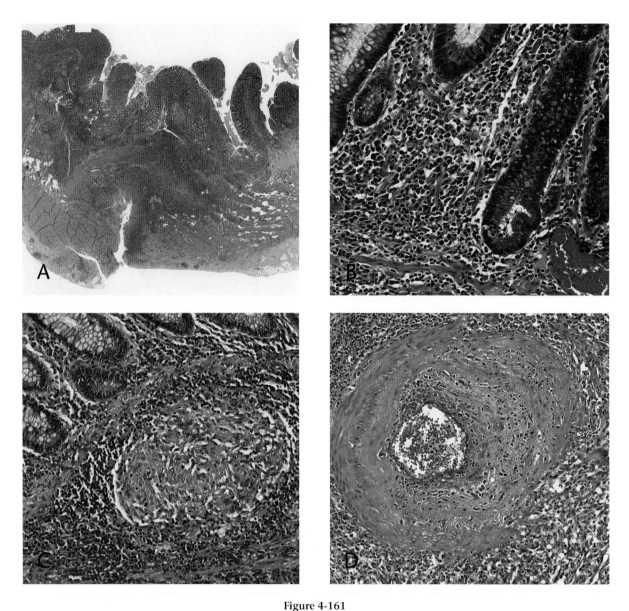

Figure 4-161

DIVERTICULAR DISEASE-ASSOCIATED COLITIS

The diverticular and interdiverticular colonic mucosa feature diffuse chronic active colitis with inflamed fistulous tracts extending through the colonic wall (A). Dense plasma cell-rich inflammation expands the mucosa and Paneth cell metaplasia is present in the crypts (B). Non-necrotic epithelioid granulomas are indistinguishable from those of Crohn disease (C). Granulomatous inflammation may also be seen in association with arteries (D).

subsides. Individuals with complicated diverticulitis, however, may undergo colectomy with a Hartmann pouch followed by delayed anastomosis. Diverticular disease-associated colitis is managed with anti-inflammatory agents, such as sulfasalazine, mesalamine, and topical corticosteroid therapy (412). Severe cases may require immunomodulatory therapy or surgery.

Diversion Colitis and Diversion-Related Changes

Definition. *Diversion-related changes* include lymphoid hyperplasia, chronic inflammation, and mucosal atrophy in a surgically diverted colonic segment. *Diversion colitis* is chronic active colitis with lymphoid hyperplasia in a surgically diverted colonic segment.

Clinical Features. Diversion-related changes represent a chronic inflammatory disorder that develops in colonic segments excluded from the fecal stream, such as a Hartmann pouch. The condition usually develops within a few months following surgical diversion. Some patients with diversion-related changes are asymptomatic, but others complain of mucoid or bloody discharge, cramping, or abdominal pain.

Pathogenesis. The etiology of diversion colitis is unknown. It may result from a deficiency in short chain fatty acids, which are required for nutritional support of colonocytes and are derived from the fermentation of dietary starches by gut flora. Altered bacterial flora presumably leads to a deficiency in short chain fatty acids and to inflammation (413). Others have postulated that surgical diversion alters mucosa-associated lymphoid tissue and cytokine production, resulting in diminished subtypes of CD3-positive T-lymphocytes, as well as decreased levels of interleukin-4 and IFN-γ (414).

Gross Findings. Longstanding diversion can result in mucosal atrophy accompanied by lymphoid hyperplasia (415). Mucosal erythema, friability, nodularity, and ulceration occur in some cases (fig. 4-162).

Microscopic Findings. Diversion of the fecal stream results in striking infiltration of the mucosa by mononuclear cell-rich inflammation accompanied by reactive lymphoid hyperplasia (416). Mild to moderate lymphoid hyperplasia with germinal centers is accompanied by atrophic or distorted crypts and variable amounts of neutrophilic inflammation (fig. 4-163) (417). Cryptitis, crypt abscesses, and aphthous-type erosions or frank ulcers are more common in symptomatic patients. Epithelioid granulomas and fissuring-type ulcers occur in diverted colonic segments from patients without a prior history of Crohn disease (418,419). Most of the inflammatory changes that occur in diverted colonic segments resolve upon re-establishment of continuity with the gastrointestinal tract (420).

Treatment and Prognosis. Some studies have shown a clinical response to the topical application of short chain fatty acid solutions, although other studies have not validated these results (413,421). Definitive treatment requires re-establishment of the continuity of the fecal stream through the diverted segment (415). Symptoms

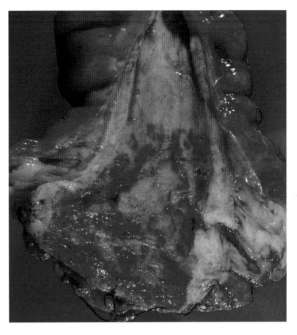

Figure 4-162

DIVERSION-RELATED CHANGES

The diverted rectosigmoid colon displays mural thickening with mucosal atrophy and loss of mucosal folds. Patchy erythema is present.

typically regress completely within 3 to 6 months of re-establishment of the fecal stream.

Stercoral Ulcer

Definition. *Stercoral ulcer* is a pressure ulcer that develops as a result of fecal impaction.

Clinical Features. Stercoral ulcers account for approximately 3 percent of colonic perforations and less than 1 percent of colorectal surgical procedures. Most patients are elderly and debilitated. They may present with acute abdominal pain preceded by obstipation or sudden onset bleeding from the lower gastrointestinal tract (422). Risk factors include chronic constipation, hemodialysis, and use of anti-cholinergic agents (423). Individuals with spinal cord injuries are also at risk for developing stercoral ulcers.

Imaging studies demonstrate a combination of findings reflecting obstruction or perforation. The proximal colon is typically dilated, whereas the distal colon may show mural thickening with fat stranding. Perforated ulcers are associated with free air in the peritoneum, stool in the peritoneum, and abscesses.

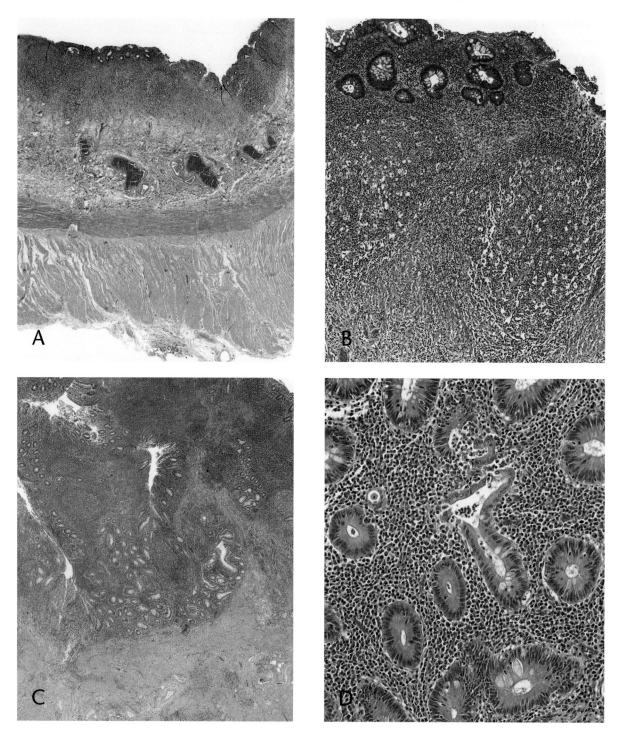

Figure 4-163

DIVERSION-RELATED CHANGES AND DIVERSION COLITIS

The mucosa is expanded by a dense mononuclear cell-rich inflammatory infiltrate with prominent lymphoid hyperplasia (A), although the crypts are atrophic and mostly uninflamed (B). Diverted colonic segments can develop mural fibrosis, lymphoid aggregates, and granulomatous inflammation that simulate features of Crohn disease (C). The amount of cryptitis and neutrophilic inflammation is often less than would be expected of patients with idiopathic inflammatory bowel disease (D).

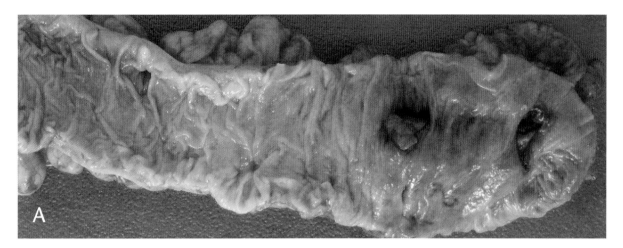

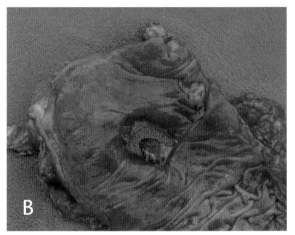

Figure 4-164

STERCORAL ULCERS

Two deep ulcers are located in the distal colorectum of an elderly patient with otherwise unremarkable colonic mucosa (A). Full-thickness necrosis is associated with mild erythema around the ulcer (B).

Pathogenesis. The rectosigmoid colon is particularly prone to development of stercoral ulcers (424). Increased luminal pressure in this region of narrow caliber and insufficient collateral blood supply leads to localized areas of ischemia that can be further damaged by hard stools with low water content (425).

Gross Findings. Stercoral ulcers tend to be large, sharply demarcated defects that may extend through the colonic wall (fig. 4-164). The mucosa immediately adjacent to the ulcer may be dusky or erythematous but the background mucosa is normal or nearly normal. Fibrinopurulent serosal plaques are often present in patients with perforated ulcers.

Microscopic Findings. The ulcer base consists of variably inflamed granulation tissue with a foreign body giant cell reaction to fecal material. Ulcers can be associated with mural necrosis, organizing serositis, and abscesses. Ischemic-type changes are often present in the adjacent mucosa.

Treatment and Prognosis. Endoscopic morcellation of impacted stools in combination with electrocoagulation of bleeding sites may be attempted in patients with non-perforated ulcers. Perforated lesions require surgical resection with pelvic irrigation. Perforation is associated with a high mortality risk, particularly in frail, elderly individuals (424).

Pneumatosis Intestinalis

Definition. *Pneumatosis intestinalis* consists of air-filled cystic spaces in the bowel wall. Synonyms include *intestinal pneumatosis, pneumatosis cystoides intestinalis,* and *pneumatosis coli.*

Clinical Features. Pneumatosis intestinalis occurs in a variety of settings; its manifestations and clinical significance depend on the situation in which it develops. Approximately 85 percent of cases are secondary to other disorders that have been previously discussed. Pneumatosis intestinalis in newborns is an important manifestation of necrotizing enterocolitis and occurs in patients with gangrenous necrosis secondary to ischemia or infection with *Clostridia* species and other organisms. The disorder is also associated with chronic obstructive pulmonary disease, mechanical ventilation, connective tissue diseases, infectious enteritis, celiac disease, idiopathic inflammatory bowel disease, leukemia, amyloidosis, and AIDS (426,427).

Approximately 15 percent of patients have idiopathic pneumatosis. Most of these patients are older adults who have asymptomatic pulmonary disease, although those with associated gastrointestinal injury present with bloody diarrhea and abdominal pain. Imaging reveals extraluminal gas in the bowel wall or mesentery. Detection of portal venous gas is associated life-threatening illness due to mural necrosis. Sonography can detect linear or focal echogenic areas in the bowel wall (428).

Pathogenesis. The mechanisms by which pneumatosis intestinalis develops are likely multifactorial. Presumably, gas dissects into the bowel wall through disruptions in the gastrointestinal mucosa that result from a combination of increased intraluminal pressure and decreased mucosal integrity. Iatrogenic causes include insufflation during endoscopy, double-contrast barium enema, and jejunostomy tube placement. Occasional cases occur in patients who take medications that cause bloating and abdominal distention.

Gross Findings. Submucosal accumulation of gas produces polypoid projections into the lumen (fig. 4-165A). Large collections appear as numerous, variably sized cysts that diffusely expand the mucosa and submucosa (fig. 4-165B,C). Occasional cases show subserosal gas accumulation as well (fig. 4-165D).

Microscopic Findings. Gas-filled cysts expand the submucosa with relative sparing of the muscularis propria. The cysts are surrounded by giant cells and macrophages, as well as scattered eosinophils (fig. 4-166). Mild forms of injury may be confined to the mucosa (fig. 4-167). Non-specific inflammatory changes, including cryptitis and crypt abscesses, may be present (429).

Treatment and Prognosis. Pneumatosis intestinalis is a clinical sign that may be seen in association with life-threatening diseases or in otherwise healthy patients. Treatment consists of managing the underlying illness in patients with gastrointestinal necrosis, infections, and ischemia. Asymptomatic pneumatosis intestinalis is observed and managed conservatively (430).

Mucosal Prolapse and Solitary Rectal Ulcer Syndrome

Definition. This spectrum of lesions is characterized by intermittent mucosal ischemia combined with mechanical forces. Entities in this spectrum include *mucosal prolapse, solitary rectal ulcer syndrome,* and *mucosal prolapse polyp.* Synonyms include *inflammatory myoglandular polyp, inflammatory cloacogenic polyp,* and *colitis cystica profunda.*

Clinical Features. Solitary rectal ulcer syndrome can occur in children and adolescents but shows a predilection for older adults, particularly women. Colitis, ulcers, polyps, and indurated masses usually develop on the anterolateral rectal wall within 4 to 10 cm of the anal verge (431). Symptoms include rectal bleeding, straining with defecation, alternating diarrhea and constipation, a sensation of incomplete rectal evacuation, and passage of mucus per rectum (432).

Prolapse-related polyps occur anywhere in the colon when the mucosa is subjected to pulsion and intermittent ischemia, such as with diverticulosis, ostomy sites, and adjacent to mass lesions or other sites of mucosal tethering (433,434). These polyps are usually asymptomatic and detected during colonoscopic examination performed for other reasons. Some patients present with hematochezia or occult blood loss.

Pathogenesis. Mucosal prolapse of the rectum is classified as complete or incomplete, depending on whether the rectal mucosa prolapses through the anus. It results from downward displacement of the partial or full thickness of the rectal wall during defecation, possibly reflecting dysfunction of the puborectalis muscle (435). Straining during defecation causes compression of the mucosa, resulting in chronic ischemic injury. Exuberant repair leads to inflammatory polyps. A similar mechanism involving mechanical forces on tethered mucosae likely accounts for the prolapse-related polyps that develop elsewhere in the colorectum.

Gross Findings. The gross and histologic features of mucosal prolapse are variable. Patients have one or more hyperemic polyps. Ulcers and

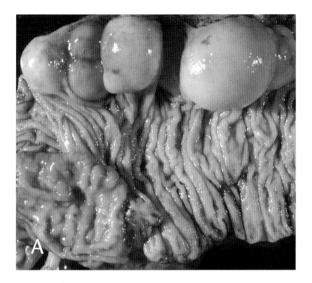

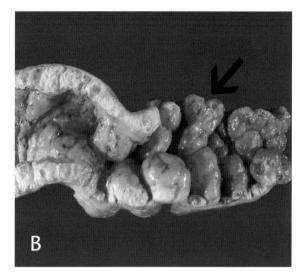

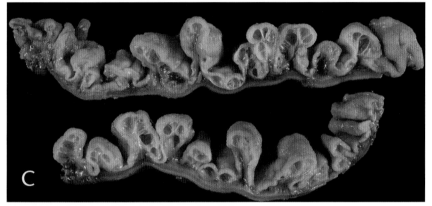

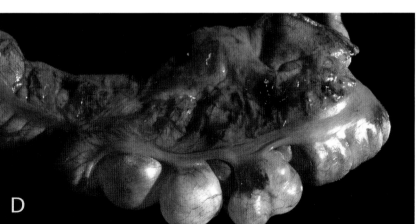

Figure 4-165

PNEUMATOSIS INTESTINALIS

Submucosal air bubbles form several yellow polyps on a background of normal mucosa (A). More diffuse disease distorts the mucosal folds, producing numerous polyps (arrow) as well as air-filled cysts in the bowel wall (B). Large cysts are most pronounced in the delicate connective tissue of the submucosa with sparing of the muscularis propria (C). Large cystic structures are present in the colonic subserosal tissues (D).

diffuse erythema simulating colitis are common and some cases are associated with partial or circumferential stenosis, mimicking malignancy (fig. 4-168) (432).

Microscopic Findings. Characteristic features include mucosal erosions with fibrin deposits associated with variably prominent crypt hyperplasia and serration (436). The epithelium is regenerative with mucin depletion, nuclear enlargement, and increased mitotic activity. The muscularis mucosae is usually prominent and displays smooth muscle cells emanating

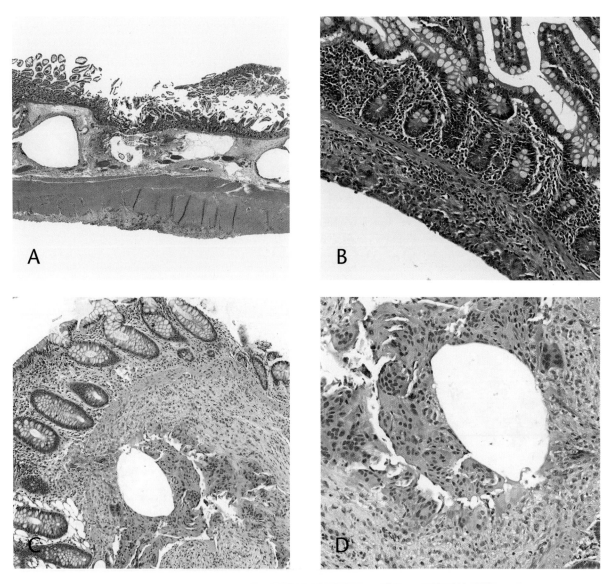

Figure 4-166

PNEUMATOSIS INTESTINALIS

Most air spaces are present in the submucosa without involvement of the muscularis propria (A). Giant cells and macrophages are associated with eosinophils at the periphery of an air space (B). Pneumatosis can simulate an intramucosal lipoma in polypectomy specimens (C), although the presence of associated granulomatous inflammation is a helpful clue (D).

into the mucosa. Bundles of smooth muscle cells are typically oriented perpendicular to the muscularis mucosae and may wrap around the crypts (437). Mucosal fibrosis, hemorrhage, and hemosiderin deposits are often prominent, particularly in patients with longstanding disease (fig. 4-169).

Treatment and Prognosis. Treatment consists of dietary modification with increased fluid and fiber intake, as well as stool softeners,

laxatives, and topical corticosteroid therapy (438). Surgery is reserved for patients with uncontrolled bleeding or refractory disease (435).

Inflammatory Cap Polyposis

Definition. *Inflammatory cap polyposis* is idiopathic inflammatory polyposis usually limited to the distal colorectum.

Clinical Features. Inflammatory cap polyposis is an uncommon disease first described by

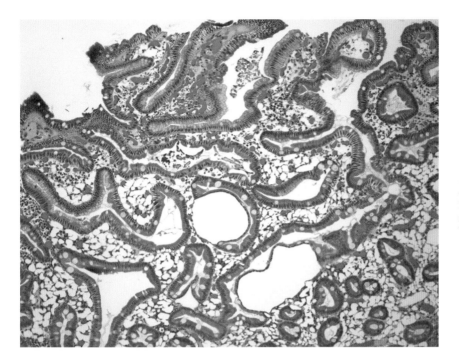

Figure 4-167

PNEUMATOSIS

Insufflation during endo-
scopic examination can intro-
duce air into the mucosa, simulating the appearance of intramucosal fat. This finding has
been termed pseudolipomatosis.

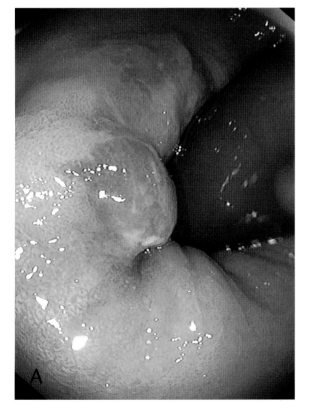

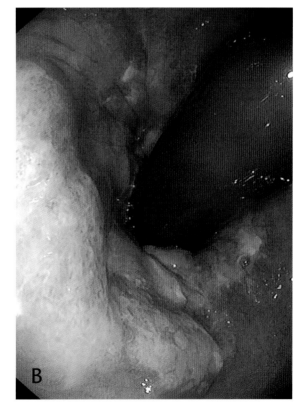

Figure 4-168

MUCOSAL PROLAPSE

Erythematous polyps are visible upon retroflexed examination of the anorectum (A). Another lesion is indurated and
nodular with patchy erythema, simulating a neoplasm (B).

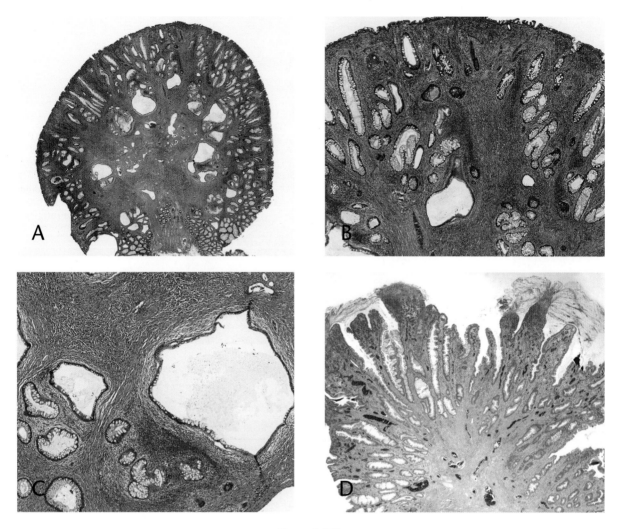

Figure 4-169

MUCOSAL PROLAPSE POLYP

A large polyp contains evenly dispersed epithelial elements embedded in inflamed, fibromuscular stroma (A). The surface shows epithelial regeneration and extravasated red blood cells with hyperplastic crypts (B). Cystically dilated crypts surrounded by lamina propria are present in the submucosa (C). Some prolapse-related polyps contain finger-like projections with erosions and pseudomembranes at their tips (D).

Williams et al. (439) in 1985, at which time it was considered a form of mucosal prolapse. It probably affects men and women with near equal frequency; variations in gender distribution in different studies likely reflect the small number of patients evaluated to date. This disorder occurs within any racial group but is more commonly reported in eastern and southeastern Asia. It also occurs within a wide age range, affecting patients as young as 12 years of age and older adults. At least 50 percent of patients do not have a history of chronic constipation or straining prior to the onset of cap polyposis (440). Symptoms include mucoid diarrhea, protein wasting, rectal bleeding, and tenesmus (441–443).

Pathogenesis. The pathogenesis of inflammatory cap polyposis is unknown. Its usual involvement of the rectum, occasional clinical association with constipation and straining upon defecation, and histologic features have led investigators to suggest a relationship to mucosal prolapse or intraluminal trauma (441,444–446). However, most patients with cap polyposis do not have a history of chronic constipation. In

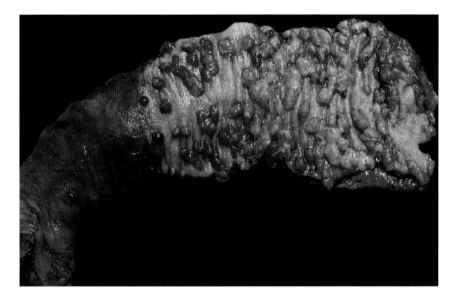

Figure 4-170

**INFLAMMATORY
CAP POLYPOSIS**

Numerous soft, sessile polyps form confluent plaques in the distal colorectum.

fact, this disease usually occurs in patients in whom mucosal prolapse is infrequent, such as younger male patients without underlying colonic motility disorders (440). Some reports have described associations with diverticular disease, colorectal carcinoma, and colitis, suggesting that it may be a non-specific mucosal response to another underlying disorder (439,447).

The most intriguing hypotheses regarding the pathogenesis of cap polyposis implicate an infectious organism in the development of this disorder (447). Although broad-spectrum antibiotics have proven ineffective in the treatment of most patients with cap polyposis, metronidazole is temporarily effective in ameliorating symptoms in some cases (445). Several investigators have independently reported successful resolution of inflammatory cap polyposis following *H. pylori* eradication therapy (448–450). Others have proposed a relationship to aberrations in the gut microbiota (451).

Gross Findings. The rectum is involved in more than 80 percent of cases, although the disease often affects the sigmoid colon and may even extend into the ascending colon in a retrograde, continuous fashion. Polyps are sessile and vary from a few millimeters to several centimeters in diameter, forming confluent friable plaques (fig. 4-170). The lesions are often erythematous with erosions (452,453).

Microscopic Findings. Inflammatory cap polyps contain elongated, hyperplastic crypts lined by mucin-depleted epithelial cells that show regenerative changes, including nuclear enlargement and increased mitotic activity (fig. 4-171A). The surface epithelium is attenuated or ulcerated, with an inflammatory "cap" of adherent mucin, fibrin, and inflammatory cells (fig. 4-171B). The lamina propria generally shows a normal degree of cellularity compared with the adjacent mucosa (fig. 4-171C). Although a small number of smooth muscle fibers may emanate from the muscularis mucosae, well-developed features of mucosal prolapse are lacking (fig. 4-171D).

Treatment and Prognosis. Inflammatory cap polyposis rarely resolves spontaneously. Most patients require some form of medical or surgical management (446,454,455). Those with fewer than 10 polyps may be managed successfully with polypectomy alone (60 percent of cases). More extensive, symptomatic disease is treated with a combination of stool softeners, anti-inflammatory agents (5-aminosalicylic acid, sulfasalazine, prednisolone), and antibiotics (metronidazole). Endoscopic and histologic resolution of disease has been reported following infliximab therapy, suggesting a role for inflammatory mediators, such as TNF-α, in the progression of this disease (456,457). Rare patients with concomitant *H. pylori* gastritis have also been successfully managed with *H. pylori* eradication therapy (448–450). Resection of the involved colon is usually reserved for patients who fail medical therapy. Recurrent symptomatic disease occurs in up to 37 percent of cases following limited resection of the affected colon (447).

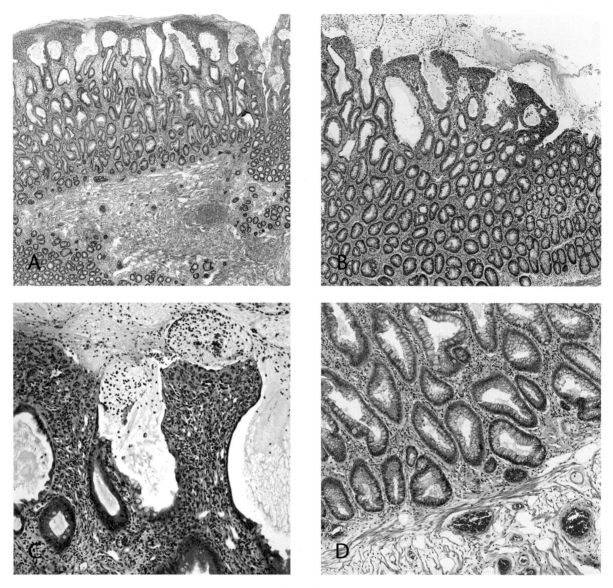

Figure 4-171

INFLAMMATORY CAP POLYPOSIS

Large sessile plaques contain superficially dilated crypts with erosions and adherent mucus (A), with more normal appearing crypts and lamina propria in the deeper mucosa, comparable to that of the adjacent nonlesional colon (B). Adherent mucus contains linear arrays of inflammatory cells (C). The muscularis mucosae and submucosa are essentially normal (D).

Stent-Related Pseudopolyposis

Self-expanding metal stents are used as a palliative or temporizing measure in patients with impending or acute bowel obstruction due to carcinoma or other obstructing lesions. These stents are deployed across the area of obstruction and cause pressure necrosis where they contact the mucosa (fig. 4-172A). Mucosa that protrudes through the stent can develop a polypoid appearance within days of stent placement (fig. 4-172B). Pseudopolyps that develop in this setting usually feature near-normal mucosa flanked by nonpolypoid ulcerated mucosa (fig. 4-172C–F). The latter displays characteristic basophilic necrosis, fibrin deposits, and eosinophil-rich inflammation, often accompanied by pseudomembranes (458).

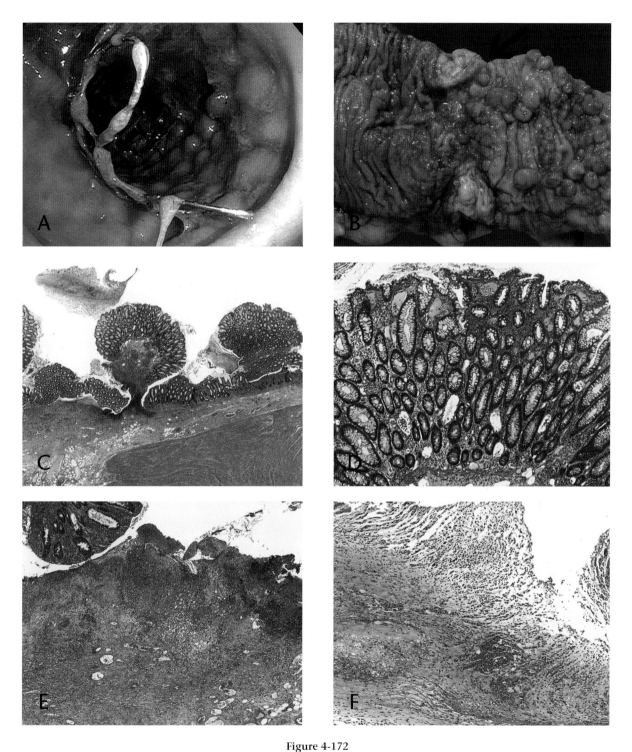

Figure 4-172

STENT-RELATED PSEUDOPOLYPOSIS

Self-expanding metal stents compress the colonic wall causing the mucosa to bulge into the lumen between areas of contact (A). A previously stented colon cancer (arrow) is surrounded by numerous erythematous pseudopolyps (B). Polypoid projections of colonic mucosa are surrounded by ulcers and ischemic mucosal changes (C). The polypoid areas contain superficially hyperplastic crypts with minimal inflammation (D). Ulcers of the nonpolypoid mucosa contain basophilic necrotic material and fibrin (E). Pseudomembranes containing streams of inflammatory cells are present in areas of ulceration (F).

REFERENCES

1. Takahashi D, Hiroma T, Takamizawa S, Nakamura T. Population-based study of esophageal and small intestinal atresia/stenosis. Pediatr Int 2014;56:838-44.
2. Kimura K, Loening-Baucke V. Bilious vomiting in the newborn: rapid diagnosis of intestinal obstruction. Am Fam Physician 2000;61:2791-8.
3. Stoll C, Dott B, Alembik Y, Roth MP. Associated congenital anomalies among cases with Down syndrome. Eur J Med Genet 2015;58:674-80.
4. Rasmussen M, Vestergaard EM, Graakjaer J, et al. 17q12 deletion and duplication syndrome in Denmark-a clinical cohort of 38 patients and review of the literature. Am J Med Genet A 2016;170:2934-42.
5. Morris G, Kennedy A Jr, Cochran W. Small bowel congenital anomalies: a review and update. Curr Gastroenterol Rep 2016;18:16.
6. Dalla Vecchia LK, Grosfeld JL, West KW, Rescorla FJ, Scherer LR, Engum SA. Intestinal atresia and stenosis: a 25-year experience with 277 cases. Arch Surg 1998;133:490-6.
7. Roberts HE, Cragan JD, Cono J, Khoury MJ, Weatherly MR, Moore CA. Increased frequency of cystic fibrosis among infants with jejunoileal atresia. Am J Med Genet 1998;78:446-9.
8. Stoll C, Alembik Y, Dott B, Roth MP. Associated malformations in patients with anorectal anomalies. Eur J Med Genet 2007;50:281-90.
9. Kim PC, Superina RA, Ein S. Colonic atresia combined with Hirschsprung's disease: a diagnostic and therapeutic challenge. J Pediatr Surg 1995;30:1216-7.
10. Paterson-Brown S, Stalewski H, Brereton RJ. Neonatal small bowel atresia, stenosis and segmental dilatation. Br J Surg 1991;78:83-6.
11. Chen R, Giliani S, Lanzi G, et al. Whole-exome sequencing identifies tetratricopeptide repeat domain 7A (TTC7A) mutations for combined immunodeficiency with intestinal atresias. J Allergy Clin Immunol 2013;132:656-64.
12. Escobar MA, Ladd AP, Grosfeld JL, et al. Duodenal atresia and stenosis: long-term follow-up over 30 years. J Pediatr Surg 2004;39:867-71.
13. Shah N, Lizardo-Escano T, Shaaban H, Dhadham G, Karki A, Spira R. Enterogenous cyst of the small bowel causing intussusception in an adult: case report and review of literature. J Nat Sci Biol Med 2015;6:208-10.
14. Chen JJ, Lee HC, Yeung CY, Chan WT, Jiang CB, Sheu JC. Meta-analysis: the clinical features of the duodenal duplication cyst. J Pediatr Surg 2010;45:1598-606.
15. Tew K, Soans BK, Millar EA. Adenocarcinoma in an ileal duplication cyst: ultrasound and computed tomography findings. Australas Radiol 2000;44:228-31.
16. Mourra N, Chafai N, Bessoud B, Reveri V, Werbrouck A, Tiret E. Colorectal duplication in adults: report of seven cases and review of the literature. J Clin Pathol 2010;63:1080-3.
17. Francis A, Kantarovich D, Khoshnam N, Alazraki AL, Patel B, Shehata BM. Pediatric Meckel's diverticulum: report of 208 cases and review of the literature. Fetal Pediatr Pathol 2016;35:199-206.
18. Ikemura M, Kunita A, Miwa Y, et al. Gut wall replacing type of gastrointestinal stromal tumor presenting as a perforation of the ileal diverticulum. Pathol Res Pract 2015;211:892-5.
19. Xue L, Qiu T, Song Y, et al. Long segmental hyperplasia of interstitial cells of Cajal with giant diverticulum formation. Int J Clin Exp Pathol 2013;6:2989-96.
20. Thirunavukarasu P, Sathaiah M, Sukumar S, et al. Meckel's diverticulum—a high-risk region for malignancy in the ileum. Insights from a population-based epidemiological study and implications in surgical management. Ann Surg 2011;253:223-30.
21. Arevalo Suarez F, Barreda C, Portugal S, et al. [Heterotopic gastric mucosa in duodenum: endoscopic and histological features]. Rev Gastroenterol Peru 2017;37:231-4. [Spanish]
22. Mannan A, Vieth M, Khararjian A, et al. The outlet patch: gastric heterotopia of the colorectum and anus. Histopathology 2018;73:220-9.
23. Iacopini F, Gotoda T, Elisei W, et al. Heterotopic gastric mucosa in the anus and rectum: first case report of endoscopic submucosal dissection and systematic review. Gastroenterol Rep (Oxf) 2016;4:196-205.
24. Borhan-Manesh F, Farnum JB. Study of helicobacter pylori colonization of patches of heterotopic gastric mucosa (HGM) at the upper esophagus. Dig Dis Sci 1993;38:142-6.
25. Emerson L, Layfield LJ, Rohr LR, Dayton MT. Adenocarcinoma arising in association with gastric heterotopic pancreas: a case report and review of the literature. J Surg Oncol 2004;87:53-7.
26. Adsay NV, Zamboni G. Paraduodenal pancreatitis: a clinico-pathologically distinct entity unifying "cystic dystrophy of heterotopic pancreas", "para-duodenal wall cyst", and "groove pancreatitis". Semin Diagn Pathol 2004;21:247-54.

27. Farris AB 3rd, Basturk O, Adsay NV. Pancreatitis, other inflammatory lesions, and pancreatic pseudotumors. Surg Pathol Clin 2011;4:625-50.

28. Goodarzi M, Rashid A, Maru D. Invasive ductal adenocarcinoma arising from pancreatic heterotopia in rectum: case report and review of literature. Hum Pathol 2010;41:1809-13.

29. Naqvi A, de la Roza G. Borderline mucinous cystic tumor in jejunal pancreatic heterotopia. Ann Diagn Pathol 2004;8:151-5.

30. Tolentino LF, Lee H, Maung T, Stabile BE, Li K, French SW. Islet cell tumor arising from a heterotopic pancreas in the duodenal wall with ulceration. Exp Mol Pathol 2004;76:51-6.

31. Engevik AC, Kaji I, Engevik MA, et al. Loss of MYO5B leads to reductions in Na(+) absorption with maintenance of CFTR-dependent Cl(-) secretion in enterocytes. Gastroenterology 2018;155:1883-97.

32. Dhekne HS, Pylypenko O, Overeem AW, et al. MYO5B, STX3, and STXBP2 mutations reveal a common disease mechanism that unifies a subset of congenital diarrheal disorders: a mutation update. Hum Mutat 2018;39:333-44.

33. Martin BA, Kerner JA, Hazard FK, Longacre TA. Evaluation of intestinal biopsies for pediatric enteropathy: a proposed immunohistochemical panel approach. Am J Surg Pathol 2014;38:1387-95.

34. Shillingford NM, Calicchio ML, Teot LA, et al. Villin immunohistochemistry is a reliable method for diagnosing microvillus inclusion disease. Am J Surg Pathol 2015;39:245-50.

35. Ruemmele FM, Schmitz J, Goulet O. Microvillous inclusion disease (microvillous atrophy). Orphanet J Rare Dis 2006;1:22.

36. Davidson GP, Cutz E, Hamilton JR, Gall DG. Familial enteropathy: a syndrome of protracted diarrhea from birth, failure to thrive, and hypoplastic villus atrophy. Gastroenterology 1978;75:783-90.

37. Reifen RM, Cutz E, Griffiths AM, Ngan BY, Sherman PM. Tufting enteropathy: a newly recognized clinicopathological entity associated with refractory diarrhea in infants. J Pediatr Gastroenterol Nutr 1994;18:379-85.

38. Sivagnanam M, Mueller JL, Lee H, et al. Identification of EpCAM as the gene for congenital tufting enteropathy. Gastroenterology 2008;135:429-37.

39. Salomon J, Espinosa-Parrilla Y, Goulet O, et al. A founder effect at the EPCAM locus in congenital tufting enteropathy in the Arabic Gulf. Eur J Med Genet 2011;54:319-22.

40. Holt-Danborg L, Vodopiutz J, Nonboe AW, et al. SPINT2 (HAI-2) missense variants identified in congenital sodium diarrhea/tufting enteropathy affect the ability of HAI-2 to inhibit prostasin but not matriptase. Hum Mol Genet 2019;28:828-41.

41. Salomon J, Goulet O, Canioni D, et al. Genetic characterization of congenital tufting enteropathy: epcam associated phenotype and involvement of SPINT2 in the syndromic form. Hum Genet 2014;133:299-310.

42. Goulet O, Salomon J, Ruemmele F, de Serres NP, Brousse N. Intestinal epithelial dysplasia (tufting enteropathy). Orphanet J Rare Dis 2007;2:20.

43. Treetipsatit J, Hazard FK. Features of gastric and colonic mucosa in congenital enteropathies: a study in histology and immunohistochemistry. Am J Surg Pathol 2014;38:1697-706.

44. Burnett JR, Hooper AJ, Hegele RA. Abetalipoproteinemia. In: Adam MP, Ardinger HH, Pagon RA, et al., eds. GeneReviews ®. Seattle: Internet; 1993.

45. Miller SA, Burnett JR, Leonis MA, McKnight CJ, van Bockxmeer FM, Hooper AJ. Novel missense MTTP gene mutations causing abetalipoproteinemia. Biochim Biophys Acta 2014;1842:1548-54.

46. Cortina G, Smart CN, Farmer DG, et al. Enteroendocrine cell dysgenesis and malabsorption, a histopathologic and immunohistochemical characterization. Hum Pathol 2007;38:570-80.

47. Wetherill C, Sutcliffe J. Hirschsprung disease and anorectal malformation. Early Hum Dev 2014;90:927-32.

48. Suita S, Taguchi T, Ieiri S, Nakatsuji T. Hirschsprung's disease in Japan: analysis of 3852 patients based on a nationwide survey in 30 years. J Pediatr Surg 2005;40:197-201.

49. Butler Tjaden NE, Trainor PA. The developmental etiology and pathogenesis of Hirschsprung disease. Transl Res 2013;162:1-15.

50. Kenny SE, Tam PK, Garcia-Barcelo M. Hirschsprung's disease. Semin Pediatr Surg 2010;19:194-200.

51. Ricciardi R, Counihan TC, Banner BF, Sweeney WB. What is the normal aganglionic segment of anorectum in adults? Dis Colon Rectum 1999;42:380-2.

52. Barshack I, Fridman E, Goldberg I, Chowers Y, Kopolovic J. The loss of calretinin expression indicates aganglionosis in Hirschsprung's disease. J Clin Pathol 2004;57:712-6.

53. Kapur RP, Reed RC, Finn LS, Patterson K, Johanson J, Rutledge JC. Calretinin immunohistochemistry versus acetylcholinesterase histochemistry in the evaluation of suction rectal biopsies for Hirschsprung disease. Pediatr Dev Pathol 2009;12:6-15.

54. Guinard-Samuel V, Bonnard A, De Lagausie P, et al. Calretinin immunohistochemistry: a simple and efficient tool to diagnose Hirschsprung disease. Mod Pathol 2009;22:1379-84.

55. Frykman PK, Short SS. Hirschsprung-associated enterocolitis: prevention and therapy. Semin Pediatr Surg 2012;21:328-35.

56. Sathe M, Houwen R. Meconium ileus in cystic fibrosis. J Cyst Fibros 2017;16(Suppl 2):S32-9.

57. Kelly T, Buxbaum J. Gastrointestinal manifestations of cystic fibrosis. Dig Dis Sci 2015;60:1903-13.

58. Rafeeq MM, Murad HAS. Cystic fibrosis: current therapeutic targets and future approaches. J Transl Med 2017;15:84.

59. van Heesewijk AE, Rush ML, Schmidt B, Kirpalani H, DeMauro SB. Agreement between study designs: a systematic review comparing observational studies and randomized trials of surgical treatments for necrotizing enterocolitis. J Matern Fetal Neonatal Med 2018:1-9.

60. Dominguez KM, Moss RL. Necrotizing enterocolitis. Clin Perinatol 2012;39:387-401.

61. Berman L, Moss RL. Necrotizing enterocolitis: an update. Semin Fetal Neonatal Med 2011;16:145-50.

62. Gephart SM, Moore EF, Fry E. Standardized feeding protocols to reduce risk of necrotizing enterocolitis in fragile infants born premature or with congenital heart disease: implementation science needed. Crit Care Nurs Clin North Am 2018;30:457-66.

63. Downard CD, Renaud E, St Peter SD, et al. Treatment of necrotizing enterocolitis: an American Pediatric Surgical Association outcomes and Clinical Trials Committee systematic review. J Pediatr Surg 2012;47:2111-22.

64. Wen J, Tang Q, Wu J, Wang Y, Cai W. Primary intestinal lymphangiectasia: four case reports and a review of the literature. Dig Dis Sci 2010;55:3466-72.

65. Vignes S, Bellanger J. [Videocapsule endoscopy as a useful tool to diagnose primary intestinal lymphangiectasia]. Rev Med Interne 2007;28:173-5. [French]

66. Vignes S, Bellanger J. [Primary intestinal lymphangiectasia (Waldmann's disease)]. Rev Med Interne 2018;39:580-5. [French]

67. Winter HS, Antonioli DA, Fukagawa N, Marcial M, Goldman H. Allergy-related proctocolitis in infants: diagnostic usefulness of rectal biopsy. Mod Pathol 1990;3:5-10.

68. Odze RD, Bines J, Leichtner AM, Goldman H, Antonioli DA. Allergic proctocolitis in infants: a prospective clinicopathologic biopsy study. Hum Pathol 1993;24:668-74.

69. DiMaio CJ, Stevens PD. Nonvariceal upper gastrointestinal bleeding. Gastrointest Endosc Clin N Am 2007;17:253-72.

70. Baxter M, Aly EH. Dieulafoy's lesion: current trends in diagnosis and management. Ann R Coll Surg Engl 2010;92:548-54.

71. Lee WS, Cho SB, Park SY, et al. Successful side-viewing endoscopic hemoclipping for Dieulafoy-like lesion at the brim of a periampullary diverticulum. BMC Gastroenterol 2010;10:24.

72. Inayat F, Ullah W, Hussain Q, Abdullah HM. Dieulafoy's lesion of the colon and rectum: a case series and literature review. BMJ Case Rep 2017;2017.

73. Jeon HK, Kim GH. Endoscopic management of Dieulafoy's lesion. Clin Endosc 2015;48:112-20.

74. Alamri Y, Tietjens J, Wakeman C. Dialysis-associated telangiectasia: case report and review of the literature. Perit Dial Int 2016;36:104-5.

75. Boley SJ, Brandt LJ. Vascular ectasias of the colon—1986. Dig Dis Sci 1986;31(Suppl):26S-42.

76. Gerson LB. Causes of gastrointestinal hemorrhage in patients with chronic renal failure. Gastroenterology 2013;145:895-7.

77. Koulaouzidis A, Yung DE, Lam JH, Smirnidis A, Douglas S, Plevris JN. The use of small-bowel capsule endoscopy in iron-deficiency anemia alone; be aware of the young anemic patient. Scand J Gastroenterol 2012;47:1094-100.

78. Benamouzig R, Benallaoua M, Saurin JC, et al. Efficacy and safety of pasireotide-LAR for the treatment of refractory bleeding due to gastrointestinal angiodysplasias: results of the ANGIOPAS multicenter phase II noncomparative prospective double-blinded randomized study. Therap Adv Gastroenterol 2018;11:1756283X18756260.

79. Nardone G, Compare D, Martino A, Rocco A. Pharmacological treatment of gastrointestinal bleeding due to angiodysplasias: a position paper of the Italian Society of Gastroenterology (SIGE). Dig Liver Dis 2018;50:542-8.

80. McFarlane M, O'Flynn L, Ventre R, Disney BR. Emerging role of thalidomide in the treatment of gastrointestinal bleeding. Frontline Gastroenterol 2018;9:98-104.

81. Tomizawa Y, Tanaka A, Kitahara H, et al. Preoperative right-sided cardiac congestion is associated with gastrointestinal bleeding in patients with continuous-flow left ventricular assist devices. Dig Dis Sci 2018;63:1518-24.

82. O'Malley M, LaGuardia L, Kalady MF, et al. The prevalence of hereditary hemorrhagic telangiectasia in juvenile polyposis syndrome. Dis Colon Rectum 2012;55:886-92.

83. Dasgupta R, Fishman SJ. Management of visceral vascular anomalies. Semin Pediatr Surg 2014;23:216-20.

84. Guttmacher AE, Marchuk DA, White RI Jr. Hereditary hemorrhagic telangiectasia. N Engl J Med 1995;333:918-24.

85. Shovlin CL, Guttmacher AE, Buscarini E, et al. Diagnostic criteria for hereditary hemorrhagic telangiectasia (Rendu-Osler-Weber syndrome). Am J Med Genet 2000;91:66-7.

86. Albinana V, Zafra MP, Colau J, et al. Mutation affecting the proximal promoter of Endoglin as the origin of hereditary hemorrhagic telangiectasia type 1. BMC Med Genet 2017;18:20.

87. McDonald J, Wooderchak-Donahue W, VanSant Webb C, Whitehead K, Stevenson DA, Bayrak-Toydemir P. Hereditary hemorrhagic telangiectasia: genetics and molecular diagnostics in a new era. Front Genet 2015;6:1.

88. Goumans MJ, Liu Z, ten Dijke P. TGF-beta signaling in vascular biology and dysfunction. Cell Res 2009;19:116-27.

89. Parra JA, Cuesta JM, Zarrabeitia R, et al. Screening pulmonary arteriovenous malformations in a large cohort of Spanish patients with hemorrhagic hereditary telangiectasia. Int J Cardiol 2016;218:240-5.

90. Zarrabeitia R, Ojeda-Fernandez L, Recio L, et al. Bazedoxifene, a new orphan drug for the treatment of bleeding in hereditary haemorrhagic telangiectasia. Thromb Haemost 2016;115:1167-77.

91. Wetzel-Strong SE, Detter MR, Marchuk DA. The pathobiology of vascular malformations: insights from human and model organism genetics. J Pathol 2017;241:281-93.

92. Feingold RM. The blue rubber bleb [corrected] nevus syndrome. J Insur Med 2009;41:67-71.

93. Fox VL. New therapies for vascular anomalies of the GI tract. Minerva Pediatr 2018;70:303-7.

94. Salloum R, Fox CE, Alvarez-Allende CR, et al. Response of blue rubber bleb nevus syndrome to sirolimus treatment. Pediatr Blood Cancer 2016;63:1911-4.

95. Ito K, Shiraki K, Sakai T, Yoshimura H, Nakano T. Portal hypertensive colopathy in patients with liver cirrhosis. World J Gastroenterol 2005;11:3127-30.

96. Diaz-Sanchez A, Nunez-Martinez O, Gonzalez-Asanza C, et al. Portal hypertensive colopathy is associated with portal hypertension severity in cirrhotic patients. World J Gastroenterol 2009;15:4781-7.

97. Higaki N, Matsui H, Imaoka H, et al. Characteristic endoscopic features of portal hypertensive enteropathy. J Gastroenterol 2008;43:327-31.

98. Smith LA, Morris AJ, Stanley AJ. The use of hemospray in portal hypertensive bleeding; a case series. J Hepatol 2014;60:457-60.

99. Branco JC, Carvalho R, Alberto SF, Reis J. Long-acting octreotide is effective in the treatment of portal hypertensive colopathy. Gastroenterol Hepatol 2017;40:536-7.

100. Brandt LJ. Intestinal ischemia. In: Sleisenger MH, Feldman M, Friedman LS, Brandt LJ, eds. Sleisenger and Fordtran's gastrointestinal and liver disease: pathophysiology, diagnosis, management. Philadelphia: Saunders; 2006:2563-885.

101. Reiner L, Jimenez FA, Rodriguez FL. Atherosclerosis in the mesenteric circulation. Observations and correlations with aortic and coronary atherosclerosis. Am Heart J 1963;66:200-9.

102. Shen L, Youssef D, Abu-Abed S, Malhotra SK, Atkinson K, Vikis E, et al. Cytomegalovirus duodenitis associated with life-threatening duodenal hemorrhage in an immunocompetent patient: a case report. Int J Surg Case Rep 2017;33:102-6.

103. Ikeda K, Nakajima S, Tanji K, et al. Intestinal perforation due to hemorrhagic cytomegalovirus enteritis in a patient with severe uncontrolled lupus nephritis: a case and review of the literature. Rheumatol Int 2017;37:1395-9.

104. Jrvinen O, Laurikka J, Salenius JP, Tarkka M. Acute intestinal ischaemia. A review of 214 cases. Ann Chir Gynaecol 1994;83:22-5.

105. Berg RD. Bacterial translocation from the gastrointestinal tract. Adv Exp Med Biol 1999;473:11-30.

106. May AG, De Weese JA, Rob CG. Hemodynamic effects of arterial stenosis. Surgery 1963;53:513-24.

107. Kairaluoma MI, Karkola P, Heikkinen D, Huttunen R, Mokka RE, Larmi TK. Mesenteric infarction. Am J Surg 1977;133:188-93.

108. Wilson C, Gupta R, Gilmour DG, Imrie CW. Acute superior mesenteric ischaemia. Br J Surg 1987;74:279-81.

109. Evans WE. Long-term evaluation of the celiac band syndrome. Surgery 1974;76:867-71.

110. Kim EN, Lamb K, Relles D, Moudgill N, DiMuzio PJ, Eisenberg JA. Median arcuate ligament syndrome-review of this rare disease. JAMA Surg 2016;151:471-7.

111. Hoang MP, Lee EL, Anand A. Histologic spectrum of arterial and arteriolar lesions in acute and chronic cocaine-induced mesenteric ischemia: report of three cases and literature review. Am J Surg Pathol 1998;22:1404-10.

112. Schoots IG, Koffeman GI, Legemate DA, Levi M, van Gulik TM. Systematic review of survival after acute mesenteric ischaemia according to disease aetiology. Br J Surg 2004;91:17-27.

113. Hoyle M, Kennedy A, Prior AL, Thomas GE. Small bowel ischaemia and infarction in young women taking oral contraceptives and progestational agents. Br J Surg 1977;64:533-7.

114. Cushman M, Kuller LH, Prentice R, et al. Estrogen plus progestin and risk of venous thrombosis. JAMA 2004;292:1573-80.

115. Arnold GL, Fawaz KA, Callow AD, Kaplan MM. Chronic intestinal ischemia associated with oral contraceptive use. Am J Gastroenterol 1982;77:32-4.

116. Hsueh W, Gonzalez-Crussi F, Arroyave JL. Platelet-activating factor-induced ischemic bowel necrosis. An investigation of secondary mediators in its pathogenesis. Am J Pathol 1986;122:231-9.

117. Michiels JJ, van Genderen PJ, Lindemans J, van Vliet HH. Erythromelalgic, thrombotic and hemorrhagic manifestations in 50 cases of thrombocythemia. Leuk Lymphoma 1996;22(Suppl 1):47-56.

118. Brandt LJ, Gomery P, Mitsudo SM, Chandler P, Boley SJ. Disseminated intravascular coagulation in nonocclusive mesenteric ischemia: the lack of specificity of fibrin thrombi in intestinal infarction. Gastroenterology 1976;71:954-7.

119. Hass DJ, Kozuch P, Brandt LJ. Pharmacologically mediated colon ischemia. Am J Gastroenterol 2007;102:1765-80.

120. Villanacci V, Casella G, Bassotti G. The spectrum of drug-related colitides: important entities, though frequently overlooked. Dig Liver Dis 2011;43:523-8.

121. Khor TS, Lauwers GY, Odze RD, Srivastava A. "Mass-forming" variant of ischemic colitis is a distinct entity with predilection for the proximal colon. Am J Surg Pathol 2015;39:1275-81.

122. Uberti G, Goldblum JR, Allende DS. Ischemic enterocolitis and its differential diagnosis. Semin Diagn Pathol 2014;31:152-64.

123. Zhou Z, Dong JF. Thrombotic thrombocytopenic purpura and anti-thrombotic therapy targeted to von Willebrand factor. Curr Vasc Pharmacol 2012;10:762-6.

124. Stein B, Everhart KK, Lacy BE. Gastroparesis: a review of current diagnosis and treatment options. J Clin Gastroenterol 2015;49:550-8.

125. Pokrovsky AV, Kasantchjan PO. Surgical treatment of chronic occlusive disease of the enteric visceral branches of the abdominal aorta. Experience with 119 operations. Ann Surg 1980;191:51-6.

126. Kim JS, Kim HJ, Hong SM, et al. Post-ischemic bowel stricture: CT features in eight cases. Korean J Radiol 2017;18:936-45.

127. Sy A, Khalidi N, Dehghan N, et al. Vasculitis in patients with Inflammatory bowel disease: a study of 32 patients and systematic review of the literature. Semin Arthritis Rheum 2016;45:475-82.

128. Guillevin L, Mahr A, Callard P, et al. Hepatitis B virus-associated polyarteritis nodosa: clinical characteristics, outcome, and impact of treatment in 115 patients. Medicine (Baltimore) 2005;84:313-22.

129. Cacoub P, Maisonobe T, Thibault V, et al. Systemic vasculitis in patients with hepatitis C. J Rheumatol 2001;28:109-18.

130. Pagnoux C, Mahr A, Cohen P, Guillevin L. Presentation and outcome of gastrointestinal involvement in systemic necrotizing vasculitides: analysis of 62 patients with polyarteritis nodosa, microscopic polyangiitis, Wegener granulomatosis, Churg-Strauss syndrome, or rheumatoid arthritis-associated vasculitis. Medicine (Baltimore) 2005;84:115-28.

131. Hiraike Y, Kodaira M, Sano M, et al. Polyarteritis nodosa diagnosed by surgically resected jejunal necrosis following acute abdomen. World J Gastroenterol 2013;19:2830-4.

132. Roikjaer O. Perforation and necrosis of the colon complicating polyarteritis nodosa. Case report. Acta Chir Scand 1987;153:385-6.

133. Tanabe J, Abe T, Okada N, et al. Massive gastrointestinal bleeding in a patient with polyarteritis nodosa. J Gastroenterol 2004;39:86-8.

134. Bourgarit A, Le Toumelin P, Pagnoux C, et al. Deaths occurring during the first year after treatment onset for polyarteritis nodosa, microscopic polyangiitis, and Churg-Strauss syndrome: a retrospective analysis of causes and factors predictive of mortality based on 595 patients. Medicine (Baltimore) 2005;84:323-30.

135. Shahedi K, Hanna RM, Melamed O, Wilson J. Wegener's granulomatosis mimicking inflammatory bowel disease and presenting with chronic enteritis. Int Med Case Rep J 2013;6:65-9.

136. Cabral DA, Canter DL, Muscal E, et al. Comparing presenting clinical features in 48 children with microscopic polyangiitis to 183 children who have granulomatosis with polyangiitis (Wegener's): an ARChiVe Cohort Study. Arthritis Rheumatol 2016;68:2514-26.

137. Ohnuki Y, Moriya Y, Yutani S, et al. Eosinophilic granulomatosis with polyangiitis (Churg-Strauss Syndrome) complicated by perforation of the small intestine and cholecystitis. Intern Med 2018;57:737-40.

138. Alberici F, Martorana D, Vaglio A. Genetic aspects of anti-neutrophil cytoplasmic antibody-associated vasculitis. Nephrol Dial Transplant 2015;30(Suppl 1):i37-45.

139. Vaglio A, Buzio C, Zwerina J. Eosinophilic granulomatosis with polyangiitis (Churg-Strauss): state of the art. Allergy 2013;68:261-73.

140. Tsurikisawa N, Oshikata C, Kinoshita A, Tsuburai T, Saito H. Longterm prognosis of 121 patients with eosinophilic granulomatosis with polyangiitis in Japan. J Rheumatol 2017;44:1206-15.

141. Navarro-Mendoza EP, Tobon GJ. Eosinophilic granulomatosis with polyangiitis: newer therapies. Curr Rheumatol Rep 2018;20:23.

142. Aguirre-Valencia D, Posso-Osorio I, Bravo JC, Bonilla-Abadia F, Tobon GJ, Canas CA. Sequential rituximab and omalizumab for the treatment of eosinophilic granulomatosis with polyangiitis (Churg-Strauss syndrome). Clin Rheumatol 2017;36:2159-62.

143. Chang WL, Yang YH, Lin YT, Chiang BL. Gastrointestinal manifestations in Henoch-Schonlein purpura: a review of 261 patients. Acta Paediatr 2004;93:1427-31.

144. Gedalia A. Henoch-Schonlein purpura. Curr Rheumatol Rep 2004;6:195-202.
145. Esaki M, Matsumoto T, Nakamura S, et al. GI involvement in Henoch-Schonlein purpura. Gastrointest Endosc 2002;56:920-3.
146. Martinez-Frontanilla LA, Haase GM, Ernster JA, Bailey WC. Surgical complications in Henoch-Schonlein purpura. J Pediatr Surg 1984;19:434-6.
147. Chetty R, Serra S. A pragmatic approach to vasculitis in the gastrointestinal tract. J Clin Pathol 2017;70:470-5.
148. Louie CY, Gomez AJ, Sibley RK, Bass D, Longacre TA. Histologic features of gastrointestinal tract biopsies in IgA vasculitis (Henoch-Schonlein Purpura). Am J Surg Pathol 2018;42:529-33.
149. Greco A, De Virgilio A, Ralli M, et al. Behcet's disease: new insights into pathophysiology, clinical features and treatment options. Autoimmun Rev 2018;17:567-75.
150. International Team for the Revision of the International Criteria for Behcet's Disease (ITR-ICBD). The International Criteria for Behcet's Disease (ICBD): a collaborative study of 27 countries on the sensitivity and specificity of the new criteria. J Eur Acad Dermatol Venereol 2014;28:338-47.
151. Arimoto J, Endo H, Kato T, et al. Clinical value of capsule endoscopy for detecting small bowel lesions in patients with intestinal Behcet's disease. Dig Endosc 2016;28:179-85.
152. Rimbas M, Nicolau A, Caraiola S, Badea CG, Voiosu MR, Baicus CR. Small bowel inflammatory involvement in Behcet's disease associated spondyloarthritis is different from other spondyloarthritides. A prospective cohort study. J Gastrointestin Liver Dis 2013;22:405-11.
153. Takada Y, Fujita Y, Igarashi M, et al. Intestinal Behcet's disease—pathognomonic changes in intramucosal lymphoid tissues and effect of a "rest cure" on intestinal lesions. J Gastroenterol 1997;32:598-604.
154. Louie CY, DiMaio MA, Charville GW, Berry GJ, Longacre TA. Gastrointestinal tract vasculopathy: clinicopathology and description of a possible "new entity" with protean features. Am J Surg Pathol 2018;42:866-76.
155. Wright CL, Cacala S. Enterocolic lymphocytic phlebitis with lymphocytic colitis, lymphocytic appendicitis, and lymphocytic enteritis. Am J Surg Pathol 2004;28:542-7.
156. Abraham SC, Solem CA, Hauser SC, Smyrk TC. Chronic antral ulcer associated with gastroduodenal lymphocytic phlebitis. Am J Surg Pathol 2004;28:1659-63.
157. Ngo N, Chang F. Enterocolic lymphocytic phlebitis: clinicopathologic features and review of the literature. Arch Pathol Lab Med 2007;131:1130-4.
158. Saraga E, Bouzourenne H. Enterocolic (lymphocytic) phlebitis: a rare cause of intestinal ischemic necrosis: a series of six patients and review of the literature. Am J Surg Pathol 2000;24:824-9.
159. Yantiss RK, Cui I, Panarelli NC, Jessurun J. Idiopathic myointimal hyperplasia of mesenteric veins: an uncommon cause of ischemic colitis with distinct mucosal features. Am J Surg Pathol 2017;41:1657-65.
160. Wangensteen KJ, Fogt F, Kann BR, Osterman MT. Idiopathic myointimal hyperplasia of the mesenteric veins diagnosed preoperatively. J Clin Gastroenterol 2015;49:491-4.
161. Abu-Alfa AK, Ayer U, West AB. Mucosal biopsy findings and venous abnormalities in idiopathic myointimal hyperplasia of the mesenteric veins. Am J Surg Pathol 1996;20:1271-8.
162. Genta RM, Haggitt RC. Idiopathic myointimal hyperplasia of mesenteric veins. Gastroenterology 1991;101:533-9.
163. Enshaei A, Hajipour B, Masoudi N. Repeated small bowel resection in a patient with Buerger's disease and intestinal involvement. J Pak Med Assoc 2016;66:467-9.
164. Cakmak A, Gyedu A, Akyol C, Kepenekci I, Koksoy C. Occlusion of the celiac trunk, the inferior mesenteric artery and stenosis of the superior mesenteric artery in peripheral thrombangiitis obliterans. Vasa 2009;38:394-6.
165. Shimizu S, Kobayashi T, Tomioka H, Ohtsu K, Matsui T, Hibi T. Involvement of herbal medicine as a cause of mesenteric phlebosclerosis: results from a large-scale nationwide survey. J Gastroenterol 2017;52:308-14.
166. Nagata Y, Watanabe T, Nagasaka K, et al. Clinical search for undiagnosed mesenteric phlebosclerosis at outpatient departments specializing in herbal (Kampo) medicine. Intern Med 2016;55:573-81.
167. Kim DW, Kang SB, Lee KH, Choe GY, Park SY, Nicholay M. Degos' disease (malignant atrophic papulosis) as a fatal cause of acute abdomen: report of a case. Surg Today 2008;38:866-70.
168. Toledo AE, Shapiro LS, Farrell JF, Magro CM, Polito J. Laparoscopy shows superiority over endoscopy for early detection of malignant atrophic papulosis gastrointestinal complications: a case report and review of literature. BMC Gastroenterol 2015;15:156.
169. Theodoridis A, Konstantinidou A, Makrantonaki E, Zouboulis CC. Malignant and benign forms of atrophic papulosis (Kohlmeier-Degos disease): systemic involvement determines the prognosis. Br J Dermatol 2014;170:110-5.
170. Farrell RJ, LaMont JT. Pathogenesis and clinical manifestations of clostridium difficile diarrhea and colitis. Curr Top Microbiol Immunol 2000;250:109-25.

171. Hogenauer C, Langner C, Beubler E, et al. Klebsiella oxytoca as a causative organism of antibiotic-associated hemorrhagic colitis. N Engl J Med 2006;355:2418-26.

172. Hannedouche T, Fillastre JP. Penicillin-induced hypersensitivity vasculitides. J Antimicrob Chemother 1987;20:3-5.

173. Nagano Y, Matsui H, Shimokawa O, et al. Bisphosphonate-induced gastrointestinal mucosal injury is mediated by mitochondrial superoxide production and lipid peroxidation. J Clin Biochem Nutr 2012;51:196-203.

174. Modi A, Siris ES, Steve Fan CP, Sajjan S. Gastrointestinal events among patients initiating osteoporosis therapy: a retrospective administrative claims database analysis. Clin Ther 2015;37:1228-34.

175. Park BJ, Clouse J, Shatin D, Stergachis A. Incidence of adverse oesophageal and gastric events in alendronate users. Pharmacoepidemiol Drug Saf 2000;9:371-6.

176. Mladenka P, Simunek T, Hubl M, Hrdina R. The role of reactive oxygen and nitrogen species in cellular iron metabolism. Free Radic Res 2006;40:263-72.

177. Abraham SC, Yardley JH, Wu TT. Erosive injury to the upper gastrointestinal tract in patients receiving iron medication: an underrecognized entity. Am J Surg Pathol 1999;23:1241-7.

178. Ji H, Yardley JH. Iron medication-associated gastric mucosal injury. Arch Pathol Lab Med 2004;128:821-2.

179. Eckstein RP, Symons P. Iron tablets cause histopathologically distinctive lesions in mucosal biopsies of the stomach and esophagus. Pathology 1996;28:142-5.

180. Hattori H. High prevalence of haemosiderin accumulation in the cytoplasm of gastric glands in patients with liver cirrhosis. J Clin Pathol 2004;57:621-4.

181. Marginean EC, Bennick M, Cyczk J, Robert ME, Jain D. Gastric siderosis: patterns and significance. Am J Surg Pathol 2006;30:514-20.

182. de Magalhaes Costa MH, Fernandes Pegado Mda G, Vargas C, et al. Pseudomelanosis duodeni associated with chronic renal failure. World J Gastroenterol 2012;18:1414-6.

183. Castellano G, Canga F, Lopez I, et al. Pseudomelanosis of the duodenum. Endoscopic, histologic, and ultrastructural study of a case. J Clin Gastroenterol 1988;10:150-4.

184. Lee HH, O'Donnell DB, Keren DF. Characteristics of melanosis duodeni: incorporation of endoscopy, pathology, and etiology. Endoscopy 1987;19:107-9.

185. Kaye P, Abdulla K, Wood J, et al. Iron-induced mucosal pathology of the upper gastrointestinal tract: a common finding in patients on oral iron therapy. Histopathology 2008;53:311-7.

186. Coogan PF, Rosenberg L, Palmer JR, et al. Phenolphthalein laxatives and risk of cancer. J Natl Cancer Inst 2000;92:1943-4.

187. Benavides SH, Morgante PE, Monserrat AJ, Zarate J, Porta EA. The pigment of melanosis coli: a lectin histochemical study. Gastrointest Endosc 1997;46:131-8.

188. Driman DK, Preiksaitis HG. Colorectal inflammation and increased cell proliferation associated with oral sodium phosphate bowel preparation solution. Hum Pathol 1998;29:972-8.

189. Ahishali E, Uygur-Bayramicli O, Dolapcioglu C, et al. Chemical colitis due to glutaraldehyde: case series and review of the literature. Dig Dis Sci 2009;54:2541-5.

190. Graham DY, Opekun AR, Willingham FF, Qureshi WA. Visible small-intestinal mucosal injury in chronic NSAID users. Clin Gastroenterol Hepatol 2005;3:55-9.

191. Gabriel SE, Jaakkimainen L, Bombardier C. Risk for serious gastrointestinal complications related to use of nonsteroidal anti-inflammatory drugs. A meta-analysis. Ann Intern Med 1991;115:787-96.

192. Watson DJ, Harper SE, Zhao PL, Quan H, Bolognese JA, Simon TJ. Gastrointestinal tolerability of the selective cyclooxygenase-2 (COX-2) inhibitor rofecoxib compared with nonselective COX-1 and COX-2 inhibitors in osteoarthritis. Arch Intern Med 2000;160:2998-3003.

193. Vane JR, Botting RM. Mechanism of action of nonsteroidal anti-inflammatory drugs. Am J Med 1998;104:2S-8.

194. Mitchell JA, Akarasereenont P, Thiemermann C, Flower RJ, Vane JR. Selectivity of nonsteroidal antiinflammatory drugs as inhibitors of constitutive and inducible cyclooxygenase. Proc Natl Acad Sci U S A 1993;90:11693-7.

195. Sumner D, Sahota J, Schofield J. Recurrence of an NSAID-induced diaphragmatic disease of the small intestine. BMJ Case Rep 2016;2016.

196. Srinivasan A, De Cruz P. Review article: a practical approach to the clinical management of NSAID enteropathy. Scand J Gastroenterol 2017;52:941-7.

197. Lang J, Price AB, Levi AJ, Burke M, Gumpel JM, Bjarnason I. Diaphragm disease: pathology of disease of the small intestine induced by non-steroidal anti-inflammatory drugs. J Clin Pathol 1988;41:516-26.

198. Zhao B, Sanati S, Eltorky M. Diaphragm disease: complete small bowel obstruction after long-term nonsteroidal anti-inflammatory drugs use. Ann Diagn Pathol 2005;9:169-73.

199. Wang YZ, Sun G, Cai FC, Yang YS. Clinical features, diagnosis, and treatment strategies of gastrointestinal diaphragm disease associated with nonsteroidal anti-inflammatory drugs. Gastroenterol Res Pract 2016;2016:3679741.

200. Lengeling RW, Mitros FA, Brennan JA, Schulze KS. Ulcerative ileitis encountered at ileo-colonoscopy: likely role of nonsteroidal agents. Clin Gastroenterol Hepatol 2003;1:160-9.

201. Courville EL, Siegel CA, Vay T, Wilcox AR, Suriawinata AA, Srivastava A. Isolated asymptomatic ileitis does not progress to overt Crohn disease on long-term follow-up despite features of chronicity in ileal biopsies. Am J Surg Pathol 2009;33:1341-7.

202. Kakar S, Nehra V, Murray JA, Dayharsh GA, Burgart LJ. Significance of intraepithelial lymphocytosis in small bowel biopsy samples with normal mucosal architecture. Am J Gastroenterol 2003;98:2027-33.

203. Harel Z, Harel S, Shah PS, Wald R, Perl J, Bell CM. Gastrointestinal adverse events with sodium polystyrene sulfonate (kayexalate) use: a systematic review. Am J Med 2013;126:264.

204. Lillemoe KD, Romolo JL, Hamilton SR, Pennington LR, Burdick JF, Williams GM. Intestinal necrosis due to sodium polystyrene (kayexalate) in sorbitol enemas: clinical and experimental support for the hypothesis. Surgery 1987;101:267-72.

205. Abraham SC, Bhagavan BS, Lee LA, Rashid A, Wu TT. Upper gastrointestinal tract injury in patients receiving kayexalate (sodium polystyrene sulfonate) in sorbitol: clinical, endoscopic, and histopathologic findings. Am J Surg Pathol 2001;25:637-44.

206. Rashid A, Hamilton SR. Necrosis of the gastrointestinal tract in uremic patients as a result of sodium polystyrene sulfonate (kayexalate) in sorbitol: an underrecognized condition. Am J Surg Pathol 1997;21:60-9.

207. Kwak HA, Hart J. The many faces of medication-related injury in the gastrointestinal tract. Surg Pathol Clin 2017;10:887-908.

208. Swanson BJ, Limketkai BN, Liu TC, et al. Sevelamer crystals in the gastrointestinal tract (GIT): a new entity associated with mucosal injury. Am J Surg Pathol 2013;37:1686-93.

209. Arnold MA, Swanson BJ, Crowder CD, et al. Colesevelam and colestipol: novel medication resins in the gastrointestinal tract. Am J Surg Pathol 2014;38:1530-7.

210. Negro A, De Marco L, Cesario V, Santi R, Boni MC, Zanelli M. A case of moderate Sprue-like enteropathy associated with telmisartan. J Clin Med Res 2017;9:1022-5.

211. Marthey L, Cadiot G, Seksik P, et al. Olmesartan-associated enteropathy: results of a national survey. Aliment Pharmacol Ther 2014;40:1103-9.

212. Ianiro G, Bibbo S, Montalto M, Ricci R, Gasbarrini A, Cammarota G. Systematic review: Sprue-like enteropathy associated with olmesartan. Aliment Pharmacol Ther 2014;40:16-23.

213. Machado I, Reolid M, Martinez de Juan F, Martinez Lapiedra C, Maia de Alcantara F. Sprue-like enteropathy associated with olmesartan in a patient with villous atrophy, HLA-DQ2 genotype and antinuclear antibodies. Rev Esp Enferm Dig 2016;108:732-3.

214. Esteve M, Temino R, Carrasco A, et al. Potential coeliac disease markers and autoimmunity in olmesartan induced enteropathy: a population-based study. Dig Liver Dis 2016;48:154-61.

215. Marco-Marques A, Sanahuja-Martinez A, Bosca-Watts MM, et al. Could HLA-DQ suggest why some patients have olmesartan-related diarrhea and others don't? Am J Gastroenterol 2015;110:1507-8.

216. Marietta EV, Nadeau AM, Cartee AK, et al. Immunopathogenesis of olmesartan-associated enteropathy. Aliment Pharmacol Ther 2015;42:1303-14.

217. Rubio-Tapia A, Herman ML, Ludvigsson JF, et al. Severe spruelike enteropathy associated with olmesartan. Mayo Clin Proc 2012;87:732-8.

218. Burbure N, Lebwohl B, Arguelles-Grande C, Green PH, Bhagat G, Lagana S. Olmesartan-associated sprue-like enteropathy: a systematic review with emphasis on histopathology. Hum Pathol 2016;50:127-34.

219. Brown I, Daveson A, Devereaux B, Laurie RM, Yantiss R, Greenson J. Sartans can cause chronic gastrointestinal injury mimicking several common conditions. Lab Invest 2018;98(Suppl 1):248-9.

220. Desruisseaux C, Bensoussan M, Desilets E, et al. Adding water to the mill: Olmesartan-induced collagenous Sprue-a case report and brief literature review. Can J Gastroenterol Hepatol 2016;2016:4837270.

221. Hruban RH, Yardley JH, Donehower RC, Boitnott JK. Taxol toxicity. Epithelial necrosis in the gastrointestinal tract associated with polymerized microtubule accumulation and mitotic arrest. Cancer 1989;63:1944-50.

222. Iacobuzio-Donahue CA, Lee EL, Abraham SC, Yardley JH, Wu TT. Colchicine toxicity: distinct morphologic findings in gastrointestinal biopsies. Am J Surg Pathol 2001;25:1067-73.

223. Torbenson M, Montgomery EA, Iacobuzio-Donahue C, Yardley JH, Wu TT, Abraham SC. Colchicine effect in a colonic hyperplastic polyp. A lesion mimicking serrated adenoma. Arch Pathol Lab Med 2002;126:615-7.

224. Behrend M. Adverse gastrointestinal effects of mycophenolate mofetil: aetiology, incidence and management. Drug Saf 2001;24:645-63.

225. Allison AC, Eugui EM. Mechanisms of action of mycophenolate mofetil in preventing acute and chronic allograft rejection. Transplantation 2005;80(Suppl):S181-90.

226. Papadimitriou JC, Drachenberg CB, Beskow CO, et al. Graft-versus-host disease-like features in mycophenolate mofetil-related colitis. Transplant Proc 2001;33:2237-8.

227. Maes BD, Dalle I, Geboes K, et al. Erosive enterocolitis in mycophenolate mofetil-treated renal-transplant recipients with persistent afebrile diarrhea. Transplantation 2003;75:665-72.

228. Parfitt JR, Jayakumar S, Driman DK. Mycophenolate mofetil-related gastrointestinal mucosal injury: variable injury patterns, including graft-versus-host disease-like changes. Am J Surg Pathol 2008;32:1367-72.

229. Star KV, Ho VT, Wang HH, Odze RD. Histologic features in colon biopsies can discriminate mycophenolate from GVHD-induced colitis. Am J Surg Pathol 2013;37:1319-28.

230. Liapis G, Boletis J, Skalioti C, et al. Histological spectrum of mycophenolate mofetil-related colitis: association with apoptosis. Histopathology 2013;63:649-58.

231. Pittman ME, Jessurun J, Yantiss RK. Differentiating posttransplant inflammatory bowel disease and other colitides in renal transplant patients. Am J Surg Pathol 2017;41:1666-74.

232. Pardoll DM. The blockade of immune checkpoints in cancer immunotherapy. Nat Rev Cancer 2012;12:252-64.

233. Zou W, Wolchok JD, Chen L. PD-L1 (B7-H1) and PD-1 pathway blockade for cancer therapy: mechanisms, response biomarkers, and combinations. Sci Transl Med 2016;8:328rv4.

234. Dilling P, Walczak J, Pikiel P, Kruszewski WJ. Multiple colon perforation as a fatal complication during treatment of metastatic melanoma with ipilimumab - case report. Pol Przegl Chir 2014;86:94-6.

235. Celli R, Kluger HM, Zhang X. Anti-PD-1 therapy-associated perforating colitis. Case Rep Gastrointest Med 2018;2018:3406437.

236. Venditti O, De Lisi D, Caricato M, et al. Ipilimumab and immune-mediated adverse events: a case report of anti-CTLA4 induced ileitis. BMC Cancer 2015;15:87.

237. Chen JH, Pezhouh MK, Lauwers GY, Masia R. Histopathologic features of colitis due to immunotherapy with anti-PD-1 antibodies. Am J Surg Pathol 2017;41:643-54.

238. Verschuren EC, van den Eertwegh AJ, Wonders J, et al. Clinical, endoscopic, and histologic characteristics of ipilimumab-associated colitis. Clin Gastroenterol Hepatol 2016;14:836-42.

239. Assarzadegan N, Montgomery E, Anders RA. Immune checkpoint inhibitor colitis: the flip side of the wonder drugs. Virchows Arch 2018;472:125-33.

240. Karamchandani DM, Chetty R. Immune checkpoint inhibitor-induced gastrointestinal and hepatic injury: pathologists' perspective. J Clin Pathol 2018;71:665-71.

241. Weidner AS, Panarelli NC, Geyer JT, et al. Idelalisib-associated colitis: histologic findings in 14 patients. Am J Surg Pathol 2015;39:1661-7.

242. Boussios S, Pentheroudakis G, Katsanos K, Pavlidis N. Systemic treatment-induced gastrointestinal toxicity: incidence, clinical presentation and management. Ann Gastroenterol 2012;25:106-18.

243. Naidu MU, Ramana GV, Rani PU, Mohan IK, Suman A, Roy P. Chemotherapy-induced and/or radiation therapy-induced oral mucositis—complicating the treatment of cancer. Neoplasia 2004;6:423-31.

244. Lee A, Ezzeldin H, Fourie J, Diasio R. Dihydropyrimidine dehydrogenase deficiency: impact of pharmacogenetics on 5-fluorouracil therapy. Clin Adv Hematol Oncol 2004;2:527-32.

245. Raida M, Schwabe W, Hausler P, et al. Prevalence of a common point mutation in the dihydropyrimidine dehydrogenase (DPD) gene within the 5'-splice donor site of intron 14 in patients with severe 5-fluorouracil (5-FU)- related toxicity compared with controls. Clin Cancer Res 2001;7:2832-9.

246. Ellis CN, McAlexander WW. Enterocolitis associated with cocaine use. Dis Colon Rectum 2005;48:2313-6.

247. Holtan SG, Pasquini M, Weisdorf DJ. Acute graft-versus-host disease: a bench-to-bedside update. Blood 2014;124:363-73.

248. Lee SJ, Flowers ME. Recognizing and managing chronic graft-versus-host disease. Hematology Am Soc Hematol Educ Program 2008:134-41.

249. Cruz-Correa M, Poonawala A, Abraham SC, et al. Endoscopic findings predict the histologic diagnosis in gastrointestinal graft-versus-host disease. Endoscopy 2002;34:808-13.

250. Ross WA, Couriel D. Colonic graft-versus-host disease. Curr Opin Gastroenterol 2005;21:64-9.

251. Narkhede M, Rybicki L, Abounader D, et al. The association of histologic grade with acute graft-versus-host disease response and outcomes. Am J Hematol 2017;92:683-8.

252. Lampert IA, Thorpe P, van Noorden S, et al. Selective sparing of enterochromaffin cells in graft versus host disease affecting the colonic mucosa. Histopathology 1985;9:875-86.

253. Washington K, Jagasia M. Pathology of graft-versus-host disease in the gastrointestinal tract. Hum Pathol 2009;40:909-17.

254. Shulman HM, Cardona DM, Greenson JK, et al. NIH consensus development project on criteria for clinical trials in chronic graft-versus-host disease: II. The 2014 Pathology Working Group report. Biol Blood Marrow Transplant 2015;21:589-603.

255. Kreft A, Mottok A, Mesteri I, et al. Consensus diagnostic histopathological criteria for acute gastrointestinal graft versus host disease improve interobserver reproducibility. Virchows Arch 2015;467:255-63.

256. Panarelli NC, Yantiss RK. Inflammatory and infectious manifestations of immunodeficiency in the gastrointestinal tract. Mod Pathol 2018;31:844-61.

257. Myerson D, Steinbach G, Gooley TA, Shulman HM. Graft-versus-host disease of the gut: a histologic activity grading system and validation. Biol Blood Marrow Transplant 2017;23:1573-9.

258. Abraham J, Janin A, Gornet JM, et al. Clinical severity scores in gastrointestinal graft-versus-host disease. Transplantation 2014;97:965-71.

259. Herrera AF, Soriano G, Bellizzi AM, et al. Cord colitis syndrome in cord-blood stem-cell transplantation. N Engl J Med 2011;365:815-24.

260. Shimoji S, Kato K, Eriguchi Y, et al. Evaluating the association between histological manifestations of cord colitis syndrome with GVHD. Bone Marrow Transplant 2013;48:1249-52.

261. Milano F, Shulman HM, Guthrie KA, Riffkin I, McDonald GB, Delaney C. Late-onset colitis after cord blood transplantation is consistent with graft-versus-host disease: results of a blinded histopathological review. Biol Blood Marrow Transplant 2014;20:1008-13.

262. Gorkiewicz G, Trajanoski S, Hogenauer C. Bradyrhizobium enterica in cord colitis syndrome. N Engl J Med 2013;369:1866-7.

263. Bhatt AS, Freeman SS, Herrera AF, et al. Sequence-based discovery of Bradyrhizobium enterica in cord colitis syndrome. N Engl J Med 2013;369:517-28.

264. Machado NO. Neutropenic enterocolitis: a continuing medical and surgical challenge. N Am J Med Sci 2010;2:293-300.

265. Sachak T, Arnold MA, Naini BV, et al. Neutropenic enterocolitis: new insights into a deadly entity. Am J Surg Pathol 2015;39:1635-42.

266. Hermsen JL, Schurr MJ, Kudsk KA, Faucher LD. Phenotyping Clostridium septicum infection: a surgeon's infectious disease. J Surg Res 2008;148:67-76.

267. Oya M, Yao T, Tsuneyoshi M. Chronic irradiation enteritis: its correlation with the elapsed time interval and morphological changes. Hum Pathol 1996;27:774-81.

268. Jessurun J. The differential diagnosis of acute colitis: clues to a specific diagnosis. Surg Pathol Clin 2017;10:863-85.

269. Greenson JK, Stern RA, Carpenter SL, Barnett JL. The clinical significance of focal active colitis. Hum Pathol 1997;28:729-33.

270. Kumar NB, Nostrant TT, Appelman HD. The histopathologic spectrum of acute self-limited colitis (acute infectious-type colitis). Am J Surg Pathol 1982;6:523-9.

271. Pacheco AR, Sperandio V. Shiga toxin in enterohemorrhagic E. coli: regulation and novel anti-virulence strategies. Front Cell Infect Microbiol 2012;2:81.

272. Mounier J, Vasselon T, Hellio R, Lesourd M, Sansonetti PJ. Shigella flexneri enters human colonic Caco-2 epithelial cells through the basolateral pole. Infect Immun 1992;60:237-48.

273. Fasano A, Noriega FR, Maneval DR Jr, et al. Shigella enterotoxin 1: an enterotoxin of Shigella flexneri 2a active in rabbit small intestine in vivo and in vitro. J Clin Invest 1995;95:2853-61.

274. Ochoa TJ, Cleary TG. Epidemiology and spectrum of disease of Escherichia coli O157. Curr Opin Infect Dis 2003;16:259-63.

275. Karmali MA, Gannon V, Sargeant JM. Verocytotoxin-producing Escherichia coli (VTEC). Vet Microbiol 2010;140:360-70.

276. Nguyen Y, Sperandio V. Enterohemorrhagic E. coli (EHEC) pathogenesis. Front Cell Infect Microbiol 2012;2:90.

277. Bagdasarian N, Rao K, Malani PN. Diagnosis and treatment of Clostridium difficile in adults: a systematic review. JAMA 2015;313:398-408.

278. Leffler DA, Lamont JT. Clostridium difficile infection. N Engl J Med 2015;372:1539-48.

279. Farooq PD, Urrunaga NH, Tang DM, von Rosenvinge EC. Pseudomembranous colitis. Dis Mon 2015;61:181-206.

280. Surawicz CM, Brandt LJ, Binion DG, et al. Guidelines for diagnosis, treatment, and prevention of Clostridium difficile infections. Am J Gastroenterol 2013;108:478-98.

281. Baker ME. Acute infectious and inflammatory enterocolitides. Radiol Clin North Am 2015;53:1255-71.

282. Dignan CR, Greenson JK. Can ischemic colitis be differentiated from C difficile colitis in biopsy specimens? Am J Surg Pathol 1997;21:706-10.

283. Yantiss RK, Odze RD. Pitfalls in the interpretation of nonneoplastic mucosal biopsies in inflammatory bowel disease. Am J Gastroenterol 2007;102:890-904.

284. Lamontagne F, Labbe AC, Haeck O, et al. Impact of emergency colectomy on survival of patients with fulminant Clostridium difficile colitis during an epidemic caused by a hypervirulent strain. Ann Surg 2007;245:267-72.

285. Parry CM, Hien TT, Dougan G, White NJ, Farrar JJ. Typhoid fever. N Engl J Med 2002;347:1770-82.

286. Kraus MD, Amatya B, Kimula Y. Histopathology of typhoid enteritis: morphologic and immunophenotypic findings. Mod Pathol 1999;12:949-55.

287. Naktin J, Beavis KG. Yersinia enterocolitica and Yersinia pseudotuberculosis. Clin Lab Med 1999;19:523-36.

288. El-Maraghi NR, Mair NS. The histopathology of enteric infection with Yersinia pseudotuberculosis. Am J Clin Pathol 1979;71:631-9.

289. Cover TL, Aber RC. Yersinia enterocolitica. N Engl J Med 1989;321:16-24.

290. Gleason TH, Patterson SD. The pathology of Yersinia enterocolitica ileocolitis. Am J Surg Pathol 1982;6:347-55.

291. Esteve M, Salas A, Fernandez-Banares F, et al. Intestinal spirochetosis and chronic watery diarrhea: clinical and histological response to treatment and long-term follow up. J Gastroenterol Hepatol 2006;21:1326-33.

292. Korner M, Gebbers JO. Clinical significance of human intestinal spirochetosis—a morphologic approach. Infection 2003;31:341-9.

293. Relman DA, Schmidt TM, MacDermott RP, Falkow S. Identification of the uncultured bacillus of Whipple's disease. N Engl J Med 1992;327:293-301.

294. Dobbins WO 3rd. HLA antigens in Whipple's disease. Arthritis Rheum 1987;30:102-5.

295. Dolmans RA, Boel CH, Lacle MM, Kusters JG. Clinical manifestations, treatment, and diagnosis of Tropheryma whipplei infections. Clin Microbiol Rev 2017;30:529-55.

296. Bai JC, Mazure RM, Vazquez H, et al. Whipple's disease. Clin Gastroenterol Hepatol 2004;2:849-60.

297. Lehmann P, Ehrenstein B, Hartung W, Dragonas C, Reischl U, Fleck M. PCR analysis is superior to histology for diagnosis of Whipple's disease mimicking seronegative rheumatic diseases. Scand J Rheumatol 2017;46:138-42.

298. Donoghue HD, Holton J. Intestinal tuberculosis. Curr Opin Infect Dis 2009;22:490-6.

299. Kirsch R, Pentecost M, Hall Pde M, Epstein DP, Watermeyer G, Friederich PW. Role of colonoscopic biopsy in distinguishing between Crohn's disease and intestinal tuberculosis. J Clin Pathol 2006;59:840-4.

300. Almadi MA, Ghosh S, Aljebreen AM. Differentiating intestinal tuberculosis from Crohn's disease: a diagnostic challenge. Am J Gastroenterol 2009;104:1003-12.

301. Solomon IH, Johncilla ME, Hornick JL, Milner DA Jr. The utility of immunohistochemistry in mycobacterial infection: a proposal for multimodality testing. Am J Surg Pathol 2017;41:1364-70.

302. Kisacik B, Pamuk ON, Onat AM, et al. Characteristics predicting tuberculosis risk under tumor necrosis factor-alpha inhibitors: report from a large multicenter cohort with high background prevalence. J Rheumatol 2016;43:524-9.

303. Lai KK, Lamps LW. Enterocolitis in immunocompromised patients. Semin Diagn Pathol 2014;31:176-91.

304. Batman PA, Kapembwa MS, Belmonte L, et al. HIV enteropathy: HAART reduces HIV-induced stem cell hyperproliferation and crypt hypertrophy to normal in jejunal mucosa. J Clin Pathol 2014;67:14-8.

305. Batman PA, Miller AR, Forster SM, Harris JR, Pinching AJ, Griffin GE. Jejunal enteropathy associated with human immunodeficiency virus infection: quantitative histology. J Clin Pathol 1989;42:275-81.

306. Cello JP, Day LW. Idiopathic AIDS enteropathy and treatment of gastrointestinal opportunistic pathogens. Gastroenterology 2009;136:1952-65.

307. Keates J, Lagahee S, Crilley P, Haber M, Kowalski T. CMV enteritis causing segmental ischemia and massive intestinal hemorrhage. Gastrointest Endosc 2001;53:355-9.

308. Shah R, Vaidya G, Kalakonda A, Manocha D, Rawlins S. Cytomegalovirus colitis mimicking rectal carcinoma in a young immunocompetent patient. ACG Case Rep J 2015;2:165-7.

309. Juric-Sekhar G, Upton MP, Swanson PE, Westerhoff M. Cytomegalovirus (CMV) in gastrointestinal mucosal biopsies: should a pathologist perform CMV immunohistochemistry if the clinician requests it? Hum Pathol 2017;60:11-5.

310. Nikkels AF, Delvenne P, Sadzot-Delvaux C, et al. Distribution of varicella zoster virus and herpes simplex virus in disseminated fatal infections. J Clin Pathol 1996;49:243-8.

311. Weidner AS, Panarelli NC, Rennert H, Jessurun J, Yantiss RK. Immunohistochemistry improves the detection of adenovirus in gastrointestinal biopsy specimens from hematopoietic stem cell transplant recipients. Am J Clin Pathol 2016;146:627-31.

312. McCurdy JD, Enders FT, Jones A, et al. Detection of cytomegalovirus in patients with inflammatory bowel disease: where to biopsy and how many biopsies? Inflamm Bowel Dis 2015;21:2833-8.

313. Yan Z, Wang L, Dennis J, Doern C, Baker J, Park JY. Clinical significance of isolated cytomegalovirus-infected gastrointestinal cells. Int J Surg Pathol 2014;22:492-8.

314. Mills AM, Guo FP, Copland AP, Pai RK, Pinsky BA. A comparison of CMV detection in gastrointestinal mucosal biopsies using immunohistochemistry and PCR performed on formalin-fixed, paraffin-embedded tissue. Am J Surg Pathol 2013;37:995-1000.

315. Baradhi KM, Aure RL, El-Amm JM. High-dose valganciclovir treatment for resistant cytomegalovirus colitis due to UL97 and UL54 mutations. Transplant Proc 2018;50:142-4.

316. Runde V, Ross S, Trenschel R, et al. Adenoviral infection after allogeneic stem cell transplantation (SCT): report on 130 patients from a single SCT unit involved in a prospective multi center surveillance study. Bone Marrow Transplant 2001;28:51-7.

317. Solomon IH, Hornick JL, Laga AC. Immunohistochemistry is rarely justified for the diagnosis of viral infections. Am J Clin Pathol 2017;147:96-104.

318. Lee YJ, Huang YT, Kim SJ, et al. Adenovirus viremia in adult CD34(+) selected hematopoietic cell transplant recipients: low incidence and high clinical impact. Biol Blood Marrow Transplant 2016;22:174-8.

319. Geramizadeh B, Foroughi R, Keshtkar-Jahromi M, Malek-Hosseini SA, Alborzi A. Gastrointestinal basidiobolomycosis, an emerging infection in the immunocompetent host: a report of 14 patients. J Med Microbiol 2012;61(Pt 12):1770-4.

320. Yousef OM, Smilack JD, Kerr DM, Ramsey R, Rosati L, Colby TV. Gastrointestinal basidiobolomycosis. Morphologic findings in a cluster of six cases. Am J Clin Pathol 1999;112:610-6.

321. Field AS, Milner DA Jr. Intestinal microsporidiosis. Clin Lab Med 2015;35:445-59.

322. Yan L, Yang C, Tang J. Disruption of the intestinal mucosal barrier in Candida albicans infections. Microbiol Res 2013;168:389-95.

323. Lamps LW, Lai KK, Milner DA Jr. Fungal infections of the gastrointestinal tract in the immunocompromised host: an update. Adv Anat Pathol 2014;21:217-27.

324. Patterson TF, Kirkpatrick WR, White M, et al. Invasive aspergillosis. Disease spectrum, treatment practices, and outcomes. I3 Aspergillus Study Group. Medicine (Baltimore) 2000;79:250-60.

325. Kazan E, Maertens J, Herbrecht R, et al. A retrospective series of gut aspergillosis in haematology patients. Clin Microbiol Infect 2011;17:588-94.

326. Petrikkos G, Skiada A, Lortholary O, Roilides E, Walsh TJ, Kontoyiannis DP. Epidemiology and clinical manifestations of mucormycosis. Clin Infect Dis 2012;54(Suppl 1):S23-34.

327. Colombo AL, Tobon A, Restrepo A, Queiroz-Telles F, Nucci M. Epidemiology of endemic systemic fungal infections in Latin America. Med Mycol 2011;49:785-98.

328. Assi MA, Sandid MS, Baddour LM, Roberts GD, Walker RC. Systemic histoplasmosis: a 15-year retrospective institutional review of 111 patients. Medicine (Baltimore) 2007;86:162-9.

329. Deng Z, Ribas JL, Gibson DW, Connor DH. Infections caused by Penicillium marneffei in China and Southeast Asia: review of eighteen published cases and report of four more Chinese cases. Rev Infect Dis 1988;10:640-52.

330. Ko CI, Hung CC, Chen MY, Hsueh PR, Hsiao CH, Wong JM. Endoscopic diagnosis of intestinal Penicilliosis marneffei: report of three cases and review of the literature. Gastrointest Endosc 1999;50:111-4.

331. Deng ZL, Connor DH. Progressive disseminated penicilliosis caused by Penicillium marneffei. Report of eight cases and differentiation of the causative organism from histoplasma capsulatum. Am J Clin Pathol 1985;84:323-7.

332. Girardin M, Greloz V, Hadengue A. Cryptococcal gastroduodenitis: a rare location of the disease. Clin Gastroenterol Hepatol 2010;8:e28-9.

333. Washington K, Gottfried MR, Wilson ML. Gastrointestinal cryptococcosis. Mod Pathol 1991;4:707-11.

334. Harris JR, Lockhart SR, Debess E, et al. Cryptococcus gattii in the United States: clinical aspects of infection with an emerging pathogen. Clin Infect Dis 2011;53:1188-95.

335. Agarwal S, Mayer L. Pathogenesis and treatment of gastrointestinal disease in antibody deficiency syndromes. J Allergy Clin Immunol 2009;124:658-64.

336. Oberhuber G, Mesteri I, Kopf W, Muller H. Demonstration of trophozoites of G. lamblia in ileal mucosal biopsy specimens may reveal giardiasis in patients with significantly inflamed parasite-free duodenal mucosa. Am J Surg Pathol 2016;40:1280-5.

337. Oberhuber G, Kastner N, Stolte M. Giardiasis: a histologic analysis of 567 cases. Scand J Gastroenterol 1997;32:48-51.

338. Robertson SA, Arnold CA, Montgomery EA, Voltaggio L. Duodenal giardiasis miss rates: lessons from a large tertiary hospital. Mod Pathol 2015;28(Suppl 2):187A.

339. Panarelli NC, Gobara N, Hoda RS, Chaump M, Jessurun J, Yantiss RK. Cytology preparations of formalin fixative aid detection of giardia in duodenal biopsy samples. Am J Surg Pathol 2017;41:570-4.

340. Herwaldt BL. Cyclospora cayetanensis: a review, focusing on the outbreaks of cyclosporiasis in the 1990s. Clin Infect Dis 2000;31:1040-57.

341. Zar FA, El-Bayoumi E, Yungbluth MM. Histologic proof of acalculous cholecystitis due to cyclospora cayetanensis. Clin Infect Dis 2001;33:E140-1.

342. Richardson RF Jr, Remler BF, Katirji B, Murad MH. Guillain-Barre syndrome after cyclospora infection. Muscle Nerve 1998;21:669-71.

343. Ortega YR, Nagle R, Gilman RH, et al. Pathologic and clinical findings in patients with cyclosporiasis and a description of intracellular parasite life-cycle stages. J Infect Dis 1997;176:1584-9.

344. Ortega YR, Sterling CR, Gilman RH, Cama VA, Diaz F. Cyclospora species—a new protozoan pathogen of humans. N Engl J Med 1993;328:1308-12.

345. Chen XM, Keithly JS, Paya CV, LaRusso NF. Cryptosporidiosis. N Engl J Med 2002;346:1723-31.

346. Ryan U, Paparini A, Monis P, Hijjawi N. It's official - cryptosporidium is a gregarine: what are the implications for the water industry? Water Res 2016;105:305-13.

347. Curry A, Smith HV. Emerging pathogens: isospora, cyclospora and microsporidia. Parasitology 1998;117(Suppl):S143-59.

348. Marcial-Seoane MA, Serrano-Olmo J. Intestinal infection with Isospora belli. P R Health Sci J 1995;14:137-40.

349. Stanley SL Jr. Amoebiasis. Lancet 2003;361:1025-34.

350. Istre GR, Kreiss K, Hopkins RS, et al. An outbreak of amebiasis spread by colonic irrigation at a chiropractic clinic. N Engl J Med 1982;307:339-42.

351. Pittman FE, Hennigar GR. Sigmoidoscopic and colonic mucosal biopsy findings in amebic colitis. Arch Pathol 1974;97:155-8.

352. Variyam EP, Gogate P, Hassan M, et al. Nondysenteric intestinal amebiasis. Colonic morphology and search for Entamoeba histolytica adherence and invasion. Dig Dis Sci 1989;34:732-40.

353. Ralston KS, Petri WA Jr. Tissue destruction and invasion by Entamoeba histolytica. Trends Parasitol 2011;27:254-63.

354. Brandt H, Tamayo RP. Pathology of human amebiasis. Hum Pathol 1970;1:351-85.

355. Schuster FL, Ramirez-Avila L. Current world status of Balantidium coli. Clin Microbiol Rev 2008;21:626-38.

356. Garcia LS. Flagellates and ciliates. Clin Lab Med 1999;19:621-38.

357. Colley DG, Bustinduy AL, Secor WE, King CH. Human schistosomiasis. Lancet 2014;383:2253-64.

358. Cao J, Liu WJ, Xu XY, Zou XP. Endoscopic findings and clinicopathologic characteristics of colonic schistosomiasis: a report of 46 cases. World J Gastroenterol 2010;16:723-7.

359. Milder JE, Walzer PD, Kilgore G, Rutherford I, Klein M. Clinical features of strongyloides stercoralis infection in an endemic area of the United States. Gastroenterology 1981;80:1481-8.

360. Levenhagen MA, Costa-Cruz JM. Update on immunologic and molecular diagnosis of human strongyloidiasis. Acta Tropica 2014;135:33-43.

361. Genta RM. Dysregulation of Strongyloidiasis: a new hypothesis. Clin Microbiol Rev 1992;5:345-55.

362. Kishimoto K, Hokama A, Hirata T, et al. Endoscopic and histopathological study on the duodenum of Strongyloides stercoralis hyperinfection. World J Gastroenterol 2008;14:1768-73.

363. Minematsu H, Hokama A, Makishi T, Arakaki K, Kinjo F, Fujita J. Colonoscopic findings and pathologic characteristics of Strongyloides colitis: a case series. Digestion 2011;83:210-4.

364. Thompson BF, Fry LC, Wells CD, et al. The spectrum of GI strongyloidiasis: an endoscopic-pathologic study. Gastrointest Endosc 2004;59:906-10.

365. Kim SG, Jo YJ, Park YS, et al. Four cases of gastric submucosal mass suspected as anisakiasis. Korean J Parasitol 2006;44:81-6.

366. Ishida M, Harada A, Egawa S, Watabe S, Ebina N, Unno M. Three successive cases of enteric anisakiasis. Dig Surg 2007;24:228-31.

367. Pravettoni V, Primavesi L, Piantanida M. Anisakis simplex: current knowledge. Eur Ann Allergy Clin Immunol 2012;44:150-6.

368. Park EY, Baek DH, Kim GH, Lee BE, Lee SJ, Park DY. Endosonographic findings and the natural course of chronic gastric anisakiasis: a single-center experience. Gastroenterol Res Pract 2018;2018:8562792.

369. Yantiss RK. Eosinophils in the GI tract: how many is too many and what do they mean? Mod Pathol 2015;28(Suppl 1):S7-21.

370. Morshed MG, Singh AE. Recent trends in the serologic diagnosis of syphilis. Clin Vaccine Immunol 2015;22:137-47.

371. Hoentjen F, Rubin DT. Infectious proctitis: when to suspect it is not inflammatory bowel disease. Dig Dis Sci 2012;57:269-73.

372. Arnold CA, Limketkai BN, Illei PB, Montgomery E, Voltaggio L. Syphilitic and lymphogranuloma venereum (LGV) proctocolitis: clues to a frequently missed diagnosis. Am J Surg Pathol 2013;37:38-46.

373. Jawale R, Lai KK, Lamps LW. Sexually transmitted infections of the lower gastrointestinal tract. Virchows Arch 2018;472:149-58.

374. Stoner BP, Cohen SE. Lymphogranuloma venereum 2015: clinical presentation, diagnosis, and treatment. Clin Infect Dis 2015;61(Suppl 8):S865-73.

375. Arnold CA, Roth R, Arsenescu R, et al. Sexually transmitted infectious colitis vs inflammatory bowel disease: distinguishing features from a case-controlled study. Am J Clin Pathol 2015;144:771-81.

376. Soni S, Srirajaskanthan R, Lucas SB, Alexander S, Wong T, White JA. Lymphogranuloma venereum proctitis masquerading as inflammatory bowel disease in 12 homosexual men. Aliment Pharmacol Ther 2010;32:59-65.

377. van Liere GA, Hoebe CJ, Dukers-Muijrers NH. Evaluation of the anatomical site distribution of chlamydia and gonorrhoea in men who have sex with men and in high-risk women by routine testing: cross-sectional study revealing missed opportunities for treatment strategies. Sex Transm Infect 2014;90:58-60.

378. McMillan A, McNeillage G, Gilmour HM, Lee FD. Histology of rectal gonorrhoea in men, with a note on anorectal infection with neisseria meningitidis. J Clin Pathol 1983;36:511-4.

379. Mayor MT, Roett MA, Uduhiri KA. Diagnosis and management of gonococcal infections. Am Fam Physician 2012;86:931-8.

380. Barbee LA, Dombrowski JC, Kerani R, Golden MR. Effect of nucleic acid amplification testing on detection of extragenital gonorrhea and chlamydial infections in men who have sex with men sexually transmitted disease clinic patients. Sex Transm Dis 2014;41:168-72.

381. Quillin SJ, Seifert HS. Neisseria gonorrhoeae host adaptation and pathogenesis. Nat Rev Microbiol 2018;16:226-40.

382. Rompalo AM. Diagnosis and treatment of sexually acquired proctitis and proctocolitis: an update. Clin Infect Dis 1999;28(Suppl 1):S84-90.

383. LeGoff J, Pere H, Belec L. Diagnosis of genital herpes simplex virus infection in the clinical laboratory. Virol J 2014;11:83.

384. Steiner I, Kennedy PG, Pachner AR. The neurotropic herpes viruses: herpes simplex and varicella-zoster. Lancet Neurol 2007;6:1015-28.

385. Kavitt RT, Lipowska AM, Anyane-Yeboa A, Gralnek IM. Diagnosis and treatment of peptic ulcer disease. Am J Med 2019;132:447-56.

386. Robert ME, Crowe SE, Burgart L, et al. Statement on best practices in the use of pathology as a diagnostic tool for celiac disease: a guide for clinicians and pathologists. Am J Surg Pathol 2018;42:e44-58.

387. Pai RK. A practical approach to small bowel biopsy interpretation: celiac disease and its mimics. Semin Diagn Pathol 2014;31:124-36.

388. Kempenich JW, Sirinek KR. Acid peptic disease. Surg Clin North Am 2018;98:933-44.

389. Brown IS, Bettington A, Bettington M, Rosty C. Tropical sprue: revisiting an underrecognized disease. Am J Surg Pathol 2014;38:666-72.

390. Quigley EM. Small intestinal bacterial overgrowth: what it is and what it is not. Curr Opin Gastroenterol 2014;30:141-6.

391. Dukowicz AC, Lacy BE, Levine GM. Small intestinal bacterial overgrowth: a comprehensive review. Gastroenterol Hepatol (NY) 2007;3:112-22.

392. Winer DA, Luck H, Tsai S, Winer S. The intestinal immune system in obesity and insulin resistance. Cell Metab 2016;23:413-26.

393. Lappinga PJ, Abraham SC, Murray JA, Vetter EA, Patel R, Wu TT. Small intestinal bacterial overgrowth: histopathologic features and clinical correlates in an underrecognized entity. Arch Pathol Lab Med 2010;134:264-70.

394. Greenson JK. The biopsy pathology of non-coeliac enteropathy. Histopathology 2015;66:29-36.

395. Lahtinen P, Mattila E, Anttila VJ, et al. Faecal microbiota transplantation in patients with clostridium difficile and significant comorbidities as well as in patients with new indications: a case series. World J Gastroenterol 2017;23:7174-84.

396. Freeman HJ, Nimmo M. Intestinal lymphangiectasia in adults. World J Gastrointest Oncol 2011;3:19-23.

397. Kishikawa H, Nishida J, Takarabe S, et al. Video capsule endoscopy findings in Ehlers-Danlos syndrome with recurrent gastrointestinal bleeding. Endoscopy 2012;44(Suppl 2):E416.

398. Kongara KR, Soffer EE. Intestinal motility in small bowel diverticulosis: a case report and review of the literature. J Clin Gastroenterol 2000;30:84-6.

399. Lebert P, Ernst O, Zins M. Acquired diverticular disease of the jejunum and ileum: imaging features and pitfalls. Abdom Radiol (NY) 2019;44:1734-43.

400. Lebert P, Millet I, Ernst O, et al. Acute jejunoileal diverticulitis: multicenter descriptive study of 33 patients. AJR Am J Roentgenol 2018;210:1245-51.

401. Robey BS, Peery AF, Dellon ES. Small bowel diverticulosis and jejunal perforation in Marfan syndrome. ACG Case Rep J 2018;5:e5.

402. Berridge FR, Dick AP. Effect of Crohn's disease on colonic diverticula. Br J Radiol 1976;49:926-9.

403. Meyers MA, Alonso DR, Morson BC, Bartram C. Pathogenesis of diverticulitis complicating granulomatous colitis. Gastroenterology 1978;74:24-31.

404. Petros JG, Happ RA. Crohn's colitis in patients with diverticular disease. Am J Gastroenterol 1991;86:247-8.

405. Sultan K, Fields S, Panagopoulos G, Korelitz BI. The nature of inflammatory bowel disease in patients with coexistent colonic diverticulosis. J Clin Gastroenterol 2006;40:317-21.

406. Schembri J, Bonello J, Christodoulou DK, Katsanos KH, Ellul P. Segmental colitis associated with diverticulosis: is it the coexistence of colonic diverticulosis and inflammatory bowel disease? Ann Gastroenterol 2017;30:257-61.

407. Klein S, Mayer L, Present DH, Youner KD, Cerulli MA, Sachar DB. Extraintestinal manifestations in patients with diverticulitis. Ann Intern Med 1988;108:700-2.

408. Imperiali G, Meucci G, Alvisi C, et al. Segmental colitis associated with diverticula: a prospective study. Gruppo di studio per le malattie infiammatorie intestinali (GSMII). Am J Gastroenterol 2000;95:1014-6.

409. Goldstein NS, Leon-Armin C, Mani A. Crohn's colitis-like changes in sigmoid diverticulitis specimens is usually an idiosyncratic inflammatory response to the diverticulosis rather than Crohn's colitis. Am J Surg Pathol 2000;24:668-75.

410. Faenza A, Spolaore R, Poggioli G, et al. [Acute tubular necrosis after kidney transplantation]. Minerva Nefrol 1983;30:221-5. [Italian]

411. Ramos GP, Papadakis KA. Mechanisms of disease: inflammatory bowel diseases. Mayo Clin Proc 2019;94:155-65.

412. Imperiali G, Terpin MM, Meucci G, Ferrara A, Minoli G. Segmental colitis associated with diverticula: a 7-year follow-up study. Endoscopy 2006;38:610-2.

413. Guillemot F, Colombel JF, Neut C, et al. Treatment of diversion colitis by short-chain fatty acids. Prospective and double-blind study. Dis Colon Rectum 1991;34:861-4.

414. Schmit A, Van Gossum A, Carol M, Houben JJ, Mascart F. Diversion of intestinal flow decreases the numbers of interleukin 4 secreting and interferon gamma secreting T lymphocytes in small bowel mucosa. Gut 2000;46:40-5.

415. Haque S, West AB. Diversion colitis—20 years a-growing. J Clin Gastroenterol 1992;15:281-3.

416. Yeong ML, Bethwaite PB, Prasad J, Isbister WH. Lymphoid follicular hyperplasia—a distinctive feature of diversion colitis. Histopathology 1991;19:55-61.

417. Grant NJ, Van Kruiningen HJ, Haque S, West AB. Mucosal inflammation in pediatric diversion colitis: a quantitative analysis. J Pediatr Gastroenterol Nutr 1997;25:273-80.

418. Lusk LB, Reichen J, Levine JS. Aphthous ulceration in diversion colitis. Clinical implications. Gastroenterology 1984;87:1171-3.

419. Ma CK, Gottlieb C, Haas PA. Diversion colitis: a clinicopathologic study of 21 cases. Hum Pathol 1990;21:429-36.

420. Korelitz BI, Cheskin LJ, Sohn N, Sommers SC. Proctitis after fecal diversion in Crohn's disease and its elimination with reanastomosis: implications for surgical management. Report of four cases. Gastroenterology 1984;87:710-3.

421. Harig JM, Soergel KH, Komorowski RA, Wood CM. Treatment of diversion colitis with short-chain-fatty acid irrigation. N Engl J Med 1989;320:23-8.

422. Huang CC, Wang IF, Chiu HH. Lower gastrointestinal bleeding caused by stercoral ulcer. CMAJ 2011;183:E134.

423. Saeed F, Kalra A, Kousar N, Pace LA, Holley JL. Stercoral ulcer as a cause of lower gastrointestinal (LGI) bleeding in chronic hemodialysis patients. Clin Nephrol 2012;77:75-8.

424. Nagar AB. Isolated colonic ulcers: diagnosis and management. Curr Gastroenterol Rep 2007;9:422-8.

425. Hussain ZH, Whitehead DA, Lacy BE. Fecal impaction. Curr Gastroenterol Rep 2014;16:404.

426. Chaudhry NS, Bi WL, Gupta S, Keraliya A, Shimizu N, Chiocca EA. Pneumatosis intestinalis after molecular targeted therapy. World Neurosurg 2019;125:312-5.

427. Gyger G, Baron M. Systemic sclerosis: gastrointestinal disease and its management. Rheum Dis Clin North Am 2015;41:459-73.

428. Sugihara Y, Okada H. Pneumatosis cystoides intestinalis. N Engl J Med 2017;377:2266.

429. Pieterse AS, Leong AS, Rowland R. The mucosal changes and pathogenesis of pneumatosis cystoides intestinalis. Hum Pathol 1985;16:683-8.

430. Wang YJ, Wang YM, Zheng YM, Jiang HQ, Zhang J. Pneumatosis cystoides intestinalis: six case reports and a review of the literature. BMC Gastroenterol 2018;18:100.

431. Saul SH, Sollenberger LC. Solitary rectal ulcer syndrome. Its clinical and pathological underdiagnosis. Am J Surg Pathol 1985;9:411-21.

432. Zhu QC, Shen RR, Qin HL, Wang Y. Solitary rectal ulcer syndrome: clinical features, pathophysiology, diagnosis and treatment strategies. World J Gastroenterol 2014;20:738-44.

433. Nakamura S, Kino I, Akagi T. Inflammatory myoglandular polyps of the colon and rectum. A clinicopathological study of 32 pedunculated polyps, distinct from other types of polyps. Am J Surg Pathol 1992;16:772-9.

434. Kelly JK. Polypoid prolapsing mucosal folds in diverticular disease. Am J Surg Pathol 1991;15:871-8.

435. Gouriou C, Chambaz M, Ropert A, et al. A systematic literature review on solitary rectal ulcer syndrome: is there a therapeutic consensus in 2018? Int J Colorectal Dis 2018;33:1647-55.

436. Saul SH. Inflammatory cloacogenic polyp: relationship to solitary rectal ulcer syndrome/ mucosal prolapse and other bowel disorders. Hum Pathol 1987;18:1120-5.

437. Lobert PF, Appelman HD. Inflammatory cloacogenic polyp. A unique inflammatory lesion of the anal transitional zone. Am J Surg Pathol 1981;5:761-6.

438. Abid S, Khawaja A, Bhimani SA, Ahmad Z, Hamid S, Jafri W. The clinical, endoscopic and histological spectrum of the solitary rectal ulcer syndrome: a single-center experience of 116 cases. BMC Gastroenterol 2012;12:72.

439. Williams GT, Bussey HJ, Morson BC. Inflamamtory 'cap' polyposis of the large intestine. Br J Surg 1985;72(Suppl):S133.

440. Ng KH, Mathur P, Kumarasinghe MP, Eu KW, Seow-Choen F. Cap polyposis: further experience and review. Dis Colon Rectum 2004;47:1208-15.

441. Oriuchi T, Kinouchi Y, Kimura M, et al. Successful treatment of cap polyposis by avoidance of intraluminal trauma: clues to pathogenesis. Am J Gastroenterol 2000;95:2095-8.

442. Oshitani N, Moriyama Y, Matsumoto T, Kobayashi K, Kitano A. Protein-losing enteropathy from cap polyposis. Lancet 1995;346:1567.

443. Peny MO, Noel JC, Haot J, et al. [Cap polyposis: a rare syndrome]. Gastroenterol Clin Biol 1998;22:349-52. [French]

444. Campbell AP, Cobb CA, Chapman RW, et al. Cap polyposis—an unusual cause of diarrhoea. Gut 1993;34:562-4.

445. Gehenot M, Colombel JF, Wolschies E, et al. Cap polyposis occurring in the postoperative course of pelvic surgery. Gut 1994;35:1670-2.

446. Konishi T, Watanabe T, Takei Y, Kojima T, Nagawa H. Confined progression of cap polyposis along the anastomotic line, implicating the role of inflammatory responses in the pathogenesis. Gastrointest Endosc 2005;62:446-7.

447. Shimizu K, Koga H, Iida M, et al. Does metronidazole cure cap polyposis by its antiinflammatory actions instead of by its antibiotic action? A case study. Dig Dis Sci 2002;47:1465-8.

448. Akamatsu T, Nakamura N, Kawamura Y, et al. Possible relationship between Helicobacter pylori infection and cap polyposis of the colon. Helicobacter 2004;9:651-6.

449. Nishiyama M, Maeda K, Aoyagi K, Sakisaka S. [Cap polyposis and Helicobacter pylori]. Nippon Rinsho 2005;63(Suppl 11):328-30. [Japanese]

450. Oiya H, Okawa K, Aoki T, Nebiki H, Inoue T. Cap polyposis cured by Helicobacter pylori eradication therapy. J Gastroenterol 2002;37:463-6.

451. Okamoto K, Watanabe T, Komeda Y, et al. Dysbiosis-associated polyposis of the colon-cap polyposis. Front Immunol 2018;9:918.

452. Esaki M, Matsumoto T, Kobayashi H, et al. Cap polyposis of the colon and rectum: an analysis of endoscopic findings. Endoscopy 2001;33:262-6.

453. Kajihara H, Uno Y, Ying H, Tanaka M, Munakata A. Features of cap polyposis by magnifying colonoscopy. Gastrointest Endosc 2000;52:775-8.

454. Ohkawara T, Kato M, Nakagawa S, et al. Spontaneous resolution of cap polyposis: case report. Gastrointest Endosc 2003;57:599-602.

455. Tomiyama R, Kinjo F, Kinjo N, Nakachi N, Kawane M, Hokama A. Gastrointestinal: cap polyposis. J Gastroenterol Hepatol 2003;18:741.

456. Maunoury V, Breisse M, Desreumaux P, Gambiez L, Colombel JF. Infliximab failure in cap polyposis. Gut 2005;54:313-4.

457. Bookman ID, Redston MS, Greenberg GR. Successful treatment of cap polyposis with infliximab. Gastroenterology 2004;126:1868-71.

458. Fulmer CG, Yantiss RK, Jessurun J. Pathologic features associated with colonic intraluminal metallic stents. Lab Inves 2018;98:263.

5 IMMUNE-MEDIATED DISEASES WITH SYSTEMIC MANIFESTATIONS

CELIAC DISEASE AND RELATED DISORDERS

Celiac Disease

Definition. *Celiac disease* is a chronic malabsorptive disorder due to an immune reaction to dietary gluten. Synonyms include *celiac sprue*, *non-tropical sprue*, and *gluten-induced enteropathy*.

Clinical Features. Celiac disease is a common malabsorptive disorder, affecting 0.05 to 0.2 percent of the population in European countries and up to 1 percent of people in the United States (1). The disease shows a predilection for females and can present at any age, although most patients are adults with a mean age of 45 years. Risk is increased in individuals with type 1 diabetes mellitus, autoimmune thyroiditis, selective IgA deficiency, Turner syndrome, and Down syndrome.

Pediatric patients first present when cereal is introduced into the diet at 1 to 2 years of age. Manifestations include diarrhea and steatorrhea, vomiting, abdominal pain, failure to thrive, short stature, and muscle wasting. Older children and adolescents can have all of these symptoms as well as delayed puberty. Adults are more likely to present with both gastrointestinal and systemic manifestations, such as infertility, recurrent fetal loss, osteopenia, anemia, and peripheral neuropathy.

Iron deficiency anemia is the most common manifestation of celiac disease, resulting from decreased iron absorption in the duodenum. Other deficiencies include calcium, selenium, copper, zinc, and vitamins A, D, E, and K. Elevated liver function tests are often present (2). Dermatitis herpetiformis, an intensely pruritic rash composed of nodules and blisters, is seen in 10 to 15 percent of patients. The rash waxes and wanes, showing a predilection for the forearms, knees, buttocks, and hairline. Only 20 percent of patients with dermatitis herpetiformis do not have underlying celiac disease (3).

Symptomatic patients with celiac disease frequently have elevated anti-gliadin, anti-endomysial, anti-deamidated gliadin-related peptide, and anti-tissue transglutaminase (TTG) autoantibodies. The overall sensitivities and specificities of these markers are over 90 percent; assays for TTG IgA antibodies are the most sensitive and specific (4). Serologic assays, however, are only valuable when patients are exposed to gluten. They are generally negative in gluten-restricted patients and may also be negative in patients with mild symptoms. Up to 5 percent of patients with celiac disease have selective IgA deficiency, in which case serum IgG antibodies need to be tested (5). False-positive serologic assays can occur in patients who have other immune-mediated disorders.

Pathogenesis. Celiac disease results from a combination of genetic and environmental factors. Virtually all patients have either HLA-DQ2 (95 percent) or HLA-DQ8 (5 percent) alleles (6). Presumably, genetically susceptible individuals develop an immune reaction to gliadin, a component of gluten that is present in wheat, barley, rye, and other cereals. Dietary exposure to gluten results in aberrant stimulation of mucosal T-cells, thereby activating adaptive and innate immune responses. The net effect is an overall increase in mucosal inflammation and epithelial cell damage. It is possible that type 12 adenovirus and some strains of rotavirus trigger symptom development; peptides present on these viruses cross-react with peptides in gliadin (7,8). Dermatitis herpetiformis develops when serum IgA antibodies bind to epidermal transglutaminase (9).

Gross Findings. At least 20 percent of patients with celiac disease have normal duodenal findings, particularly children. When present, endoscopic abnormalities include loss of villi, scalloped mucosal folds, or a mosaic pattern (fig. 5-1) (1). Chronic, severe disease can result in complete mucosal atrophy and increasingly

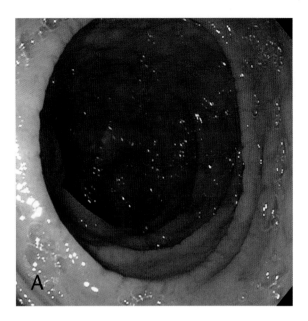
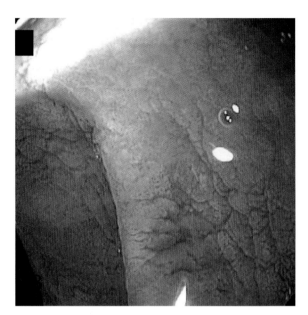

Figure 5-1

CELIAC DISEASE

Thickened duodenal folds have a scalloped appearance and the background mucosa is nodular (A). Loss of mucosal folds and a mosaic pattern are evident (B).

visible vasculature. Erythema and ulcers are not typical; their presence should prompt consideration of other entities or neoplastic progression of celiac disease. Mucosal abnormalities are most pronounced in the duodenum and proximal jejunum but are often patchy (10).

Optimal sampling includes tissues obtained from the duodenal bulb, proximal duodenum, and distal duodenum submitted in separate containers (1). Sampling of the gastric antrum and colon can also be informative, especially if intraepithelial lymphocytosis is present at those sites.

Microscopic Findings. Celiac disease produces variably severe villous architectural abnormalities ranging from normal villous architecture to complete blunting with crypt hyperplasia (fig. 5-2). Virtually all symptomatic patients with celiac disease have increased intraepithelial T-cells in their duodenal mucosae. Lymphocytes are evenly distributed throughout the epithelium, or they are more numerous in the villous tips than their lateral aspects (fig. 5-3). Celiac disease generally features at least 25 intraepithelial lymphocytes per 100 duodenal enterocytes and more than 40/100 enterocytes in most cases (1). Immunostains against CD3 and CD8 are of no value in assessing biopsy material for celiac disease

and can, in some cases, lead to overestimation of the number of intraepithelial lymphocytes in otherwise healthy patients (11).

Other common changes of celiac disease include variable villous shortening, crypt hyperplasia, and plasma cell-rich inflammation in the lamina propria (fig. 5-4). Neutrophils and eosinophils are more common in cases that show substantial villous blunting but are present in low numbers; numerous crypt abscesses should prompt consideration of peptic injury, infection, or other immune-mediated disorders (12). Injured surface epithelial cells typically display some degree of cytoplasmic depletion and may contain vacuoles (13). Although several classification schemes have been proposed to grade severity of histologic abnormalities, these schemes lack clinical utility and reproducibility; their use is largely limited to investigative studies (1,14).

Celiac disease often elicits intraepithelial lymphocytosis throughout the gastrointestinal tract. It is one consideration in patients with lymphocytic esophagitis and is strongly associated with lymphocytic gastritis, particularly in pediatric patients, as described in chapters 2 and 3. Intraepithelial lymphocytes may also be detected in ileal biopsy samples, often in

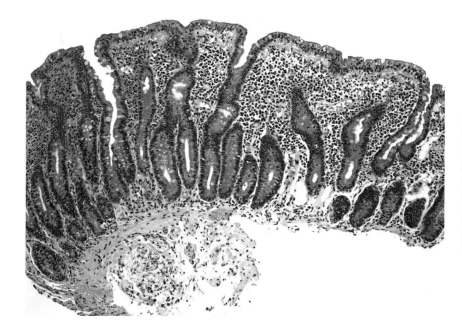

Figure 5-2

CELIAC DISEASE

Marked villous blunting and crypt hyperplasia produce the appearance of a flat mucosa, resembling that of the colon. Although some may classify villous blunting as a form of atrophy, it is best considered to represent mucosal remodeling since the overall thickness is near normal. Plasma cells expand the mucosa and are present in both superficial and deep locations.

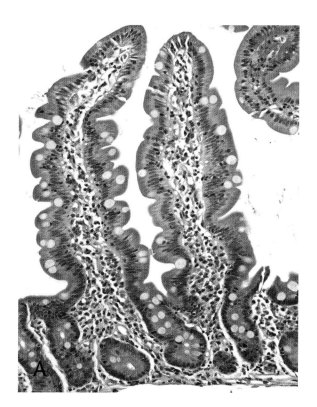

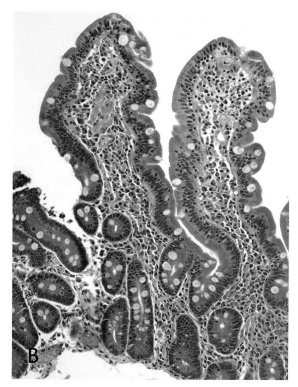

Figure 5-3

INTRAEPITHELIAL LYMPHOCYTOSIS WITH NORMAL VILLOUS ARCHITECTURE

Normal duodenal villi contain a few intraepithelial lymphocytes that are more numerous on their deep and lateral aspects (A). Biopsy samples from some patients with celiac disease display normal villous architecture with increased intraepithelial lymphocytes dispersed over the entire villus, particularly at the villous tips (B).

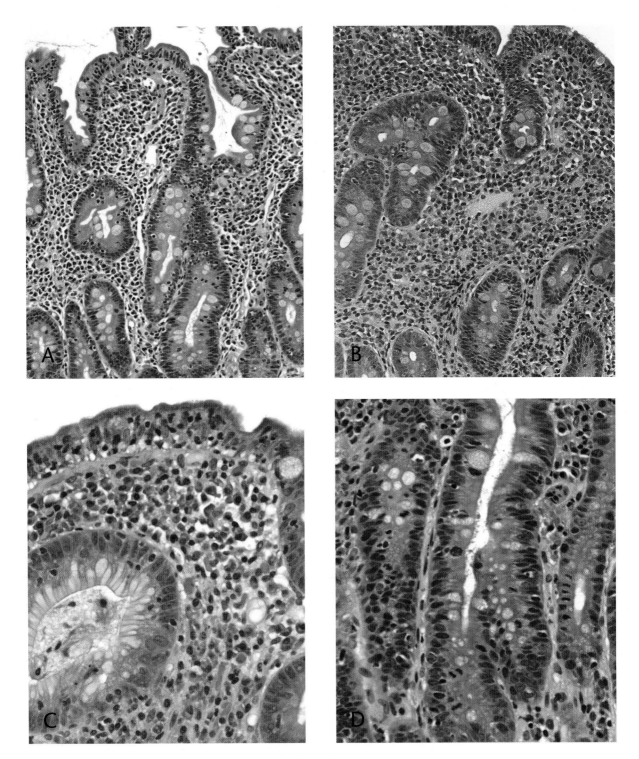

Figure 5-4

CELIAC DISEASE

Villous architectural abnormalities secondary to celiac disease are always accompanied by intraepithelial lymphocytosis (A) and mononuclear cell-rich lamina propria infiltrates with numerous plasma cells (B). Neutrophils may be present in small numbers, particularly in the duodenal bulb (C). Intraepithelial lymphocytes tend to be less numerous in the crypts and apoptotic debris is inconspicuous (D).

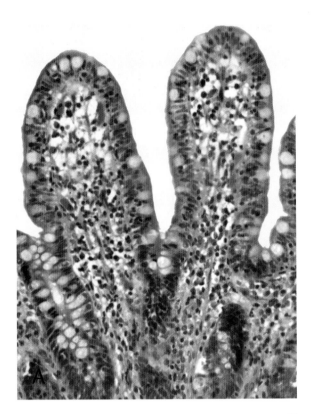
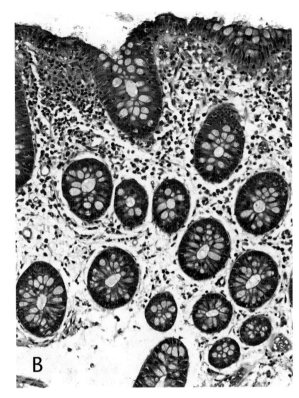

Figure 5-5

GASTROINTESTINAL LYMPHOCYTOSIS ASSOCIATED WITH CELIAC DISEASE

Intraepithelial lymphocytosis of the ileum (A) and colon (B) can occur in patients with celiac disease. Epithelial inflammation is unaccompanied by mucosal architectural abnormalities, although some cases show increased cellularity of the lamina propria.

association with preserved villous architecture and normal lamina propria cellularity (fig. 5-5A). Both lymphocytic colitis and colonic lymphocytosis occur in patients with celiac disease (fig. 5-5B). Thus, evaluation of the upper gastrointestinal tract should be considered whenever patients with diarrheal symptoms have intraepithelial lymphocytosis in samples from the lower gastrointestinal tract.

Differential Diagnosis. Intraepithelial lymphocytosis is a sensitive, but non-specific, histologic marker of celiac disease. It occurs in patients with other immune-mediated disorders, including thyroiditis, rheumatoid arthritis, and microscopic colitis. Other diseases that elicit mononuclear cell infiltrates and villous architectural abnormalities are peptic duodenitis, small intestinal bacterial overgrowth, medication-related injury, tropical sprue, hypersensitivity to non-gluten dietary proteins, autoimmune enterocolitis, idiopathic

inflammatory bowel disease, infections, and common variable immunodeficiency. Features that differentiate celiac disease from some of its mimics are summarized in Table 5-1.

Treatment and Prognosis. Most patients respond well to gluten withdrawal and 10 to 20 percent of children even become gluten tolerant over time. However, approximately 10 percent of patients do not respond to gluten restriction or develop recurrent symptoms after an initial response to gluten withdrawal. Most of these cases can be explained by intentional or inadvertent non-compliance with dietary restrictions or disease due to other causes, such as disaccharide intolerance, irritable bowel syndrome, small intestinal bacterial overgrowth, food allergies, pancreatic insufficiency, and microscopic colitis (15). Gluten restriction decreases lymphoma risk in patients with celiac disease, although individuals with longstanding exposure to gluten are at risk for both B- and T-cell lymphomas, most notably,

Table 5-1

DISTINGUISHING FEATURES OF ENTITIES THAT CAUSE INTRAEPITHELIAL LYMPHOCYTOSIS OF THE DUODENUM

Entity	Clinical Associations	Endoscopic Findings	Disease Distribution	Distinguishing Histologic Features
Topical injury				
Peptic duodenitis	*H. pylori* gastritis Chemical gastropathy	Ulcers and erythema	Duodenal bulb	Foveolar cell metaplasia Intraepithelial lymphocytosis often patchy Neutrophils
Immune injury				
Celiac disease	Immune disorders Endomysial, tissue transglutaminase, and gliadin antibodies	Normal or malabsorptive pattern	Duodenum Proximal jejunum	Surface intraepithelial lymphocytosis more prominent than crypt inflammation Plasma cell-rich inflammation Rare crypt abscesses and granulocytes
Crohn disease	Arthralgias Oral aphthous ulcers Anti-*Saccharomyces cerevisiae* antibodies	Malabsorptive pattern Ulcers, strictures	Entire GI tract, mostly small bowel and colon	Grossly and microscopically patchy disease Neutrophilic cryptitis Non-necrotic granulomas Intraepithelial lymphocytosis often patchy
Autoimmune enteropathy	IPEX[a] syndrome APECED/APS1 Antienterocyte and goblet cell antibodies Immune disorders	Malabsorptive pattern	Entire GI tract, mostly small bowel and colon	Crypt injury greater than surface injury Crypt-predominant intraepithelial lymphocytosis Numerous crypt abscesses Apoptotic crypt epithelial cells Paneth, endocrine, and goblet cells may be decreased
Common variable immunodeficiency	Hemolytic anemia Recurrent infections Decreased serum immunoglobulin	Malabsorptive pattern Ulcers	Entire GI tract, mostly small bowel and colon	Crypt injury greater than surface injury Intraepithelial lymphocytosis often patchy Granulocytes and apoptotic debris Decreased or absent lamina propria plasma cells Cytomegalovirus, lymphoid aggregates, giardiasis
Eosinophilic gastroenteritis	Atopy and asthma	Malabsorptive patterm	Entire GI tract	Eosinophils in lamina propria and epithelium
Medications				
Checkpoint inhibitors/ targeted agents	History of malignancy	Normal or erythema and erosions	Entire GI tract, mostly small bowel and colon	Neutrophilic cryptitis Apoptotic crypt epithelial cells Intraepithelial lymphocytosis often patchy
Angiotensin receptor blockers	History of hypertension	Normal or malabsorptive pattern	Entire GI tract, mostly small bowel and colon	Intraepithelial lymphocytosis Numerous crypt abscesses Apoptotic crypt epithelial cells Variably decreased Paneth, endocrine, and goblet cells
NSAIDs	Numerous clinical associations	Occasional ulcers	Entire GI tract	Mild villous blunting Intraepithelial lymphocytosis often patchy

		Endoscopic	Disease	Distinguishing
Entity	Clinical Associations	Findings	Distribution	Histologic Features

Table 5-1, continued

		Endoscopic Findings	Disease Distribution	Distinguishing Histologic Features
Infection				
Tropical sprue	Vitamin B12 deficiency	Normal or mal-absorptive pattern	Ileum>duodenum	Mild villous blunting Mild intraepithelial lymphocytosis
Bacterial overgrowth	Impaired gut motility Postsurgical patient	Normal or mal-absorptive pattern	Small bowel	Partial villous blunting Intraepithelial lympho-cytosis with neutrophils
Viruses	Immunocompromise	Variable ranging from normal to extensive ulcers	Entire GI tract	Viral cytopathic changes Neutrophils, apoptotic debris Intraepithelial lymphocytosis often patchy
Protozoans	Immunocompromise	Often normal with mild changes	Entire GI tract, mostly small bowel and colon	Organisms may be detected in samples Intraepithelial lympho-cytosis often patchy Ulcers with invasive infections

[a]IPEX = immune dysregulation, polyendocrinopathy, and X-linked syndrome; APECED = autoimmune polyendocrinopa-thies, mucocutaneous candidiasis, and ectodermal dystropy; GI = gastrointestinal.

enteropathy-associated T-cell lymphoma (16,17). Patients are also at risk for carcinomas of the oropharynx, esophagus, and small bowel.

Refractory Sprue

Refractory sprue is defined as persistent malab-sorptive symptoms and villous blunting despite strict adherence to a gluten-free diet for at least 6 months and exclusion of other etiologies (15). Some patients have relapsed symptoms after an initial period of improvement, whereas others never completely respond to gluten restriction. Endoscopic findings may resemble those of ce-liac disease or feature mucosal atrophy, erythe-ma, and ulcers. Enlarged, cavitating mesenteric lymph nodes and splenic atrophy occur in 30 percent of patients (18).

Refractory sprue is classified based on the immunophenotypic and molecular features of the T-cell infiltrate present in the duodenal mucosa. *Type 1 refractory sprue* features villous blunting and crypt hyperplasia with intraepi-thelial lymphocytosis. It is morphologically and immunophenotypically indistinguishable from celiac disease. Intraepithelial T-cells express CD8 as well as surface CD3, CD7, CD103, and TCR-β. These cells display polyclonal T-cell receptor gene rearrangements, although clinically insig-nificant clones are occasionally identified (19). Type 1 refractory sprue is associated with other autoimmune diseases and typically responds

well to corticosteroids or azathioprine-based immunosuppressive therapy.

Type 2 refractory sprue is also morphologically similar to celiac disease, although infiltrating T-cells are immunophenotypically abnormal. They show frequent loss of surface CD3, CD7, and/or CD8 staining with or without cytoplas-mic CD3 staining (fig. 5-6). Type 2 refractory sprue is defined by loss of multiple surface T-cell markers in over 20 percent of the T-cell population by flow cytometric analysis and immunohistochemical loss of CD8 in over 50 percent of intraepithelial lymphocytes. Patients with Type 2 refractory sprue frequently have abnormal T-cell populations in gastric and colonic biopsies as well, indicating that the disorder is a diffuse process. Molecular studies demonstrate monoclonal T-cell receptor gene rearrangements. Type 2 refractory sprue is es-sentially a precursor to enteropathy-associated T-cell lymphoma: nearly 50 percent of patients ultimately develop lymphoma (20).

Ulcerative Jejunoileitis

Ulcers are rarely seen in patients with un-complicated celiac disease. When present, they are usually related to superimposed peptic or medication-related injury when located in the proximal duodenum near the bulb. However, some patients with established celiac disease develop *ulcerative jejunitis* characterized by

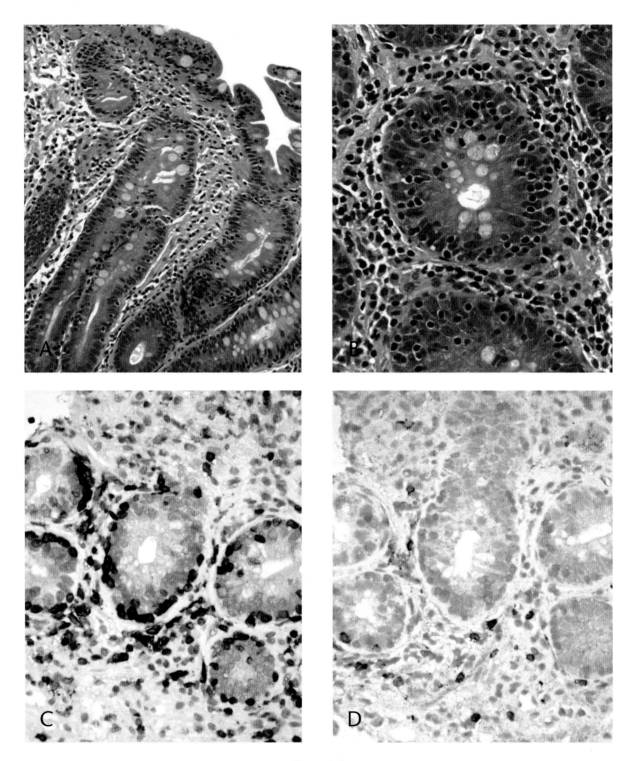

Figure 5-6

TYPE 2 REFRACTORY CELIAC DISEASE

Refractory celiac disease is morphologically indistinguishable from celiac disease. It usually produces partial or complete villous blunting (A) with intraepithelial lymphocytosis (B). The intraepithelial lymphocytes show abnormal immunophenotypic expression of T-cell markers: CD3 may be preserved (C) but CD8 is typically lost (D).

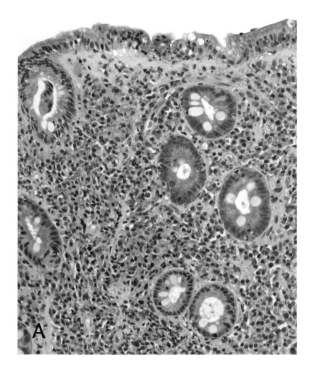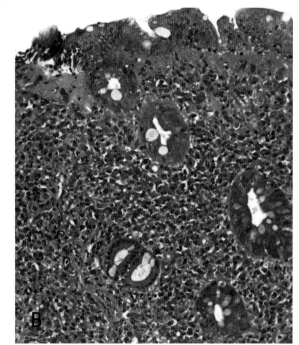

Figure 5-7

COLLAGENOUS SPRUE

Marked villous blunting and plasma cell-rich lamina propria inflammation are accompanied by an irregular layer of subepithelial collagen (A). A trichrome stain demonstrates inflammatory cells and entrapped capillaries in the thickened collagen layer (B).

multiple ulcers of the distal duodenum and jejunum. They present with iron deficiency anemia, hemorrhage, perforation, or bowel obstruction.

In *ulcerative jejunoileitis*, ulcers are accompanied by celiac sprue-like changes or subepithelial collagen deposits in the adjacent mucosa. Intraepithelial T-cells show an aberrant phenotype and monoclonal T-cell receptor gene rearrangements, similar to those of type 2 refractory sprue (18). Ulcerative jejunoileitis is widely considered to represent a T-cell neoplasm and, in fact, many mass-forming cases reported in the older literature likely represent enteropathy-associated T-cell lymphoma.

Collagenous Sprue

Collagenous sprue occurs in patients with chronic mucosal injury due to a variety of etiologies. Although most cases are idiopathic, development of this disorder may explain persistent malabsorptive symptoms in patients with a prior history of celiac disease. Less than 25 percent of patients with collagenous sprue

have elevated celiac disease-related antibody titers (21). Occasional cases have been reported in patients with tropical sprue, non-gluten protein intolerance, and medication effects, particularly sartans and related agents (22,23).

The histologic features include sprue-like inflammatory changes accompanied by subepithelial collagen deposits with entrapped inflammatory cells and capillaries (fig. 5-7). The collagen deposits tend to be less pronounced than those of collagenous gastritis and collagenous colitis. Treatment consists of immunosuppressive therapy, which generally results in symptomatic improvement (21).

IDIOPATHIC INFLAMMATORY BOWEL DISEASE

Ulcerative Colitis

Definition. *Ulcerative colitis* is a chronic immune-mediated inflammatory condition of the colorectum resulting from environmental influences and genetically susceptibility.

341

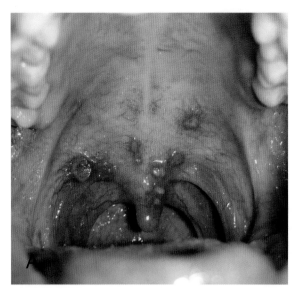
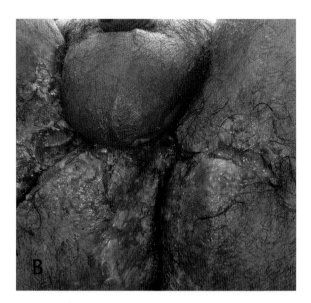

Figure 5-8

IDIOPATHIC INFLAMMATORY BOWEL DISEASE

Discrete and confluent aphthous ulcers are present on the mucosa of the soft palate and uvula (A). Pyoderma gangrenosum of the perineum appears as large ulcers on a background of tissue necrosis and chronic skin changes (B). (Courtesy of Dr. K. Garrett, New York, NY.)

Clinical Features. Ulcerative colitis develops in 40 to 240 per 100,000 individuals each year and its incidence is increasing; it is estimated that up to 1 percent of the United States population will develop this disease (24). Ulcerative colitis demonstrates a bimodal age distribution, with a large peak in adolescence/young adulthood and a smaller peak in older adults. Men and women are equally affected.

Patients present with recurrent fevers, chills, abdominal pain, cramps, tenesmus, and bloody diarrhea with pus or mucus. Extraintestinal manifestations include arthralgias, pyoderma gangrenosum, erythema nodosum, uveitis, and oral aphthous ulcers (fig. 5-8). Some individuals develop primary sclerosing cholangitis or, less commonly, primary biliary cholangitis.

Serum pANCA titers may be elevated and stool studies from symptomatic patients generally feature elevated inflammatory markers, including calprotectin (25,26). Imaging results vary depending on the severity of disease. Mild changes include edema and ulcers in the distal colon, whereas severe colitis produces radiographically visible submucosal edema and colonic dilation accompanied by ulcers. The submucosa is often prominent due to diffuse accumulation of adipose tissue. Mesenteric adenopathy may be present.

Pathogenesis. Ulcerative colitis results from the complex interplay between environmental influences and microbial exposures in genetically susceptible patients. Ashkenazi Jews are at increased risk compared with the general population and susceptibility has been linked to HLA-DRB and IL-10 variants (27,28). Presumably, genetic factors underlie an aberrant Th2 cell-mediated inflammatory response to abnormal intestinal flora (29). Several lines of evidence suggest that the intestinal microbiomes of patients with ulcerative colitis consist of a disproportionate number of pro-inflammatory and mucolytic bacteria, such as *Proteobacteria* and *Bacteroidetes*, although it is not clear whether this is an initiating abnormality or a consequence of intestinal inflammation (24). Other environmental risk factors are poorly defined. Both prior smoking history and appendectomy appear to be protective against the development of colitis and, in fact, appendectomy after disease onset may abrogate therapy-refractory symptoms (30). Weak associations with prior infectious enterocolitis, diet, climate, and physical activity have also been described.

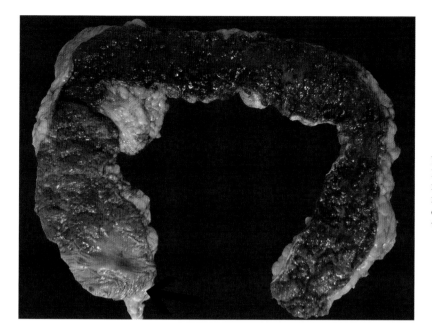

Figure 5-9

ULCERATIVE COLITIS

The colon is slightly shortened but of similar caliber in all areas. Diffuse mucosal erythema, ulcers, and nodularity extend from the distal aspect more proximally. The most proximal colonic mucosa is finely granular and the ileal mucosa (arrow) is spared.

Figure 5-10

ULCERATIVE COLITIS

Severely active chronic colitis features mucosal edema and erythema accompanied by extensive ulcers. Residual islands of mucosa have a nodular appearance.

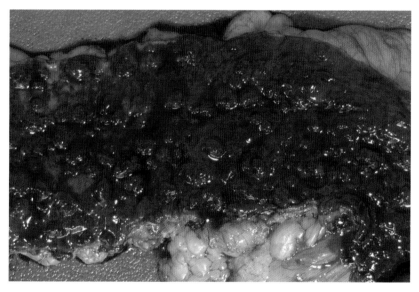

Gross Findings. Classic ulcerative colitis is a superficial, diffuse disease that affects the mucosa in a continuous fashion, extending from the rectum into the abdominal colon (fig. 5-9). Flares of disease feature erythema, edema, and friable, granular mucosa with ulcers (fig. 5-10). Typical changes of longstanding colitis include loss of the mucosal vascular pattern, flattened folds, and pseudopolyps that may be sessile, pedunculated, or filiform in appearance (fig. 5-11). Approximately 30 percent of patients have pancolitis and 20 percent have left-sided disease. The remainder have inflammation confined to the distal colorectum. The ileum is typically spared, although some patients develop granularity and erythema in its distal few centimeters.

Microscopic Findings. Ulcerative colitis is a waxing and waning disorder characterized by variation in the severity of histologic abnormalities and clinical symptoms. The disease is confined to the mucosa and superficial submucosa with rare exception (fig. 5-12). Biopsy samples from symptomatic patients feature a dense plasma cell-rich inflammatory infiltrate that expands the mucosa and extends into the deep mucosa between the crypt bases and the

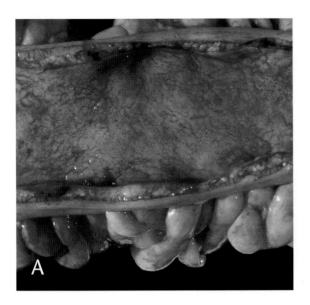
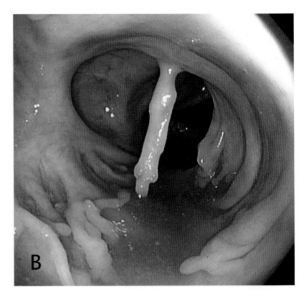

Figure 5-11

ULCERATIVE COLITIS

Longstanding ulcerative colitis results in mucosal atrophy with loss of the transverse folds, as well as erythema and erosions (A). Elongated, filiform pseudopolyps are commonly present (B).

Figure 5-12

ULCERATIVE COLITIS

Ulcerative colitis is a superficial chronic inflammatory condition. Dense mononuclear cell-rich inflammation expands the architecturally distorted mucosa but the muscularis propria is spared.

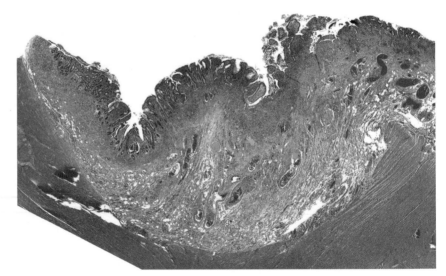

muscularis mucosae (fig. 5-13A). Eosinophils are invariably present and may be numerous, particularly in the proximal colon. Neutrophilic inflammation is concentrated in and around crypts (fig. 5-13B). Mild active colitis features crypt infiltration by neutrophils, whereas crypt abscesses and erosions are seen in moderately active disease (fig. 5-13C). Clinically severe disease usually correlates with the presence of crypt destruction and ulcers. Similar findings are often seen in the appendix (fig. 5-13D).

Mucosal remodeling tends to be most pronounced in patients with persistent symptoms for long periods of time. It is characterized by short, branched, or horizontal crypts and an undulating or villous mucosal surface (fig. 5-14A,B). Paneth cell metaplasia and hyperplasia are frequently present; pseudopyloric glandular metaplasia can occur but is uncommon (fig. 5-14C,D). The superficial submucosa may show hyperplasia of the muscularis mucosae but the deeper submucosa displays prominent

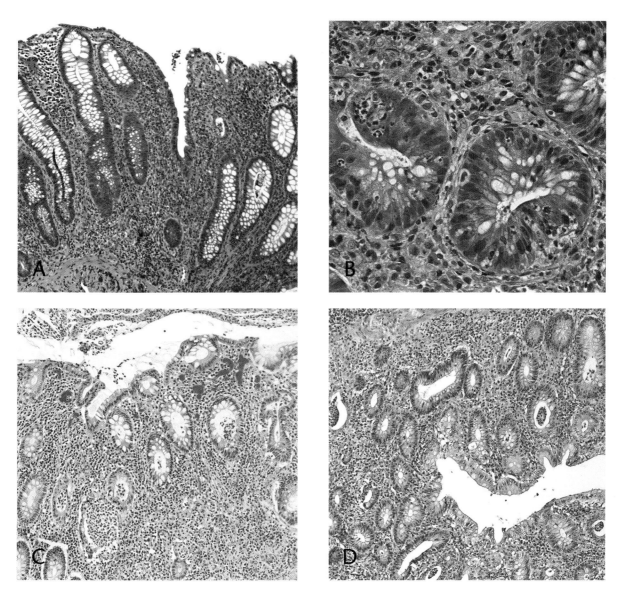

Figure 5-13

ULCERATIVE COLITIS

Symptomatic ulcerative colitis features plasma cell-rich inflammation that expands the mucosa and extends to its deepest aspect (i.e., basal plasmacytosis) even when crypt architectural distortion is not well developed (A). Neutrophilic inflammation is centered on the crypts; cryptitis is surrounded by a few neutrophils in the immediate vicinity but diffuse neutrophilia of the lamina propria is not typical (B). Severe disease activity features numerous crypt abscesses, crypt destruction, and ulcers with exudates (C). Chronic active appendicitis is frequently present in patients who undergo colectomy for refractory disease (D).

fat accumulation. Importantly, crypt abnormalities, surface architectural distortion, and cellular metaplasia are not specific features of ulcerative colitis. These changes can occur as a result of any type of persistent injury (31).

Ileal inflammation is present in nearly 20 percent of patients with ulcerative colitis. It usually consists of mild, patchy neutrophilic inflammation in the crypt epithelium and is limited to the distal few centimeters of ileum. Ileitis may be related to luminal stasis in the inflamed gut, medications, or involvement by the same immune-mediated inflammatory process affecting the colon, as described below.

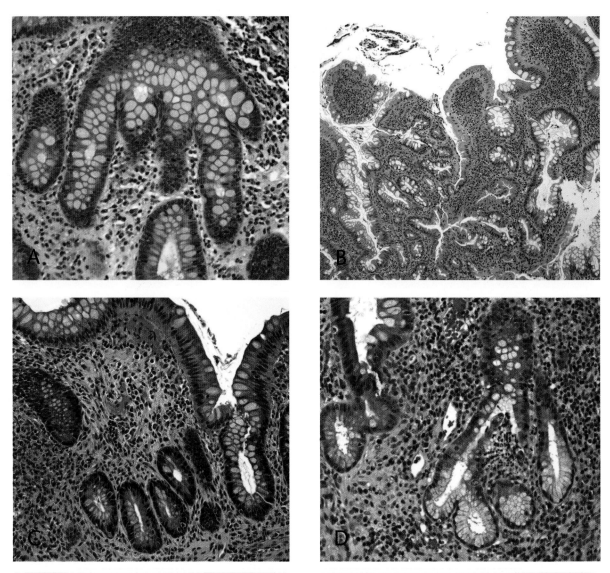

Figure 5-14

ULCERATIVE COLITIS

Crypt architectural distortion results from repetitive bouts of crypt destruction. Crypts are often short and branched, stopping short of the muscularis mucosae (A). The surface may assume a villiform appearance over time, with broad, frond-like projections containing plasma cell-rich inflammation (B). Mucosal healing manifests with disorganized repopulation of the mucosa by regenerative-appearing crypts that show increased numbers of Paneth cells in the proximal colon (i.e., Paneth cell hyperplasia) or Paneth cell metaplasia in the distal colon (C). Metaplasia to a gastric phenotype (i.e., pseudopyloric metaplasia) is uncommon in the colon (D).

Less Common (Crohn-Like) Features of Ulcerative Colitis. There are several circumstances in which the "classic" morphologic features of ulcerative colitis are accompanied by atypical features that have been historically attributed to Crohn disease. For example, ulcerative colitis need not appear as retrograde, continuous inflammation extending from the rectum. Disease is often discontinuous or patchy in patients who respond to medical therapy, as well as in patients with new-onset colitis; nearly 50 percent of pediatric patients have some degree of rectal sparing or patchy disease at initial presentation (32). Pediatric and adult patients may have left-sided proctosigmoiditis with sparing of the transverse colon and inflammation

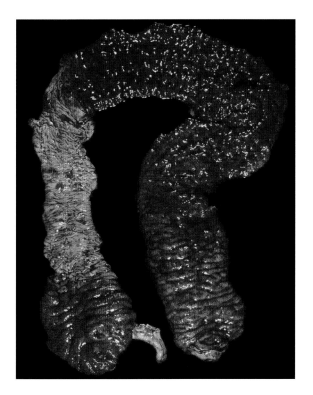

Figure 5-15

ULCERATIVE COLITIS

Skip lesions are common in patients with ulcerative colitis. Patients may have diffuse continuous disease in the distal colorectum, sparing of the mid colon, and inflammation of the cecum, appendix, or appendiceal orifice.

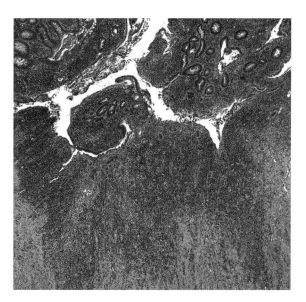

Figure 5-16

FULMINANT ULCERATIVE COLITIS

Severe ulcerative colitis features extensive ulcers lined by chronically inflamed granulation tissue that extends into the muscularis propria.

in the cecum or peri-appendiceal mucosa (fig. 5-15). This type of "skip lesion" occurs in up to 86 percent of ulcerative colitis cases and is not associated with ultimate development of Crohn disease (33).

Patients with fulminant ulcerative colitis can develop deep ulcers that extend into the muscularis propria (34,35). These crack-like ulcers are lined by granulation tissue and surrounded by dense chronic inflammation (fig. 5-16). Ruptured crypts and extruded mucin commonly elicit granulomatous inflammation, simulating the granulomas of Crohn disease (fig. 5-17). Mucin granulomas contain neutrophils, lymphocytes, and foamy macrophages, none of which is typical of Crohn disease-related granulomas (32). Multiple tissue levels that demonstrate the relationship between granulomatous inflammation and crypt epithelium can facilitate a diagnosis in challenging cases.

Some patients with ulcerative colitis develop extra-colonic inflammation in the gastrointestinal tract. Diffuse erosions, increased plasma cells, and pseudopyloric gland metaplasia can be detected in the distal several centimeters of the ileum (fig. 5-18). These findings tend to be more common in patients with severe pancolitis but also occur in patients with relative or complete sparing of the cecum and ascending colon (36). Patchy asymptomatic inflammation of the upper gastrointestinal tract is a common finding in patients with ulcerative colitis; some individuals even develop diffuse, chronic active enteritis in the duodenum and jejunum, particularly following colectomy (37,38).

Differential Diagnosis. Distinction between ulcerative colitis and acute colitis may be problematic in the early phases of disease when crypt and cellular changes of chronic injury are mild or absent. Dense plasma cell-rich inflammation in the lamina propria, particularly in the deep mucosa, is a helpful diagnostic feature of chronic colitis and is universally present in patients with clinically symptomatic ulcerative colitis. In contrast, plasma cell-rich inflammation is accompanied by macrophages and granulocytes when detected in patients with resolving acute colitis.

347

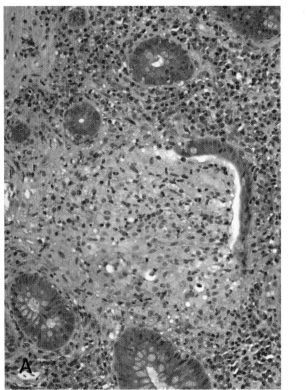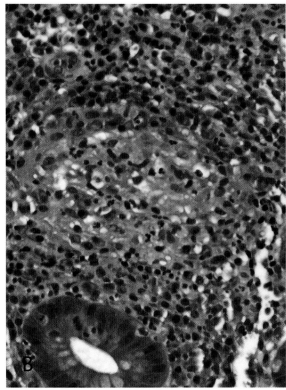

Figure 5-17

ULCERATIVE COLITIS

Crypt rupture with extrusion of mucin into the lamina propria elicits a granulomatous tissue reaction. Aggregates of macrophages contain bubbly cytoplasm and are intimately associated with other types of inflammatory cells. The close proximity of the inflammatory reaction to an injured crypt is a clue to the diagnosis (A). As the inflammatory process heals, granulomatous foci organize so that there are fewer macrophages containing mucin. Unlike Crohn-type granulomas, however, those related to crypt rupture contain granulocytes (B).

Figure 5-18

CHRONIC ILEITIS RELATED TO ULCERATIVE COLITIS

Severe ileal injury with architectural abnormalities, dense plasma cell-rich inflammation, and erosions raise the possibility of Crohn disease. However, these changes are confined to the distal few centimeters of ileum and are superficial, similar to the pattern of ulcerative colitis in the colon. They likely represent an immune-mediated ileitis related to ulcerative colitis.

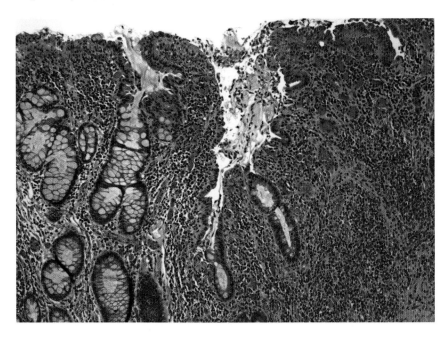

Infections that develop in patients with established inflammatory bowel disease can simulate a colitis flare or masquerade as refractory disease. The two most common organisms causing infections that mimic flares of chronic colitis are cytomegalovirus (CMV) and *Clostridium difficile*. CMV reactivation usually occurs in patients recently exposed to corticosteroid therapy and has become less common in an era of better medical management (39). When present, scattered viral inclusions in endothelial cells are often obscured by dense inflammation; immunohistochemical stains facilitate a diagnosis in areas of intense inflammation (fig. 5-19). Superimposed *C. difficile* infection can elicit characteristic pseudomembranes and necrotic crypts or feature an acute pattern of injury (fig. 5-20).

Treatment and Prognosis. Mild colitic symptoms are commonly managed with topical and/or oral mesalamine or other anti-inflammatory agents. More severe colitis usually requires corticosteroid or tacrolimus therapy to induce remission followed by transition to other medications in order to avoid systemic toxicity (40). Azathioprine and 6-mercaptopurine effectively maintain remission in many patients with moderately active pancolitis, whereas targeted biologic agents are increasingly used to manage severe disease. The latter include antagonists to TNF-α (e.g., infliximab, adalimumab, golimumab, certolizumab) and adhesion molecules (e.g., vedolizumab, natalizumab, etrolizumab), although a number of other drugs are currently under investigation (41). Use of these agents has drastically improved therapeutic response compared with corticosteroids and, as a result, most patients achieve remission in the modern era. Surgical treatment is reserved for patients with medically refractory or fulminant disease, some of whom can develop toxic megacolon and perforation. Inflammation-induced colorectal carcinoma occurs in approximately 5 percent of patients.

Crohn Disease

Definition. *Crohn disease* (also termed *regional enteritis*) is a systemic immune-mediated inflammatory condition with dominant gastrointestinal manifestations that results from a combination of environmental and genetic influences.

Clinical Features. Crohn disease develops in approximately 20 per 100,000 persons in the United States each year and, like ulcerative colitis, is increasing in incidence (42). It displays a bimodal age distribution, with peak incidences in young adulthood and older adults. Patients with Crohn disease typically present with abdominal pain, weight loss, failure to thrive, chronic malabsorption, loose stools, and non-bloody diarrhea, although those with colonic involvement may have bloody diarrhea. Disease of the upper gastrointestinal tract manifests with post-prandial pain, dysphagia, dyspepsia, obstructive symptoms, or bleeding from duodenal-enteric fistulae. Patients with disease of the proximal small intestine have malabsorption of zinc and fat-soluble vitamins. Fibrostenosing ileal disease can produce a tender mass in the right lower quadrant or cause malabsorption of B12 and bile salts.

Extraintestinal manifestations are similar to those of ulcerative colitis. Oral and genital aphthous ulcers tend to be more common in patients with Crohn disease, whereas liver disease is less frequent compared with ulcerative colitis patients.

Patients with active Crohn disease have abnormal laboratory and radiographic findings. Elevated erythrocyte sedimentation rates and C-reactive protein levels reflect gastrointestinal inflammation. Serum anti-*Saccharomyces cerevisiae* antibodies (ASCA) can be detected, especially in patients with severe disease activity or *NOD2* polymorphisms (43,44). Abdominal imaging reveals aphthous and deep ulcers, mucosal abnormalities, obstruction, abscesses, strictures, fistulae, and inflammatory masses. These changes are often accompanied by mesenteric fat stranding and lymphadenopathy.

Pathogenesis. Crohn disease shows familial clustering with a predilection for specific ethnic groups. It is also associated with smoking, increased intake of animal and milk proteins, and an increased ratio of omega-6 to omega-3 polyunsaturated fatty acids (45). The mechanisms by which Crohn disease develops are poorly understood. Most evidence suggests that it occurs following an environmental stimulus in a genetically susceptible host. Presumably, episodes of infectious gastroenteritis due to *Escherichia coli*, mycobacteria, or other bacterial pathogens

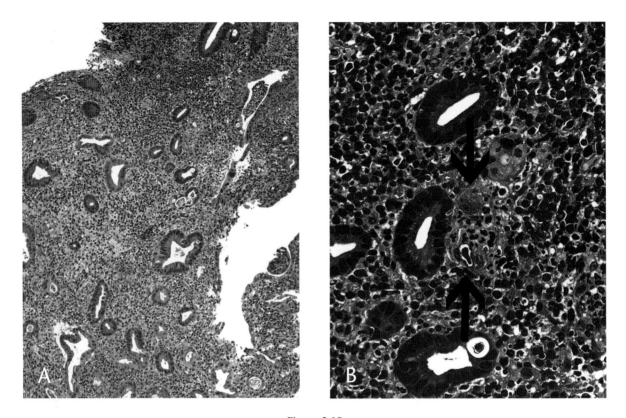

Figure 5-19

CYTOMEGALOVIRUS REACTIVATION IN ULCERATIVE COLITIS

Biopsy samples display diffuse plasma cell-rich inflammation of the lamina propria with a disproportionate amount of crypt destruction and injury (A). Closer examination reveals scattered viral inclusions in endothelial cells (arrows) with characteristic intranuclear inclusions and amphophilic cytoplasm (B).

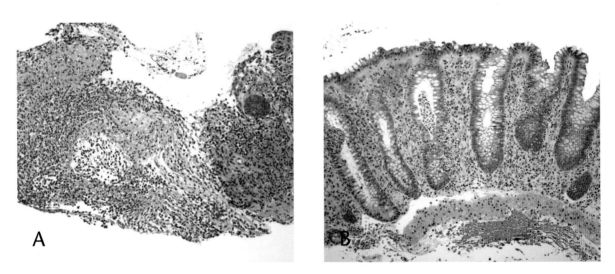

Figure 5-20

CLOSTRIDIUM DIFFICILE SUPERINFECTION IN ULCERATIVE COLITIS

Pseudomembranes are not typical of ulcerative colitis, and when present, should prompt consideration of a superimposed infection (A). *C. difficile* can also elicit an acute pattern of injury in colitic patients (B).

act as a trigger for immune dysregulation in susceptible hosts, resulting in elaboration of pro-inflammatory cytokines that increase mucosal permeability and facilitate transmigration of bacteria and antigens across the mucosa.

Many patients with Crohn disease have underlying polymorphisms affecting *NOD2 (CARD15)* on chromosome 16. This gene encodes nucleotide-binding oligomerization domain-containing protein 2. Monocytes that express this protein enhance B-cell activation through NF-κB signaling upon exposure to bacterial peptidoglycans (46). Other genes implicated in the pathogenesis of Crohn disease include *OCTN3, IL23R, ATG16L1, IRGM,* and *SLC11A1,* which play important roles in macrophage activation, inflammation mediation, and autophagy (47–50). All of these genetic alterations affect adaptive and innate immune responses, particularly those mediated by Th1 cells (51).

Gross Findings. Crohn disease can affect any part of the gastrointestinal tract and displays a patchy distribution. Clinically significant esophageal disease is rare, affecting approximately 1 percent of patients. Gastric erythema is frequently identified, particularly in the antrum; more severe gastric disease may cause gastric outlet obstruction, ulceration, or bleeding. Patchy or segmental ulcers and erythema can occur throughout the duodenum, although involvement of the distal small bowel is most common. Typical features include erythematous, granular mucosa with aphthous erosions or deep longitudinal ulcers with intervening ridges of intact mucosa that impart a cobblestone appearance (fig. 5-21). Pseudopolyps, mural fibrosis, fistulae, and strictures are commonly present.

At least 80 percent of patients with Crohn disease have ileal involvement, most of whom have inflammation confined to the distal ileum and proximal right colon (fig. 5-22). One-fifth of patients have colonic disease alone, which may appear as segmental colitis or superficial pancolitis that simulates ulcerative colitis (fig. 5-23). Patients with anal disease develop large, often multiple, perianal skin tags, as well as fistulous openings onto the skin surface.

Microscopic Findings. Biopsy samples frequently show patchy, variably active chronic inflammation with expansion of the lamina propria by plasma cell-rich inflammation.

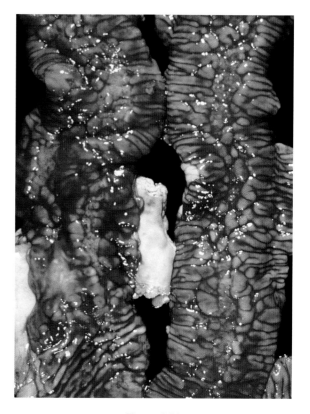

Figure 5-21

SMALL INTESTINAL CROHN DISEASE

A long segment shows mostly preserved mucosal folds along the antimesenteric border, with ulcers and nodularity on the mesenteric aspect of the small bowel.

Approximately 30 percent of cases, particularly those from younger patients, contain non-necrotic epithelioid granulomas that consist of clustered macrophages surrounded by a cuff of lymphocytes (fig. 5-24). Gastric involvement typically features foci of chronic inflammation surrounding individual glands and pits infiltrated by neutrophils. Crohn disease of the duodenum displays variable villous architectural abnormalities; multiple tissue fragments show a spectrum of inflammatory changes (fig. 5-25). Neutrophilic inflammation and ulcers are always accompanied by dense, plasma cell-rich inflammation of the lamina propria (fig. 5-26). Ileal samples show villous architectural abnormalities and patchy chronic inflammation with pseudopyloric metaplasia, goblet cell hyperplasia, and increased Paneth cells in an abnormal distribution (fig. 5-27) (31). Aphthous ulcers appear as thin erosions overlying lymphoid

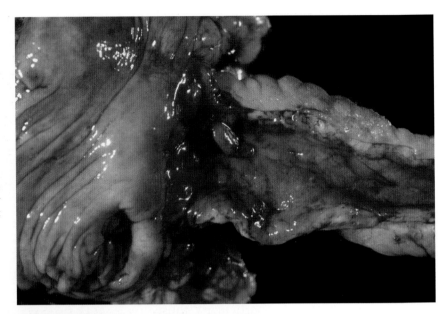

Figure 5-22

FIBROSTENOSING TERMINAL ILEITIS DUE TO CROHN DISEASE

The ileal wall is thickened and surrounded by creeping fat. The mucosal folds are effaced; patchy ulcers are present. The adjacent colonic mucosa (left) is normal.

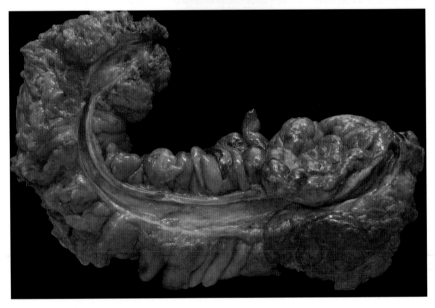

Figure 5-23

CROHN COLITIS

This segment of narrowed sigmoid colon shows abundant creeping fat and loss of the transverse mucosal folds. A stricture is present in the upper rectum (right).

aggregates (fig. 5-28). Features of Crohn disease in colonic biopsy samples are similar to those of ulcerative colitis, although the infiltrates tend to be patchy in tissue samples obtained from different sites, multiple samples obtained from the same region, or even in a single tissue fragment (fig. 5-29).

Although some patients with Crohn disease develop superficial colitis with limited involvement of the muscularis propria, most resection specimens show evidence of mural injury (32). Deep ulcers, fissures, and fistulae are lined by granulation tissue and granulomatous in-

flammation associated with fecal material (fig. 5-30A,B). The wall displays variable fibrosis, neuronal hypertrophy, and fibromuscularization of the submucosa. The muscularis mucosae and muscularis propria are often thicker than normal; the former may show splaying around the deep crypts (fig. 5-30C). Mural lymphoid aggregates are present around ulcers, subjacent to intact mucosae, and in subserosal fat (fig. 5-30D). Occasional cases show granulomatous vasculitis with giant cells and fibrinoid necrosis; this finding is generally unaccompanied by systemic manifestations of vasculitis (fig. 5-31) (52).

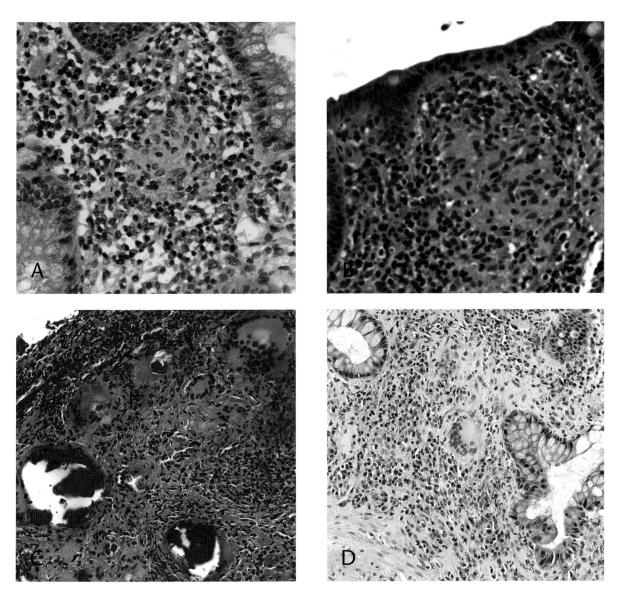

Figure 5-24

CROHN DISEASE

Non-necrotic epithelioid granulomas consist of tight macrophage aggregates surrounded by lymphocytes (A). Granulomas may be located anywhere in the mucosa, bowel wall, or regional lymph nodes (B). Older granulomas contain round calcifications, which are often numerous (C). Isolated giant cells may be present in the mucosae of patients with Crohn disease but are non-specific; they may also be seen in association with any type of colonic injury that causes crypt rupture (D).

Differential Diagnosis. Crohn disease is a diagnosis of exclusion and should only be considered after eliminating the possibilities of infection, medication-related injury, and other immune-mediated disorders. Bacterial or parasitic infections, medications (e.g., NSAIDs), radiation injury, and ischemia may cause patchy or segmental enterocolitis and mimic the histologic appearance of Crohn disease in biopsy or resection specimens. *Salmonella* and *Yersinia* produce a predominantly right-sided colitis characterized by mononuclear cell-rich inflammation of the lamina propria. Chronic radiation and ischemic injury induce mucosal atrophy, pseudopyloric metaplasia, fissures, fibrosis, and lymphoid aggregates.

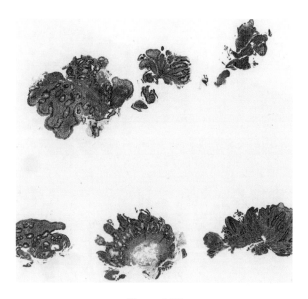

Figure 5-25

CROHN DISEASE OF THE DUODENUM

Multiple tissue fragments obtained from the same area show variability with respect to mucosal inflammation and architectural distortion.

Treatment and Prognosis. Similar to ulcerative colitis, aminosalicylates may adequately control mild Crohn disease. Remission of moderate to severe enterocolitis is induced with corticosteroids or cyclosporine. Most patients are then offered more powerful immunomodulatory and biologic agents that can profoundly alter the natural history of disease. Antagonists to TNF-α (e.g., infliximab, adalimumab, golimumab, certolizumab), adhesion molecules (e.g., vedolizumab, natalizumab, etrolizumab), and interleukins (e.g., ustekinumab) are highly effective in maintaining remission in affected patients, especially when combined with azathioprine or mercaptopurine (53,54). Surgery is reserved for patients with complex fistulae, organizing abscesses, perforation, obstruction, dysplasia, and carcinoma. Localized stenosing disease can be managed with stricturoplasty or endoscopic techniques to preserve the small bowel mucosa (55,56).

Patients with Crohn disease are at risk for internal and external fistulae to the bowel, vagina, bladder, anus, or abdominal wall. Complications of poorly controlled symptoms are related to chronic malabsorption and poor nutritional status, which may result in death. Patients treated with long-term biologic agents are at increased risk for disseminated infections due to mycobacteria and histoplasmosis (57,58). Those managed with a combination of biologic agents and immunomodulatory therapy may develop hepatosplenic gamma-delta T-cell lymphoma (58). Short-gut syndrome and extensive abdominal adhesions are more common in individuals who undergo multiple abdominal surgeries and extensive removal of the small bowel. Patients with Crohn disease may also develop dysplasia and carcinoma, albeit the risk is generally lower than that of patients with ulcerative colitis.

Pouch Inflammation Following Ileal Pouch-Anal Anastomosis

Definition. A constellation of clinical symptoms, endoscopic abnormalities, and histologic active (i.e., neutrophilic) inflammation of ileal pouch mucosa can occur after ileal pouch anastomosis.

Clinical Features. Ileal pouch-anal anastomosis is a common procedure performed following complete proctocolectomy for ulcerative colitis and familial adenomatous polyposis. The procedure entails creation of an ileal reservoir that mimics the rectal ampulla. This pouch usually has a "J" configuration. The afferent ileal limb represents the long arm and the short arm is the blind-ended efferent limb. The base of the reservoir is sewn to the proximal aspect of the anal sphincter, which is surfaced by a thin cuff of rectal mucosa. Inflammation can occur in the afferent limb (i.e., *pre-pouch ileitis*), the pouch mucosa (i.e., *pouchitis*), or residual rectal mucosa (i.e., *cuffitis*). Inflammation of the rectal cuff is usually attributed to underlying ulcerative colitis.

Pouchitis occurs almost exclusively in patients with ulcerative colitis; clinically significant inflammation of the pouch mucosa in patients with familial adenomatous polyposis is usually secondary to infection, medication-related injury, tension on the pouch, vascular compromise, or post-surgical strictures (60). Crohn disease is generally considered a contraindication to this procedure because it is associated with high complication rates. Overall, at least 50 percent of ulcerative colitis patients develop at least one episode of pouchitis following ileal pouch construction and 10 to 15 percent develop severe or recurrent pouchitis (61).

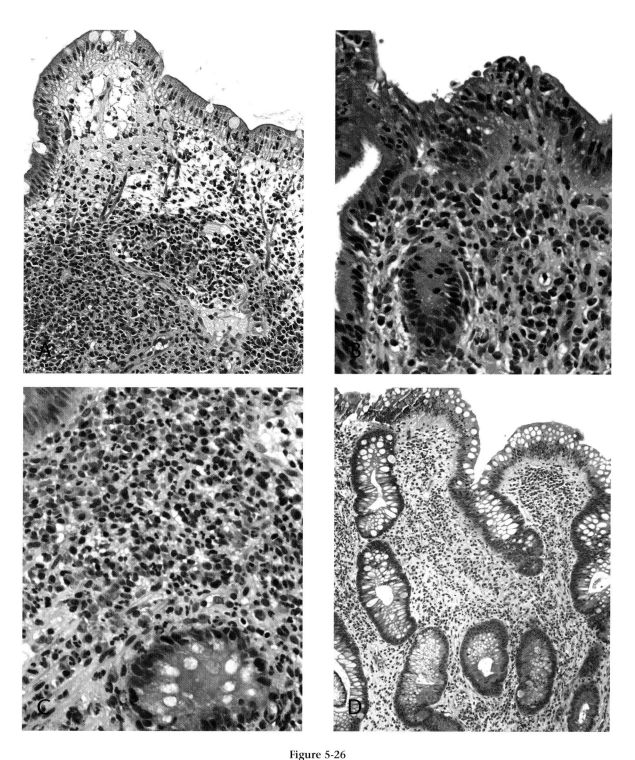

Figure 5-26

CROHN DISEASE OF THE DUODENUM

Active disease can cause villous architectural abnormalities accompanied by mucosal edema and plasma cell-rich lamina propria inflammation (A). Neutrophilic inflammation of the surface epithelium is associated with crypt injury (B). Lamina propria neutrophils tend to be more pronounced around crypts (C). Villous abnormalities are accompanied by goblet cell hyperplasia, Paneth cell hyperplasia, and variability in crypt architecture (D).

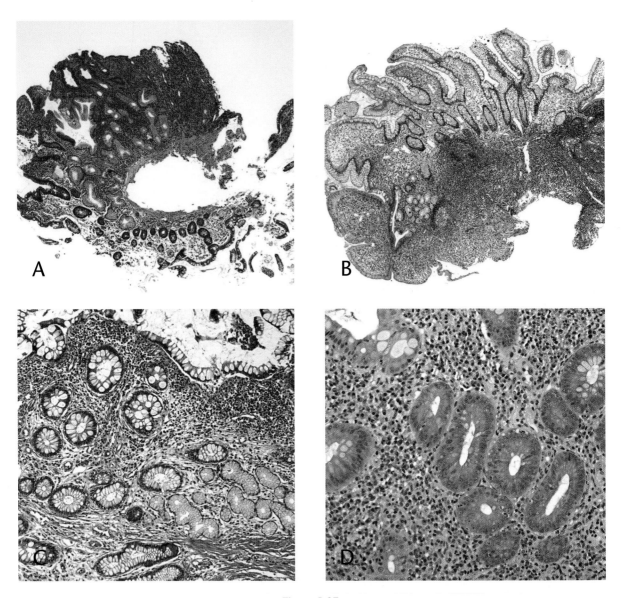

Figure 5-27

CROHN DISEASE OF THE ILEUM

Inflammation is often patchy, even in a single tissue fragment. Part of the tissue fragment is infiltrated by dense plasma cell-rich inflammation and shows pseudopyloric metaplasia, whereas other areas are spared (A). Villous abnormalities include broad, distended villi lined by increased numbers of goblet cells. Hyperplasia of the muscularis mucosae with splaying of its inner layer into the lamina propria is accompanied by pseudopyloric metaplasia of the crypts (B). Some crypts have a horizontal configuration and contain increased numbers of Paneth cells (C). Plasma cell-rich inflammation expands the mucosa and is associated with neutrophilic cryptitis (D).

Risk factors include severe pancolitis with fissuring ulcers, inflammation of the terminal ileum or appendix in colectomy specimens, primary sclerosing cholangitis, tobacco use, and elevated serum ANCA levels (34,35). Symptoms include increased frequency of bowel movements, which are often loose, tenesmus, and bloody stools, accompanied by fevers and malaise. Pre-pouch ileitis is a common finding, occurring in 13 percent of patients with pouchitis. It may reflect a medication injury or recurrence of inflammatory bowel disease in the ileal mucosa, but does not imply a diagnosis of Crohn disease or have any association with pouch failure (62).

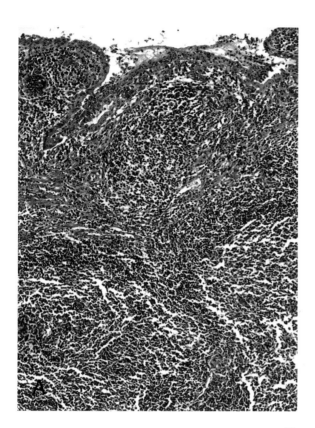
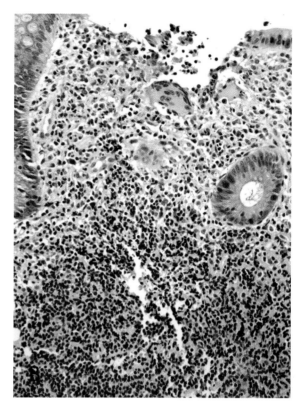

Figure 5-28

APHTHOUS ULCERS OF CROHN DISEASE

Aphthous erosions appear as a thin layer of inflamed granulation tissue overlying lymphoid aggregates (A). Right: Some contain scattered giant cells and scant inflammatory debris (B).

Pathogenesis. Pouchitis develops as a result of host and environmental influences. Immunologic alterations associated with luminal stasis alter the composition of bacterial flora in the pouch. Patients with acute pouchitis have increased *Clostridia* species, whereas those with chronic pouchitis have more numerous *Staphylococcus aureus* in stool samples (63). Presumably, increased numbers of pro-inflammatory bacterial species cause direct mucosal injury and alter homeostasis with respect to metabolism of intraluminal sugars to short-chain fatty acids, the primary nutrients of enterocytes. Mucosal inflammation leads to increased pouch output, further diluting short-chain fatty acids in the pouch reservoir and promoting enterocyte injury.

Gross Findings. The inflamed ileal pouch is lined by erythematous, granular mucosa with increased friability and edema. More severe disease manifests with hemorrhage, superficial erosions, and ulcers that may be surfaced with pseudomem-branes (fig. 5-32A). Pseudopolyps and loss of the mucosal vascular pattern can develop in patients with persistent inflammation (fig. 5-32B).

Microscopic Findings. Biopsy samples from ileal pouches of asymptomatic patients with ulcerative colitis often show mucosal remodeling, which does not necessarily imply the presence of pouchitis. The villi tend to be blunter than those of the normal ileum and contain increased mononuclear cell-rich inflammation (fig. 5-33). Pseudopyloric metaplasia of the crypt epithelium and increased numbers of Paneth cells are common, especially in samples obtained from patients with recurrent bouts of pouch inflammation (fig. 5-34A). Patients with pouchitis have increased plasma cell-rich inflammation in the lamina propria as well as neutrophilic cryptitis. Moderate to severe pouchitis features more extensive neutrophilic infiltration of the surface epithelium, erosions, and crypt abscesses with destruction (fig. 5-34B).

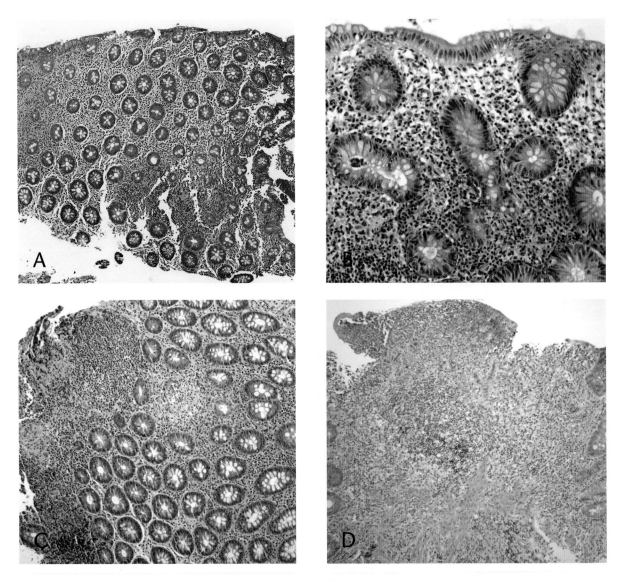

Figure 5-29

CROHN COLITIS

Unlike ulcerative colitis, which generally involves tissue fragments in a diffuse fashion, Crohn disease is often patchy. Several foci of enhanced lamina propria cellularity surround crypts (A) and contain a combination of mononuclear cells and neutrophils associated with cryptitis (B). Microscopic areas of crypt destruction are surrounded by nearly normal crypts (C). Aphthous ulcers are often present in severe disease (D).

Treatment and Prognosis. Initial treatment of pouchitis and pre-pouch ileitis consists of antibiotic therapy (64). Antibiotic-resistant cases may be treated with anti-inflammatory agents and corticosteroids, although azathioprine and biologic agents can also be used for long-term maintenance (65,66). Short-chain fatty acids and stool transplantation are variably successful in reducing symptoms of patients with mild inflammation.

Pouch failure is an uncommon occurrence, affecting less than 1 percent of patients who undergo ileal pouch-anal anastomosis. Dysplasia and adenocarcinoma of the pouch mucosa are extremely uncommon but well-recognized complications. The residual cuff of rectal mucosa is

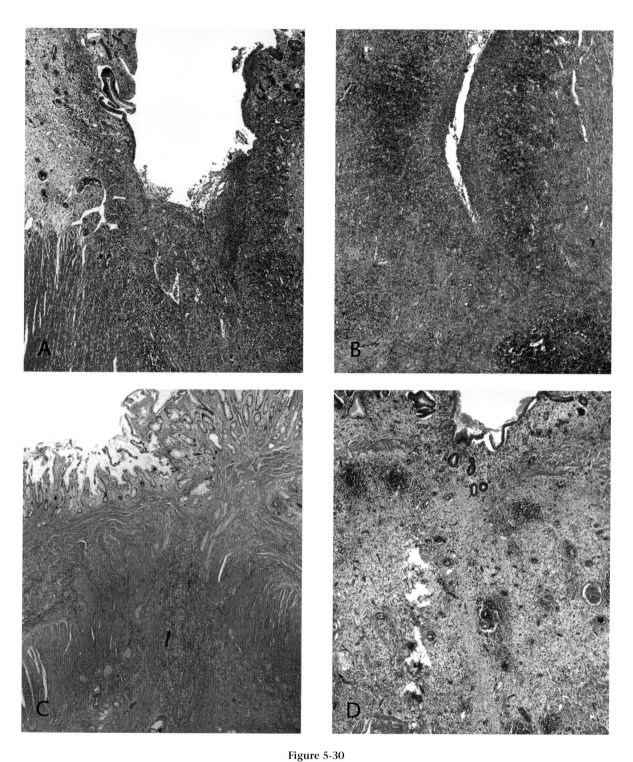

Figure 5-30

CROHN DISEASE

Resection specimens from patients with Crohn disease demonstrate the mural nature of disease. Sharply demarcated ulcers extend into the muscularis propria (A). Fissures and fistulae are lined by chronically inflamed granulation tissue (B). Ulcers heal with fibrosis and smooth muscle hyperplasia of the submucosa with loss of the muscularis propria (C). Lymphoid aggregates are present at all levels in the bowel wall (D).

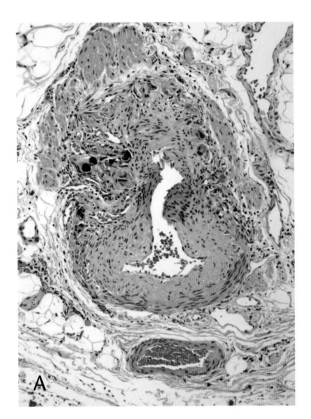
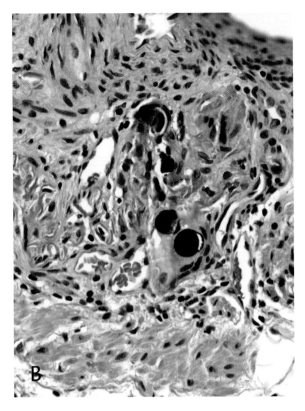

Figure 5-31

CROHN DISEASE

Occasional resection specimens from patients with Crohn disease display a localized vasculitis that affects medium-sized and large arteries. Calcifications are associated with inflammation of the arterial wall (A) with scattered giant cells (B).

also at increased risk for neoplasia, and thus, requires regular surveillance.

Collagenous Colitis

Definition. *Collagenous colitis (microscopic colitis)* is a clinicopathologic entity characterized by normal colonoscopic findings and microscopically visible chronic colitis with subepithelial collagen deposition.

Clinical Features. Collagenous colitis is a fairly common disorder, affecting approximately 5 per 100,000 persons in the United States each year (67). The disease is more common in middle-aged adults and shows a striking predilection for women. Patients typically present with chronic, watery, non-bloody diarrhea with a mean of eight stools per day, increased urgency and incontinence, and frequent nocturnal stooling. Other symptoms include crampy abdominal pain, weight loss, fatigue, and bloating. Many cases masquerade as irritable bowel syndrome, resulting in a delayed diagnosis. Laboratory studies are frequently normal, although some patients have increased fecal white blood cells.

Pathogenesis. Collagenous colitis is classified as one of the non-destructive chronic colitides. It is likely the result of an immune-mediated phenomenon, although a unifying pathogenetic mechanism for all cases is lacking. Many patients report taking NSAIDs, selective serotonin reuptake inhibitors, or sartans (68). There is clearly an association between collagenous colitis and idiopathic inflammatory bowel disease; patients with collagenous colitis who progress to ulcerative colitis or Crohn disease have similar immune cell populations in their colonic mucosae (69).

Gross Findings. Colonoscopy typically reveals normal colonic mucosa, although mild abnormalities may be seen in some patients. Approximately 33 percent of patients have endoscopically apparent erythema, mucosal

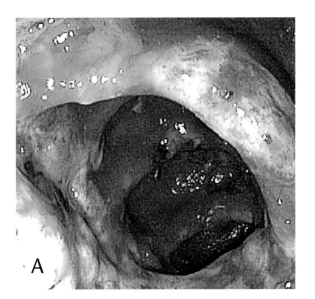
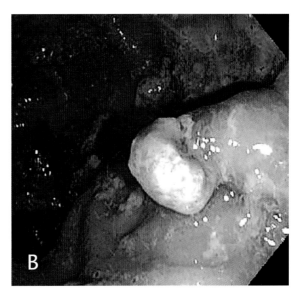

Figure 5-32

POUCHITIS

The diagnosis of pouchitis requires a combination of clinical and histologic abnormalities. Endoscopy reveals shallow ulcers and exudates (A). Pseudopolyps are present in some cases, especially when patients have recurrent bouts of inflammation (B).

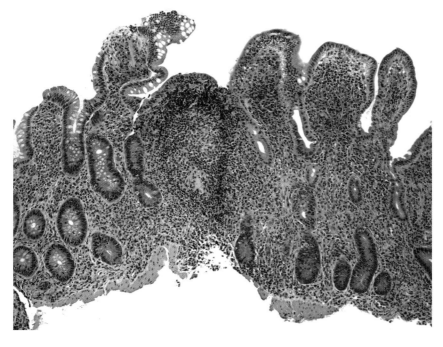

Figure 5-33

ILEAL POUCH MUCOSA

Patients who undergo ileal pouch-anal anastomosis for ulcerative colitis often have biopsy samples that show mucosal remodeling. The villi tend to be short and expanded by mononuclear cell-rich inflammation. The presence of these changes in the absence of cryptitis should not be interpreted as pouchitis.

friability, or ulcers (70). Linear mucosal tears may be evident in some cases, presumably reflecting the fragility of the fibrotic mucosa. Pseudomembranes are occasionally identified, even in patients without *C. difficile* infection.

Microscopic Findings. The histologic abnormalities of collagenous colitis tend to be more prominent in the proximal colon and include a diffuse mixed inflammatory infiltrate in the lamina propria, crypt and surface epithelial cell injury, and expansion of the subepithelial collagen layer (fig. 5-35). The collagen layer is usually over 10 μm thick and has an irregular interface with the lamina propria. It contains capillaries, inflamma-

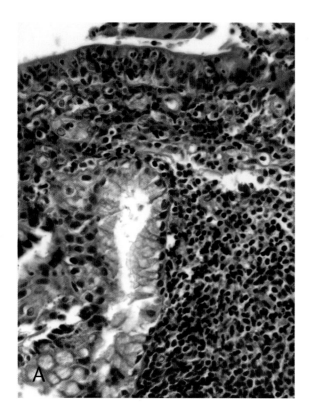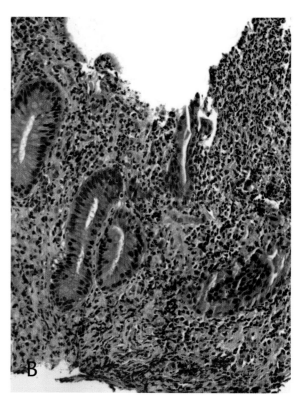

Figure 5-34

POUCHITIS

A histologic diagnosis of pouchitis requires neutrophilic inflammation of crypt and surface epithelium. Pseudopyloric metaplasia is commonly present in samples obtained from patients with recurrent or chronic pouchitis but this feature should not be interpreted as evidence of Crohn disease (A). Severe pouchitis features erosions, cryptitis, and crypt destruction (B).

tory cells, and apoptotic debris. Patchy mononuclear cell inflammation in crypt epithelium is accompanied by eosinophils and neutrophils. The surface epithelium is frequently inflamed, attenuated, or detached from the lamina propria. Neutrophilic inflammation, pseudomembranes, and ulcers have been described in association with NSAID use, *C. difficile* infection, and other bacterial pathogens, but their presence does not necessarily imply the presence of a superimposed process (fig. 5-36) (71). Paneth cell metaplasia and occasional branched crypts may be present but are of no prognostic significance (72).

Differential Diagnosis. Collagenous colitis is an idiopathic disorder and, thus, the diagnosis is one of exclusion. It should be distinguished from the prominent basement membrane-like material that is commonly encountered in biopsy samples from the left colon and hyperplastic polyps (fig. 5-37A). Samples from the left colon

can normally feature a thick, glassy band of eosinophilic material that has a smooth interface with the subjacent lamina propria.

Radiation-induced mucosal injury can result in subepithelial collagen deposition with entrapped vessels and inflammatory cells (fig. 5-37B). However, collagen is also present throughout the lamina propria, particularly around ectatic mucosal vessels. It is unaccompanied by mononuclear cell-rich infiltrates in the lamina propria and lacks inflammatory cells in the surface epithelium.

Occasional cases of systemic amyloidosis show a predominantly subepithelial distribution of deposits that simulates the appearance of collagen. These deposits have a nodular appearance and smooth interface with the lamina propria (fig. 5-37C). A Congo red histochemical stain facilitates distinction from subepithelial collagen (fig. 5-37D).

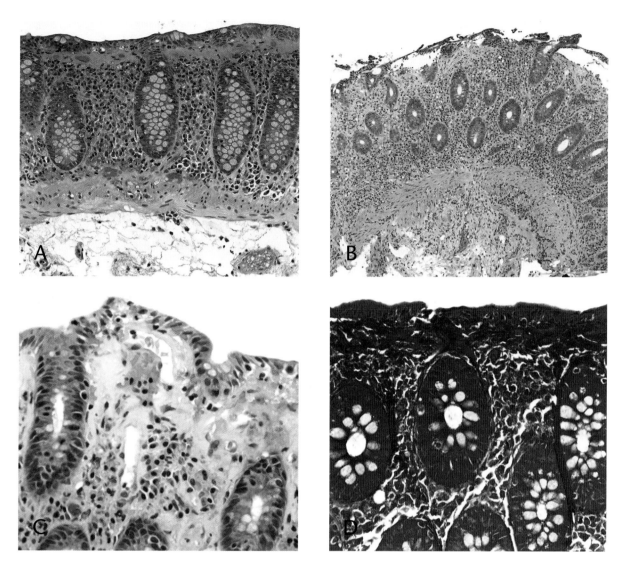

Figure 5-35

COLLAGENOUS COLITIS

Collagenous colitis features mononuclear cell-rich infiltrates that expand the lamina propria, particularly the upper mucosa, accompanied by subepithelial collagen deposition (A). Damage to the superficial epithelium leads to its frequent detachment from the rest of the mucosa (B). The subepithelial collagen layer displays an irregular interface with the subjacent lamina propria and contains entrapped capillaries and inflammatory cells (C). Trichrome histochemical stains highlight collagen deposits and entrapped elements (D).

Treatment and Prognosis. Patients with mild symptoms are managed with cholestyramine, loperamide, diphenoxylate/atropine, and bismuth subsalicylate. Budesonide is generally reserved for patients with moderate to severe symptoms, and patients with severe debilitating diarrhea can be offered immunomodulatory or biologic agents similar to regimens used to control idiopathic inflammatory bowel disease (73). Some patients with collagenous colitis develop colonic perforation at the time of, or soon after, colonoscopic examination (fig. 5-38) (70,74).

There is an association between collagenous colitis and idiopathic inflammatory bowel disease. Some patients with collagenous colitis develop ulcerative colitis or Crohn disease and some with established idiopathic inflammatory

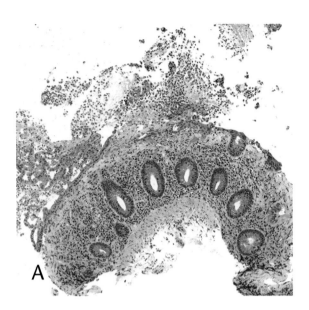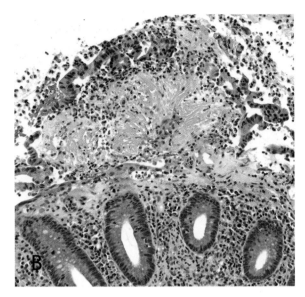

Figure 5-36

COLLAGENOUS COLITIS WITH PSEUDOMEMBRANES

Inflammatory exudates and pseudomembranes are present over an erosion (A). Exudates contain detached degenerated epithelial cells, fibrin, and inflammatory cells (B).

bowel disease have collagenous colitis-type changes in individual biopsy samples (69).

Lymphocytic Colitis

Definition. *Lymphocytic colitis* is characterized by normal colonoscopic findings and microscopically evident chronic colitis with intraepithelial lymphocytosis. Synonyms include *microscopic colitis* and *Brainerd diarrhea*.

Clinical Features. Lymphocytic colitis occurs at rates comparable to those of collagenous colitis, affecting 3 to 6 per 100,000 persons in the United States each year (67). The disease is more common in older adults; cases in young adults and children are usually related to celiac disease. Lymphocytic colitis affects men more commonly than collagenous colitis but still shows a predilection for women (75).

Patients present with chronic, watery, nonbloody diarrhea similar to individuals affected by collagenous colitis. Many have coexisting immune-mediated thyroiditis, arthritis, or other autoimmune disorders. Approximately 30 percent of patients have celiac disease. Laboratory studies are frequently normal, although some patients have increased fecal white blood cells.

Pathogenesis. Lymphocytic colitis is a nondestructive chronic colitis of unclear etiology.

Most cases are idiopathic and immune-mediated, whereas others have been attributed to unidentified infectious causes. Occasional outbreaks of colitis with clinical and pathologic features of lymphocytic colitis have been described and are likely related to an infectious agent, although no causative organism has been reported to date (76,77). Lymphocytic colitis can also develop following an episode of infectious diarrhea secondary to *Campylobacter*, *Yersinia*, and other organisms (78). Rare cases progress to destructive chronic colitis (i.e., ulcerative colitis and Crohn disease) over time (32).

Medications have been implicated in the pathogenesis of lymphocytic colitis. Some authors suggest that NSAIDs and proton pump inhibitors increase mucosal permeability, allowing passage of antigens into the mucosa and recruitment of intraepithelial lymphocytes (79). Other reported medication associations include selective serotonin reuptake inhibitors, β-blockers, HMG-CoA reductase inhibitors, and bisphosphonates (68).

Gross Findings. Most patients have normal endoscopic findings. Patchy erythema or granularity may be detected in a minority of patients (fig. 5-39). Similar to collagenous colitis, lymphocytic colitis tends to affect the abdominal

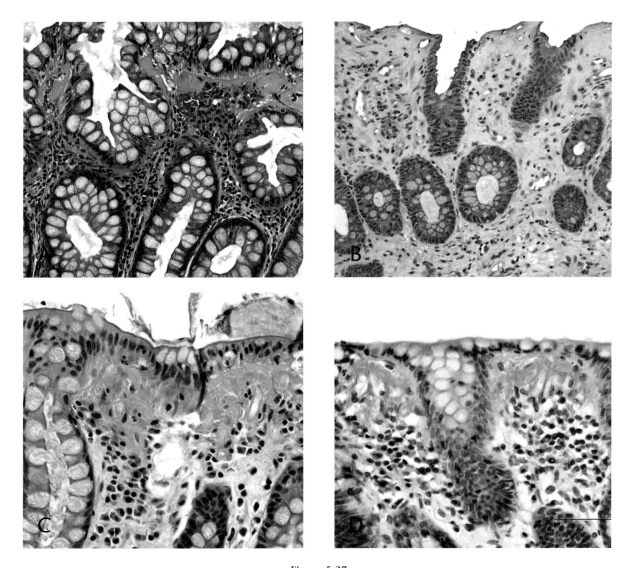

Figure 5-37

DIFFERENTIAL DIAGNOSIS OF COLLAGENOUS COLITIS

The colonic basement membrane is often prominent in the distal colorectum of left-sided hyperplastic polyps. Unlike collagenous colitis, these samples feature a homogeneous band of eosinophilic material that shows a smooth interface with the underlying lamina propria (A). Radiation-induced colopathy features lamina propria fibrosis that can be more pronounced around crypts and under the surface epithelium. However, there is no abrupt transition between these areas and the rest of the lamina propria, which tends to be pauci-inflammatory (B). Amyloid deposits are rarely confined to a subepithelial location. They tend to have a nodular appearance and lack vascular ingrowth (C). A Congo red stain helps distinguish amyloid from collagen (D). (C,D: courtesy of Dr. J. Hart, Chicago, IL.)

colon, particularly the proximal colon. Failure to detect the disease upon flexible sigmoidoscopy does not exclude the diagnosis.

Microscopic Findings. The diagnosis of lymphocytic colitis requires two components: mononuclear cell-rich inflammation of the lamina propria with numerous plasma cells and intraepithelial lymphocytosis. Intraepithelial lymphocytes tend to be most pronounced in the surface epithelium where they are associated with cytoplasmic depletion and other features of epithelial cell injury. There is no subepithelial collagen deposition. Lamina propria inflammation is more pronounced beneath the surface, producing a "blue band" upon low-power examination (fig. 5-40). The crypts are of normal

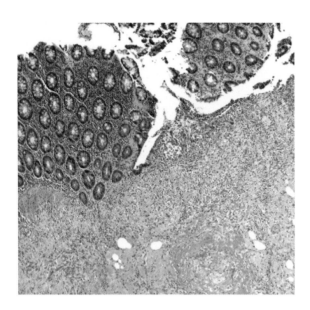

Figure 5-38

COLLAGENOUS COLITIS

Perforation is a rare complication of collagenous colitis. It tends to occur following colonoscopy or other instrumentation. Deep, sharply demarcated ulcers are associated with an inflammatory reaction. Subepithelial collagen and lamina propria inflammation are evident in the adjacent mucosa.

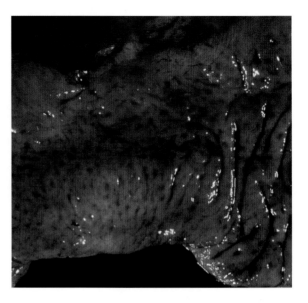

Figure 5-39

LYMPHOCYTIC COLITIS

This patient underwent colectomy for intractable diarrhea due to lymphocytic colitis. The mucosa shows patchy erythema and slightly flattened folds but is otherwise unremarkable.

length and distribution. Although occasional branched crypts and foci of cellular metaplasia may be observed, they are not prominent and their presence does not predict ultimate development of idiopathic inflammatory bowel disease (72). Neutrophils may be present in low numbers in the lamina propria and rarely within the crypts. More than occasional foci of neutrophilic cryptitis should prompt concern for an alternative diagnosis.

Differential Diagnosis. Lymphocytic colitis should be distinguished from colonic lymphocytosis, which features increased intraepithelial lymphocytes unassociated with chronic colitis. Colonic lymphocytosis is a non-specific finding that may be seen in patients with celiac disease, resolving acute colitis, and a variety of medication-related injuries (fig. 5-41). As discussed in chapter 4, several medications, particularly targeted agents and checkpoint inhibitors, can cause colonic injury that simulates lymphocytic colitis. Most of these also induce crypt cell apoptosis, which is not a prominent feature of lymphocytic colitis.

Treatment and Prognosis. Patients are managed similar to those with collagenous colitis. Cholestyramine, loperamide, diphenoxylate/atropine, and bismuth subsalicylate are used to control mild diarrheal symptoms. Budesonide is an effective alternative for patients with moderate symptoms, whereas severe debilitating diarrhea may require more powerful medications such as immunomodulatory or biologic agents (73). Similar to collagenous colitis, some patients with lymphocytic colitis may develop other forms of chronic colitis, including collagenous colitis, ulcerative colitis, and Crohn disease (69).

Eosinophilic Gastroenteritis

Definition. *Eosinophilic gastroenteritis* is a hypersensitivity disorder characterized by eosinophil-rich inflammation in one or more segments of the gastrointestinal tract. It is also termed *allergic gastroenteritis*.

Clinical Features. Eosinophilic gastroenteritis affects males more than females, and particularly children and young adults. Most patients have a history of hypersensitivity with atopic dermatitis, asthma, and allergies. Presenting symptoms include dysphagia, abdominal pain,

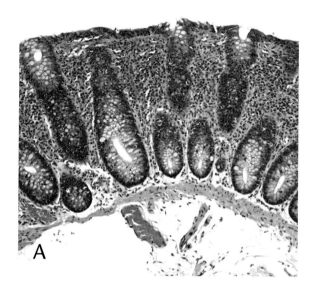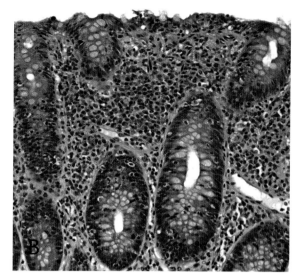

Figure 5-40

LYMPHOCYTIC COLITIS

The lamina propria is expanded by a plasma cell-rich infiltrate that is most prominent in the superficial mucosa. The crypt architecture is preserved (A). Numerous intraepithelial lymphocytes are present in the crypt and surface epithelium (B).

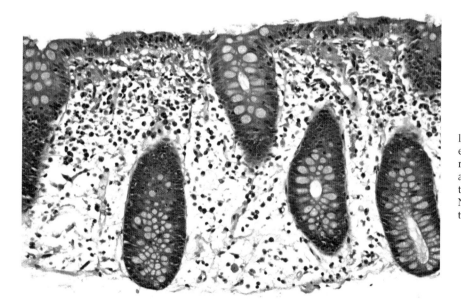

Figure 5-41

COLONIC LYMPHOCYTOSIS

Increased intraepithelial lymphocytes in the surface epithelium is a nonspecific response to a variety of injuries and should not be considered to represent lymphocytic colitis. Note the normal cellularity of the lamina propria.

nausea, vomiting, malabsorptive diarrhea, and rectal bleeding. Infants and small children may present with failure to thrive. Some patients with mural involvement of the gastrointestinal tract present with ascites and abdominal distention (80). Peripheral eosinophilia, elevated serum IgE levels, positive skin test responses to food antigens, and iron deficiency anemia are common laboratory abnormalities.

Pathogenesis. Eosinophilic gastroenteritis has been historically classified as mucosal, mural, or serosal, although these variants are likely unrelated (81). Mucosal eosinophilic gastroenteritis is a hypersensitivity disorder similar to eosinophilic esophagitis and, despite its name, may involve the full thickness of the intestinal wall (82). Most examples of eosinophilic gastroenteritis that spare the mucosa (i.e., mural

367

and serosal variants) can be attributed to other etiologies, as described below (83,84).

Gross Findings. Esophageal involvement by eosinophilic gastroenteritis is endoscopically similar to eosinophilic esophagitis; distinguishing these entities requires sampling of the remaining gastrointestinal tract. Eosinophilic gastroenteritis frequently involves the gastric antrum and small bowel, causing mild inflammatory changes. Colorectal involvement is less common and features mild, non-specific abnormalities with patchy erythema or erosions.

Microscopic Findings. Extensive sampling is often required to establish a diagnosis of eosinophilic gastroenteritis because eosinophils show a patchy distribution. Clustered and degranulated eosinophils expand the lamina propria and infiltrate the epithelium (fig. 5-42A,B). Their presence in the muscularis mucosae is a helpful clue (fig. 5-42C). Small bowel biopsy samples may also feature partial or complete villous blunting with crypt hyperplasia and intraepithelial lymphocytosis, simulating the features of celiac disease. Resection specimens feature diffuse eosinophilic infiltration of the submucosa and muscularis propria accompanied by edema (fig. 5-42D).

In contrast to mucosal eosinophilic gastroenteritis, the mural and serosal forms are not associated with hypersensitivity. Most reported cases of "mural eosinophilic gastroenteritis" show a predilection for the pre-pyloric antrum and many have been reported to respond to *H. pylori* therapy, suggesting they are related to peptic ulcer disease (84–86). Other cases represent inflammatory fibroid polyps, Crohn disease, radiation injury, or infections with parasites or specific fungi that elicit eosinophilia.

Reported cases of the serosal variant describe eosinophil-rich ascites and variable bowel wall thickening. A lack of cohesive clinical and laboratory findings suggests that "serosal eosinophilic gastroenteritis" results from multiple different etiologies. Anisakiasis and metal allergies that manifest following abdominal surgery with stapling devices are common causes of serosal eosinophilia (fig. 5-43) (87–90). For these reasons, other entities should be rigorously excluded before considering a diagnosis of mural or serosal eosinophilic gastroenteritis.

Treatment and Prognosis. The diagnosis of eosinophilic gastroenteritis should be made in the appropriate clinical setting and supported by laboratory findings. Treatment consists of an elimination diet with, or without, systemic corticosteroid therapy. Leukotriene receptor antagonists have shown promise as second-line agents for patients with relapsing disease (91).

Autoimmune Enteropathy

Definition. *Autoimmune enteropathy* is an immune-mediated gastroenteritis characterized by destruction of specialized epithelial cells.

Clinical Features. Autoimmune enteropathy is an umbrella term encompassing a heterogeneous group of disorders that share similar symptoms, laboratory findings, and pathologic features in biopsy samples. Its overall incidence is less than 1 per 100,000 children and it is even rarer in adults. The disease usually manifests in young children but can present at any age, including older adults. More than 80 percent of patients have other immune-mediated disorders, such as rheumatoid arthritis, myasthenia gravis, psoriatic arthritis, hypothyroidism, autoimmune myopathies, idiopathic thrombocytopenic purpura, and Raynaud phenomenon (92). Approximately 80 percent of patients have autoantibodies to enterocytes, goblet cells, parietal cells, and islet cells; antinuclear antibodies are commonly present (93). Five diagnostic criteria for autoimmune enteropathy have been proposed: 1) chronic diarrhea (over 6 weeks), 2) malabsorption, 3) characteristic histologic abnormalities in duodenal biopsy samples, 4) exclusion of other causes of enteritis, and 5) anti-enterocyte or anti-goblet cell antibodies (93,94).

Autoimmune enteropathies are classified by their clinical presentations and associated disorders (95). Pediatric disease generally presents within the first 6 months of life with life-threatening diarrhea (96,97). Pediatric autoimmune enteropathy can be confined to the gastrointestinal tract (i.e., primary disease) or manifest as one component of a syndrome. *Immune dysregulation, polyendocrinopathy,* and *X-linked* (IPEX) *syndrome* are due to *FOXP3* mutations on the X chromosome (i.e., *autoimmune polyendocrinopathy syndrome-type 3)*, whereas *autoimmune polyendocrinopathies, mucocutaneous candidiasis,* and *ectodermal dystrophy* (APECED) *syndrome* (i.e., *autoimmune polyendocrinopathy syndrome-type 1)* are usually inherited as an

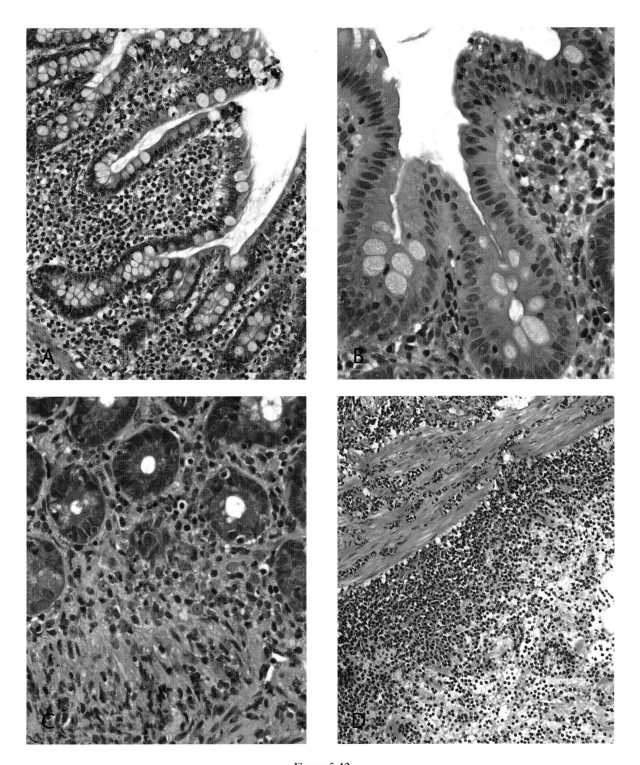

Figure 5-42

EOSINOPHILIC GASTROENTERITIS

Numerous intact and degranulated eosinophils are present in the small bowel (A) and colonic mucosa (B). Eosinophilic infiltration of the muscularis mucosae is a helpful diagnostic clue (C). The disorder usually causes more severe inflammatory changes in the mucosa but can involve the muscularis propria and subserosa (D).

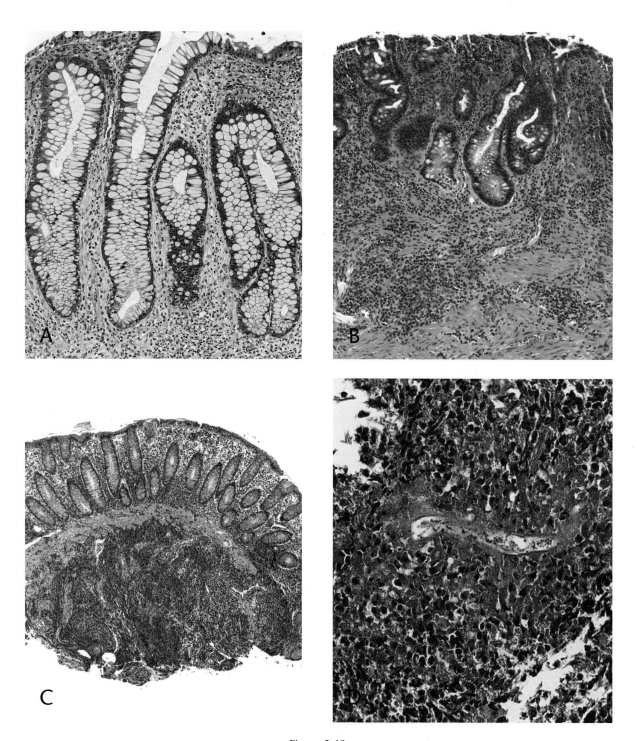

Figure 5-43

DIFFERENTIAL DIAGNOSIS OF EOSINOPHILIC GASTROENTERITIS

Eosinophilic gastroenteritis is a diagnosis of exclusion. Biopsy samples from this patient were initially interpreted to represent eosinophilic gastroenteritis but ultimately proved to represent strongyloidiasis due to underlying common variable immunodeficiency. There is diffuse mucosal eosinophilia without plasma cells (A). Eosinophils are often present in patients with ulcerative colitis, particularly in the right colon. Plasma cells are prominent in the background (B). Aggregates of eosinophils should suggest parasitic infection, especially when located in the deep mucosa or submucosa (C). Deeper tissue levels demonstrated strongyloidiasis in this case (D).

autosomal recessive disorders due to defective *AIRE* (98,99). Both of these genetic variants of autoimmune polyendocrinopathy syndromes feature other immune-mediated diseases, including thyroiditis, Addison disease, diabetes mellitus, hemolytic anemia, mucocutaneous manifestations, and recurrent infections (100). The classification of autoimmune polyendocrinopathy syndromes is summarized in Table 5-2.

Autoimmune enteropathy can occur in adult patients. Some patients with germline *AIRE* mutations develop symptoms in adolescence or young adulthood. However, most older patients with clinical and pathologic features of adult-onset autoimmune enteropathy ultimately prove to have a medication-related injury. Offending drugs include olmesartan and related agents, immunomodulators and checkpoint inhibitors, and some immunosuppressive drugs, as described in chapter 4. Adults may also develop autoimmune enteropathy as a paraneoplastic condition or in association with thymoma. The latter has been termed *thymoma-associated multiorgan autoimmunity* (TAMA), although nearly 25 percent of reported cases have been confined to the gastrointestinal tract (101).

Pathogenesis. The pathogenesis of autoimmune enteropathy is not entirely clear, although inappropriate T-cell activation and loss of self-tolerance have been implicated, particularly with respect to regulatory T-cell function. The transcription factor encoded by *FOXP3* is required for the development and function of regulatory T-cells; loss of function results in hyperactivation of immune cells. Abnormalities in other genes that modulate regulatory T-cells, such as *CTLA4, CD25, STAT1, STAT3, STAT5B,* and *ITCH*, may account for some cases of autoimmune enteropathy. Aberrant expression of HLA class II molecules by crypt epithelial cells can also elicit T-cell mediated injury in some cases (102). On the other hand, autoantibodies probably represent an epiphenomenon related to underlying immune dysregulation and are unlikely to be pathogenic. Autoantibodies directed against goblet cells and enterocytes are not specific for autoimmune enteropathy; they can develop in patients with human immunodeficiency virus infection, inflammatory bowel disease, and even celiac disease. Titers wane with successful treatment.

Gross Findings. Endoscopic findings are variable, mimicking celiac disease and idiopathic inflammatory bowel disease in some cases. Occasional patients have mild abnormalities or normal-appearing mucosae. Complete mucosal flattening, scalloped folds, and a mosaic pattern can be seen in patients with duodenal disease. Erythema, ulcers, and mucosal granularity may occur in patients with extensive colonic involvement.

Microscopic Findings. Some authors have classified the histologic patterns of autoimmune enteropathy as chronic active enteritis, celiac disease-like, and graft-versus-host disease-like (103). However, these patterns of injury do not correlate well with clinical manifestations or mechanisms of disease, and are often present in various combinations. Most duodenal biopsy samples from patients with autoimmune enteropathy feature moderate to severe villous blunting and crypt hyperplasia accompanied by plasma cell-rich inflammation that expands the lamina propria (fig. 5-44A). Neutrophils are invariably present, often with crypt abscesses. Intraepithelial lymphocytosis is usually patchy, and when present, tends to be more pronounced in the crypts than surface epithelium (fig. 5-44B). Occasional cases feature prominent surface intraepithelial lymphocytosis, closely simulating celiac disease. Crypt cell apoptosis is always present and can be striking, affecting multiple cells within single crypts or forming luminal aggregates of necrotic cellular debris (fig. 5-44C). Goblet cells, endocrine cells, and Paneth cells are often decreased in number or absent, although some cases show preservation of these cell types. Occasional cases show only mild mucosal inflammation and preserved villous architecture with decreased goblet and Paneth cells (fig. 5-44D).

Many cases affect multiple sites in the gastrointestinal tract. Chronic active gastritis and colitis can simulate idiopathic inflammatory bowel disease or feature intraepithelial lymphocytosis with, or without, subepithelial collagen deposits.

Treatment and Prognosis. Patients do not respond to gluten withdrawal. Untreated patients may die as a result of severe malabsorptive diarrhea. Immunosuppressive therapy with corticosteroids alone is often insufficient; treatment typically requires azathioprine,

Table 5-2

FEATURES OF HERITABLE AUTOIMMUNE POLYENDOCRINOPATHY SYNDROMES[a]

Entity	Type 1 (APECED[b] Syndrome)	Type 2	Type 3 (IPEX Syndrome)
Primary manifestations	Addison disease, chronic mucocutaneous candidiasis, hypoparathyroidism	Addison disease, autoimmune thyroiditis, type 1 diabetes mellitus	Autoimmune enteropathy, neonatal type 1 diabetes mellitus, eczema
Other manifestations	Autoimmune thyroiditis, pneumonitis, pancreatitis, nephritis autoimmune gastroenteropathy, type 1 diabetes mellitus, vitiligo, alopecia, nail dystrophy, keratitis, enamel hypoplasia, retinitis, primary ovarian insufficiency	Autoimmune gastroenteropathy, celiac disease alopecia, vitiligo, primary ovarian insufficiency	Autoimmune thyroiditis, hemolytic anemia, thrombocytopenia
Age at presentation	Childhood, adolescence	Adolescence, young adulthood	Infancy
Prevalence	1:100,000	1:1,000	1:1,000,000
Treatment	Immunosuppression Symptom relief	Hormone replacement	Hormone replacement Bone marrow transplantation
Complications	Adrenal insufficiency, hypocalcemia, oropharyngeal and esophageal carcinoma	Adrenal insufficiency	Infections
Mode of inheritance	Autosomal recessive or dominant	None established	X-linked
Affected gene	*AIRE*	Major histocompatibility complex and others	*FOXP3*
Serologic abnormalities	Autoantibodies to interferon-α, interferon-φ cytokines, and intracellular proteins	Autoantibodies to 21-hydroxylase, glutamic acid decarboxylase-65, islet antigen-2, thyroid perioxidase, thyrotropin receptor	Autoantibodies to glutamic acid decarboxylase-65, as well as lymphocytosis, eosinophilia, increased IgE, and increased cytokine production

[a]Modified from Table 1 from Husebye, ES, Anderson, MS, Kampe, O. Autoimmune polyendocrine syndromes. N Engl J Med 2018;378:1132-41.
[b]APECED = autoimmune polyendocrinopathies, mucocutaneous candidiasis, and ectodermal dystrophy; IPEX = immune dysregulation, polyendocrinopathy, and X-linked.

methotrexate, mycophenolate, tacrolimus, cyclosporine, or combinations of these agents (93). Infliximab, rituximab and abatacept have also been used with some success. Bone marrow transplantation may be considered for patients with germline mutations (104). Resolution of symptoms is accompanied by reconstitution of the mucosa by its normal components.

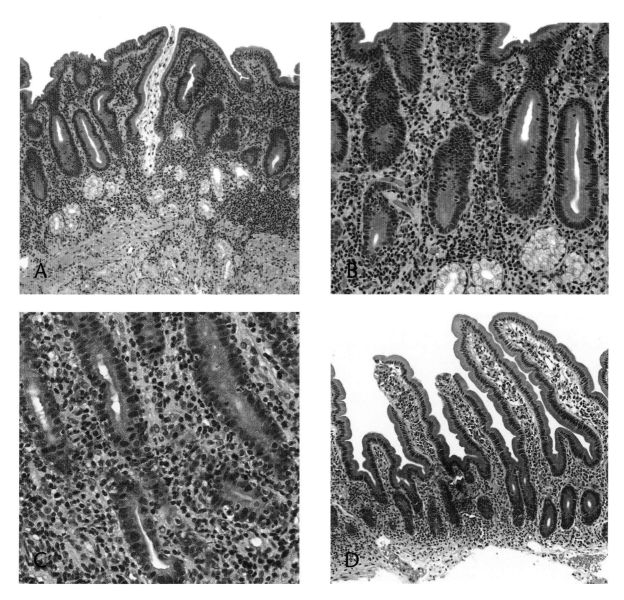

Figure 5-44

AUTOIMMUNE ENTEROPATHY

Moderate to severe villous blunting is accompanied by striking crypt hyperplasia and plasma cell-rich lamina propria inflammation (A). Goblet and Paneth cells are decreased in number (B). Crypts show patchy infiltration by lymphocytes and granulocytes with scattered apoptotic epithelial cells (C). Some cases show partial or complete preservation of villous architecture without substantial lamina propria inflammation or intraepithelial lymphocytosis. Goblet cells, however, are lacking in both surface and crypt epithelia (D).

REFERENCES

1. Robert ME, Crowe SE, Burgart L, et al. Statement on best practices in the use of pathology as a diagnostic tool for celiac disease: a guide for clinicians and pathologists. Am J Surg Pathol 2018;42:e44-58.

2. Majumdar K, Sakhuja P, Puri AS, et al. Coeliac disease and the liver: spectrum of liver histology, serology and treatment response at a tertiary referral centre. J Clin Pathol 2018;71:412-9.

3. Rodrigo S, Abboud G, Oh D, et al. High intraepithelial eosinophil counts in esophageal squamous epithelium are not specific for eosinophilic esophagitis in adults. Am J Gastroenterol 2008;103:435-42.

4. Thawani SP, Brannagan TH 3rd, Lebwohl B, Green PH, Ludvigsson JF. Risk of neuropathy among 28,232 patients with biopsy-verified celiac disease. JAMA Neurol 2015;72:806-11.

5. Leonard MM, Sapone A, Catassi C, Fasano A. Celiac disease and nonceliac gluten sensitivity: a review. JAMA 2017;318:647-56.

6. Fasano A, Berti I, Gerarduzzi T, et al. Prevalence of celiac disease in at-risk and not-at-risk groups in the united states: a large multicenter study. Arch Intern Med 2003;163:286-92.

7. Bouziat R, Hinterleitner R, Brown JJ, et al. Reovirus infection triggers inflammatory responses to dietary antigens and development of celiac disease. Science 2017;356:44-50.

8. Fasano A, Catassi C. Clinical practice. Celiac disease. N Engl J Med 2012;367:2419-26.

9. Karpati S, Sardy M, Nemeth K, et al. Transglutaminases in autoimmune and inherited skin diseases: the phenomena of epitope spreading and functional compensation. Exp Dermatol 2018;27:807-14.

10. Panarelli NC, Yantiss RK. The importance of biopsy sampling practices in the pathologic evaluation of gastrointestinal disorders. Curr Opin Gastroenterol 2016;32:374-81.

11. Hudacko R, Kathy Zhou X, Yantiss RK. Immunohistochemical stains for CD3 and CD8 do not improve detection of gluten-sensitive enteropathy in duodenal biopsies. Mod Pathol 2013;26:1241-5.

12. Corazza GR, Villanacci V, Zambelli C, et al. Comparison of the interobserver reproducibility with different histologic criteria used in celiac disease. Clin Gastroenterol Hepatol 2007;5:838-43.

13. Greenson JK. The biopsy pathology of non-coeliac enteropathy. Histopathology 2015;66:29-36.

14. Oberhuber G, Granditsch G, Vogelsang H. The histopathology of coeliac disease: time for a standardized report scheme for pathologists. Eur J Gastroenterol Hepatol 1999;11:1185-94.

15. Rishi AR, Rubio-Tapia A, Murray JA. Refractory celiac disease. Expert Rev Gastroenterol Hepatol 2016;10:537-46.

16. Ondrejka S, Jagadeesh D. Enteropathy-associated t-cell lymphoma. Curr Hematol Malig Rep 2016;11:504-13.

17. Delabie J, Holte H, Vose JM, et al. Enteropathy-associated T-cell lymphoma: clinical and histological findings from the international peripheral T-cell lymphoma project. Blood 2011;118:148-55.

18. Rubio-Tapia A, Murray JA. Classification and management of refractory coeliac disease. Gut 2010;59:547-57.

19. Celli R, Hui P, Triscott H, et al. Clinical insignficance of monoclonal T-cell populations and duodenal intraepithelial T-cell phenotypes in celiac and non-celiac patients. Am J Surg Pathol 2019;43:151-60.

20. Malamut G, Verkarre V, Suarez F, et al. The enteropathy associated with common variable immunodeficiency: the delineated frontiers with celiac disease. Am J Gastroenterol 2010;105:2262-75.

21. Lan N, Shen B, Yuan L, Liu X. Comparison of clinical features, treatment, and outcomes of collagenous sprue, celiac disease, and collagenous colitis. J Gastroenterol Hepatol 2017;32:120-7.

22. Rubio-Tapia A, Herman ML, Ludvigsson JF, et al. Severe spruelike enteropathy associated with olmesartan. Mayo Clin Proc 2012;87:732-8.

23. Vakiani E, Arguelles-Grande C, Mansukhani MM, et al. Collagenous sprue is not always associated with dismal outcomes: a clinicopathological study of 19 patients. Mod Pathol 2010;23:12-26.

24. Ramos GP, Papadakis KA. Mechanisms of disease: inflammatory bowel diseases. Mayo Clin Proc 2019;94:155-65.

25. Duerr RH, Targan SR, Landers CJ, Sutherland LR, Shanahan F. Anti-neutrophil cytoplasmic antibodies in ulcerative colitis. Comparison with other colitides/diarrheal illnesses. Gastroenterology 1991;100:1590-6.

26. Walsham NE, Sherwood RA. Fecal calprotectin in inflammatory bowel disease. Clin Exp Gastroenterol 2016;9:21-9.

27. Glocker EO, Kotlarz D, Boztug K, et al. Inflammatory bowel disease and mutations affecting the interleukin-10 receptor. N Engl J Med 2009;361:2033-45.

28. Venkateswaran S, Prince J, Cutler DJ, et al. Enhanced contribution of HLA in pediatric onset ulcerative colitis. Inflamm Bowel Dis 2018;24:829-38.

29. Bouma G, Strober W. The immunological and genetic basis of inflammatory bowel disease. Nat Rev Immunol 2003;3:521-33.
30. Sahami S, Wildenberg ME, Koens L, et al. Appendectomy for therapy-refractory ulcerative colitis results in pathological improvement of colonic inflammation: short-term results of the PASSION study. J Crohns Colitis 2019;13:165-71.
31. Choi EK, Appelman HD. Chronic colitis in biopsy samples: is it inflammatory bowel disease or something else? Surg Pathol Clin 2017;10:841-61.
32. Yantiss RK, Odze RD. Diagnostic difficulties in inflammatory bowel disease pathology. Histopathology 2006;48:116-32.
33. Mutinga ML, Odze RD, Wang HH, Hornick JL, Farraye FA. The clinical significance of right-sided colonic inflammation in patients with left-sided chronic ulcerative colitis. Inflamm Bowel Dis 2004;10:215-9.
34. Yantiss RK, Farraye FA, O'Brien MJ, et al. Prognostic significance of superficial fissuring ulceration in patients with severe "indeterminate" colitis. Am J Surg Pathol 2006;30:165-70.
35. Yantiss RK, Sapp HL, Farraye FA, et al. Histologic predictors of pouchitis in patients with chronic ulcerative colitis. Am J Surg Pathol 2004;28:999-1006.
36. Haskell H, Andrews CW Jr, Reddy SI, et al. Pathologic features and clinical significance of "backwash" ileitis in ulcerative colitis. Am J Surg Pathol 2005;29:1472-81.
37. Lin J, McKenna BJ, Appelman HD. Morphologic findings in upper gastrointestinal biopsies of patients with ulcerative colitis: a controlled study. Am J Surg Pathol 2010;34:1672-7.
38. Valdez R, Appelman HD, Bronner MP, Greenson JK. Diffuse duodenitis associated with ulcerative colitis. Am J Surg Pathol 2000;24:1407-13.
39. Hissong E, Chen Z, Yantiss RK. Cytomegalovirus reactivation in inflammatory bowel disease: an uncommon occurrence related to corticosteroid dependence. Mod Pathol 2019;32:1210-6.
40. Komaki Y, Komaki F, Ido A, Sakuraba A. Efficacy and safety of tacrolimus therapy for active ulcerative colitis; a systematic review and meta-analysis. J Crohns Colitis 2016;10:484-94.
41. Arora Z, Shen B. Biological therapy for ulcerative colitis. Gastroenterol Rep (Oxf) 2015;3:103-9.
42. Molodecky NA, Soon IS, Rabi DM, et al. Increasing incidence and prevalence of the inflammatory bowel diseases with time, based on systematic review. Gastroenterology 2012;142:46-54.
43. Walker LJ, Aldhous MC, Drummond HE, et al. Anti-saccharomyces cerevisiae antibodies (ASCA) in Crohn's disease are associated with disease severity but not nod2/card15 mutations. Clin Exp Immunol 2004;135:490-6.
44. Cruyssen BV, Peeters H, Hoffman IE, et al. CARD15 polymorphisms are associated with anti-saccharomyces cerevisiae antibodies in caucasian Crohn's disease patients. Clin Exp Immunol 2005;140:354-9.
45. Shoda R, Matsueda K, Yamato S, Umeda N. Epidemiologic analysis of Crohn disease in Japan: increased dietary intake of n-6 polyunsaturated fatty acids and animal protein relates to the increased incidence of Crohn disease in Japan. Am J Clin Nutr 1996;63:741-5.
46. Ogur, Y, Inohara N, Benito A, Chen FF, Yamaoka S, Nunez G. Nod2, a NOD1/APAF-1 family member that is restricted to monocytes and activates NF-kappab. J Biol Chem 2001;276:4812-8.
47. Chermesh I, Azriel A, Alter-Koltunoff M, Eliakim R, Karban A, Levi BZ. Crohn's disease and SLC11A1 promoter polymorphism. Dig Dis Sci 2007;52:1632-5.
48. Diegelmann J, Czamara D, Le Bras E, et al. Intestinal dmbt1 expression is modulated by Crohn's disease-associated IL23R variants and by a DMBT1 variant which influences binding of the transcription factors CREB1 and ATF-2. PLoS One 2013;8:e77773.
49. Prescott NJ, Dominy KM, Kubo M, et al. Independent and population-specific association of risk variants at the IRGM locus with Crohn's disease. Hum Mol Genet 2010;19:1828-39.
50. Prescott NJ, Fisher SA, Franke A, et al. A nonsynonymous SNP in ATG16L1 predisposes to ileal Crohn's disease and is independent of CARD15 and IBD5. Gastroenterology 2007;132:1665-71.
51. Cobrin GM, Abreu MT. Defects in mucosal immunity leading to Crohn's disease. Immunol Rev 2005;206:277-95.
52. Colombat M, Imbert A, Bruneval P, Chatelain D, Gontier MF. Giant cell arteritis localized to the colon associated with Crohn's disease. Histopathology 2001;38:21-4.
53. Eustace GJ, Melmed GY. Therapy for Crohn's disease: a review of recent developments. Curr Gastroenterol Rep 2018;20:19.
54. Armuzzi A, Ardizzone S, Biancone L, et al. Ustekinumab in the management of Crohn's disease: expert opinion. Dig Liver Dis 2018;50:653-60.
55. Bessissow T, Reinglas J, Aruljothy A, Lakatos PL, Van Assche G. Endoscopic management of Crohn's strictures. World J Gastroenterol 2018;24:1859-67.
56. Michelassi F, Balestracci T, Chappell R, Block GE. Primary and recurrent Crohn's disease. Experience with 1379 patients. Ann Surg 1991;214:230-8.
57. Cao BL, Qasem A, Sharp RC, Abdelli LS, Naser SA. Systematic review and meta-analysis on the association of tuberculosis in Crohn's disease patients treated with tumor necrosis factor -α inhibitors (anti-TNFα). World J Gastroenterol 2018;24:2764-75.

58. Seminerio JL, Loftus EV Jr, Colombel JF, Thapa P, Sandborn WJ. Infliximab for Crohn's disease: the first 500 patients followed up through 2009. Dig Dis Sci 2013;58:797-806.

59. Kelsen J, Dige A, Schwindt H, et al. Infliximab induces clonal expansion of γδ-T cells in Crohn's disease: a predictor of lymphoma risk? PLoS One 2011;6:e17890.

60. Romanos J, Samarasekera DN, Stebbing JF, Jewell DP, Kettlewell MG, Mortensen NJ. Outcome of 200 restorative proctocolectomy operations: the John Radcliffe Hospital experience. Br J Surg 1997;84:814-8.

61. Persborn M, Gerritsen J, Wallon C, Carlsson A, Akkermans LM, Söderholm JD. The effects of probiotics on barrier function and mucosal pouch microbiota during maintenance treatment for severe pouchitis in patients with ulcerative colitis. Aliment Pharmacol Ther 2013;38:772-83.

62. McLaughlin SD, Clark SK, Bell AJ, Tekkis PP, Ciclitira PJ, Nicholls RJ. Incidence and short-term implications of prepouch ileitis following restorative proctocolectomy with ileal pouch-anal anastomosis for ulcerative colitis. Dis Colon Rectum 2009;52:879-83.

63. Segal JP, Oke S, Hold GL, Clark SK, Faiz OD, Hart AL. Systematic review: ileoanal pouch microbiota in health and disease. Aliment Pharmacol Ther 2018;47:466-77.

64. McLaughlin SD, Clark SK, Bell AJ, Tekkis PP, Ciclitira PJ, Nicholls RJ. An open study of antibiotics for the treatment of pre-pouch ileitis following restorative proctocolectomy with ileal pouch-anal anastomosis. Aliment Pharmacol Ther 2009;29:69-74.

65. Greuter T, Rogler G. Alicaforsen in the treatment of pouchitis. Immunotherapy 2017;9:1143-52.

66. Herfarth HH, Long MD, Isaacs KL. Use of biologics in pouchitis: a systematic review. J Clin Gastroenterol 2015;49:647-54.

67. Tong J, Zheng Q, Zhang C, Lo R, Shen J, Ran Z. Incidence, prevalence, and temporal trends of microscopic colitis: a systematic review and meta-analysis. Am J Gastroenterol 2015;110:265-76.

68. Fernandez-Banares F, Esteve M, Espinos JC, et al. Drug consumption and the risk of microscopic colitis. Am J Gastroenterol 2007;102:324-30.

69. Li J, Yan Y, Meng Z, et al. Microscopic colitis evolved into inflammatory bowel diseases is characterized by increased th1/tc1 cells in colonic mucosal lamina propria. Dig Dis Sci 2017;62:2755-67.

70. Marlicz W, Skonieczna-Zydecka K, Yung DE, Loniewski I, Koulaouzidis A. Endoscopic findings and colonic perforation in microscopic colitis: a systematic review. Dig Liver Dis 2017;49:1073-85.

71. Yuan S, Reyes V, Bronner MP. Pseudomembranous collagenous colitis. Am J Surg Pathol 2003;27:1375-9.

72. Ayata G, Ithamukkala S, Sapp H, et al. Prevalence and significance of inflammatory bowel disease-like morphologic features in collagenous and lymphocytic colitis. Am J Surg Pathol 2002;26:1414-23.

73. Gentile N, Yen EF. Prevalence, pathogenesis, diagnosis, and management of microscopic colitis. Gut Liver 2018;12:227-35.

74. Allende DS, Taylor SL, Bronner MP. Colonic perforation as a complication of collagenous colitis in a series of 12 patients. Am J Gastroenterol 2008;103:2598-604.

75. Gentile NM, Khanna S, Loftus EV Jr, et al. The epidemiology of microscopic colitis in Olmsted county from 2002 to 2010: a population-based study. Clin Gastroenterol Hepatol 2014;12:838-42.

76. Osterholm MT, MacDonald KL, White KE, et al. An outbreak of a newly recognized chronic diarrhea syndrome associated with raw milk consumption. JAMA 1986;256:484-90.

77. Vugia, DJ, Abbott, S, Mintz, ED, et al. A restaurant-associated outbreak of brainerd diarrhea in california. Clin Infect Dis 2006;43:62-4.

78. Perk G, Ackerman Z, Cohen P, Eliakim R. Lymphocytic colitis: a clue to an infectious trigger. Scand J Gastroenterol 1999;34:110-2.

79. Masclee GM, Coloma PM, Kuipers EJ, Sturkenboom MC. Increased risk of microscopic colitis with use of proton pump inhibitors and non-steroidal anti-inflammatory drugs. Am J Gastroenterol 2015;110:749-59.

80. Cheng LJ, Zhang SC. Abdominal ascites in children as the presentation of eosinophilic gastroenteritis: a surgeon's perspective. Clin Res Hepatol Gastroenterol 2019;43:e12-7.

81. Talley NJ, Shorter RG, Phillips SF, Zinsmeister AR. Eosinophilic gastroenteritis: a clinicopathological study of patients with disease of the mucosa, muscle layer, and subserosal tissues. Gut 1990;31:54-8.

82. Rothenberg ME. Eosinophilic gastrointestinal disorders (EGID). J Allergy Clin Immunol 2004;113:11-28.

83. Yantiss RK. Eosinophils in the GI tract: how many is too many and what do they mean? Mod Pathol 2015;28(Suppl 1):S7-21.

84. Yun MY, Cho YU, Park IS, et al. Eosinophilic gastroenteritis presenting as small bowel obstruction: a case report and review of the literature. World J Gastroenterol 2007;13:1758-60.

85. Furuta K, Adachi K, Aimi M, et al. Case-control study of association of eosinophilic gastrointestinal disorders with helicobacter pylori infection in Japan. J Clin Biochem Nutr 2013;53:60-2.

86. Manatsathit W, Sermsathanasawadi R, Pongpaiboon A, Pongprasobchai S. Mucosal-type eosinophilic gastroenteritis in Thailand: 12-year retrospective study. J Med Assoc Thai 2013;96(Suppl 2):S194-202.

87. Couture C, Measures L, Gagnon J, Desbiens C. Human intestinal anisakiosis due to consumption of raw salmon. Am J Surg Pathol 2003;27:1167-72.

88. Walker NI, Croese J, Clouston AD, Parry M, Loukas A, Prociv P. Eosinophilic enteritis in northeastern Australia. Pathology, association with ancylostoma caninum, and implications. Am J Surg Pathol 1995;19:328-37.

89. Lim CB, Goldin RD, Darzi A, Hanna GB. Characterization of materials eliciting foreign body reaction in stapled human gastrointestinal anastomoses. Br J Surg 2008;95:1044-50.

90. Valentine-Thon E, Muller K, Guzzi G, Kreisel S, Ohnsorge P, Sandkamp M. LTT-MELISA is clinically relevant for detecting and monitoring metal sensitivity. Neuro Endocrinol Lett 2006;27(Suppl 1):17-24.

91. Schwartz DA, Pardi DS, Murray JA. Use of montelukast as steroid-sparing agent for recurrent eosinophilic gastroenteritis. Dig Dis Sci 2001;46:1787-90.

92. Singhi AD, Goyal A, Davison JM, Regueiro MD, Roche RL, Ranganathan S. Pediatric autoimmune enteropathy: an entity frequently associated with immunodeficiency disorders. Mod Pathol 2014;27:543-53.

93. Akram S, Murray JA, Pardi DS, et al. Adult autoimmune enteropathy: Mayo clinic Rochester experience. Clin Gastroenterol Hepatol 2007;5:1282-90.

94. Unsworth DJ, Walker-Smith JA. Autoimmunity in diarrhoeal disease. J Pediatr Gastroenterol Nutr 1985;4:375-80.

95. Umetsu SE, Brown I, Langner C, Lauwers GY. Autoimmune enteropathies. Virchows Arch 2018; 472:55-66.

96. Goulet OJ, Brousse N, Canioni D, Walker-Smith JA, Schmitz J, Phillips AD. Syndrome of intractable diarrhoea with persistent villous atrophy in early childhood: a clinicopathological survey of 47 cases. J Pediatr Gastroenterol Nutr 1998;26:151-61.

97. Catassi C, Fabiani E, Spagnuolo MI, Barera G, Guarino A. Severe and protracted diarrhea: results of the 3-year SIGEP multicenter survey. Working group of the Italian Society of Pediatric Gastroenterology and Hepatology (SIGEP). J Pediatr Gastroenterol Nutr 1999;29:63-8.

98. d'Hennezel E, Ben-Shoshan M, Ochs HD, et al. FOXP3 forkhead domain mutation and regulatory T cells in the IPEX syndrome. N Engl J Med 2009;361:1710-3.

99. Blanco Quiros A, Arranz Sanz E, Bernardo Ordiz D, Garrote Adrados JA. From autoimmune enteropathy to the IPEX (immune dysfunction, polyendocrinopathy, enteropathy, x-linked) syndrome. Allergol Immunopathol (Madr) 2009;37:208-15.

100. Husebye ES, Anderson MS, Kampe O. Autoimmune polyendocrine syndromes. N Engl J Med 2018;378:1132-41.

101. Slavik T, Potgieter FM, Brittain D. Thymoma-associated multiorgan autoimmunity with exclusive gastrointestinal tract involvement: case report and review of the literature. Virchows Arch 2018;473:121-5.

102. Mirakian R, Hill S, Richardson A, Milla PJ, Walker-Smith JA, Bottazzo GF. HLA product expression and lymphocyte subpopulations in jejunum biopsies of children with idiopathic protracted diarrhoea and enterocyte autoantibodies. J Autoimmun 1988;1:263-77.

103. Masia R, Peyton S, Lauwers GY, Brown I. Gastrointestinal biopsy findings of autoimmune enteropathy: a review of 25 cases. Am J Surg Pathol 2014;38:1319-29.

104. Patey-Mariaud de Serre N, Canioni D, Ganousse S, et al. Digestive histopathological presentation of ipex syndrome. Mod Pathol 2009;22:95-102.

6 SYSTEMIC DISORDERS WITH GASTROINTESTINAL MANIFESTATIONS

PRIMARY IMMUNODEFICIENCIES

Common Variable Immunodeficiency

Definition. *Common variable immunodeficiency* (CVID) is an umbrella term for a heterogeneous group of disorders characterized by failed plasma cell maturation. It encompasses several types of immunoglobulin deficiencies associated with defective mononuclear cells that cannot suppress immune responses (1).

Clinical Features. CVID can present at any age with different types of recurrent, persistent, and opportunistic infections, autoimmune disorders, and gastrointestinal complaints (2). This disease is the second most common immunodeficiency disorder to involve the gastrointestinal tract. Affected patients are at risk for lymphoma and gastrointestinal infection, particularly giardiasis and cytomegalovirus (3). The authors have also seen several cases of chronic strongyloidiasis in this patient population, presumably reflecting decreased mucosal IgA-secreting plasma cells. Abdominal pain, malabsorption, and diarrhea are common gastrointestinal symptoms.

Gross Findings. The gastrointestinal mucosa is often normal. Mucosal nodularity in the proximal small bowel commonly reflects lymphoid hyperplasia (fig. 6-1A) (4). Involvement of the lower gastrointestinal tract can simulate the endoscopic appearance of inflammatory bowel diseases with patchy or diffuse ulcers, erythema, and friability (fig. 6-1B) (5).

Microscopic Findings. Any part of the gastrointestinal tract may be affected by CVID (5). Duodenal changes range from preserved villous

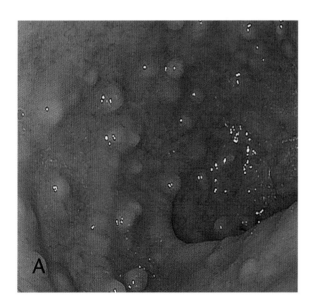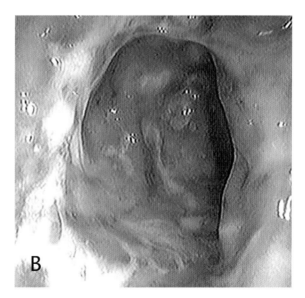

Figure 6-1

COMMON VARIABLE IMMUNODEFICIENCY

The duodenal mucosa is nodular, reflecting prominent lymphoid aggregates (A). The terminal ileum displays flattened mucosal folds with nodularity and ulcers (B).

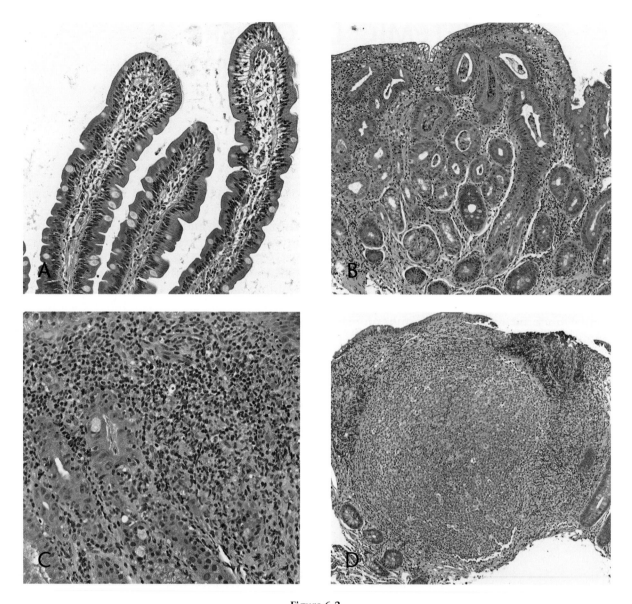

Figure 6-2

COMMON VARIABLE IMMUNODEFICIENCY

Duodenal biopsy samples feature intraepithelial lymphocytosis with normal villous architecture and rare plasma cells in the lamina propria (A). Another case displays complete villous flattening with crypt hyperplasia and increased mononuclear cell-rich inflammation of the lamina propria; intraepithelial lymphocytosis is not as striking as would be expected of celiac disease (B). Numerous apoptotic crypt epithelial cells are present in association with neutrophilic infiltration and crypt destruction (C). Large lymphoid follicles with germinal centers distort the mucosal architecture (D).

architecture with intraepithelial lymphocytosis to complete villous flattening with diffuse chronic inflammation and poorly formed granulomas (fig. 6-2A,B). Villous architectural abnormalities are accompanied by scattered apoptotic crypt epithelial cells and neutrophilic cryptitis (fig. 6-2C). Lymphoid nodules with germinal centers are characteristically present (fig. 6-2D). Plasma cells are usually decreased in number or absent. A paucity of plasma cells is a helpful diagnostic clue since most inflammatory conditions that cause villous architectural abnormalities and mucosal lymphocytosis also elicit plasma cell-rich inflammation. Nevertheless,

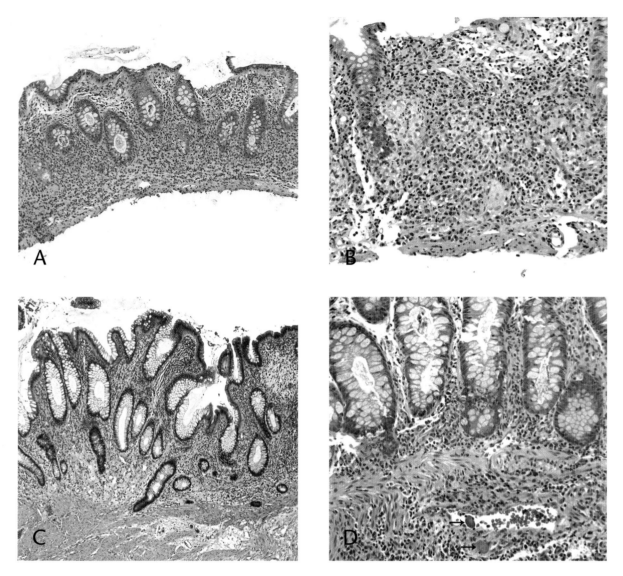

Figure 6-3

COMMON VARIABLE IMMUNODEFICIENCY

Colonic biopsy samples often display diffuse mononuclear cell-rich inflammation, predominantly in the deep mucosa (A). Foci of cryptitis, pericryptal granulomatous inflammation (B), and crypt architectural distortion (C) simulate changes of idiopathic inflammatory bowel disease, although the conspicuous lack of plasmacytosis is a helpful diagnostic clue. Many patients have concomitant cytomegalovirus inclusions (arrows) (D).

the detection of plasma cells in biopsy samples does not exclude the possibility of CVID; some patients have normal numbers of plasma cells that simply do not secrete immunoglobulin (5).

Colonic biopsy samples from patients with CVID frequently show changes that simulate those of idiopathic inflammatory bowel disease. Patchy or diffuse mononuclear cell-rich inflammation is accompanied by apoptotic debris in

the crypts, crypt abscesses, and neutrophilic cryptitis, as well as pericryptal granulomatous inflammation (fig. 6-3). Crypt architectural abnormalities tend to be patchy. Intraepithelial lymphocytosis or subepithelial collagen deposits are present in some cases.

Differential Diagnosis. Disease in the upper gastrointestinal tract may simulate the features of celiac disease, particularly when villous

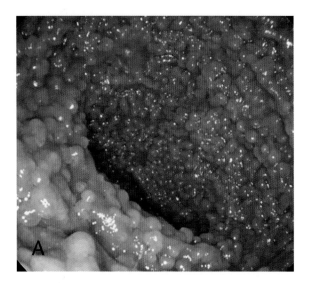 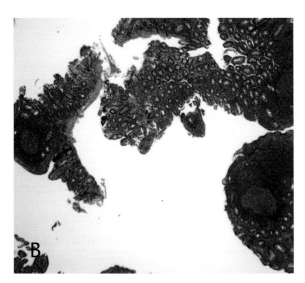

Figure 6-4

SELECTIVE IGA DEFICIENCY

The duodenum is carpeted by polypoid lymphoid aggregates (A) associated with germinal centers that expand the lamina propria (B).

blunting and intraepithelial lymphocytosis are prominent. However, lymphoid hyperplasia, neutrophilic cryptitis, and crypt cell apoptosis are not typical of celiac disease. Villous architectural abnormalities secondary to celiac disease are also accompanied by dense plasma cell-rich inflammatory infiltrates in the lamina propria.

Involvement of the lower gastrointestinal tract often produces an active colitis with granulomatous inflammation that simulates inflammatory bowel disease. Crypt architectural abnormalities are often present but tend to be patchy. An absence of numerous plasma cells accompanying neutrophilic cryptitis in combination with cytomegalovirus inclusions is not expected in idiopathic inflammatory bowel disease, especially if not recently treated with corticosteroid therapy (6).

Treatment and Prognosis. Patients with CVID are managed with immunoglobulin replacement. Antibiotic agents are used to control infections, although patients typically require extended courses of therapy. Most treated patients have a normal life expectancy provided they are treated before end-organ damage or malignancies develop (7).

Selective IgA Deficiency

Selective IgA deficiency is the most common primary immunodeficiency. This disorder re-

sults from defects in maturation of IgA-bearing B-cells to IgA-secreting plasma cells (8). Symptomatic patients develop recurrent sinopulmonary and gastrointestinal infections, reflecting a deficiency in the most important class of secreted mucosal immunoglobulin (8). They have an increased risk for celiac disease, as well as chronic giardiasis and strongyloidiasis.

Serologic screening tests for celiac disease that use IgA antibodies yield false negative results; IgG antibodies to deaminated gliadin peptides and other markers should be used to detect celiac disease in this patient population (9). Gastrointestinal biopsy samples are often normal or show lymphoid hyperplasia (fig. 6-4). Inflammatory changes, such as granulomas and chronic mucosal injury, can simulate idiopathic inflammatory bowel disease, but are uncommon (6).

Chronic Granulomatous Disease

Chronic granulomatous disease is a rare genetic disorder characterized by severe, recurrent bacterial and fungal infections. Patients inherit either X-linked or autosomal recessive defects in genes encoding components of the NADPH oxidase complex. Resultant attenuated digestion of exogenous materials causes chronic granulomatous inflammation (10).

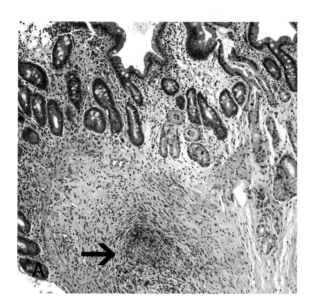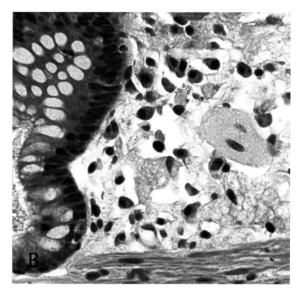

Figure 6-5

CHRONIC GRANULOMATOUS DISEASE

A submucosal granuloma (arrow) is present in otherwise normal duodenal mucosa from a toddler with failure to thrive (A). Lamina propria macrophages contain granular material and are a clue to the diagnosis of chronic granulomatous disease (B).

Gastrointestinal involvement may manifest with histologic features that overlap with those of idiopathic inflammatory bowel disease, particularly Crohn disease (fig. 6-5A). Chronic active enterocolitis with granulomas is accompanied by variable villous blunting and mucosal eosinophilia. Pigmented macrophages are often present in tissue samples from patients with chronic granulomatous disease (fig. 6-5B) (11).

CONNECTIVE TISSUE DISORDERS

Ehlers-Danlos Syndrome Type IV

Definition. *Ehlers-Danlos syndrome type IV* is an inherited connective tissue disorder due to abnormalities in type III procollagen. Synonyms include *Sack-Barabas syndrome* and *vascular-type Ehlers-Danlos syndrome*.

Clinical Features. Ehlers-Danlos syndrome has a prevalence of 1/10,000 to 1/25,000 persons; approximately 5 to 10 percent of patients have type IV disease (12). Variants were historically classified using Roman numerals and disease phenotype but most recent criteria are based on specific genetic alterations. We now recognize 13 variants of Ehlers-Danlos syndrome (13).

Patients with the disorder have characteristic facies with prominent cheekbones and sunken cheeks, premature aging of the skin (acrogeria), translucent skin, and easy bruisability (14). Those with the vascular variant (type IV) are at increased risk for arterial rupture or dissection, perforation of the gastrointestinal tract, and uterine rupture, especially during pregnancy (15). Most gastrointestinal perforations occur in the sigmoid colon and are increasingly common with advanced age. Spontaneous rupture of the splenic and hepatic capsules also occur.

Pathogenesis. Type IV Ehlers-Danlos syndrome is an autosomal dominant inherited disorder resulting from *COL3A1* mutations, the gene encoding type III procollagen (16). Type III collagen is an important component of the intestinal wall, investing aggregates of smooth muscle cells in the muscularis propria (14). Rare patients have an autosomal recessive pattern of inheritance due to specific *COL1A1* mutations that affect type I collagen production.

Gross Findings. Invasive imaging techniques are often contraindicated when intestinal perforation is suspected. Resection specimens display one or more perforation sites on a background of otherwise normal-appearing colonic mucosa.

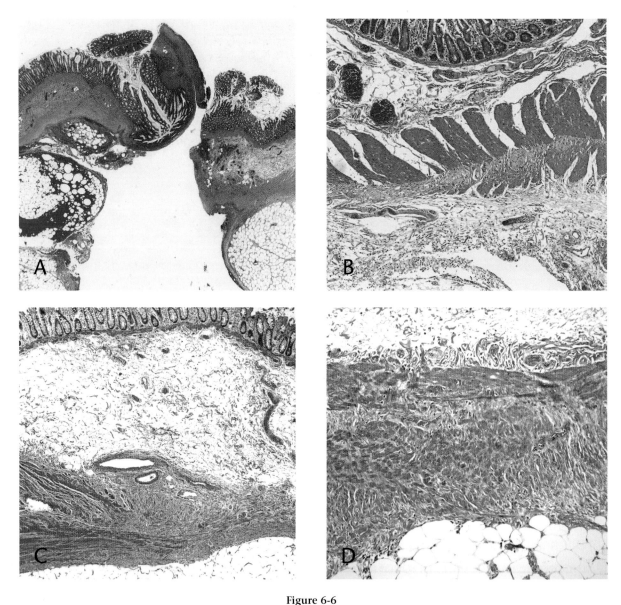

Figure 6-6

EHLERS-DANLOS SYNDROME

A resected segment of perforated colon contains a diverticulum-like area where the mucosal components protrude (A) through the muscularis propria, the outer layer of which is markedly attenuated (B). A trichrome stain demonstrates near-complete fibrosis of the muscularis propria (C) and an intimate admixture of collagen and smooth muscle cell bundles (D).

The bowel wall features thin, fragile areas that simulate diverticula.

Microscopic Findings. The mucosal and submucosal layers are usually normal, whereas the muscularis propria is often attenuated with areas of variable thickness and fibrosis. Perforation sites are surrounded by irregularly organized bundles of smooth muscle cells (fig. 6-6A,B). Trichrome and reticulin stains demonstrate col-

lagenous replacement of the muscularis propria with irregular and fragmented collagen fibrils (fig. 6-6C,D).

Treatment and Prognosis. Vascular rupture and dissection are more likely to cause death than gastrointestinal perforation and are often managed with a conservative approach (17). Nearly 80 percent of affected patients have a serious episode of gastrointestinal bleeding by

40 years of age and up to one-third develop multiple enterocolic perforations requiring surgical resection (17–19). Intestinal rupture requires urgent surgical attention, although the mortality rate is only 2 percent (20). The treatment of choice generally includes resection of the affected bowel with ileostomy, rather than a primary anastomosis, due to the risk of complications following a primary anastomosis (21). Some advocate for total colectomy with ileostomy or ileo-rectal anastomosis due to a lower risk of small intestinal perforation than colonic rupture.

Collagen Vascular Diseases

Definition. *Collagen vascular diseases* are a heterogeneous group of immune-mediated disorders that are characterized by inflammation and fibrosis of blood vessels and connective tissues. These include *systemic lupus erythematosus, rheumatoid arthritis, Sjögren syndrome, progressive systemic sclerosis* (*scleroderma*), *CREST* (calcinosis, Raynaud phenomenon, esophageal dysmotility, sclerodactyly, and telangiectasia) *syndrome*, and *mixed connective tissue disease.*

Clinical Features. With the exceptions of progressive systemic sclerosis and CREST syndrome, most patients with connective tissue disorders do not have striking gastrointestinal manifestations. Approximately one-third of patients with systemic lupus erythematosus develop ischemic enterocolitis as a result of small vessel vasculitis (22–24). Progressive systemic sclerosis and CREST syndrome are frequently associated with mucosal telangiectasias, and some patients have vasculitis-related gastrointestinal injury. Less than 0.5 percent of patients with rheumatoid arthritis have vasculitis of the gastrointestinal tract (25–27). Patients with high rheumatoid factor titers and cutaneous disease manifestations are more likely to develop ischemia-related enterocolitis and ulcers (28). Nearly 25 percent of patients with Sjögren syndrome experience esophageal symptoms related to inadequate oral secretions (29).

Approximately 90 percent of patients with progressive systemic sclerosis or CREST syndrome have symptoms related to the gastrointestinal tract; it is the most commonly affected extracutaneous site in patients with these disorders (30). Patients present with symptoms related to mural fibrosis and dysmotility (31). Presenting manifestations are usually related to esophageal disease and include dysphagia, odynophagia, and severe gastroesophageal reflux disease (32). Gastric involvement causes delayed emptying, early satiety, bloating, and obstructive symptoms. Poor intestinal motility promotes small intestinal bacterial overgrowth, leading to malabsorptive diarrhea.

Pathogenesis. Progressive systemic sclerosis and CREST syndrome probably cause a vasculopathy that leads to neural damage and muscle fibrosis. Autoantibodies to myenteric nerve components are present in most patients with progressive systemic sclerosis, although it is not clear whether they cause injury or merely represent an epiphenomenon (33). Systemic lupus erythematosus and rheumatoid arthritis feature a variety of autoantibodies that can affect any organ system. Vascular injury results from inflammation and complement deposition that activate endothelial cells, causing thrombosis and damage to the muscularis propria and autonomic nervous system (34). These changes may lead to decreased intestinal motility and lymphangiectasia that result in altered intestinal flora and protein-losing enteropathy (35–37). Dysregulated lymphocytes infiltrate glandular epithelium in Sjögren syndrome, although the mechanisms are poorly understood (29).

Gross Findings. Progressive systemic sclerosis and CREST syndrome are frequently associated with mucosal telangiectasias and vascular ectasias throughout the gastrointestinal tract (30,38). Wide-mouthed diverticula develop as a result of increased intraluminal pressures (39). Fibrosis at the gastroesophageal junction results in incompetence of the lower esophageal sphincter and severe gastroesophageal reflux disease. Esophageal webs are reported in Sjögren syndrome (29).

Microscopic Findings. Progressive systemic sclerosis typically causes mural fibrosis, particularly affecting the inner layer of the muscularis propria (fig. 6-7). Mural vessels often show proliferative endarteritis (40). Vasculitis due to systemic lupus erythematosus features fibrinoid necrosis of small vessels with mixed inflammation accompanied by ischemic mucosal changes (fig. 6-8) (41). Rheumatoid arthritis causes necrotizing inflammation of medium-sized

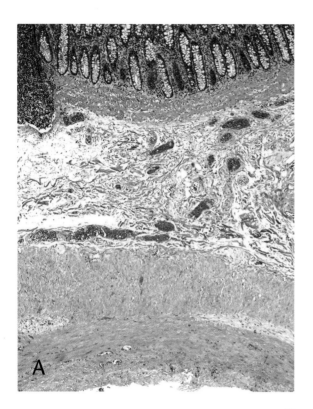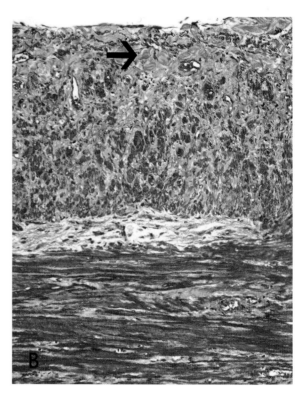

Figure 6-7

PROGRESSIVE SYSTEMIC SCLEROSIS

Smooth muscle of the muscularis propria is replaced by fibrosis (A). A trichrome stain demonstrates a predilection of fibrosis for the inner layer (arrow) of the muscularis propria (B).

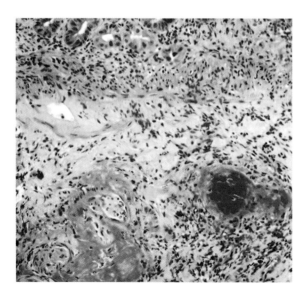

Figure 6-8

SYSTEMIC LUPUS ERYTHEMATOSUS

Biopsy samples from the small intestine reveal ischemic enteritis and small vessel vasculitis with fibrinoid necrosis and mixed inflammation.

arteries (42). Atrophic gastritis and chronic inflammation of esophageal glands and ducts may be seen in Sjögren syndrome (29).

Treatment and Prognosis. Connective tissue diseases are systemic disorders that require immunosuppressive therapy. Treatment of gastrointestinal manifestations is aimed at symptomatic relief and maintaining nutrition. Dysmotility and small intestinal bacterial overgrowth are managed with various combinations of prokinetic and probiotic agents (43,44). Patients with malabsorption are maintained with high-protein diets, although some require either enteral or parenteral nutrition (45). Esophageal strictures can be endoscopically dilated but intestinal surgery carries a risk of prolonged ileus (46). Therapy for Sjögren syndrome is aimed at increasing salivary gland secretions to improve passage of food through the upper digestive tract (47).

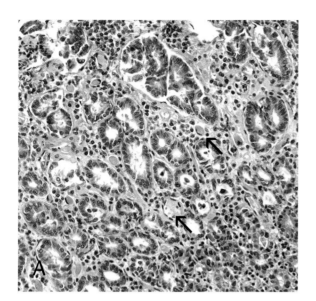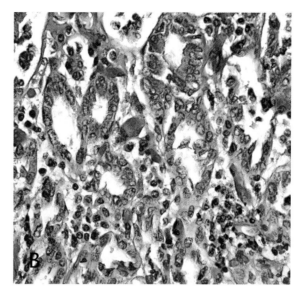

Figure 6-9

CRYOGLOBULINEMIA

Hyalinized thrombi (arrows) occlude small vessels in the jejunal mucosa of a patient with mixed cryoglobulinemia (A). A periodic acid–Schiff plus diastase (PAS-D) stain highlights thrombi (B).

DEPOSITION DISEASES

Cryoglobulinemia

Definition. Cryoglobulins are circulating immunoglobulins that precipitate when cooled and resolubilize upon warming. *Cryoglobulinemia* is systemic small vessel vasculitis caused by immunoglobulin deposition

Clinical Features. Cryoglobulinemia primarily affects the skin, joints, kidneys, and peripheral nervous system. Patients present with purpura, glomerulonephritis, peripheral neuropathy, and arthritis. Involvement of the gastrointestinal tract occurs in less than 5 percent of affected patients, producing abdominal pain and gastrointestinal bleeding. Cardiac involvement, including valve damage and myocardial infarction, is also rare (48).

Pathogenesis. Cryoglobulins are classified by the type of precipitating immunoglobulin and nature of underlying condition. Type I cryoglobulins are monoclonal immunoglobulins linked to B-cell lymphoproliferative disorders (49). Type II cryoglobulins feature polyclonal IgG and monoclonal IgM with rheumatoid factor. Type III cryoglobulins consist of polyclonal IgG and polyclonal IgM with rheumatoid factor (50). Types II and III cryoglobulins are considered mixed cryoglobulinemias and are often associated with hepatitis C virus infection (48). Cryoglobulins cause injury when they deposit in capillaries and activate complement, resulting in neutrophilic infiltrates, endothelial damage, and thrombosis (51).

Gross Findings. Cryoglobulinemia-associated vasculitis can induce sloughing of intestinal mucosa with contact bleeding, mucosal friability, and ulcers (52,53).

Microscopic Findings. Biopsy samples show active mucosal inflammation or erosions and congested capillaries that contain hyalinized thrombi composed of fibrin and immunoglobulin (fig. 6-9). Patients can develop leukocytoclastic angiitis which features neutrophilic infiltration and fibrinoid necrosis of arterioles and capillaries.

Treatment and Prognosis. Treatment of cryoglobulinemia is aimed at controlling the underlying inflammatory disorder. Corticosteroid therapy may alleviate vasculitic flares but high doses are contraindicated in patients with hematopoietic malignancies and hepatitis C virus infection (54). Severe disease and gastrointestinal involvement are associated with worse outcomes (55).

Amyloidosis

Definition. *Amyloidosis* is a heterogeneous group of disorders featuring abnormal accumulation of extracellular misfolded proteins or immunoglobulins.

Clinical Features. Amyloidosis frequently involves the gastrointestinal tract. Approximately 70 percent of patients with AL amyloidosis (κ or λ immunoglobulin light chains) and 55 percent of those with AA amyloidosis (serum amyloid A) have gastrointestinal involvement (56). Although most individuals with limited disease are asymptomatic, those with extensive amyloidosis develop gastrointestinal symptoms. Esophageal amyloidosis leads to reflux and dysphagia. Gastric involvement may manifest with bloating, pain, gastric outlet obstruction, and hematemesis. Diarrhea results from malabsorption secondary to mucosal deposits, as well as luminal stasis due to impaired gut motility. Gastrointestinal bleeding and ischemic enterocolitis may result from vascular fragility. Weight loss, nausea, vomiting, diarrhea, constipation, and melena occur in patients with both primary and secondary amyloidosis (56).

Pathogenesis. Acquired amyloidosis usually results from an underlying inflammatory or neoplastic condition. Misfolded proteins aggregate into amyloid fibrils and precipitate with a β-pleated sheet structure. More than 30 such proteins have been identified (57). Plasma cell dyscrasias give rise to AL (immunoglobulin light chains) and AH (immunoglobulin heavy chains) amyloidosis, whereas AA occurs in patients with rheumatoid arthritis, idiopathic inflammatory bowel disease, familial Mediterranean fever, and other chronic inflammatory conditions. Senile amyloidosis results from the accumulation of ATTR (tissue transthyretin) and is usually asymptomatic. Accumulation of Aβ2M (β2-microglobulin) used to be a frequent consequence of chronic kidney disease because the abnormal protein was not removed by hemodialysis, although this abnormality is much less common in the modern era (58). Defects in genes encoding several proteins underlie hereditary forms of amyloidosis, such as ATTR and ApoAI (apolipoprotein AI) (59). Systemic amyloidosis causes multisystem organ dysfunction due to mechanical effects of tissue distortion (60).

Gross Findings. Amyloid deposits cause mucosal granularity and friability. Strictures, ulcers, and mucosal atrophy also occur. The small bowel may feature nodularity and scalloped mucosal folds; yellow-white polyps can occur in the small intestine and colon. Abundant amyloid deposition can produce thickened, indurated folds (fig. 6-10). Patients may also have esophagitis and retained gastric contents due to decreased motility (56).

Microscopic Findings. Amyloid deposits consist of amorphous, waxy, pink material with characteristic cracking artifact. Vascular and perivascular deposits around submucosal arteries are most common, although more extensive deposits can be seen in the muscularis propria and myenteric nerves. Mucosal deposits are less common and may simulate fibrosis (fig. 6-11). Some have suggested that AA amyloid is more often present in the lamina propria compared with AL, although both types of amyloid can be seen in all layers of the bowel wall and around vessels (61). Deposits typically have a nodular or globular appearance (fig. 6-12).

Rectal and gastric biopsies are often employed to diagnose gastrointestinal amyloidosis, although biopsy samples obtained from multiple sites are more likely to yield a diagnosis (fig. 6-13) (61). Tissue samples should be sufficiently deep to include superficial submucosal vessels, as these are often the most heavily involved regions in the gut.

Immunohistochemical and Ultrastructural Findings. Amyloid stains bright red with Congo red histochemical stains and displays apple-green birefringence under polarized light (fig. 6-14) (62). Immunofluorescence for thioflavin can also be used to detect amyloid, and immunohistochemical stains for κ and λ can identify immunoglobulin light chain-derived amyloid.

Electron microscopy demonstrates a characteristic fibrillary structure consisting of twisted β-pleated sheets; the interlocking fibrils form unbranched structures that measure 7.5 to 10.0 μm in width (60). Immunohistochemistry is of limited use for subtyping amyloid. Mass spectrometry can be used to determine amyloid protein composition (63).

Differential Diagnosis. Amyloid occasionally deposits in a subepithelial distribution, simulating collagenous colitis, as discussed in

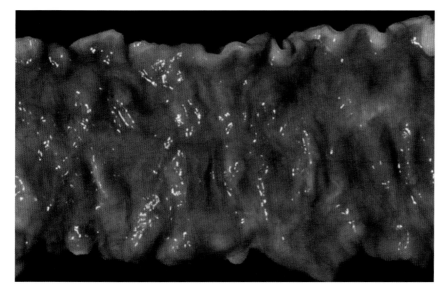

Figure 6-10

AMYLOIDOSIS

A segment of colon removed at autopsy has indurated mucosal folds. The thickened colonic wall is rigid upon opening.

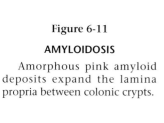

Figure 6-11

AMYLOIDOSIS

Amorphous pink amyloid deposits expand the lamina propria between colonic crypts.

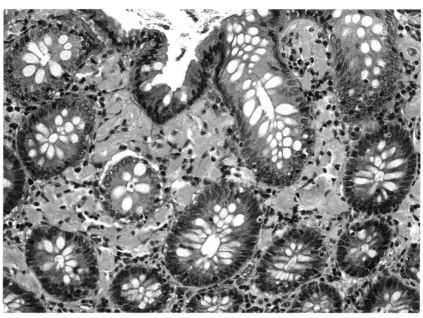

chapter 5. In contrast to amyloid, subepithelial collagen deposits display an irregular interface with the subjacent lamina propria, are more deeply eosinophilic, and contain proliferating blood vessels, inflammatory cells, and apoptotic debris as well as other features of microscopic colitis (64). Collagen can be highlighted with a trichrome stain and is not congophilic. Other entities in the differential diagnosis are lymphoplasmacytic lymphoma and light chain deposition disease, described below.

Treatment and Prognosis. Treatment of patients with hematopoietic neoplasms con-sists of systemic chemotherapy targeting the plasma cell dyscrasia. Immunosuppression improves outcome in patients with rheumato-logic disorders and serum amyloid A deposition. Therapeutic options are limited for those with hereditary amyloidosis, who often must rely on organ transplantation. Emerging treatment modalities include RNA-inhibiting agents and monoclonal antibodies directed against amyloid deposits (65). Prognosis is heavily influenced by the extent of organ damage; patients with poor cardiac function can succumb to the disease within months of diagnosis (66).

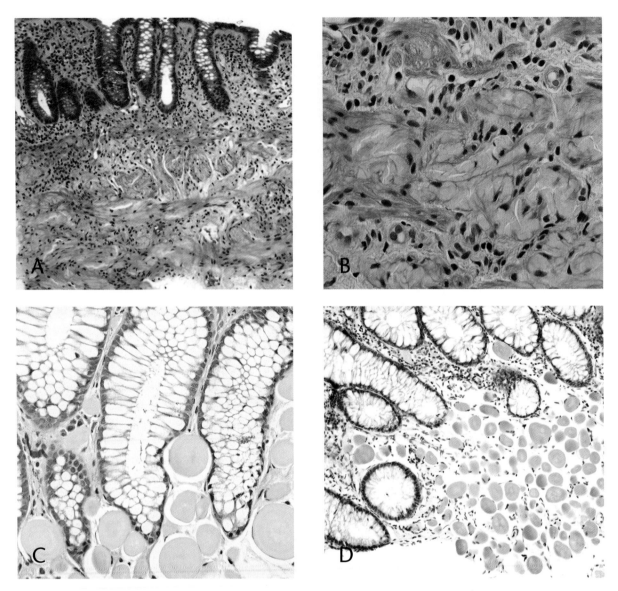

Figure 6-12

AMYLOIDOSIS

Colonic biopsy samples from a patient with primary amyloidosis display amyloid deposits in the submucosa (A). Amorphous vascular deposits expand the vessel walls and occlude their lumens (B). Occasional cases feature round deposits that lack a waxy appearance and simulate other proteinaceous deposits (C). Congo red stains help establish a diagnosis (D).

Lymphoplasmacytic Lymphoma

Lymphoplasmacytic lymphoma with immunoglobulin deposits (*Waldenström macroglobulinemia*) and light chain deposition disease can produce eosinophilic extracellular material that simulates amyloid. Monoclonal IgM deposits occur in patients with lymphoplasmacytic lymphomas that secrete immunoglobulin.

Clinical findings include hepatosplenomegaly, lymphadenopathy, and increased blood viscosity in combination with 10 percent or more clonal lymphoplasmacytic cells in bone marrow samples (67). Most patients have an established IgM monoclonal gammopathy of undetermined significance (MGUS).

The small intestine is the most frequent site of protein deposition, which imparts a nodular

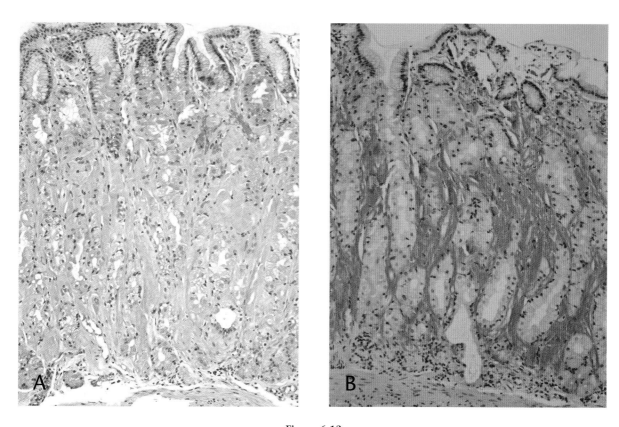

Figure 6-13

AMYLOIDOSIS

Amyloid deposits expand the mucosa and obliterate oxyntic glands in this gastric sample from a hemodialysis patient (A). A Congo red stain highlights extensive mucosal involvement and characteristic cracks in amyloid deposits (B).

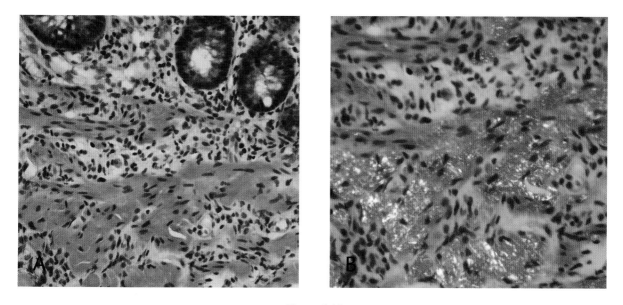

Figure 6-14

AMYLOIDOSIS

Amyloid deposits are congophilic (A) and display "apple-green" birefringence under polarized light (B).

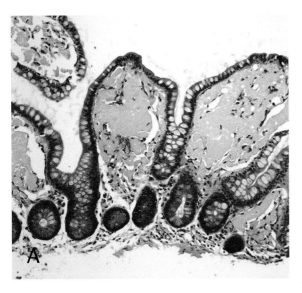
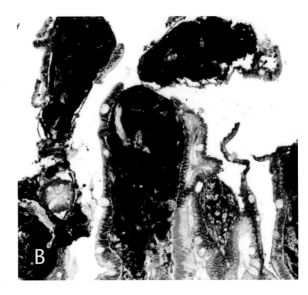

Figure 6-15

IMMUNOGLOBULIN DEPOSITS DUE TO LYMPHOPLASMACYTIC LYMPHOMA

The villi are distended by immunoglobulin deposits that are more dense and eosinophilic than amyloid (A). The deposits stain strongly with antibodies against IgM and are Congo red negative (B).

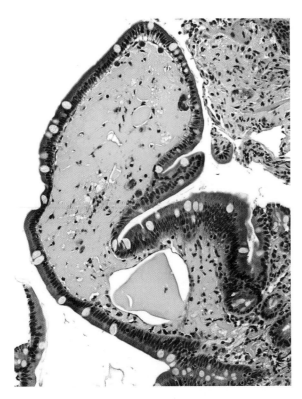

Figure 6-16

LIGHT CHAIN DEPOSITION DISEASE

Light chain immunoglobulins expand the villi and are morphologically similar to IgM deposits. (Courtesy of Dr. S. Owens, Ann Arbor, MI.)

white-gray appearance that is most pronounced on the crests of folds (68). Dense, eosinophilic immunoglobulin deposits expand the lamina propria and cause villous blunting (fig. 6-15A). Lymphangiectasia and foamy macrophages are frequently associated findings. Immunoglobulin deposits are periodic acid-Schiff (PAS) positive and diastase resistant, with strong, diffuse IgM immunostaining and light chain restriction (fig. 6-15B) (67).

Light Chain Deposition Disease

Light chain deposition disease results from a clonal expansion of plasma cells. The kidneys and heart are almost always affected, whereas gastrointestinal involvement is rare (69). Light chains form eosinophilic deposits in and around blood vessels and expand the lamina propria, similar to IgM (fig. 6-16). They show either κ or λ restriction, tend to have a more granular ultrastructural appearance than amyloid, and lack typical apple-green birefringence upon polarization of Congo red stains (62).

NON-NEOPLASTIC POLYPOSIS SYNDROMES

A short synopsis of the hamartomatous syndromes is presented. The reader is referred to reference 70 for a comprehensive discussion of this topic.

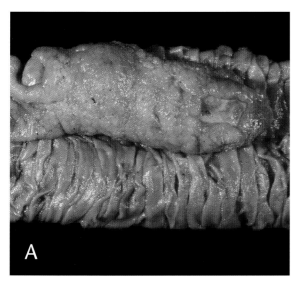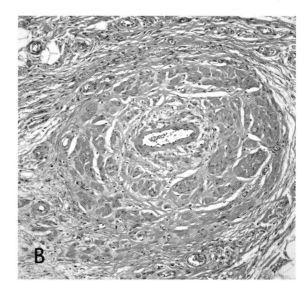

Figure 6-17

SPORADIC HAMARTOMA

A sausage-shaped polypoid mass is attached to the small bowel by a thick pedicle. The overlying mucosa is granular, with patchy ulcers related to luminal trauma (A). The hamartoma contains aggregates of fibroadipose tissue and blood vessels surrounded by disorganized bundles of smooth muscle cells (B).

Sporadic Hamartomatous Polyps

Gastrointestinal hamartomas contain a combination of nondysplastic mucosal elements, lymphoid tissue, and mesenchymal tissue (fig. 6-17). Sporadic hamartomas are uncommon in the upper gastrointestinal tract. Disorganized aggregates of fibroadipose tissue, smooth muscle, and abnormal blood vessels comprise esophageal hamartomas (71,72). Gastric polyps contain variable numbers of pyloric glands, foveolar or oxyntic epithelium, and supportive stroma. Intestinal hamartomas feature the normal elements of the wall but the components are somewhat disorganized, and may feature abnormally thick-walled vessels. Supportive lamina propria is variably inflamed and the crypts are often dilated.

Sporadic juvenile polyps occur in 1 to 2 percent of the pediatric population (73). They have a sessile or pedunculated appearance with a smooth, erythematous surface. Juvenile polyps of the distal colorectum readily auto-amputate, presenting with hematochezia or passage of tissue per rectum. They contain cystically dilated crypts and inflamed, edematous stroma with numerous eosinophils. Other colonic hamartomas are subcentimeter polyps containing thick-walled blood vessels, fat, and irregularly distributed ganglion cells.

Juvenile Polyposis Syndrome

Juvenile polyposis syndrome is an autosomal dominant disorder affecting 1/100,000 persons. It is classified as *infantile juvenile polyposis, juvenile polyposis coli,* or *generalized juvenile polyposis* depending on its phenotypic manifestations. Diagnostic clinical criteria include: 1) at least five colorectal juvenile polyps, 2) any number of extracolonic juvenile polyps, and 3) juvenile polyps in patients with affected family members (74).

Juvenile polyposis results from TGF-β–mediated signaling abnormalities; alterations in *SMAD4* or *BMBR1A* are detected in nearly 50 percent of patients (75,76). The nature of the underlying molecular defect is related to phenotypic manifestations. For example, patients with upper gastrointestinal tract polyposis and hereditary hemorrhagic telangiectasia usually have *SMAD4* mutations, whereas cardiac defects are associated with *BMBR1A* mutations (77,78). Infantile juvenile polyposis is often the result of large deletions involving *BMBR1A* and *PTEN* (79). The cumulative colorectal cancer risk is 68 percent by 60 years of age (80). Carcinomas of the stomach, pancreas,

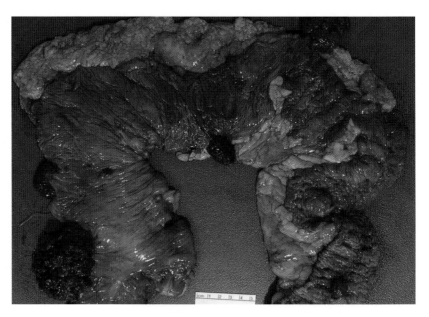

Figure 6-18

JUVENILE POLYPOSIS SYNDROME

Several mulberry-like pedunculated polyps are present in a colectomy specimen from a patient with juvenile polyposis syndrome.

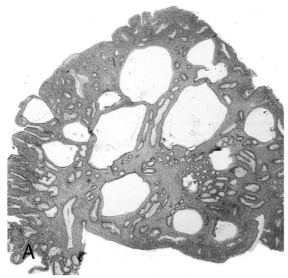

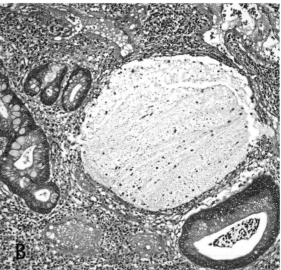

Figure 6-19

JUVENILE POLYPOSIS SYNDROME

Typical juvenile polyps contain cystically dilated crypts surrounded by inflamed, edematous stroma (A). The lamina propria is expanded by a mixed inflammatory cell infiltrate rich in eosinophils (B).

and proximal small intestine also occur in combination with the syndrome (81,82).

Most juvenile polyps have a smooth, granular surface, although larger lesions often have a mulberry-like appearance (fig. 6-18). Syndromic colorectal polyps often resemble sporadic juvenile polyps or inflammatory-type polyps. They contain cystically dilated crypts and inflamed lamina propria with numerous eosinophils

and occasional ganglion cells or neuromatous elements (fig. 6-19) (83).

Atypical juvenile polyps occur exclusively in association with juvenile polyposis syndrome. They tend to contain more crowded crypts that vary in size and shape rather than evenly distributed dilated crypts embedded in eosinophil-rich lamina propria (fig. 6-20). Atypical juvenile polyps can develop conventional-type dysplasia

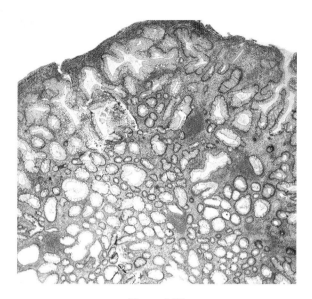

Figure 6-20

JUVENILE POLYPOSIS SYNDROME

Atypical juvenile polyps have a higher gland to stroma ratio than typical polyps. Crypts are crowded and branched and are irregularly distributed in the lamina propria.

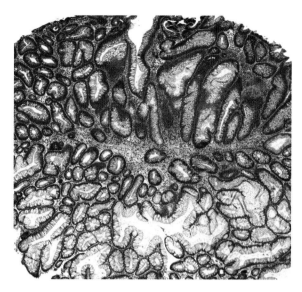

Figure 6-21

JUVENILE POLYPOSIS SYNDROME

Some atypical juvenile polyps develop dysplasia, which generally resembles that of conventional tubular or villous adenomas. Crowded cells with enlarged, hyperchromatic nuclei populate the crypts and surface of the polyp.

similar to that seen in tubular and villous colorectal adenomas (fig. 6-21). Gastric juvenile polyps resemble hyperplastic polyps. Numerous juvenile polyps of the stomach can grow in a confluent fashion, causing diffuse expansion of the gastric mucosa that mimics Menetrier disease (fig. 6-22) (84).

Peutz-Jeghers Syndrome

Peutz-Jeghers syndrome affects 1/200,000 persons with an autosomal dominant pattern of inheritance. The syndrome features numerous gastrointestinal hamartomatous polyps in combination with mucocutaneous pigmentation and an overall increased risk for cancer of 93 percent by 65 years of age (85,86). Risk is highest for colorectal cancer (35 to 40 percent), followed by carcinomas of the pancreas (35 percent) and stomach (28 percent). Malignancies outside the gastrointestinal tract occur in the breast, testes, and gynecologic tract.

Children and young adults typically present with abdominal pain or bleeding related to intussusception or trauma to benign polyps, whereas older patients more often manifest disease with malignant complications (87). More than 50 percent of patients with Peutz-Jeghers syndrome have *LKB1* (*STK11*) mutations;

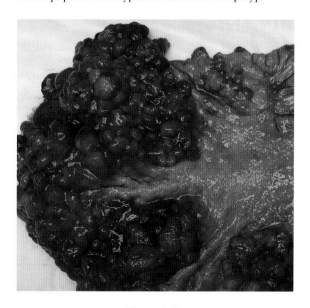

Figure 6-22

JUVENILE POLYPOSIS SYNDROME

Clusters of polyps carpet the distal stomach. The uninvolved rugae appear normal. (Courtesy of Dr. D. Lewin, Charleston, SC.)

this gene encodes a serine threonine kinase responsible for regulating cell growth and *p27* transcription (88–91).

395

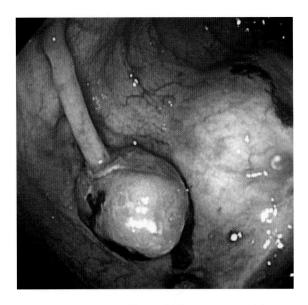

Figure 6-23

PEUTZ-JEGHERS SYNDROME

Most Peutz-Jeghers polyps are pedunculated, with a thick stalk and round smooth surface.

Hamartomatous polyps show a predilection for the small intestine, although at least 50 percent of affected patients have lesions in the stomach, colorectum, appendix, gallbladder, bladder, or nasopharynx (92,93). Peutz-Jeghers polyps generally have a multinodular smooth surface and thick stalk reflecting large aggregates of smooth muscle cells (fig. 6-23). Polyps contain aggregates of non-dysplastic mucosal elements surrounded by bundles of smooth muscle cells that emanate from the muscularis mucosae (fig. 6-24). Lesional crypts are normal or show slight serration or dilatation. Occasional polyps contain foci of dysplasia. Up to 10 percent of small bowel hamartomas are associated with aggregates of epithelium and lamina propria extending through the muscularis propria (fig. 6-25).

Virtually all Peutz-Jeghers polyps occur in patients with the syndrome. Solitary lesions are associated with cancer risk similar to that of syndromic lesions, and they likely represent a *forme fruste* of the syndrome (94).

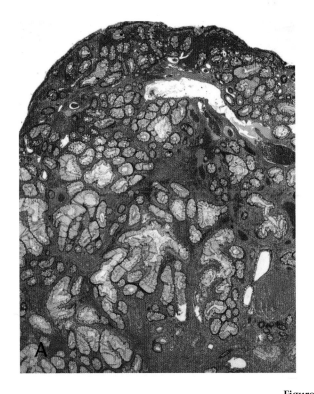
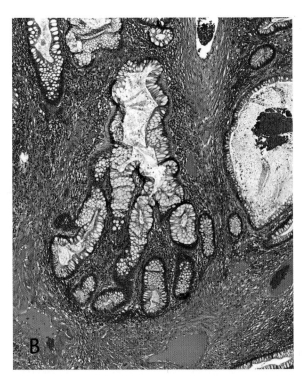

Figure 6-24

PEUTZ-JEGHERS SYNDROME

A colonic polyp contains bundles of smooth muscle cells emanating from the muscularis mucosae, entrapping lobules of non-dysplastic mucosal elements (A). Colonic crypts often have a slightly hyperplastic appearance or contain numerous goblet cells. They are invested by a rim of lamina propria (B).

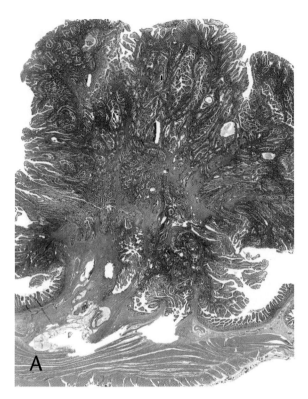
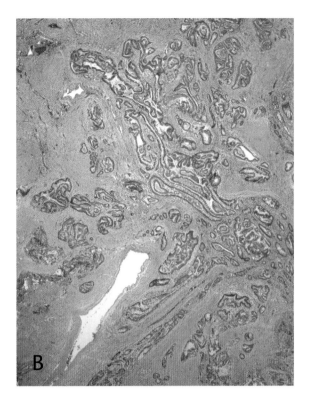

Figure 6-25

PEUTZ-JEGHERS SYNDROME

Small intestinal polyps usually display well-developed arborizing bundles of smooth muscle cells emanating from the muscularis mucosae into the polyp head (A). Lobules of mucosal elements are present in the polyp stalk or the muscularis propria (B).

PTEN Hamartoma-Tumor Syndrome

PTEN hamartoma-tumor syndrome is an autosomal dominant disorder affecting 1/200,000 persons (95). It features various types of hamartomatous polyps throughout the gastrointestinal tract, oral and cutaneous hamartomatous lesions, benign and malignant diseases of the breast and thyroid gland, and macrocephaly; it encompasses Cowden syndrome, Bannayan-Riley-Ruvalcaba syndrome, and related disorders (96,97).

Mucocutaneous manifestations occur in virtually all patients, although hamartomatous polyps develop in only 35 to 40 percent. Patients are at increased risk for both colonic adenomas and carcinomas but lifetime risk is highest for carcinomas of the breast (25 to 50 percent in women) and thyroid gland (10 percent) (92,98).

PTEN is a tumor suppressor gene that encodes a lipid phosphatase important to cell cycling, apoptosis, and genomic stability. Some patients have phenotypic manifestations of disease but lack germline *PTEN* mutations; they may have mutations affecting dehydrogenase complex subunits B (*SDHB*) or D (*SDHD*) (99).

Gastrointestinal manifestations of *PTEN* hamartoma-tumor syndrome are variable. Multifocal esophageal glycogenic acanthosis is virtually pathognomonic, although it is not present in all patients with the syndrome (fig. 6-26). Gastric hamartomas contain dilated, regenerative-appearing pits and edematous lamina propria, similar to hyperplastic polyps of the stomach (100). Some intestinal polyps resemble juvenile polyps or inflammatory polyps with cystic crypts and mucosal edema. Others resemble normal mucosa but contain myofibroblastic proliferations, Schwann cells, or ganglion cells in the lamina propria. Affected patients also have prominent lymphoid aggregates, ganglioneuromas, lipomas, and adenomas elsewhere in the colon (fig. 6-27) (101,102).

Cronkhite-Canada Syndrome

Cronkhite-Canada syndrome is a rare, acquired condition characterized by gastrointestinal polyposis, skin hyperpigmentation, alopecia, onychodystrophy, and malabsorptive diarrhea

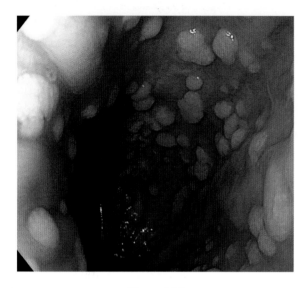

Figure 6-26

PTEN **HAMARTOMA-TUMOR SYNDROME**

Multifocal glycogenic acanthosis is a common esophageal manifestation.

(103). Most cases have been reported in older adults from Europe, the United States, and Japan (104).

The etiology of Cronkhite-Canada syndrome is unknown but the disorder is best considered a form of non-heritable inflammatory polyposis; extraintestinal manifestations of disease are mostly the result of mucosal abnormalities in the gastrointestinal tract. It may represent an immune-mediated disorder: some patients have elevated serum IgG4 and increased IgG4-bearing plasma cell infiltrates in gastrointestinal polyps; others have systemic lupus erythematosus, thyroiditis, rheumatoid arthritis, or antinuclear antibodies (105).

Patients with Cronkhite-Canada syndrome develop inflammatory polyps throughout the gastrointestinal tract. Most are hyperemic, slightly translucent nodules coated by mucin (fig. 6-28A) (106). They contain hyperplastic and cystically dilated glands or crypts supported by edematous lamina propria with mixed inflammation and prominent eosinophils (fig. 6-28B). Similar inflammatory changes are often detected in the non-polypoid mucosa, allowing for distinction from hamartomatous polyposis syndromes.

Up to 25 percent of affected patients have gastrointestinal cancers at the time of diagnosis, although this relationship may be influenced

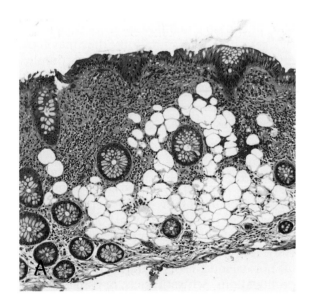
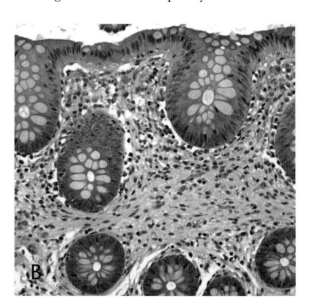

Figure 6-27

PTEN **HAMARTOMA-TUMOR SYNDROME**

Many colonic hamartomas feature a lipomatous component (A) or ganglioneuromatous elements (B).

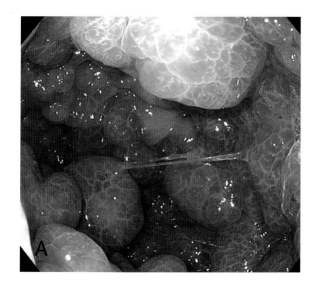 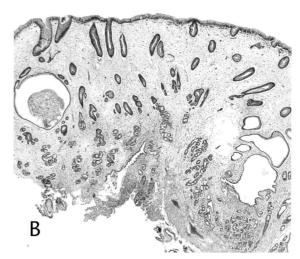

Figure 6-28

CRONKHITE-CANADA SYNDROME

The gastric folds are effaced by innumerable erythematous polyps, some of which are surfaced by adherent mucin (A). (Courtesy of Dr. M. Feely, Gainesville, FL.) Gastric polyps feature cystically dilated glands supported by edematous lamina propria (B). (Courtesy of Dr. E. Montgomery, Baltimore, MD.)

by reporting bias of this rare disorder combined with the overall incidence of gastrointestinal carcinomas in older patients (107). Treatment consists of correction of electrolyte imbalances, nutritional supplementation, rehydration, antibiotics, antihistamines, and immunosuppressive therapies. Patients undergo regular surveillance for colorectal cancer and may be referred for colectomy in the event of dysplasia development (106). Cronkhite-Canada syndrome is associated with high mortality; nearly 50 percent of patients die from malnutrition, bleeding, or infection (108).

Ganglioneuromas and Ganglioneuromatosis

Ganglioneuromas and *ganglioneuromatosis* are hamartomatous proliferations of ganglion cells, nerve fibers, Schwann cells, and fibroblasts. They affect the intestine in a localized or diffuse fashion. Multifocal ganglioneuromas may reflect underlying *PTEN* hamartoma-tumor syndrome or juvenile polyposis syndrome, whereas ganglioneuromatosis is almost always associated with multiple endocrine neoplasia (MEN) IIB or type I neurofibromatosis. Any intestinal segment may be affected, although disease is most common in the colon. Large lesions can cause dysmotility, obstruction, or megacolon (109).

Ganglioneuromas usually appear as small polypoid protrusions surfaced by normal-appearing mucosa, whereas ganglioneuromatosis presents as an ill-defined diffuse mural thickening (fig. 6-29A). Larger lesions are centered in the muscularis propria or submucosa and form ill-defined, nodular aggregates that displace normal elements and penetrate the mucosa (fig. 6-29B,C). They consist of disorganized bundles of nerves and Schwann cells that contain clustered and singly dispersed mature ganglion cells (fig. 6-29D) (110).

Ganglioneuromas and ganglioneuromatosis are benign. Surgical resection is limited to patients with obstructive symptoms or bleeding complications (109).

MISCELLANEOUS DISORDERS

Malakoplakia

Definition. *Malakoplakia* is an intracytoplasmic accumulation of partially digested microbes within mononuclear phagocytic cells.

Clinical Features. The colon is the second most common site affected by malakoplakia, following the genitourinary tract. Other sites less commonly affected include the skin, gynecologic tracts, visceral organs, and extra-colonic gastrointestinal

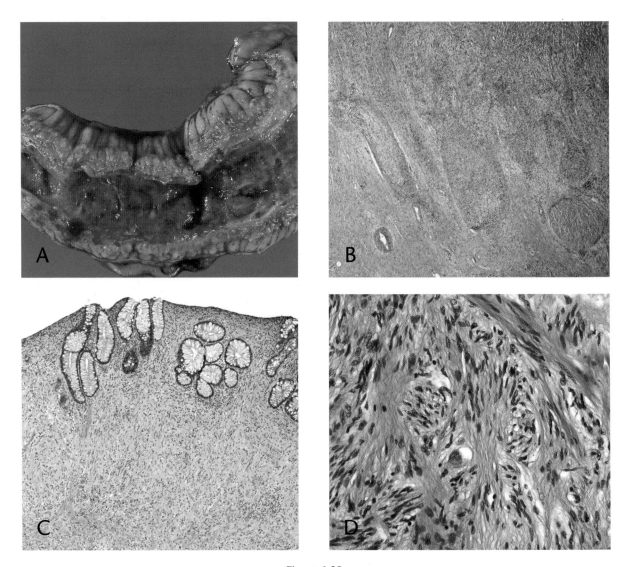

Figure 6-29

GANGLIONEUROMATOSIS OF THE APPENDIX

The appendix from a patient with type 1 neurofibromatosis is diffusely thickened (A). The same case features a multinodular proliferation of ganglioneuromatous elements that distorts and expands the muscularis propria (B). Infiltration of the appendiceal mucosa effaces the lamina propria and displaces the crypts (C). The proliferation consists of disorganized bundles of nerves, ganglion cells, and Schwann cells (D).

organs (111,112). Gastrointestinal malakoplakia may be asymptomatic or cause abdominal pain, diarrhea, rectal bleeding, and fever. It occurs in immunosuppressed patients and may be seen in combination with concomitant colonic adenocarcinoma (113).

Pathogenesis. Malakoplakia results from defective digestion of phagocytosed bacteria within macrophages and monocytes due to impaired lysosomal enzyme release. Ultrastructural analyses reveal Gram-negative bacteria, such as *Escherichia coli* and *Klebsiella* sp. in various stages of degradation within phagolysosomes (62). Bacterial breakdown products become mineralized by iron and calcium deposits.

Gross Findings. Malakoplakia produces soft yellow plaques or raised gray lesions with central depressions and peripheral hyperemia (114). It usually displays segmental distribution in the rectosigmoid colon. Fibrosis and extracellular calcification may occur in patients with long-standing disease.

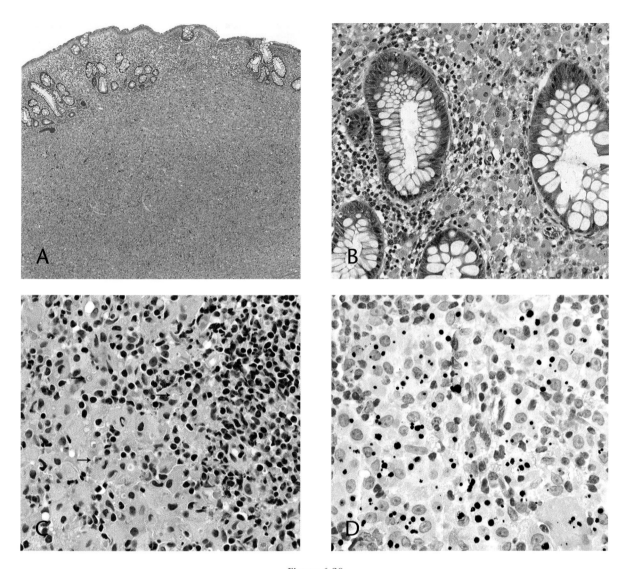

Figure 6-30

MALAKOPLAKIA

The colonic wall is diffusely infiltrated by sheets of macrophages (A) accompanied by scattered eosinophils and lymphocytes (B). (A,B: courtesy of Dr. J. Greenson, Ann Arbor, MI.) Numerous macrophages contain targetoid inclusions (arrows) representing Michaelis-Gutmann bodies (C). A von Kossa stain highlights the calcium content (D).

Microscopic Findings. Malakoplakia features sheets of macrophages permeating all layers of the bowel wall, often with effacement of mucosal architecture (fig. 6-30). Macrophages contain targetoid intracytoplasmic inclusions, called Michaelis-Gutmann bodies, which represent mineralized phagosome remnants or calcospherites (fig. 6-30C). Giant cells, eosinophils, and lymphocytes are frequently present. Michaelis-Gutmann bodies are highlighted with PAS-D, Prussian blue, and von Kossa histochemical stains (fig. 6-30D).

Differential Diagnosis. The differential diagnosis includes a variety of organisms that elicit macrophage-rich inflammatory infiltrates, such as *Histoplasma capsulatum*, *Mycobacterium avium intracellulare* (MAI) complex, *Tropheryma whipplei*, and *Leishmania donovani*. Morphologic assessment and histochemical stains reliably distinguish these organisms from malakoplakia. Fungi and mycobacteria stain with Gomori methenamine silver (GMS) and acid-fast stains, respectively, whereas leishmaniasis can be highlighted with

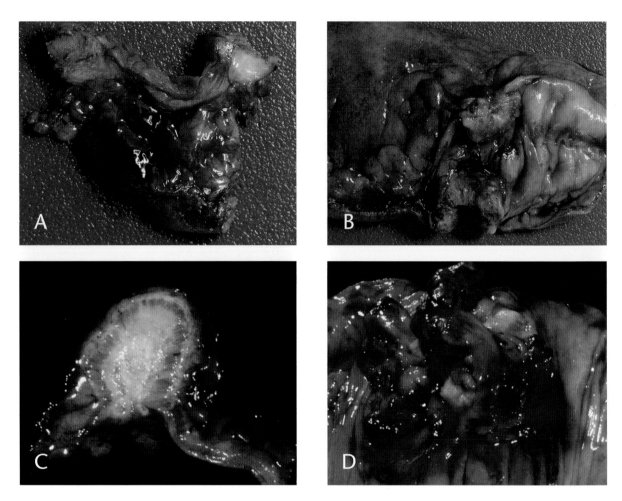

Figure 6-31

ENDOMETRIOSIS

Red-black serosal discoloration reflects hemorrhage in endometriotic foci (A). Mural infiltration induces smooth muscle hyperplasia and fibrosis resulting in strictures (B). Endometriosis forms a smooth submucosal mass projecting into the lumen (C). Inflammatory polyps and ulcers are associated with mucosal disease (D).

Giemsa stains. None of these organisms stain with iron or calcium preparations.

Treatment and Prognosis. Antibiotic therapy with quinolones and trimethoprim-sulfamethoxazole generally results in decreased symptoms. Surgical resection is rarely necessary (114).

Endometriosis

Definition. *Endometriosis* is the presence of endometrioid glands and/or stroma in extrauterine sites.

Clinical Features. Intestinal endometriosis shows a predilection for the rectosigmoid colon, particularly the rectovaginal septum, followed by the appendix and ileocecal region. Patients with limited intestinal involvement are usually asymptomatic but those with extensive disease can present with symptoms related to bowel obstruction, perforation, and bleeding (115). Catamenial abdominal pain and diarrhea are occasionally reported (116). Neoplastic transformation to mullerian-type carcinomas and sarcomas is an uncommon occurrence that is usually associated with unopposed hormonal therapy (117). Appendiceal endometriosis may clinically and radiographically simulate acute appendicitis or act as a lead point for an intussusception (118).

Pathogenesis. The mechanism by which gastrointestinal endometriosis develops is not clear. Some have suggested that it results from retrograde

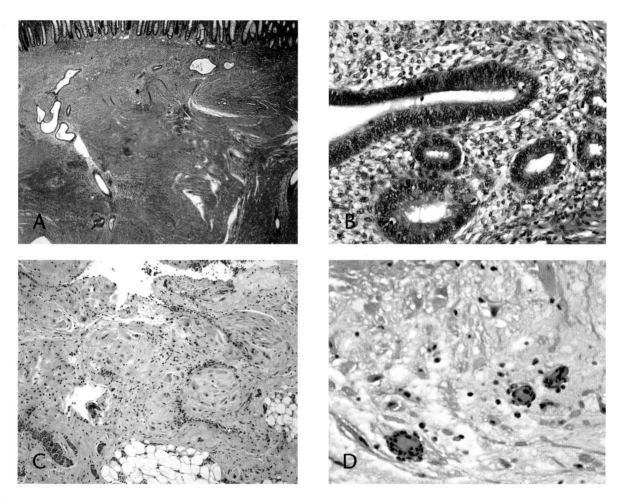

Figure 6-32

ENDOMETRIOSIS

Aggregates of endometrioid glands and stroma are present in the muscularis propria and submucosa in combination with irregular hyperplasia of smooth muscle cells and mural fibrosis (A). Endometrioid glands are enmeshed in cellular stroma (B). Lobules of decidualized stroma contain polygonal cells with abundant amphophilic cytoplasm (C). Myxoid endometrioid stroma simulates mucin and may raise the possibility of a mucinous neoplasm, particularly in the appendix (D).

flow of uterine contents into the peritoneum during menstruation. Symptoms are related to a mass effect and cyclic hormonal influences on ectopic tissue (119). Endometriosis can sometimes harbor mutations that are typically associated with neoplasms, namely alterations affecting *ARID1A*, *PIK3CA*, *KRAS*, and *PPP2R1A* (120).

Gross Findings. Serosal endometriosis can produce gray or black patches (powder burns) that reflect remote hemorrhage (fig. 6-31A). Mural endometriosis elicits hypertrophy and hyperplasia of smooth muscle cells with fibrosis, distorting the muscularis propria and causing strictures that simulate malignancy (fig. 6-31B,C). Mucosal in-

volvement can cause solitary or clustered polyps or ulcerated masses (fig. 6-31D) (116).

Microscopic Findings. Endometriotic foci contain variable proportions of endometrioid glands and stroma, often with hemorrhage and hemosiderin deposits (fig. 6-32A). Glands are often inactive or attenuated with tubal metaplasia, although proliferative changes, cystic dilatation, hyperplasia, and neoplastic transformation are well described (fig. 6-32B) (117). Stromal cells are usually plump spindle cells. Decidualized stromal cells are polygonal with abundant eosinophilic cytoplasm and well-defined cell membranes; myxoid degeneration can simulate mucin (fig. 6-32C,D).

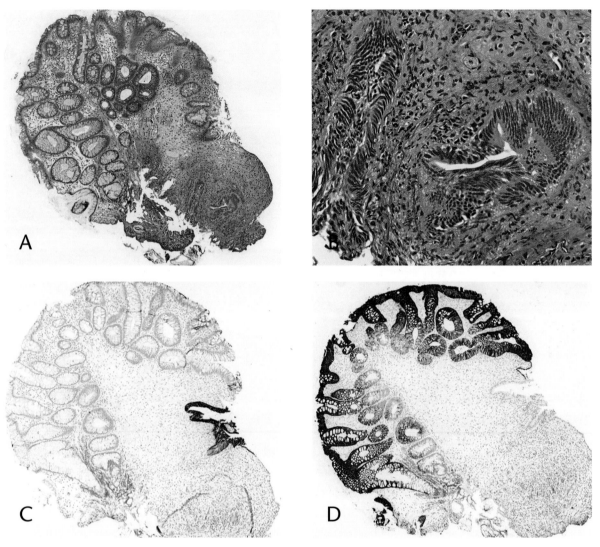

Figure 6-33

ENDOMETRIOSIS

Endometriosis can produce colonic polyps. A focus of endometrioid glands in the stalk of this polyp simulates a tubular adenoma (A). Glands lack cytoplasmic mucin and are associated with decidualized endometrioid stroma that is rich in capillaries (B). An immunostain for CK7 highlights endometrioid glands (C), whereas colonic crypts are positive for CK20 (D).

Endometriosis can induce reactive epithelial cell changes that mimic inflammatory conditions and neoplasia. It can simulate Crohn disease when it causes segmental enterocolitis because chronic mucosal changes, such as crypt hyperplasia, architectural distortion, and pyloric metaplasia occur in combination with mural fibrosis and neuronal hypertrophy. Fibromuscularization of the lamina propria accompanied by regenerative and hyperplastic crypts can simulate features of mucosal prolapse (116). Inflammatory polyps overlying endometriotic foci can feature regenerative cytologic atypia and simulate neoplasia, especially when present in association with endometrioid glands that show nuclear enlargement and an absence of cytoplasmic mucin (fig. 6-33).

The diagnosis of endometriosis is usually made following routine evaluation of histologic sections, although endometrioid glands can simulate neoplastic intestinal epithelia, particularly when they show reactive changes (fig. 6-33A,B). Endometrioid glands label with

CK7, PAX8, and estrogen receptor (fig. 6-33C,D). Endometrioid stroma can be highlighted with CD10 immunostains.

Treatment and Prognosis. Symptomatic intestinal endometriosis is usually treated with hormone therapy and analgesics (120). Extensive intestinal involvement that causes severe bleeding, obstructive symptoms, or a mass lesion often requires surgical resection.

REFERENCES

1. Bonilla FA, Barlan I, Chapel H, et al. International consensus document (ICON): common variable immunodeficiency disorders. J Allergy Clin Immunol Pract 2016;4:38-59.
2. Patuzzo G, Barbieri A, Tinazzi E, et al. Autoimmunity and infection in common variable immunodeficiency (CVID). Autoimmunity Rev 2016;15:877-82.
3. Mortaz E, Tabarsi P, Mansouri D, et al. Cancers related to immunodeficiencies: update and perspectives. Front Immunol 2016;7:365.
4. Molaei M, Kaboli A, Fathi AM, Mashayekhi R, Pejhan S, Zali MR. Nodular lymphoid hyperplasia in common variable immunodeficiency syndrome mimicking familial adenomatous polyposis on endoscopy. Indian J Pathol Microbiol 2009;52:530-3.
5. Daniels JA, Lederman HM, Maitra A, Montgomery EA. Gastrointestinal tract pathology in patients with common variable immunodeficiency (CVID): a clinicopathologic study and review. Am J Surg Pathol 2007;31:1800-12.
6. Panarelli NC, Yantiss RK. Inflammatory and infectious manifestations of immunodeficiency in the gastrointestinal tract. Mod Pathol 2018;31:844-61.
7. Park MA, Li JT, Hagan JB, Maddox DE, Abraham RS. Common variable immunodeficiency: a new look at an old disease. Lancet 2008;372:489-502.
8. Aghamohammadi A, Cheraghi T, Gharagozlou M, et al. IgA deficiency: correlation between clinical and immunological phenotypes. J Clin Immunol 2009;29:130-6.
9. Pallav K, Xu H, Leffler DA, Kabbani T, Kelly CP. Immunoglobulin a deficiency in celiac disease in the United States. J Gastroenterol Hepatol 2016;31:133-7.
10. Marciano BE, Rosenzweig SD, Kleiner DE, et al. Gastrointestinal involvement in chronic granulomatous disease. Pediatrics 2004;114:462-8.
11. Alimchandani M, Lai JP, Aung PP, et al. Gastrointestinal histopathology in chronic granulomatous disease: a study of 87 patients. Am J Surg Pathol 2013;37:1365-72.
12. Beighton P, De Paepe A, Steinmann B, Tsipouras P, Wenstrup RJ. Ehlers-Danlos syndromes: revised nosology, villefranche, 1997. Ehlers-Danlos National Foundation (USA) and Ehlers-Danlos support group (UK). Am J Med Genet 1998;77:31-7.
13. Malfait F, Francomano C, Byers P, et al. The 2017 international classification of the Ehlers-Danlos syndromes. Am J Med Genet C Semin Med Genet 2017;175:8-26.
14. Germain DP. Ehlers-Danlos syndrome type IV. Orphanet J Rare Dis 2007;2:32.
15. Germain, DP, Herrera-Guzman, Y. Vascular Ehlers-Danlos syndrome. Ann Genet 2004;47:1-9.
16. Pepin M, Schwarze U, Superti-Furga A, Byers PH. Clinical and genetic features of Ehlers-Danlos syndrome type IV, the vascular type. N Engl J Med 2000;342:673-80.
17. Prahlow JA, Wagner SA. Death due to Ehlers-Danlos syndrome type IV. Am J Forensic Med Pathol 2005;26:78-82.
18. Silva R, Cogbill TH, Hansbrough JF, Zapata-Sirvent RL, Harrington DS. Intestinal perforation and vascular rupture in Ehlers-Danlos syndrome. Int Surg 1986;71:48-50.
19. Sykes EM Jr. Colon perforation in Ehlers-Danlos syndrome. Report of two cases and review of the literature. Am J Surg 1984;147:410-3.
20. Oderich GS, Panneton JM, Bower TC, et al. The spectrum, management and clinical outcome of Ehlers-Danlos syndrome type IV: a 30-year experience. J Vasc Surg 2005;42:98-106.
21. Berney T, La Scala G, Vettorel D, et al. Surgical pitfalls in a patient with type IV Ehlers-Danlos syndrome and spontaneous colonic rupture. Report of a case. Dis Colon Rectum 1994;37:1038-42.
22. Hoffman BI, Katz WA. The gastrointestinal manifestations of systemic lupus erythematosus: a review of the literature. Semin Arthritis Rheum 1980;9:237-47.
23. Weiser MM, Andres GA, Brentjens Jr, Evans JT, Reichlin M. Systemic lupus erythematosus and intestinal venulitis. Gastroenterology 1981;81:570-9.
24. Papa MZ, Shiloni E, McDonald HD. Total colonic necrosis. A catastrophic complication of systemic lupus erythematosus. Dis Colon Rectum 1986;29:576-8.
25. Bienenstock H, Minick CR, Rogoff B. Mesenteric arteritis and intestinal infarction in rheumatoid disease. Arch Intern Med 1967;119:359-64.
26. Lindsay MK, Tavadia HB, Whyte AS, Lee P, Webb J. Acute abdomen in rheumatoid arthritis due to necrotizing arteritis. Br Med J 1973;2:592-3.

27. Louie CY, DiMaio MA, Charville GW, Berry GJ, Longacre TA. Gastrointestinal tract vasculopathy: clinicopathology and description of a possible "new entity" with protean features. Am J Surg Pathol 2018;42:866-76.

28. Babian M, Nasef S, Soloway G. Gastrointestinal infarction as a manifestation of rheumatoid vasculitis. Am J Gastroenterol 1998;93:119-20.

29. Popov Y, Salomon-Escoto K. Gastrointestinal and hepatic disease in Sjogren syndrome. Rheum Dis Clin North Am 2018;44:143-51.

30. Forbes A, Marie I. Gastrointestinal complications: the most frequent internal complications of systemic sclerosis. Rheumatology 2009;48 (Suppl 3):iii36-9.

31. Bassel K, Harford W. Gastrointestinal manifestations of collagen-vascular diseases. Semin Gastrointest Dis 1995;6:228-40.

32. Denaxas K, Ladas SD, Karamanolis GP. Evaluation and management of esophageal manifestations in systemic sclerosis. Ann Gastroenterol 2018;31:165-70.

33. Kawaguchi Y, Nakamura Y, Matsumoto I, et al. Muscarinic-3 acetylcholine receptor autoantibody in patients with systemic sclerosis: contribution to severe gastrointestinal tract dysmotility. Ann Rheum Dis 2009;68:710-4.

34. Alves SC, Fasano S, Isenberg DA. Autoimmune gastrointestinal complications in patients with systemic lupus erythematosus: case series and literature review. Lupus 2016;25:1509-19.

35. Al-Mogairen SM. Lupus protein-losing enteropathy (LUPLE): a systematic review. Rheumatol Int 2011;31:995-1001.

36. Abdollahi-Roodsaz S, Joosten LA, Koenders MI, et al. Stimulation of TLR2 and TLR4 differentially skews the balance of T cells in a mouse model of arthritis. J Clin Invest 2008;118:205-16.

37. Wu HJ, Ivanov II, Darce J, et al. Gut-residing segmented filamentous bacteria drive autoimmune arthritis via T helper 17 cells. Immunity 2010;32:815-27.

38. Kirby DF, Chatterjee S. Evaluation and management of gastrointestinal manifestations in scleroderma. Curr Opin Rheumatol 2014;26:621-9.

39. Ingegnoli F, Schioppo T. Zenker diverticulum in systemic sclerosis-related achalasic megaesophagus. J Clin Rheumatol 2017;23:444.

40. Pattanaik D, Brown M, Postlethwaite BC, Postlethwaite AE. Pathogenesis of systemic sclerosis. Front Immunol 2015;6:272.

41. Barile-Fabris L, Hernandez-Cabrera MF, Barragan-Garfias JA. Vasculitis in systemic lupus erythematosus. Curr Rheumatol Rep 2014;16:440.

42. Bartels CM, Bridges AJ. Rheumatoid vasculitis: vanishing menace or target for new treatments? Curr Rheumatol Rep 2010;12:414-9.

43. Soifer LO, Peralta D, Dima G, Besasso H. [Comparative clinical efficacy of a probiotic vs. an antibiotic in the treatment of patients with intestinal bacterial overgrowth and chronic abdominal functional distension: a pilot study]. Acta Gastroenterol Latinoam 2010;40:323-7. [Spanish]

44. Boeckxstaens GE, Bartelsman JF, Lauwers L, Tytgat GN. Treatment of GI dysmotility in scleroderma with the new enterokinetic agent prucalopride. Am J Gastroenterol 2002;97:194-7.

45. Baron M, Hudson M, Steele R, Canadian Scleroderma Research Group. Malnutrition is common in systemic sclerosis: results from the Canadian scleroderma research group database. J Rheumatol 2009;36:2737-43.

46. Gyger G, Baron M. Systemic sclerosis: gastrointestinal disease and its management. Rheum Dis Clin North Am 2015;41:459-73.

47. Ramos-Casals M, Tzioufas AG, Stone JH, Sisó A, Bosch X. Treatment of primary Sjogren syndrome: a systematic review. JAMA 2010;304:452-60.

48. Cacoub P, Comarmond C, Domont F, Savey L, Saadoun D. Cryoglobulinemia vasculitis. Am J Med 2015;128:950-5.

49. Terrier B, Karras A, Kahn JE, et al. The spectrum of type I cryoglobulinemia vasculitis: new insights based on 64 cases. Medicine (Baltimore) 2013;92:61-8.

50. Ferri C, Sebastiani M, Giuggioli D, et al. Mixed cryoglobulinemia: demographic, clinical, and serologic features and survival in 231 patients. Semin Arthritis Rheum 2004;33:355-74.

51. Fine GD, Trainer TD, Krawitt EL. Gastrointestinal bleeding, cryoglobulinemia, and hepatitis C. Am J Gastroenterol 2004;99:964-5.

52. Berera S, Gomez A, Dholaria K, et al. A rare case of hepatitis C-associated cryoglobulinemic duodenal vasculitis. ACG Case Rep J 2016;3:e134.

53. Kawano S, Torisu T, Esaki M. A rare cause of gastrointestinal ulcers. Gastroenterology 2016;151:403-4.

54. Terrier B, Krastinova E, Marie I, et al. Management of noninfectious mixed cryoglobulinemia vasculitis: data from 242 cases included in the cryovas survey. Blood 2012;119:5996-6004.

55. Terrier B, Semoun O, Saadoun D, Sène D, Resche-Rigon M, Cacoub P. Prognostic factors in patients with hepatitis C virus infection and systemic vasculitis. Arthritis Rheum 2011;63:1748-57.

56. Iida T, Yamano H, Nakase H. Systemic amyloidosis with gastrointestinal involvement: diagnosis from endoscopic and histological views. J Gastroenterol Hepatol 2018;33:583-90.

57. Sipe JD, Benson MD, Buxbaum JN, et al. Nomenclature 2014: amyloid fibril proteins and clinical classification of the amyloidosis. Amyloid 2014;21:221-4.

58. Mineshima M. Intensive hemodialysis: effects of treatment time and frequency on time-averaged concentrations of solutes. Contrib Nephrol 2018;196:184-7.

59. Merlini G, Dispenzieri A, Sanchorawala V, et al. Systemic immunoglobulin light chain amyloidosis. Nat Rev Dis Primers 2018;4:38.

60. Knowles TP, Vendruscolo M, Dobson CM. The amyloid state and its association with protein misfolding diseases. Nat Rev Mol Cell Biol 2014;15:384-96.

61. Freudenthaler S, Hegenbart U, Schonland S, Behrens HM, Kruger S, Rocken C. Amyloid in biopsies of the gastrointestinal tract-a retrospective observational study on 542 patients. Virchows Arch 2016;468:569-77.

62. Fitzgibbons PL. Histochemistry in the diagnosis of non-neoplastic gastrointestinal disorders. Semin Diagn Pathol 2018;35:370-80.

63. Winter M, Tholey A, Kristen A, Rocken C. MALDI mass spectrometry imaging: a novel tool for the identification and classification of amyloidosis. Proteomics 2017;17.

64. Groisman GM, Lachter J, Vlodavsky E. Amyloid colitis mimicking collagenous colitis. Histopathology 1997;31:201-2.

65. Wechalekar AD, Gillmore JD, Hawkins PN. Systemic amyloidosis. Lancet 2016;387:2641-54.

66. Kourelis TV, Kumar SK, Gertz MA, et al. Coexistent multiple myeloma or increased bone marrow plasma cells define equally high-risk populations in patients with immunoglobulin light chain amyloidosis. J Clin Oncol 2013;31:4319-24.

67. Gertz MA. Waldenstrom macroglobulinemia: 2017 update on diagnosis, risk stratification, and management. Am J Hematol 2017;92:209-17.

68. Pratz KW, Dingli D, Smyrk TC, Lust JA. Intestinal lymphangiectasia with protein-losing enteropathy in waldenstrom macroglobulinemia. Medicine (Baltimore) 2007;86:210-4.

69. Jimenez-Zepeda VH. Light chain deposition disease: novel biological insights and treatment advances. Int J Lab Hematol 2012;34:347-55.

70. Montgomery EA, Yantis YK, Snover DC, Tang LH. Tumors of the intestines. AFIP Atlas of Tumor Pathology, 4th Series, Fascicle 26. Washington DC: American Registry of Pathology; 2017.

71. Trindade AJ, Fan C, Bienstock B. Endoscopic resection of a rare subepithelial esophageal hamartoma. Dig Liver Dis 2018;50:617.

72. Wu WM, Wang XD, Sun G, Qiang LH, Yang YS. Adult asymptomatic hamartoma in the distal esophagus: a rare case. Intern Med 2014;53:1945-8.

73. Johncilla M, Yantiss RK. Malformations, choristomas, and hamartomas of the gastrointestinal tract and pancreas. Semin Diagn Pathol 2019;36:24-38.

74. Giardiello FM, Hamilton SR, Kern SE, et al. Colorectal neoplasia in juvenile polyposis or juvenile polyps. Arch Dis Child 1991;66:971-5.

75. Howe Jr, Sayed MG, Ahmed AF, et al. The prevalence of MADH4 and BMPR1A mutations in juvenile polyposis and absence of BMPR2, BMPR1B, and ACVR1 mutations. J Med Genet 2004;41:484-91.

76. Zhou XP, Woodford-Richens K, Lehtonen R, et al. Germline mutations in BMPR1A/ALK3 cause a subset of cases of juvenile polyposis syndrome and of Cowden and Bannayan-Riley-Ruvalcaba syndromes. Am J Hum Genet 2001;69:704-11.

77. Friedl W, Uhlhaas S, Schulmann K, et al. Juvenile polyposis: massive gastric polyposis is more common in MADH4 mutation carriers than in BMPR1A mutation carriers. Hum Genet 2002;111:108-11.

78. Gallione CJ, Repetto GM, Legius E, et al. A combined syndrome of juvenile polyposis and hereditary haemorrhagic telangiectasia associated with mutations in MADH4 (SMAD4). Lancet 2004;363:852-9.

79. Delnatte C, Sanlaville D, Mougenot JF, Stoppa-Lyonnet D. [Contiguous gene deletion within chromosome arm 10q is associated with juvenile polyposis of infancy, reflecting cooperation between the BMPR1A and PTEN tumor-suppressor genes]. Med Sci (Paris) 2006;22:912-3. [French]

80. Jarvinen H, Franssila KO. Familial juvenile polyposis coli; increased risk of colorectal cancer. Gut 1984;25:792-800.

81. Heiss KF, Schaffner D, Ricketts RR, Winn K. Malignant risk in juvenile polyposis coli: increasing documentation in the pediatric age group. J Pediatr Surg 1993;28:1188-93.

82. Howe JR, Mitros FA, Summers RW. The risk of gastrointestinal carcinoma in familial juvenile polyposis. Ann Surg Oncol 1998;5:751-6.

83. Arnout van Hattem WA, Langeveld D, de Leng WW, et al. Histologic variations in juvenile polyp phenotype correlate with genetic defect underlying juvenile polyposis. Am J Surg Pathol 2011;35:530-6.

84. Gonzalez RS, Adsay V, Graham RP, et al. Massive gastric juvenile-type polyposis: a clinicopathologic analysis of 22 cases. Histopathology 2017;70:918-28.

85. McGarrity TJ, Kulin HE, Zaino RJ. Peutz-Jeghers syndrome. Am J Gastroenterol 2000;95:596-604.

86. Hearle N, Schumacher V, Menko FH, et al. Frequency and spectrum of cancers in the Peutz-Jeghers syndrome. Clin Cancer Res 2006;12:3209-15.

87. Hinds R, Philp C, Hyer W, Fell JM. Complications of childhood Peutz-Jeghers syndrome: implications for pediatric screening. J Pediatr Gastroenterol Nutr 2004;39:219-20.

88. Nelen MR, Padberg GW, Peeters EA, et al. Localization of the gene for Cowden disease to chromosome 10q22-23. Nat Genet 1996;13:114-6.

89. Xie X, Wang Z, Chen Y. Association of LKB1 with a WD-repeat protein WDR6 is implicated in cell growth arrest and p27(Kip1) induction. Mol Cell Biochem 2007;301:115-22.

90. Trojan J, Brieger A, Raedle J, Roth WK, Zeuzem S. Peutz-Jeghers syndrome: molecular analysis of a three-generation kindred with a novel defect in the serine threonine kinase gene STK11. Am J Gastroenterol 1999;94:257-61.

91. Trojan J, Raedle J, Zeuzem S. [Mutated serine-threonine kinase gene (STK11) is the cause of Peutz-Jeghers syndrome]. Z Gastroenterol 1998;36:871-3. [German]

92. Wirtzfeld DA, Petrelli NJ, Rodriguez-Bigas MA. Hamartomatous polyposis syndromes: molecular genetics, neoplastic risk, and surveillance recommendations. Ann Surg Oncol 2001;8:319-27.

93. Latchford AR, Phillips RK. Gastrointestinal polyps and cancer in Peutz-Jeghers syndrome: clinical aspects. Fam Cancer 2011;10:455-61.

94. Burkart AL, Sheridan T, Lewin M, Fenton H, Ali NJ, Montgomery E. Do sporadic Peutz-Jeghers polyps exist? Experience of a large teaching hospital. Am J Surg Pathol 2007;31:1209-14.

95. Spoto CP, Gullo I, Carneiro F, Montgomery EA, Brosens LA. Hereditary gastrointestinal carcinomas and their precursors: an algorithm for genetic testing. Semin Diagn Pathol 2018;35:170-83.

96. Lam-Himlin D, Park JY, Cornish TC, Shi C, Montgomery E. Morphologic characterization of syndromic gastric polyps. Am J Surg Pathol 2010;34:1656-62.

97. DiLiberti JH. Inherited macrocephaly-hamartoma syndromes. Am J Med Genet 1998;79:284-90.

98. Starink TM, van der Veen JP, Arwert F, et al. The Cowden syndrome: a clinical and genetic study in 21 patients. Clin Genet 1986;29:222-33.

99. Bayley JP. Succinate dehydrogenase gene variants and their role in Cowden syndrome. Am J Hum Genet 2011;88:674-5.

100. Rosty C. The role of the surgical pathologist in the diagnosis of gastrointestinal polyposis syndromes. Adv Anat Pathol 2018;25:1-13.

101. Caliskan A, Kohlmann WK, Affolter KE, Downs-Kelly E, Kanth P, Bronner MP. Intramucosal lipomas of the colon implicate Cowden syndrome. Mod Pathol 2018;31:643-51.

102. Ngeow J, Heald B, Rybicki LA, et al. Prevalence of germline PTEN, BMPR1A, SMAD4, STK11, and ENG mutations in patients with moderate-load colorectal polyps. Gastroenterology 2013;144:1402-9.

103. Vashistha N, Chakravarty S, Singhal D. Cronkhite-Canada syndrome. Gastrointest Endosc 2017;86:922-3.

104. Sweetser S, Boardman LA. Cronkhite-Canada syndrome: an acquired condition of gastrointestinal polyposis and dermatologic abnormalities. Gastroenterol Hepatol (N Y) 2012;8:201-3.

105. Sweetser S, Ahlquist DA, Osborn NK, et al. Clinicopathologic features and treatment outcomes in Cronkhite-Canada syndrome: support for autoimmunity. Dig Dis Sci 2012;57:496-502.

106. Zhao R, Huang M, Banafea O, et al. Cronkhite-Canada syndrome: a rare case report and literature review. BMC Gastroenterol 2016;16:23.

107. Watanabe C, Komoto S, Tomita K, et al. Endoscopic and clinical evaluation of treatment and prognosis of Cronkhite-Canada syndrome: a Japanese nationwide survey. J Gastroenterol 2016;51:327-36.

108. Ward E, Wolfsen HC, Ng C. Medical management of Cronkhite-Canada syndrome. South Med J 2002;95:272-4.

109. Iwamuro M, Omote R, Tanaka T, et al. Diffuse intestinal ganglioneuromatosis showing multiple large bowel ulcers in a patient with neurofibromatosis type 1. Intern Med 2017;56:3287-91.

110. Rittershaus AC, Appelman HD. Benign gastrointestinal mesenchymal BUMPS: a brief review of some spindle cell polyps with published names. Arch Pathol Lab Med 2011;135:1311-9.

111. Wick MR. Granulomatous & histiocytic dermatitides. Semin Diagn Pathol 2017;34:301-11.

112. Vitkovski T, Costales C, Chen S, Saltman B, Kahn L. Malakoplakia of the thyroid gland: a case report and review of literature. Int J Surg Pathol 2015;23:308-12.

113. Weinrach DM, Wang KL, Cisler JJ, Diaz LK. Pathologic quiz case: a 54-year-old liver transplant recipient with diffuse thickening of the sigmoid colon. Malakoplakia of the colon associated with liver transplant. Arch Pathol Lab Med 2004;128:e133-4.

114. Yen JM, Soh NW, Petersson F, Pandya G. Rectosigmoid malakoplakia. BMJ Case Rep 2017;2017.

115. Rossini R, Lisi G, Pesci A, et al. Depth of intestinal wall infiltration and clinical presentation of deep infiltrating endometriosis: evaluation of 553 consecutive cases. J Laparoendosc Adv Surg Tech A 2018;28:152-6.

116. Yantiss RK, Clement PB, Young RH. Endometriosis of the intestinal tract: a study of 44 cases of a disease that may cause diverse challenges in clinical and pathologic evaluation. Am J Surg Pathol 2001;25:445-54.

117. Yantiss RK, Clement PB, Young RH. Neoplastic and pre-neoplastic changes in gastrointestinal endometriosis: a study of 17 cases. Am J Surg Pathol 2000;24:513-24.

118. Birkness J, Lam-Himlin D, Byrnes K, Wood L, Voltaggio L. The inverted appendix - a potentially problematic diagnosis: clinicopathologic analysis of 21 cases. Histopathology 2019;74:853-60.

119. Vercellini P, Frattaruolo MP, Rosati R, et al. Medical treatment or surgery for colorectal endometriosis? Results of a shared decision-making approach. Hum Reprod 2018;33:202-11.

120. Anglesio MS, Papadopoulos N, Ayhan A, et al. Cancer-associated mutations in endometriosis without cancer. N Engl J Med 2017;376:1835-48.

121. Abrao MS, Petraglia F, Falcone T, Keckstein J, Osuga Y, Chapron C. Deep endometriosis infiltrating the recto-sigmoid: critical factors to consider before management. Hum Reprod Update 2015;21:329-39.

7 DISEASES OF THE VERMIFORM APPENDIX

CONGENITAL AND ACQUIRED STRUCTURAL ANOMALIES

Appendiceal Agenesis

Appendiceal agenesis is the congenital absence of the appendix. Congenital anomalies involving the appendix are rare and most cases are clinically asymptomatic (1,2). The incidence of appendiceal agenesis is approximately 1/100,000 appendices examined at autopsy (3).

Appendiceal agenesis may occur in the presence of a normal cecum or in association with either cecal dysgenesis or ileal atresia (4). Most cases are unaccompanied by other developmental abnormalities. However, appendiceal agenesis has been reported in combination with maternal thalidomide ingestion, in patients with trisomy 18, and in individuals with multiple congenital abnormalities of the gastrointestinal tract (3,5).

Appendiceal Duplication

Appendiceal duplication is the partial or complete duplication of the appendix. The incidence of appendiceal duplication is 0.004 to 0.009 percent and it occurs with similar frequencies among men and women (6).

Duplications are classified in three groups based on their anatomy (7). Incomplete (type A) duplications feature two appendices that share a common base. Complete (type B) duplications consist of two appendices that each arise at a different location on the cecum. Type C duplications feature two complete appendices, each of which is associated with a duplicated cecum (8). Triplication of the appendix can also occur (9).

Appendiceal Diverticula and Diverticulitis

Definition. *Appendiceal diverticula* are congenital or acquired mucosa-lined outpouchings of the appendiceal wall.

Clinical Features. The incidence of appendiceal diverticula is reportedly less than 2 percent (2). Congenital diverticula are much less common than acquired diverticula, with a reported incidence of 0.014 percent compared with acquired lesions, which have an incidence ranging from 0.2 to 1.7 percent (1,2).

Most diverticula are asymptomatic lesions discovered following incidental appendectomy for unrelated surgical indications. Diverticula affect both sexes equally and can be single or multifocal. Inflamed diverticula elicit right lower quadrant pain that mimics the features of acute appendicitis, although the former tends to occur in older patients and have a more insidious onset of symptoms (10,11).

Pathogenesis. Similar to congenital diverticula that develop elsewhere in the gastrointestinal tract, those of the appendix are lined by all layers of the normal appendiceal wall. Acquired diverticula represent herniations of mucosa and submucosa through the appendix. They presumably result from luminal obstruction that leads to appendiceal distention, muscular hypertrophy, and increased intraluminal pressure. These changes promote pulsion of the inner appendiceal layers through weak points in the muscularis propria, such as sites of penetration by vascular bundles and areas injured by previous episodes of inflammation or necrosis.

Increased intraluminal pressures due to mucus accumulation can also lead to diverticula. Approximately 14 percent of appendectomy specimens from patients with cystic fibrosis contain diverticula associated with thick mucoid secretions (12,13). Non-neoplastic diverticula occur in patients with appendiceal mucinous neoplasms and other obstructive lesions (14).

Gross Findings. Diverticula typically appear as one or more outpouchings along the antimesenteric and mesenteric borders of the

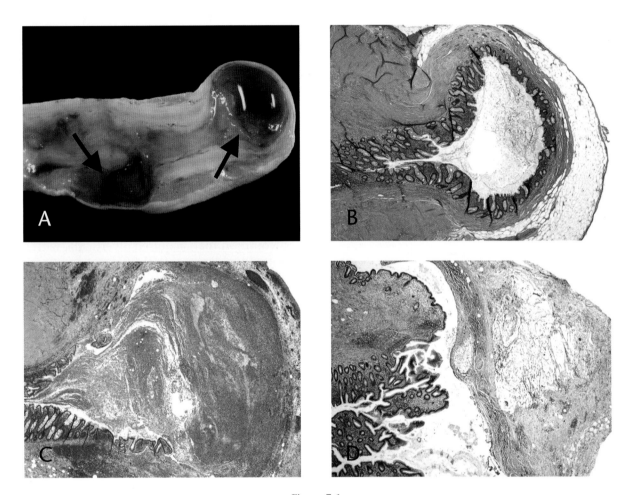

Figure 7-1

APPENDICEAL DIVERTICULA AND ASSOCIATED DIVERTICULITIS

This appendectomy specimen contains two diverticula (arrows) at the appendiceal tip and along its lateral border (A). An acquired diverticulum features mucosa and submucosa herniated through the muscularis propria (B). Perforated diverticulitis is associated with organizing inflammation and mucin around the diverticulum (C). Organizing mucin, fibrosis, and chronic inflammation surround a previously ruptured diverticulum (D).

distal appendix (fig. 7-1A). Most are small, ranging from 2 to 5 mm, and they impart a beaded appearance to the outer appendix when multiple. Inflamed diverticula often contain stool.

Microscopic Findings. Congenital diverticula contain all layers of the appendiceal wall; the mucosa may display mild, nonspecific inflammatory changes or be entirely normal. Acquired diverticula lack a muscularis propria (fig. 7-1B). Uninflamed acquired diverticula are lined by normal-appearing or slightly attenuated mucosa. Mild epithelial cell hyperplasia may be present, but it overlies evenly distributed crypts supported by lamina propria.

Diverticulitis is initially associated with localized neutrophil-rich inflammation that can spread to the appendix proper, causing appendicitis or periappendicitis (fig. 7-1C). Persistent inflammation leads to mononuclear cell-rich inflammation and fibrosis. Extensive inflammatory changes distort, obliterate, or disrupt diverticula, resulting in extrusion of mucin into the appendiceal wall (fig. 7-1D).

Differential Diagnosis. Appendiceal diverticula can simulate appendiceal mucinous neoplasms, especially when they rupture or display post-inflammatory mucosal hyperplasia (15). Unlike mucinous neoplasms, however,

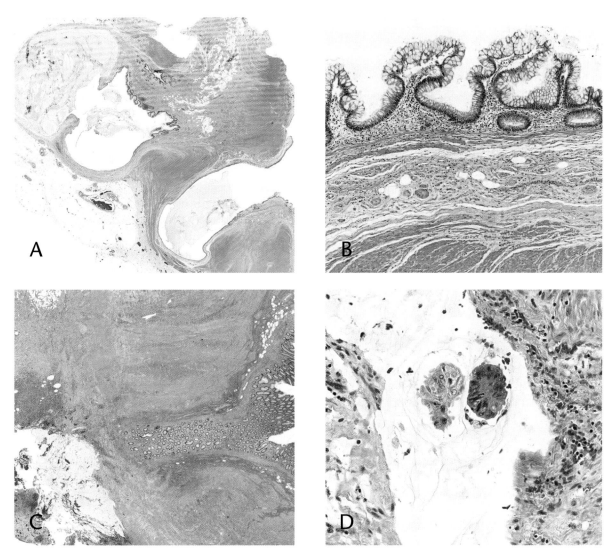

Figure 7-2

APPENDICEAL DIVERTICULA SIMULATE MUCINOUS NEOPLASIA

Diverticula may dilate and rupture, extruding mucus into the periappendiceal soft tissue (A). The slightly flattened mucosa shows mild surface epithelial hyperplasia with numerous goblet cells and normal crypts separated by abundant lamina propria (B). Another ruptured diverticulum is associated with pools of extruded mucin (C) that contain rare clusters of non-neoplastic epithelial cells (D).

diverticula feature normal-appearing crypts separated by preserved lamina propria (fig. 7-2). Crypts may contain Paneth cells or endocrine cells, neither of which is prominent in most mucinous neoplasms. Mucosal hyperplasia characteristically features mature-appearing goblet cells and non-mucinous epithelial cells, rather than the barrel-shaped, acid mucin-containing epithelial cells typical of mucinous neoplasms. Diverticula generally lack hyalinized fibrosis and obliteration

of the muscularis mucosae, which are usually present in appendiceal mucinous neoplasms.

MECHANICAL ABNORMALITIES OF THE APPENDIX

Intussusception

Definition. *Intussusception* (*inverted appendix*) is the invagination or telescoping of the distal appendix into the proximal appendix or cecum.

411

Clinical Features. Appendiceal intussusception is detected in 0.1 percent of patients undergoing appendectomy (2). This condition occurs at all ages and, contrary to prior notions, is more common in adults (16–18). Symptoms typically include nausea, vomiting, diarrhea, lower gastrointestinal bleeding, and episodic lower abdominal pain over the course of weeks, although some patients have a more acute presentation that simulates acute appendicitis (19). Occasional patients are asymptomatic.

Imaging reveals a "target" lesion that reflects two concentric layers of bowel wall. Barium enema displays a filling defect that appears as a "coiled spring sign" (20).

Pathogenesis. Anatomic variants, such as a cone-shaped appendix or thin mesoappendix, predispose to appendiceal intussusception. Other risk factors include endometriosis, lymphoid hyperplasia, and appendiceal neoplasms (21–23). Pediatric cases tend to be associated with lymphadenopathy and viral infection, especially adenovirus (24). Presumably, mural irritation or tethering of the mucosa and submucosa to a mural lesion leads to abnormal peristalsis and telescoping of the appendix into its lumen (19). Intussusception can also occur in patients without any underlying condition.

Gross Findings. The appendix may intussuscept into itself or serve as a lead point for invagination into the cecum (19,25). Intussusception of part, or all, of the appendix into the cecum produces an edematous polypoid mass (fig. 7-3).

Microscopic Findings. The intussuscepted appendix is externally surfaced by normal mucosa that surrounds the submucosa and muscularis propria (26). Its epithelium may be hyperplastic, inflamed, or eroded, especially when superimposed ischemic changes are present. The submucosa is often edematous and accompanied by a thick or fibrotic muscularis propria (fig. 7-4). Appendices occasionally undergo autoamputation following intussusception.

Treatment and Prognosis. Appendiceal intussusception is treated surgically, with options ranging from appendectomy to ileocecectomy depending on the amount of affected appendix (27). Additional treatment may be required in cases associated with mural abnormalities contributing to the intussusception.

INFLAMMATORY CONDITIONS OF THE APPENDIX

Acute Appendicitis

Definition. *Acute appendicitis* is acute appendiceal inflammation due to a combination of factors.

Clinical Features. Acute appendicitis is one of the most common inflammatory conditions of the gastrointestinal tract resulting in surgical resection specimens. It develops less frequently among populations that consume diets rich in fiber, and is more common in Western countries (28–31). Although its incidence has declined in recent years, up to 12 percent of the population of the United States develops acute appendicitis (32–36).

The disease occurs at any age with peak incidences in the second and third decades of life (33,37,38). Acute appendicitis affects males slightly more commonly than females, particularly during early childhood, and displays seasonal variation with a peak in the summer months (33,37–40). It is also more common among human immunodeficiency virus (HIV)-infected patients than the general population (41).

Classic signs of acute appendicitis include acute-onset periumbilical, colicky pain that later localizes to the right lower quadrant, nausea, vomiting, and localized ileus. Some patients have a palpable mass on rectal examination. Fever and leukocytosis accompany the peritoneal inflammatory signs. These classic symptoms are less common in elderly patients who tend to present with protracted abdominal pain and fewer systemic manifestations (40,42). Aberrant location of the inflamed appendix can also cause urogenital symptoms with right renal colic, dysuria, frequency, and urinary retention (43).

Pathogenesis. Acute appendicitis is not regularly associated with any specific pathogen or mechanism of development; multiple etiologic factors are of more, or less, importance in any individual patient (44). The likely precipitating factor in most cases is luminal obstruction followed by mucosal ischemia, loss of mucosal integrity, and bacterial infection. Occasional patients develop appendicitis following barium enema examinations and colonoscopic procedures (45–47).

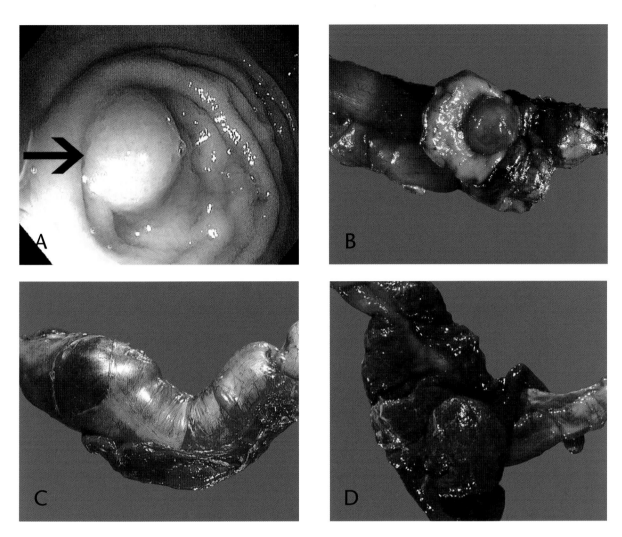

Figure 7-3

APPENDICEAL INTUSSUSCEPTION

The intussuscepted proximal appendix forms a polypoid mass (arrow) at the appendiceal orifice (A). The inverted appendix appears as an indurated polyp surrounded by a cuff of cecum (B). Another intussuscepted appendix is distended and erythematous with prominent serosal vasculature (C). Upon opening, the appendiceal mucosa is extensively hemorrhagic; the intussusceptum forms a polypoid mass (D).

Appendiceal obstruction can result from several mechanisms. Fecaliths and calculi composed of inspissated feces and mucus can obstruct the appendix when trapped in the lumen. Fecaliths consist of hard, but crushable, fecal material (fig. 7-5). They are detected in 2 percent of appendices and 11 percent of appendices removed for appendicitis symptoms (48). Calculi are mineralized, noncrushable stones detected in 1 to 2 percent of appendices (49). They are more likely than fecaliths to occur in combination with appendiceal perforation and periappendiceal abscesses. Gallstones, helminthic aggregates, barium, pins, nails, bubble gum, teeth, seeds, and other material can cause appendicitis due to luminal obstruction (50). Partial obstruction may occur as a result of neoplasia at the appendiceal orifice or reactive lymphoid hyperplasia (fig. 7-6). The latter is a common manifestation of viral infection, particularly in young patients (51).

Secretions accumulate behind the obstruction, resulting in increased intraluminal pressure that compromises perfusion and promotes

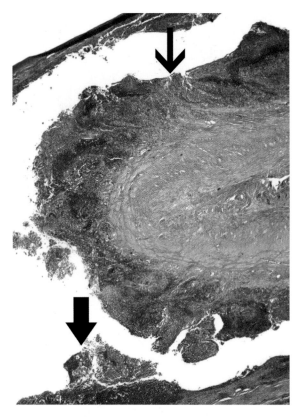

Figure 7-4

APPENDICEAL INTUSSUSCEPTION

The intussuscepted appendiceal tip (arrow) has an "inside-out" appearance within the intussuscipiens (block arrow).

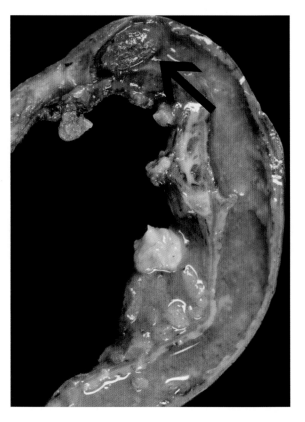

Figure 7-5

FECALITH

A fecalith (arrow) is lodged in the proximal appendix, obstructing the lumen. The distal appendix is slightly dilated and contains mucoid material.

mucosal ischemia. Progressive mucosal injury leads to loss of barrier integrity and impairs defenses, such that pathogens invade the tissue and elicit an inflammatory response (52–55). Some data suggest that acutely inflamed appendices contain higher numbers of *Fusobacteria sp.* relative to other microbes (56). Other organisms implicated in the pathogenesis of acute appendicitis are enumerated in Table 7-1. Local tissue injury promotes capillary and arteriolar occlusion by thrombi and edema, furthering ischemic injury, gangrene, and peritonitis. The appendix may also become secondarily infected when patients suffer from generalized bacterial enterocolitis (57).

Gross Findings. Appendicitis may involve the entire appendix or only part of it. Limited involvement is most common in the appendiceal tip (44). Acute appendicitis is broadly classified as simple, gangrenous, or perforated based on operative and pathologic features. The earliest visible signs of acute appendicitis include dilatation and congestion of serosal vessels, localized or generalized hyperemia, and a dull serosal appearance (fig. 7-7A). Well-developed acute appendicitis features marked vascular engorgement, serosal congestion, and a granular, fibrinous, or purulent coating on the outer appendix (fig. 7-7B). The mesoappendix is often edematous and contiguous structures are occasionally inflamed. The appendix itself contains purulent material that may be accompanied by an impacted fecalith or calculus. The gangrenous appendix is soft, purple-gray, and hemorrhagic; thrombi may be visible in the mesoappendix.

Microscopic Findings. The histologic features of acute appendicitis depend on the

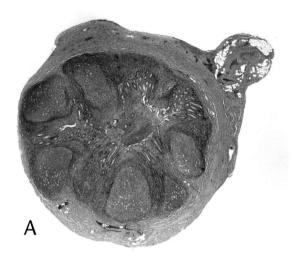 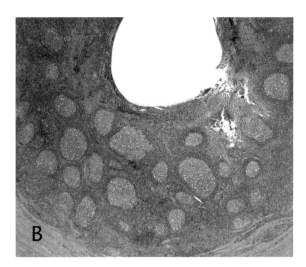

Figure 7-6

LYMPHOID HYPERPLASIA

Marked mucosal lymphoid hyperplasia can obstruct the lumen of the appendix (A). Numerous lymphoid follicles contain large germinal centers (B).

duration and severity of the disease, and range from minimal inflammation to extensive mural necrosis and perforation (58). Neutrophilic infiltration of the lamina propria and crypts progress to crypt abscesses, erosions, and aggregates of luminal neutrophils, as well as marginating inflammatory cells in and around the vasculature. Progressive injury causes extensive ulcers, striking submucosal edema with patchy necrosis of the muscularis propria, and subserosal inflammation (fig. 7-8). Neutrophils predominate for the first few days after symptom onset, but eosinophils become progressively more numerous when the interval between the onset of symptoms and appendectomy exceeds more than 72 hours (59). Severe injury features confluent ulcers, destruction of the muscularis propria, and neutrophil-rich inflammation extending through the appendiceal wall into periappendiceal soft tissue.

Minimal histologic criteria for a diagnosis of acute appendicitis have never been clearly established. The presence of mural neutrophils is widely considered a requirement for the diagnosis, but compelling evidence supporting this view is lacking. Experimental data suggest even mild mucosal injury can progress to gangrenous appendicitis, and some patients with clinically

Table 7-1
ORGANISMS ASSOCIATED WITH ACUTE APPENDICITIS
Bacteroides fragilis
Bilophila wadsworthia
Campylobacter jejuni
Eggerthelia lenta
Fusobacterium nucleatum
Haemophilus influenzae
Klebsiella sp.
Lactobacillus sp.
Peptostreptococcus micros
Pseudomonas sp.
Shigella sp.
Staphylococcus aureus
β-Hemolytic *Streptococcus* group A
Streptococcus milleri
Streptococcus pneumoniae
Streptococcus anginosus
Yersinia enterocolitica
Yersinia pseudotuberculosis

suspected appendicitis have increased levels of pro-inflammatory cytokines in histologically normal appendices (60,61).

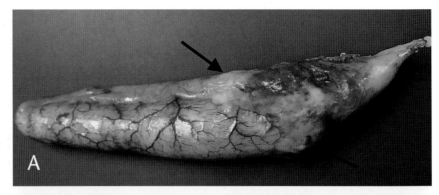

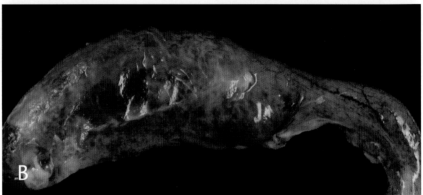

Figure 7-7

ACUTE APPENDICITIS

The serosa has a dull appearance, with scattered exudates (arrows) and injected vessels (A). Progressive injury leads to appendiceal dilatation, increased hyperemia, vascular engorgement, and plaque-like white-yellow exudates (B).

Salmonella, Shigella, Clostridium difficile, and *Campylobacter* infections characteristically elicit only superficial appendiceal injury (fig. 7-9) (62). Thus, inflammation limited to the mucosa should not be dismissed when patients present with clinical features of appendicitis. Submission of the entire appendix is recommended when initial sections are histologically normal, thereby ensuring that foci of inflammation, small polyps, and neoplasms are not overlooked.

Differential Diagnosis. The clinical differential diagnosis of acute appendicitis includes infectious gastroenteritis, pelvic inflammatory disease, ovarian cysts, small bowel obstruction, intussusception, right-sided diverticulitis, omental infarction, kidney stones, mesenteric lymphadenopathy, Meckel diverticulitis, and right lower quadrant malignancy. Entities that produce similar histologic changes include several infections, appendiceal diverticulitis, and involvement by idiopathic inflammatory bowel disease. Specific features of these disorders are described in prior and subsequent sections of this chapter.

Treatment and Prognosis. Most patients with signs and symptoms of appendicitis are treated with appendectomy owing to the historically high mortality rate associated with appendiceal perforation. In fact, many patients who presented with vague symptoms used to be treated with appendectomy, even when the clinical suspicion was low (63). As a result, the frequency with which pathologists encountered histologically normal appendices ranged as high as 30 percent in some centers (64). More recent data suggest that active observation of patients with suspected acute appendicitis leads to fewer appendectomy procedures for uninflamed appendices (63,65). A growing body of data also supports a more conservative approach to management of acute appendicitis. Select patients may be treated with antibiotic therapy alone; those presenting with appendiceal perforation are routinely treated with antibiotic agents prior to surgery (66,67).

The most common complications of acute appendicitis are related to appendiceal perforation. These include generalized peritonitis, periappendiceal or subdiaphragmatic abscesses, pneumatosis coli, and adhesions. Risk of

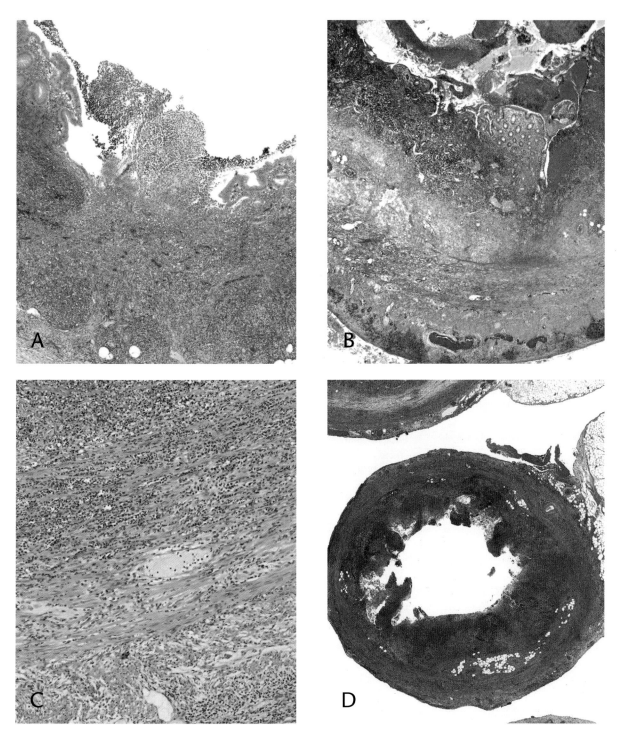

Figure 7-8

ACUTE APPENDICITIS

Early appendicitis features patchy ulcers and exudates unassociated with inflammation of the submucosa and muscular wall (A). Progressive injury leads to extensive ulcers, submucosal edema, congestion, and destruction of the muscularis propria (B). Neutrophil-rich inflammatory infiltrates permeate the muscularis propria (C). Well-developed acute appendicitis features extensive ulcers, mural neutrophil-rich inflammatory infiltrates, and periappendicitis accompanied by serositis (D).

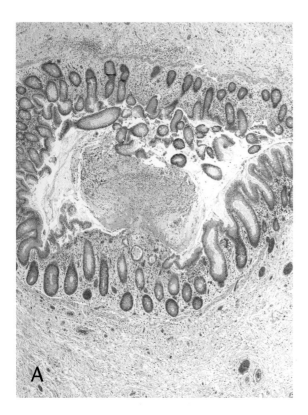
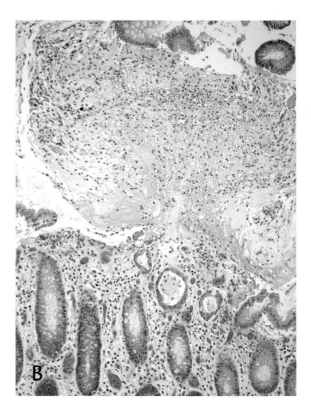

Figure 7-9

PSEUDOMEMBRANOUS APPENDICITIS

The appendix can be involved by any infection that causes colitis. This patient with *Clostridium difficile* infection also had appendiceal inflammation with striking submucosal edema (A). Pseudomembranous exudates composed of necrotic cells, mucus, and fibrin overlie withered, regenerative-appearing crypts (B).

perforation is highest in infants and patients over 75 years of age: at least 50 percent of patients in these groups develop appendiceal perforation compared with only 10 to 29 percent of patients 10 to 40 years of age (42,58,68). Suppurative pyelophlebitis of serosal and appendiceal vessels can extend to distant sites or embolize the liver with infected thrombi, causing secondary bacterial infections, hepatic abscesses, and cholangitis. Thrombophlebitis may also lead to sepsis, shock, and disseminated intravascular coagulopathy. Fistulae between the appendix and other gastrointestinal organs, vagina, bladder, or skin develop in some patients. Lumbar abscesses occur, but are infrequent. Appendicitis among elderly patients is associated with higher mortality and complication rates, possibly reflecting its more frequent association with appendiceal or cecal malignancies (40,44,58,69,70).

Stump Appendicitis

Some patients develop inflammation in residual appendiceal tissue following an appendectomy procedure (71). They present with vague abdominal pain, nausea, vomiting, or fevers that do not clearly implicate appendicitis as the cause of symptoms. Not surprisingly, more than one-third of patients with *stump appendicitis* develop a perforation by the time they undergo re-exploration (72). Inversion of the appendiceal stump following surgery leads to ileocolic intussusception in some patients (73).

Eosinophilic Appendicitis

Eosinophil-rich inflammatory infiltrates in the appendix usually reflect resolving acute appendicitis, rather than a hypersensitivity disorder or parasitic infection (fig. 7-10). Eosinophils are commonly observed in appendectomy specimens when symptoms persist for

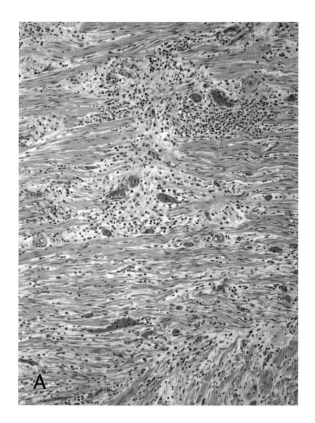 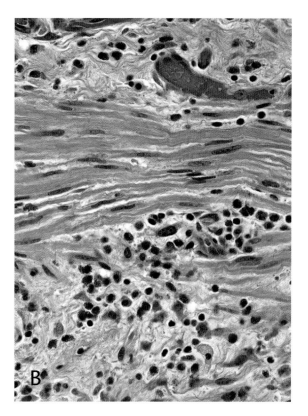

Figure 7-10

SUBACUTE APPENDICITIS

Eosinophils are progressively more numerous as the interval between symptom onset and appendectomy increases. Mural eosinophils are accompanied by lymphocytes and a few neutrophils approximately 1 week after symptom onset (A). Eosinophils are evenly dispersed in the muscularis propria and show minimal degranulation (B).

more than 24 hours prior to surgery (59). Mural eosinophils are present in nearly 40 percent of appendices removed within 12 to 84 hours of symptom onset and increase in number thereafter (74). Their presence rarely represents a primary eosinophilic disorder, especially when accompanied by other cell types (75).

Eosinophilic gastroenteritis can involve the appendix, but it is always accompanied by extra-appendiceal disease and generally features clustered eosinophils in the mucosa and epithelium. Aggregates of eosinophils that show degranulation and Splendore-Hoeppli phenomenon raise the possibility of infection. When present, additional tissue sections may reveal an organism or ova.

Interval Appendicitis

Patients with perforated appendicitis are increasingly treated with antibiotic therapy fol-

lowed by elective appendectomy several weeks after symptom onset, rather than immediate appendectomy. These delayed appendectomy specimens show mural fibrosis and irregularly distributed lymphoid aggregates (fig. 7-11A,B). More than 50 percent of cases contain non-necrotic granulomas (fig. 7-11C,D). They are usually located in follicles, but may be distributed throughout the appendiceal wall (66,76). Adhesions, acellular mucin pools containing inflammatory cells, xanthogranulomatous inflammation, diverticula, and mucosal hyperplasia may also be present.

Chronic Appendicitis

Definition. *Chronic appendicitis* is mononuclear cell-rich appendicitis with variable fibrosis.

Clinical Features. Chronic appendicitis is a descriptive term applied to situations that do not fit clinical or histologic features of acute appendicitis. Most examples likely reflect delayed

419

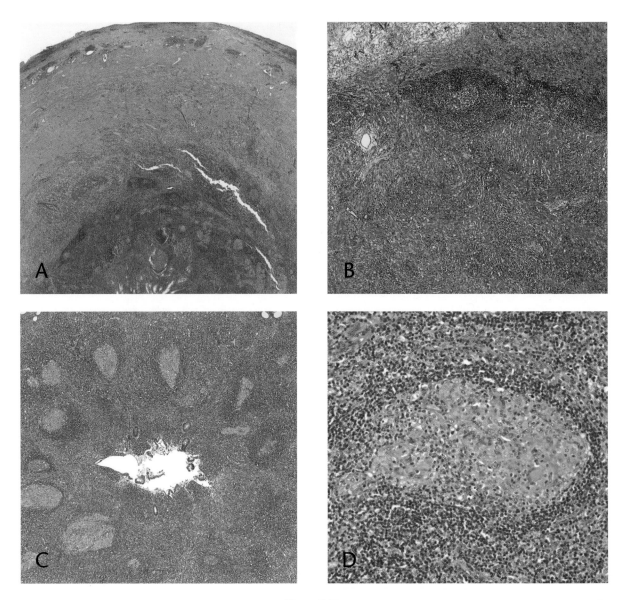

Figure 7-11

INTERVAL APPENDICITIS

Delayed appendectomy specimens often display mural lymphoid aggregates (A) with frequent germinal centers, dispersed chronic inflammation, and mural fibrosis (B). Epithelioid granulomas are often present, especially in mucosal and submucosal lymphoid follicles (C). Granulomas are composed of plump macrophages surrounded by lymphocytes, similar to granulomas associated with Crohn disease (D).

appendectomy, recurrent appendicitis, idiopathic inflammatory bowel disease or other immune-mediated disorders, or specific types of infectious appendicitis. Older patients may present with large inflammatory masses termed ligneous cecitis, appendicular granuloma, and pseudo-neoplastic appendicitis. This finding likely reflects incomplete resolution of retrocecal appendicitis.

Gross Findings. The appendix is usually indurated and fibrotic. Some cases feature localized periappendiceal mucin accumulation that simulates the radiographic and gross appearance of a mucinous neoplasm.

Microscopic Findings. The histologic features of chronic appendicitis are nonspecific. The epithelium may be hyperplastic, with a

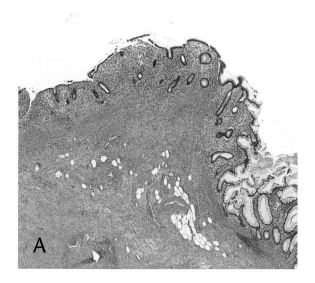 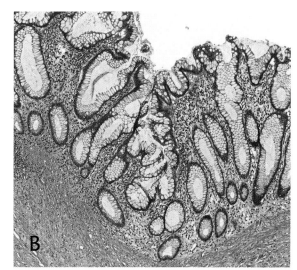

Figure 7-12

CHRONIC APPENDICITIS AND POSTINFLAMMATORY APPENDIX

An area of mucosal hyperplasia shows a gradual transition to more normal-appearing mucosa (A). The surface epithelium is slightly undulating and contains increased numbers of mature goblet cells supported by abundant lamina propria (B).

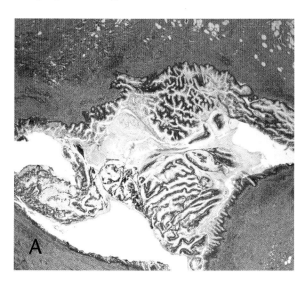 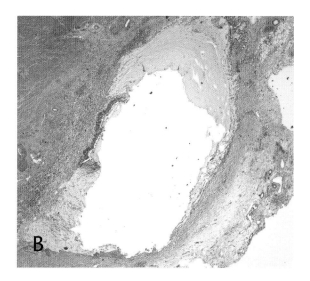

Figure 7-13

CHRONIC APPENDICITIS AND POSTINFLAMMATORY APPENDIX

Appendectomy specimens from patients with recurrent, or remote, appendicitis symptoms may show mild appendiceal dilatation accompanied by mucosal hyperplasia (A) and organizing periappendiceal mucin (B).

slightly serrated surface and increased numbers of distended goblet cells (fig. 7-12). Increased lymphoplasmacytic inflammation, mural lymphoid aggregates, and mural fibrosis with destruction of the muscularis propria are occasionally present. Mild appendiceal dilatation, diverticula, and loculated mucoid material in periappendiceal soft tissues reflect remote perforated appendicitis (fig. 7-13) (12).

Differential Diagnosis. Low-grade appendiceal mucinous neoplasm is the most important entity to consider in the differential diagnosis of the chronically inflamed appendix, especially when it is associated with organizing

Table 7-2

CAUSES OF GRANULOMATOUS APPENDICITIS

Entity	Distinguishing Features	Associated Features
Crohn Disease	Non-necrotic granulomas Chronic active mucosal injury Sinus tracts or fistulae Mural fibrosis, lymphoid aggregates	Involvement of ileum and/or colon History of Crohn disease
Interval appendectomy	Mucosal granulomas often in lymphoid follicles Mural fibrosis, lymphoid aggregates Xanthogranulomatous inflammation	History of prior appendicitis or recurrent appendicitis symptoms
Yersinia infection	Suppurative granulomas Lymphoid hyperplasia Mural fibrosis, lymphoid aggregates	Ileocolic inflammation Mesenteric lymphadenopathy
Mycobacterial infection	Necrotic and non-necrotic granulomas, often confluent Dense fibrosis with adhesions Acid fast and PAS-D stains can be helpful	Ileocolic inflammation Mesenteric lymphadenopathy Immunosuppression is common
Actinomyces infection	*Actinomyces* colonies in lumen and/or tissue Non-necrotic epithelioid granulomas Sinus tracts, fibrosis, and lymphoid aggregates	Appendicitis with fistulae Abdominal abscesses Perforated viscus
Histoplasmosis	Non-necrotic granulomas Sheets of large macrophages containing organisms	Systemic infection Immunocompromised patient
Schistosomiasis	Granulomas obliterate veins containing eggs Peripheral rim of eosinophils	Peripheral eosinophilia
Sarcoidosis	Non-necrotic granulomas Mural fibrosis, lymphoid aggregates	Other stigmata of sarcoidosis

periappendiceal mucin and diverticula. Post-inflammatory epithelial cell hyperplasia displays a gradual transition to clearly non-neoplastic epithelium and contains well-formed, mature-appearing goblet cells, rather than the barrel-shaped, nongoblet mucinous cells of a neoplasm. Goblet cell-rich epithelium is supported by lamina propria, which is almost always decreased or obliterated in mucinous neoplasms. The mucosa also contains evenly spaced crypts lined by bland goblet cells as well as scattered Paneth cells and endocrine cells, neither of which is prominent in most mucinous neoplasms (77). Post-inflammatory appendices often contain non-necrotic granulomas and likely account for most cases of granulomatous appendicitis in the United States, although a variety of infectious and immune-mediated disorders can cause similar changes (Table 7-2) (78,79).

Chronic Idiopathic Inflammatory Bowel Disease

Crohn Disease. The appendix is involved in approximately 20 percent of patients with established Crohn disease, most of whom have ileocolic involvement and mesenteric lymphadenopathy (80). The affected appendix is enlarged and thickened, and is often adherent to the terminal ileum or cecum. Transmural lymphoid aggregates, sinus tracts, neuronal hyperplasia, and fibrosis occur in combination with ulcers, crypt architectural distortion, and mural fibrosis (fig. 7-14A). Epithelioid granulomas frequently display a perivascular distribution, but may also occur in the mucosa and lymphoid nodules (fig. 7-14B).

All of the features of Crohn disease can be seen in granulomatous appendicitis due to a variety of infections, delayed appendectomy specimens, and patients with sarcoidosis; isolated appendiceal Crohn disease accounts for less than 10 percent of granulomatous appendicitis cases (81,82). Thus, a diagnosis of appendiceal Crohn disease should not be based on evaluation of the appendix alone, especially when patients do not already have a diagnosis of idiopathic inflammatory bowel disease.

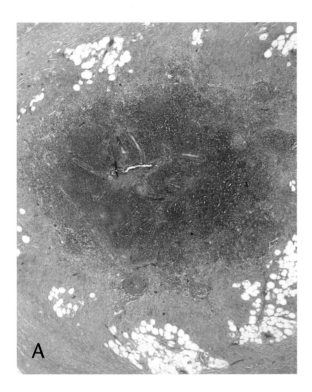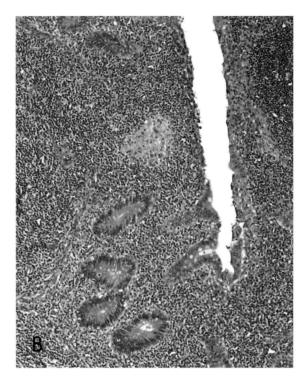

Figure 7-14

APPENDICEAL CROHN DISEASE

Lymphoid aggregates and neutrophilic inflammation surround the lumen; lymphoid aggregates and submucosal fibrosis are present (A). A small epithelioid granuloma is associated with the lymphoid tissue (B).

Ulcerative Colitis. Appendiceal involvement occurs in at least 50 percent of ulcerative colitis patients, and up to 86 percent of those with pancolitis (83,84). In fact, the appendix plays an immunomodulatory role in the evolution of ulcerative colitis (85). Prior appendectomy is protective against the development of ulcerative colitis and is associated with decreased disease severity in patients who later develop ulcerative colitis (86). Patients with ulcerative colitis and appendiceal involvement are also at risk for developing symptomatic inflammation in the ileal pouch after an anal anastomosis procedure (83).

Appendiceal inflammation in the setting of ulcerative colitis is usually continuous with cecal disease activity, but inflammation of the appendix or peri-appendiceal colonic mucosa accompanied by left-sided colitis and sparing of the intervening colon is a well-recognized phenomenon (87–89). Similar to colonic disease, the mucosa is expanded by dense plasma cell-rich inflammation and features crypt abscesses with ulcers (fig. 7-15).

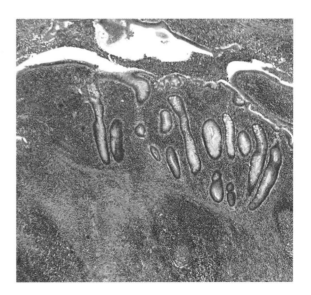

Figure 7-15

ULCERATIVE COLITIS INVOLVING APPENDIX

Dense plasma cell-rich inflammation expands the mucosa; the latter shows crypt architectural disarray and erosions with luminal neutrophils, similar to features of colonic disease.

Specific Bacterial Causes of Appendicitis

Campylobacter. Patients with *Campylobacter* infection may present with the clinical features of acute appendicitis. The appendix is often grossly normal, but mesenteric lymph nodes are enlarged and swollen (90). The histologic features are reminiscent of *Campylobacter*-related colitis: the mucosa is infiltrated by neutrophils and eosinophils associated with crypt abscesses, edema, and hemorrhage. Although some cases involve the entire appendiceal wall, most are limited to the mucosa and superficial submucosa. Curved rod-shaped organisms are rarely identified with silver impregnation stains; microbiological cultures or stool polymerase chain reaction (PCR) assays are more sensitive for organism detection (57,91).

Yersinia. Yersinia enterocolitica and *Y. pseudotuberculosis* are gram-negative coccobacilli detected in a variety of meat and dairy products, fish, and shellfish. These organisms account for approximately 25 percent of cases of isolated granulomatous appendicitis (52,92). Patients present with symptoms of acute appendicitis or enterocolitis. Individuals with underlying immunodeficiency and those receiving desferrioxamine for iron overload are at increased risk for a protracted disease course requiring therapy with fluoroquinolones or other agents (62).

Yersinia show a predilection for the ileocolic region and appendix; infection is accompanied by mesenteric lymphadenopathy that may show central necrosis. The appendix is typically enlarged and indurated due to striking lymphoid hyperplasia and mural lymphoid aggregates. Irregularly shaped granulomas with coagulative or suppurative necrosis are located in follicles or the appendiceal wall (fig. 7-16A) (92). Non-necrotic epithelioid granulomas are surrounded by a cuff of lymphocytes, closely simulating the features of Crohn disease (fig. 7-16B). Suppurative granulomas are more common in patients with *Y. pseudotuberculosis* (fig. 7-16C,D). However, this organism elicits overlapping histologic features with those of *Y. enterocolitica* infection; molecular confirmation may be considered, if necessary (93,94).

Mycobacterium Tuberculosis. Most patients with tuberculous appendicitis in the United States are immunocompromised individuals with secondary involvement of the appendix by ileocolic disease or disseminated infection (95). Patients present with symptoms of acute appendicitis or vague, intermittent symptoms. Mesenteric lymphadenopathy and matted lymph nodes are typically present (96). Treatment consists of resection followed by several months of antibiotic therapy.

The appendix is distorted by granulomatous inflammation and fibrosis, or embedded in an inflammatory mass along with the terminal ileum and cecum (97). Confluent granulomas show central coagulative necrosis. Organisms are short, acid-fast rods with a slightly beaded appearance. They are often numerous in immunodeficient patients, but tend to be scarce in immunocompetent patients; cultures and molecular assays may be required to establish a diagnosis (62).

Some immunocompromised patients develop appendicitis due to atypical mycobacterial infections. These cases feature epithelioid granulomas as well as poorly formed aggregates of macrophages that expand the lamina propria. Acid fast and periodic acid–Schiff-diastase (PAS-D) stains demonstrate innumerable thin, delicate rods. The features of these infections are further discussed in chapter 4.

Actinomycosis. Approximately 5 percent of the population in the United States harbors *Actinomyces israelii* as part of the normal intestinal flora, yet the same organism can cause an invasive infection. The incidence of *Actinomyces*-related appendicitis has decreased over time, mirroring that of perforated appendicitis and the widespread use of broad-spectrum antibiotics (98). Luminal organisms can be detected in normal appendices; a diagnosis of infection requires infiltrating organisms in the appendix or luminal bacteria associated with mural changes, as described below.

Actinomyces israelii are anaerobic, filamentous bacteria that are gram-positive, acid fast-negative, and black with silver impregnation stains. Organisms show a predilection for the ileocecal area, sometimes forming an inflammatory mass with multiple sinus tracts. Infection elicits exuberant fibrosis that imparts an indurated or wooden appearance to the appendix (99,100). Yellow or brown sulfur granules are detected in 50 percent of cases. These structures consist of bacterial colonies cemented together by polysaccharides and surrounded by club-shaped

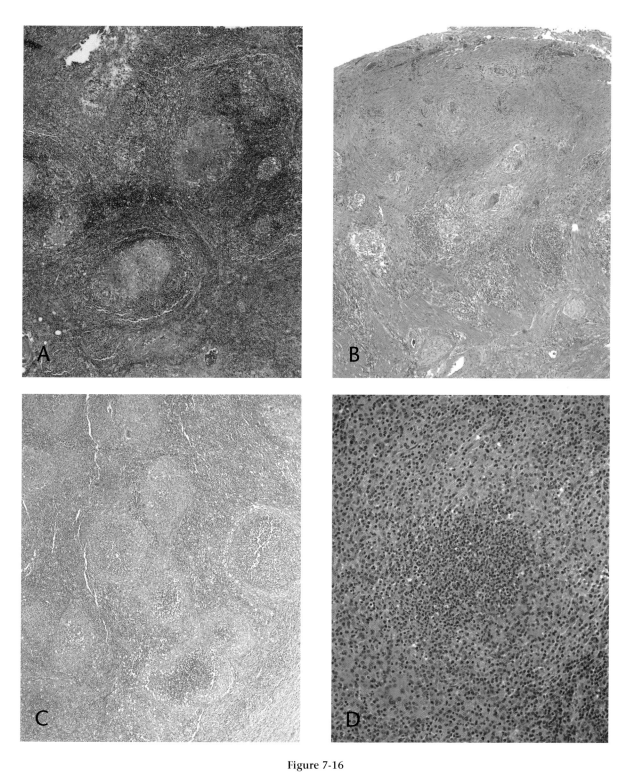

Figure 7-16

YERSINIA **APPENDICITIS**

Epithelioid granulomas with variable necrosis and surrounding lymphoid cuffs are typical of *Yersinia* enterocolitica (A). Some cases feature granulomas, transmural lymphoid aggregates, and neuronal hyperplasia in the outer half of the appendix that mimic Crohn disease (B). *Y. pseudotuberculosis* organisms elicit granulomas centered on follicles (C) with central suppurative necrosis (D).

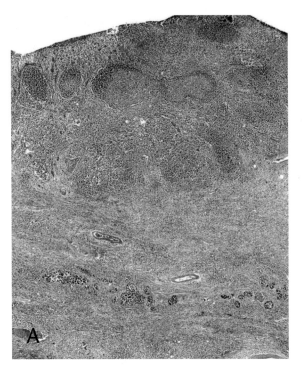
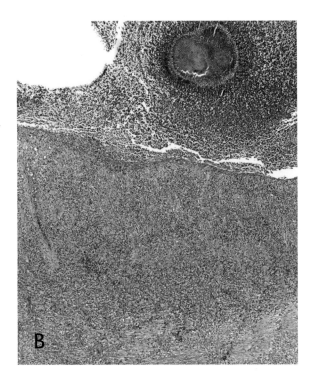

Figure 7-17

ACTINOMYCOSIS

Mural fibrosis is accompanied by mixed suppurative and lymphocytic inflammation, resulting in a markedly thickened appendix (A). Organisms are surrounded by radiating, club-like processes of Splendore-Hoeppli protein and intense neutrophil-rich inflammation in the lumen (B).

projections of radially arranged Splendore-Hoeppli protein (fig. 7-17).

The inflammatory reaction is predominantly suppurative, but granulomas, linear arrays of lymphoid aggregates, and fibrosis are prominent (101). Inflammation can extend across serosal surfaces, producing fistulae between the appendix, viscera, and skin (62).

Unrecognized actinomycosis can spread to mesenteric veins and embolize the liver, producing hepatic abscesses. It can also cause intra-abdominal or pelvic abscesses. Thus, the possibility of actinomycosis should be considered any time patients develop postappendectomy fistulae or when a diagnosis of Crohn disease is entertained based on pathologic findings in the appendix (102). Treatment consists of antibiotic therapy with or without, surgical resection.

Viral Appendicitis

Adenovirus. Adenovirus infection causes striking lymphoid hyperplasia of the ileocolic region and associated lymph nodes, leading to ileocecal intussusception (103,104). Appendiceal changes include marked lymphoid hyperplasia with surface epithelial cell degeneration and apoptotic nuclear debris. Infected epithelial cells contain smudgy or glassy eosinophilic nuclear inclusions and display indistinct nuclear membranes (fig. 7-18) (51). They tend to be clustered or singly scattered in surface and crypt epithelia or present in degenerated epithelial cells of the exudates.

The diagnosis is confirmed with immunohistochemical stains, PCR, and viral cultures. Serologic and fecal studies are sensitive, but viral detection by these methods does not always imply active infection (62).

Cytomegalovirus. Cytomegalovirus (CMV) is the most common viral infection of immunosuppressed patients; occasional cases occur in immunocompetent patients (105–107). Presenting symptoms of appendiceal disease include diarrhea, fever, and vague abdominal pain that ultimately localizes to the right lower quadrant (108). Patients with CMV-associated appendicitis have systemic infection that

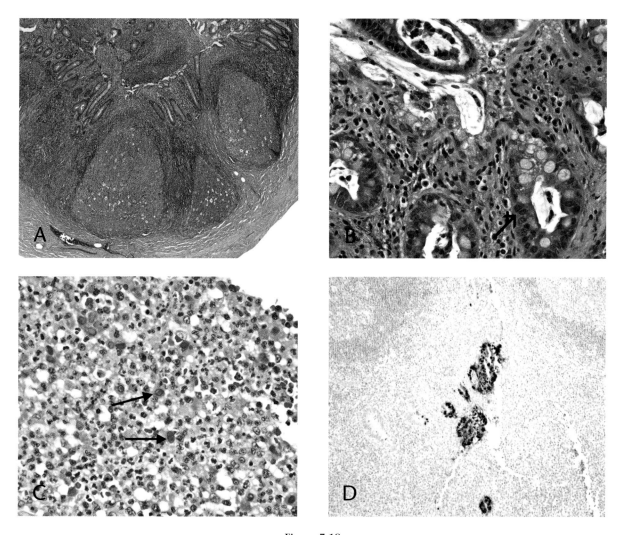

Figure 7-18

ADENOVIRUS INFECTION OF THE APPENDIX

Adenovirus elicits striking lymphoid hyperplasia (A) with crypt epithelial cell injury, smudgy nuclear inclusions in crypt cells, and degenerated epithelial cells in the crypt lumina (B). Degenerated epithelial cells with nuclear inclusions (arrows) are present in the exudate of an infected appendix (C). Immunohistochemistry highlights the infected cells (D).

requires antiviral therapy following surgical resection (109).

Appendiceal injury features epithelial cell degeneration, necrosis, and ulcers with mixed, macrophage-rich inflammation in the wall. Multifocal crypt epithelial cell apoptosis, perivascular neutrophil clusters, and macrophage-rich infiltrates are clues to the diagnosis. The virus infects endothelial cells and glandular epithelial cells; both feature abundant amphophilic cytoplasm as well as cytoplasmic or nuclear inclusions.

Cytoplasmic inclusions are variably sized, brightly eosinophilic granules. Intranuclear inclusions are associated with peripheral chromatin clearing that imparts an owl's eye appearance. Molecular assays and serologic studies can facilitate a diagnosis, but may be negative in patients with limited involvement of one, or a few, organs.

Other Viral Causes of Appendicitis. Any pathogenic virus that causes gastroenteritis can infect the appendix. Most patients present with a viral prodrome, fever and malaise, sore throat and rash, or gastrointestinal distress, rather than symptoms of appendicitis. Epstein-Barr virus elicits striking lymphoid hyperplasia and

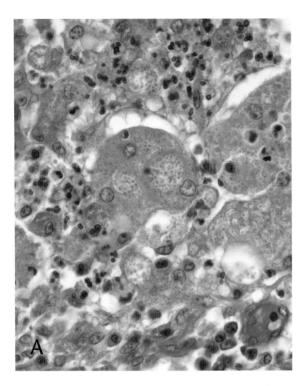 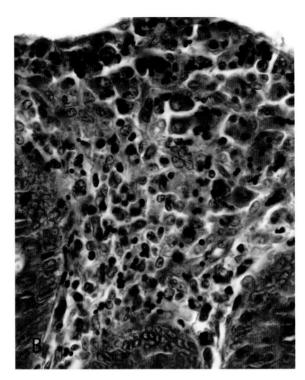

Figure 7-19

HISTOPLASMOSIS OF APPENDIX

The lamina propria is expanded by macrophages and multinucleated giant cells that contain numerous round-to-ovoid organisms (A). Fungi are highlighted with methenamine silver counterstained with hematoxylin and eosin (H&E) (B).

lymphocyte-rich inflammation accompanied by scattered aggregates of immunoblasts (110). Measles infection of the appendix occurs in patients with gastrointestinal symptoms, which may precede the viral exanthem (111,112). This virus also elicits lymphoid hyperplasia; multinucleated Warthin-Finkeldey cells may be detected in germinal centers and the lamina propria (113).

Fungal Infection

Fungal appendicitis is infrequent and most cases develop in immunocompromised or debilitated patients. *Histoplasma capsulatum* is the most common fungus to infect the appendix. It generally affects individuals living in endemic areas, and appendiceal involvement is part of a disseminated process (114). Infection elicits a lymphohistiocytic or granulomatous inflammatory response with variable neutrophilic infiltrates; intracellular organisms are readily apparent in tissue macrophages and stain with PAS, PAS-D, and silver impregnation (fig. 7-19).

Mucor are ubiquitous saprophytic fungi with broad, pauci-septate hyphae that branch haphazardly and have optically clear centers on cross section. This branching pattern is in sharp contrast to the regular branched pattern of *Aspergillus* and similar filamentous fungi. *Mucor* and *Aspergillus* show a tendency to invade blood vessels, causing thrombosis and vascular dissemination as well as ulcers, extensive tissue necrosis, and inflammatory masses in some cases (fig. 7-20) (115).

Candida sp. rarely infect the appendix. Affected patients are generally immunosuppressed and gastrointestinal involvement is secondary to fungal sepsis (116).

Parasitic Infection

Enterobius Vermicularis. *Enterobius vermicularis* (*Oxyuris vermicularis*), also known as pinworm or threadworm, has a worldwide distribution. It is the most common appendiceal parasite in patients from temperate and cold climates, and is found in approximately 1 to 4 percent of appendectomy specimens (117–119).

Poor sanitation and crowded living conditions enhance transmission, and children are particularly susceptible to infection (120).

Adult female worms measure 6 to 12 mm, whereas males span only 2 to 5 mm. Ova hatch in the duodenum, where the larvae molt and become sexually mature. Mating occurs in the cecum, appendix, or ileum. The males die soon after copulation; females migrate to the perianal skin and perineum to lay eggs, and die shortly after. The eggs are highly contagious and resistant to common disinfectants.

Adult worms reside in the lumen of the appendix (fig. 7-21A,B). They are usually non-invasive and do not elicit an inflammatory response. Rare invasive examples elicit eosinophil-rich inflammatory infiltrates, neutrophils, and occasional granulomas (119). Pinworms have easily visible lateral ala and internal organs; eggs can be seen in the females (fig. 7-21C,D) (62).

Schistosomiasis. Schistosomiasis is one of the most widespread parasitic diseases, affecting approximately 300 million people worldwide; infection rates are highest in Africa, Asia, and Puerto Rico (121,122). Infection results from exposure to contaminated water that harbors snail species necessary to the trematode life cycle (123). Worms penetrate the skin and make their way to the veins of the gastrointestinal tract (*S. mansoni*), liver (*S. japonicum, S. mekongi,* and *S. intercalatum*), or urinary bladder (*S. haemotobium*). They mate in the venous system where females shed eggs that embolize the viscera, causing granulomatous inflammation.

Schistosomes are found in 1 to 15 percent of appendectomy specimens from endemic areas (121,124). Acute appendiceal symptoms are more common in children, presumably reflecting the presence of viable ova and new-onset infection.

Intravascular eggs do not cause an inflammatory reaction, but those that erode through the vascular wall are surrounded by granulomatous inflammation with a peripheral cuff of eosinophils (fig. 7-22). Granulomas become fibrotic and hyalinized over time and ova typically calcify (125). Some patients develop suppurative bacterial infections secondary to the inflammation and fibrosis accompanying calcified ova. Calcified eggs are intensely basophilic; speciation can be facilitated by the recognition of characteristic spines. Eggs are

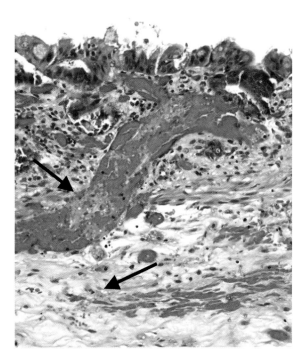

Figure 7-20

INVASIVE *ASPERGILLUS* INFECTION

Fungal forms are present within vessels and the wall of the appendix (arrows). There is essentially no associated inflammation in this extremely immunosuppressed patient.

acid fast, although histochemical stains are not required to establish a diagnosis.

Strongyloides Stercoralis. *Strongyloides stercoralis* is a nematode endemic to tropical climates. Infectious filariform larvae are contracted from contaminated soil. Most infected patients are asymptomatic. Immunosuppressed patients, particularly those receiving corticosteroid therapy or with HTLV-1 infection, are at risk for chronic disease and are more likely to have gastrointestinal symptoms (126). Appendiceal involvement produces symptoms of acute appendicitis accompanied by leukocytosis and peripheral eosinophilia.

Adult worms are curved with sharply pointed tails (127). Larvae are smaller, with a thin cuticle that contains rows of small nuclei. Invasive larvae are accompanied by eosinophil aggregates with degranulation and Splendore-Hoeppli phenomenon. Stool examinations and serologic tests can facilitate a diagnosis, although the morphologic features present in histologic sections are essentially pathognomonic.

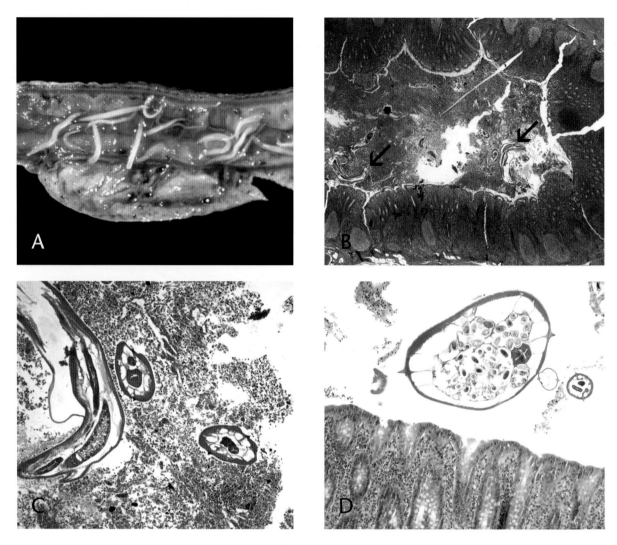

Figure 7-21

ENTEROBIASIS OF APPENDIX

Multiple worms are present in the lumen (A). Worms (arrows) are associated with fecal material in the lumen (B). Transverse and longitudinal sections demonstrate internal organs and lateral ala of several worms (C). A female worm contains many eggs (D).

Other Parasitic Infections. Virtually any parasite that infects the gastrointestinal tract can involve the appendix. *Trichuris* and *Ascaris* are usually limited to the appendiceal lumen, whereas whipworms often invade the wall. *Entamoeba* and *Balantidium coli* are detected in the appendices of patients with ileocolic infection. The organisms are usually located in the lumen and contain bubbly cytoplasm with small, eccentric nuclei, although the *Balantidium* are much larger than *Entamoeba* (fig. 7-23). Amebae can be highlighted with trichrome and PAS stains. *E. histolytica* contain ingested red blood cells or cell fragments.

MISCELLANEOUS CONDITIONS

Mucocele

Neoplastic and non-neoplastic conditions can lead to appendiceal dilatation and mucin accumulation, which has historically been classified under the umbrella of a *mucocele*. Although it is important to exclude neoplasia when an appendix with this appearance is encountered, a variety of non-neoplastic conditions can cause cystic dilatation of the appendix with abundant mucin, including cystic fibrosis, obstruction by fecalith, and retention cysts. The

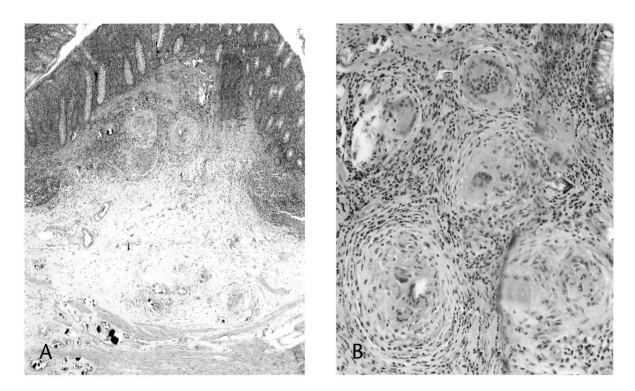

Figure 7-22

SCHISTOSOMIASIS OF APPENDIX

Calcified schistosome eggs are present within hyalinized, fibrotic granulomas in the submucosa and muscularis propria, as well as more cellular granulomas in the superficial submucosa (A). Cellular granulomas are associated with calcified schistosome eggs and prominent eosinophilia (B).

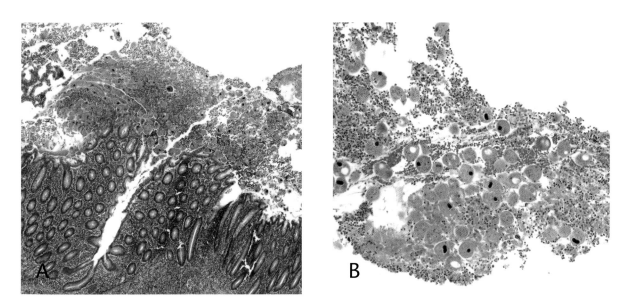

Figure 7-23

BALANTIDIUM COLI

Numerous *B. coli* are present in the lumen of the appendix (A). The parasites have characteristic large, kidney bean-shaped nuclei (B).

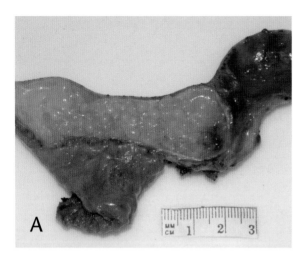
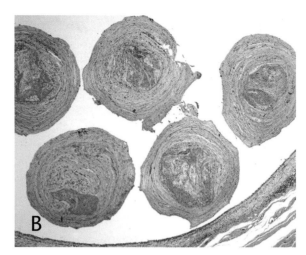

Figure 7-24

MYXOGLOBULOSIS

The distended appendix contains numerous translucent spheres (A) composed of lamellated mucin with a central eosinophilic, granular core (B). Although previously reported in association with non-neoplastic and neoplastic appendiceal lesions, most of these cases are related to low-grade mucinous neoplasms. (Courtesy of Dr. I. Brown, Brisbane, Australia.)

term "mucocele" is best avoided as a pathologic diagnosis because it simply denotes the gross appearance of a mucin-filled appendix, regardless of the underlying histologic diagnosis.

Myxoglobulosis

Myxoglobulosis has been described in association with mucin-filled, non-neoplastic appendices. This abnormality features numerous discrete globules of translucent mucin resembling frog spawn; they consist of lamellated mucin with a central eosinophilic, granular core (fig. 7-24) (128). However, virtually all examples of well-documented myxoglobulosis occur in the setting of appendiceal mucinous neoplasia. Thus, this finding should prompt submission of the entire appendix in order to exclude the possibility of a neoplasm.

Fibrous Obliteration

Fibrous obliteration is mucosal and submucosal obliteration by disorganized fibroblasts, Schwann cells, and axons. Synonyms include *fibrous occlusion of the appendix, appendiceal neuroma, neurogenic appendicopathy, neurogenic appendicitis,* and *neurotization of appendix.*

Fibrous obliteration of the appendix is almost always an incidental finding in patients who undergo appendectomy for other reasons. It may be found in patients with, or without, symptoms of acute appendicitis.

Fibrous obliteration may occur as a result of aging or represent a consequence of resolved appendicitis (129). Affected appendices contain increased levels of substance P, vasoactive intestinal peptide, tumor necrosis factor-alpha, interleukin-2, cyclo-oxygenases 1 and 2, and prostaglandin E2, leading some investigators to suggest that elaboration of these agents in the uninflamed appendix produces appendicitis symptoms (60,130,131). Others have failed to demonstrate a relationship between fibrous obliteration of the appendix and clinical symptoms (132).

The obliterative process starts in the distal appendix and progresses over time, eventually effacing the mucosa, submucosa, and Peyer patches (fig. 7-25). Fibrosis is accompanied by admixed nerve fibers, Schwann cells, endocrine cells, and smooth muscle cells. Neural elements and Schwann cells are often associated with eosinophils and lymphocytes. They may be highlighted by S-100 protein immunostains. Pathologic distinction between fibrous obliteration, neural hyperplasia, and neuroma is subjective and arbitrary.

Periappendicitis

Periappendicitis is inflammation confined to the appendiceal serosa and periappendiceal soft tissues. It is detected in up to 5 percent of patients with clinically suspected acute appendicitis. It occurs most commonly in boys

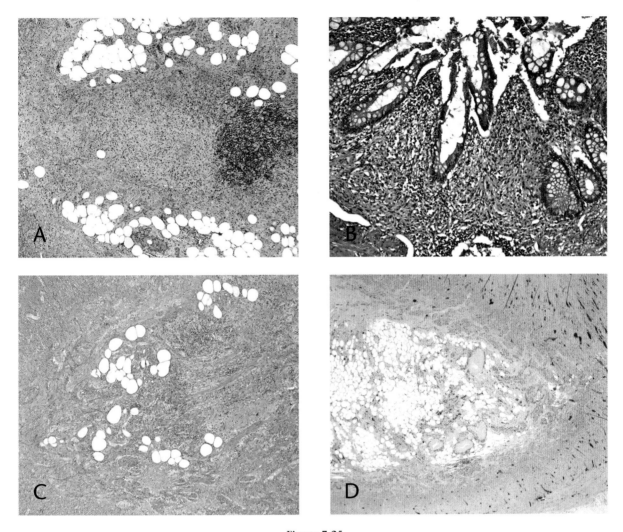

Figure 7-25

FIBROUS OBLITERATION

The tip of the appendix is initially involved, then the process spreads proximally, obliterating the mucosa, lymphoid aggregates, and submucosa (A). Spindle cells are present in the appendiceal mucosa (B). Fibrosis is usually accompanied by admixed nerve fibers, Schwann cells, endocrine cells, and muscle (C). An S-100 protein immunostain highlights the Schwann cells (D).

younger than 12 years of age and in females ages 17 to 21 years (133). Most cases reflect serosal inflammation secondary to pelvic inflammatory disease, intra-abdominal abscesses, diverticulitis, inflammatory bowel disease, or intestinal tumors (Table 7-3). Surgical manipulation may induce neutrophilic margination in the serosa.

Histologic features include neutrophil-rich inflammation and edema limited to the periappendiceal soft tissues, serosa, and outermost muscularis propria (fig. 7-25). Some cases display accumulation of fibrin unaccompanied by abundant inflammation. Periappendicitis

Table 7-3

DIFFERENTIAL DIAGNOSIS OF PERIAPPENDICITIS

Pelvic inflammatory disease

Ectopic pregnancy

Urologic diseases

Inflammatory bowel disease

Colonic neoplasms

Colitis

Colonic diverticulitis

Abdominal aortic aneurysm

Chlamydial infection

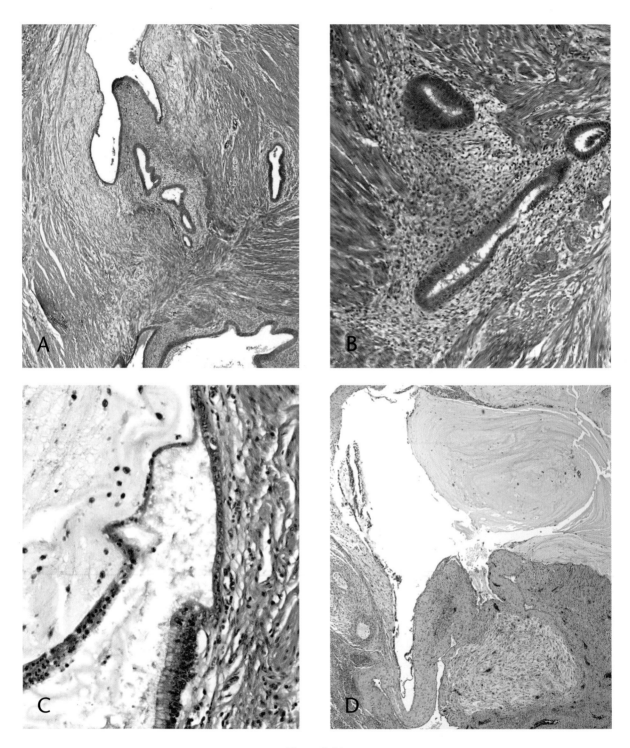

Figure 7-26

APPENDICEAL ENDOMETRIOSIS

Endometriosis elicits hypertrophy of the muscularis propria (A). Endometrioid glands and stroma are present in association with macrophages and hemosiderin (B). Endometriotic glands may undergo mucinous metaplasia that simulates a mucinous neoplasm (C). Decidualized endometriosis has a myxoid appearance and may be associated with abundant mucin, simulating a neoplasm (D).

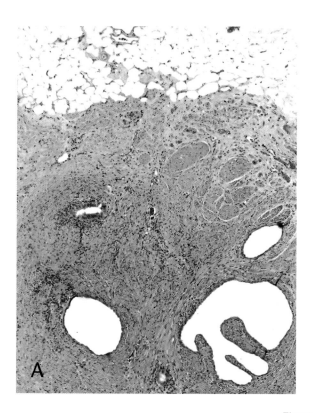 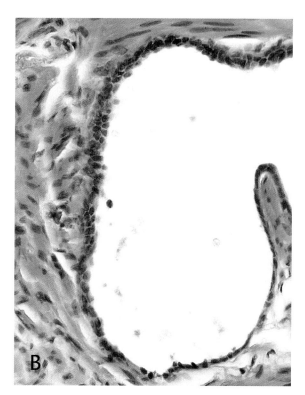

Figure 7-27

ENDOSALPINGIOSIS INVOLVING APPENDIX

Glands of endosalpingiosis are located in the outer muscularis propria (A). The epithelium resembles that of the fallopian tube. There is no associated endometrial-type stroma (B).

resolves with fibrosis, fibrous adhesions, and chronic inflammation that may extend into the mesoappendix. The entire appendix should be submitted to exclude the possibility of acute appendicitis whenever a diagnosis of periappendicitis is considered because the finding of periappendicitis alone necessitates further evaluation to exclude an extra-appendiceal process.

Endometriosis

Endometriosis is detected in approximately 1 percent of appendectomy specimens (134–136). It can cause symptoms of acute or chronic appendicitis, or manifest with abdominal pain due to appendiceal intussusception (26,137,138). Endometriosis usually involves the serosal surface or the muscular layers of the appendix, and rarely extends to the mucosa. It may produce discrete brown-red or hemorrhagic foci, although most cases are not appreciated grossly.

Variable amounts of endometrioid epithelium and stroma are present in association with hemorrhage and hemosiderin deposits (fig. 7-26A,B). Occasional cases show mucinous metaplasia or decidual change that simulates a mucinous neoplasm (fig. 7-26C,D) (139). Immunostains directed against PAX-8 and estrogen receptors highlight mullerian glands and facilitate a diagnosis in challenging cases (140).

Endosalpingiosis

Endosalpingiosis features benign ciliated tubal-type glands derived from peritoneal mesothelial cells (fig. 7-27). It usually occurs as an incidental finding on the outer aspect of the appendix, but rare cases produce mass lesions that can mimic malignancy (141,142). Distinction from endometriosis is straightforward: endosalpingiosis lacks endometrioid stroma, macrophages, and hemorrhage. Immunostains directed against PAX-8 and WT1 can facilitate distinction from other mimics, such as mesothelial inclusions and mesonephric remnants (143).

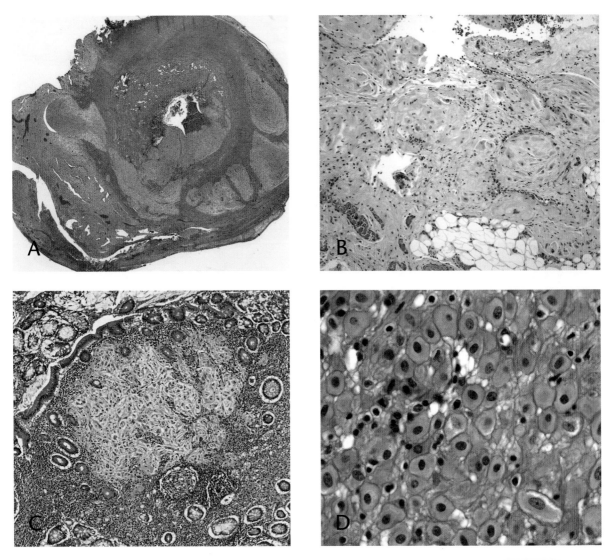

Figure 7-28

APPENDICEAL DECIDUOSIS

Multiple nodules of decidualized stroma involve the full thickness of the appendiceal wall (A), forming small nodules in the mesoappendix (B) and mucosa (C). Decidualized cells contain abundant eosinophilic cytoplasm with small nuclei and prominent cell membranes (D).

Deciduosis of the Appendix

Nodules of decidualized stromal cells are frequently detected in the subserosal connective tissue of appendectomy specimens obtained from reproductive-age women, especially those who are pregnant or undergoing a post-partum tubal ligation. Most patients are asymptomatic, although this finding has been reported as the only abnormality in patients with symptoms of acute appendicitis (144). It is not clear whether these foci of deciduosis represent ectopic uterine stromal cells or decidualized mesenchymal cells of another process. Regardless, they resemble decidua found elsewhere and feature tight aggregates of polygonal cells with slightly basophilic or eosinophilic cytoplasm (fig. 7-28) (145).

Non-Neoplastic Appendiceal Polyps

Hyperplastic polyps are occasionally observed in the appendix. They are small, sessile nodules that do not involve the circumference of the

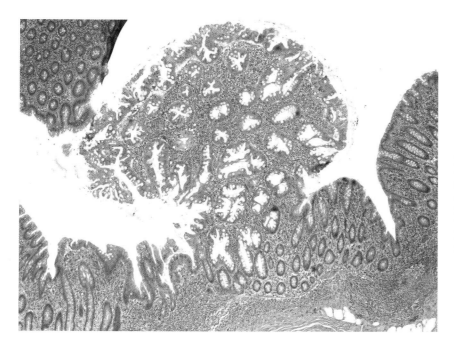

Figure 7-29

HYPERPLASTIC POLYP OF APPENDIX

Appendiceal hyperplastic polyps resemble their colonic counterparts. This lesion is small and does not spread circumferentially along the mucosa; crypts are narrow at their bases and do not show lateral branching in the deep mucosa.

appendix. They resemble colorectal hyperplastic polyps, containing non-dysplastic crypts lined by serrated epithelium that features both goblet and non-goblet mucinous epithelial cells (fig. 7-29) (146,147). These lesions should be distinguished from appendiceal neoplasms that resemble sessile serrated polyps of the colon. The latter tend to be large, circumferential proliferations of elongated and dilated crypts that display serration along the full length of the crypt as well as lateral budding or branching of the deep crypts.

Other non-neoplastic polyps, such as Peutz-Jeghers polyps and vascular lesions, also occur in the appendix, although most of these are uncommon. These polyps are discussed further in chapter 4 (148,149).

REFERENCES

1. Collins DC. A study of 50,000 specimens of the human vermiform appendix. Surg Gynecol Obstet 1955;101:437-45.
2. Misdraji J, Graeme-Cook FM. Miscellaneous conditions of the appendix. Semin Diagn Pathol 2004;21:151-63.
3. Collins DC. Agenesis of the vermiform appendix. Am J Surg 1951;82:689-96.
4. Yokose Y, Maruyama H, Tsutsumi M, Uchida K, Shiraiwa K, Konishi Y. Ileal atresia and absence of appendix. Acta Pathol Jpn 1986;36:1403-10.
5. Bremner DN, Mooney G. Agenesis of appendix: a further thalidomide anomaly. Lancet 1978;1:826.
6. Varshney M, Shahid M, Maheshwari V, Mubeen A, Gaur K. Duplication of appendix: an accidental finding. BMJ Case Rep 2011;2011.
7. Cave AJ. Appendix vermiformis duplex. J Anat 1936;70(Pt 2):283-92.
8. Wallbridge PH. Double appendix. Br J Surg 1962;50:346-7.
9. Tinckler LF. Triple appendix vermiformis—a unique case. Br J Surg 1968;55:79-81.
10. Payan HM. Diverticular disease of the appendix. Dis Colon Rectum 1977;20:473-6.
11. Phillips BJ, Perry CW. Appendiceal diverticulitis. Mayo Clin Proc 1999;74:890-2.
12. Martens M, De Boeck K, Van Der Steen K, Smet M, Eggermont E. A right lower quadrant mass in cystic fibrosis: a diagnostic challenge. Eur J Pediatr 1992;151:329-31.
13. George DH. Diverticulosis of the vermiform appendix in patients with cystic fibrosis. Hum Pathol 1987;18:75-9.

14. Dupre MP, Jadavji I, Matshes E, Urbanski SJ. Diverticular disease of the vermiform appendix: a diagnostic clue to underlying appendiceal neoplasm. Hum Pathol 2008;39:1823-6.

15. Hsu M, Young RH, Misdraji J. Ruptured appendiceal diverticula mimicking low-grade appendiceal mucinous neoplasms. Am J Surg Pathol 2009;33:1515-21.

16. Fink VH, Santos AL, Goldberg SL. Intussusception of the appendix. Case reports and reviews of the literature. Am J Gastroenterol 1964;42:431-41.

17. Forshall I. Intussusception of the vermiform appendix with a report of seven cases in children. Br J Surg 1953;40:305-12.

18. Chaar CI, Wexelman B, Zuckerman K, Longo W. Intussusception of the appendix: comprehensive review of the literature. Am J Surg 2009;198:122-8.

19. Samuk I, Nica A, Iakovski Y, Freud E. Appendiceal intussusception: a diagnostic challenge. Eur J Pediatr Surg 2018;28:30-3.

20. Hines JJ, Paek GK, Lee P, Wu L, Katz DS. Beyond appendicitis; radiologic review of unusual and rare pathology of the appendix. Abdom Radiol (NY) 2016;41:568-81.

21. Ho L, Rosenman LD. Complete invagination of the vermiform appendix with villous adenoma, intussuscepting to the splenic flexure of the colon. Surgery 1975;77:505-6.

22. Lauwers GY, Prendergast NC, Wahl SJ, Bagchi S. Invagination of vermiform appendix. Dig Dis Sci 1993;38:565-8.

23. Rodriguez MA, Wasdahl WA. Mucinous carcinoid and endometriosis in an inside-out appendix. Am J Gastroenterol 1978;69:199-202.

24. Grynspan D, Rabah R. Adenoviral appendicitis presenting clinically as acute appendicitis. Pediatr Dev Pathol 2008;11:138-41.

25. Ozuner G, Davidson P, Church J. Intussusception of the vermiform appendix: preoperative colonoscopic diagnosis of two cases and review of the literature. Int J Colorectal Dis 2000;15:185-7.

26. Sakaguchi N, Ito M, Sano K, Baba T, Koyama M, Hotchi M. Intussusception of the appendix: a report of three cases with different clinical and pathologic features. Pathol Int 1995;45:757-61.

27. Park BS, Shin DH, Kim DI, Son GM, Kim HS. Appendiceal intussusception requiring an ileocecectomy: a case report and comment on the optimal surgery. BMC Surg 2018;18:48.

28. Rode J, Dhillon AP, Hutt MS. Appendicitis revisited: a comparative study of Malawian and English appendices. J Pathol 1987;153:357-63.

29. Lee JA. The influence of sex and age on appendicitis in children and young adults. Gut 1962;3:80-4.

30. Brender JD, Weiss NS, Koepsell TD, Marcuse EK. Fiber intake and childhood appendicitis. Am J Public Health 1985;75:399-400.

31. Adamidis D, Roma-Giannikou E, Karamolegou K, Tselalidou E, Constantopoulos A. Fiber intake and childhood appendicitis. Int J Food Sci Nutr 2000;51:153-7.

32. Hardin DM Jr. Acute appendicitis: review and update. Am Fam Physician 1999;60:2027-34.

33. Addiss DG, Shaffer N, Fowler BS, Tauxe RV. The epidemiology of appendicitis and appendectomy in the United States. Am J Epidemiol 1990;132:910-25.

34. Arnbjornsson E. Acute appendicitis and dietary fiber. Arch Surg 1983;118:868-70.

35. Kang JY, Hoare J, Majeed A, Williamson RC, Maxwell JD. Decline in admission rates for acute appendicitis in England. Br J Surg 2003;90:1586-92.

36. Williams NM, Jackson D, Everson NW, Johnstone JM. Is the incidence of acute appendicitis really falling? Ann R Coll Surg Engl 1998;80:122-4.

37. Al-Omran M, Mamdani M, McLeod RS. Epidemiologic features of acute appendicitis in Ontario, Canada. Can J Surg 2003;46:263-8.

38. Korner H, Sondenaa K, Soreide JA, et al. Incidence of acute nonperforated and perforated appendicitis: age-specific and sex-specific analysis. World J Surg 1997;21:313-7.

39. Luckmann R, Davis P. The epidemiology of acute appendicitis in California: racial, gender, and seasonal variation. Epidemiology 1991;2:323-30.

40. Hui TT, Major KM, Avital I, Hiatt JR, Margulies DR. Outcome of elderly patients with appendicitis: effect of computed tomography and laparoscopy. Arch Surg 2002;137:995-8.

41. Klein DB, Hurley LB, Horberg MA, et al. Increased rates of appendicitis in HIV-infected men: 1991-2005. J Acquir Immune Defic Syndr 2009;52:139-40.

42. Storm-Dickerson TL, Horattas MC. What have we learned over the past 20 years about appendicitis in the elderly? Am J Surg 2003;185:198-201.

43. Gardikis S, Touloupidis S, Dimitriadis G, et al. Urological symptoms of acute appendicitis in childhood and early adolescence. Int Urol Nephrol 2002;34:189-92.

44. Carr NJ. The pathology of acute appendicitis. Ann Diagn Pathol 2000;4:46-58.

45. Jacob H, Toyonaga T, Ohara Y, et al. Endoscopic submucosal dissection of cecal lesions in proximity to the appendiceal orifice. Endoscopy 2016;48:829-36.

46. Basson MD, Persinger D, Newman WP. Association of colonoscopy with risk of appendicitis. JAMA Surg 2018;153:90-1.

47. Katagiri H, Lefor AK, Kubota T, Mizokami K. Barium appendicitis: a single institution review in Japan. World J Gastrointest Surg 2016;8:651-5.

48. Nitecki S, Karmeli R, Sarr MG. Appendiceal calculi and fecaliths as indications for appendectomy. Surg Gynecol Obstet 1990;171:185-8.

49. Shin MS, Ho KJ. Appendicolith. Significance in acute appendicitis and demonstration by computed tomography. Dig Dis Sci 1985;30:184-7.

50. Balch CM, Silver D. Foreign bodies in the appendix. Report of eight cases and review of the literature. Arch Surg 1971;102:14-20.

51. Lynch DT, Lott L, Cebe K, McDonald JM, Abplanalp A, Tully C, et al. Adenovirus-associated acute appendicitis: an under-recognized relationship? Mil Med 2017;182:e1765-8.

52. Bennion RS, Thompson JE Jr, Gil J, Schmit PJ. The role of Yersinia enterocolitica in appendicitis in the southwestern United States. Am Surg 1991;57:766-8.

53. Astagneau P, Goldstein FW, Francoual S, Baviera E, Barthalon M, Acar JF. Appendicitis due to both Streptococcus pneumoniae and haemophilus influenzae. Eur J Clin Microbiol Infect Dis 1992;11:559-60.

54. Lau WY, Teoh-Chan CH, Fan ST, Yam WC, Lau KF, Wong SH. The bacteriology and septic complication of patients with appendicitis. Ann Surg 1984;200:576-81.

55. Madden NP, Hart CA. Streptococcus milleri in appendicitis in children. J Pediatr Surg 1985;20:6-7.

56. Rogers MB, Brower-Sinning R, Firek B, Zhong D, Morowitz MJ. Acute appendicitis in children is associated with a local expansion of fusobacteria. Clin Infect Dis 2016;63:71-8.

57. Chan FT, Stringel G, Mackenzie AM. Isolation of campylobacter jejuni from an appendix. J Clin Microbiol 1983;18:422-4.

58. Kraemer M, Franke C, Ohmann C, Yang Q, Acute Abdominal Pain Study G. Acute appendicitis in late adulthood: incidence, presentation, and outcome. Results of a prospective multicenter acute abdominal pain study and a review of the literature. Langenbecks Arch Surg 2000;385:470-81.

59. Yantiss RK. Eosinophils in the GI tract: how many is too many and what do they mean? Mod Pathol 2015;28(Suppl 1):S7-21.

60. Wang Y, Reen DJ, Puri P. Is a histologically normal appendix following emergency appendicectomy alway normal? Lancet 1996;347:1076-9.

61. Buirge RE, Dennis C, Varco RL, Wangensteen OH. Histology of experimental appendiceal obstruction (rabbit, ape and man). Arch Pathol Lab Med 1940;30:481.

62. Lamps LW. Infectious causes of appendicitis. Infect Dis Clin North Am 2010;24:995-1018.

63. Jones PF. Suspected acute appendicitis: trends in management over 30 years. Br J Surg 2001;88:1570-7.

64. Blair NP, Bugis SP, Turner LJ, MacLeod MM. Review of the pathologic diagnoses of 2,216 appendectomy specimens. Am J Surg 1993;165:618-20.

65. Kosloske AM, Love CL, Rohrer JE, Goldthorn JF, Lacey SR. The diagnosis of appendicitis in children: outcomes of a strategy based on pediatric surgical evaluation. Pediatrics 2004;113(Pt 1):29-34.

66. Guo G, Greenson JK. Histopathology of interval (delayed) appendectomy specimens: strong association with granulomatous and xanthogranulomatous appendicitis. Am J Surg Pathol 2003;27:1147-51.

67. Wagner M, Tubre DJ, Asensio JA. Evolution and current trends in the management of acute appendicitis. Surg Clin North Am 2018;98:1005-23.

68. Koepsell TD, Inui TS, Farewell VT. Factors affecting perforation in acute appendicitis. Surg Gynecol Obstet 1981;153:508-10.

69. Campbell KL, De Beaux AC. Non-steroidal anti-inflammatory drugs and appendicitis in patients aged over 50 years. Br J Surg 1992;79:967-8.

70. Horattas MC, Guyton DP, Wu D. A reappraisal of appendicitis in the elderly. Am J Surg 1990;160:291-3.

71. Giesen LJ, van den Boom AL, van Rossem CC, den Hoed PT, Wijnhoven BP. Retrospective multicenter study on risk factors for surgical site infections after appendectomy for acute Appendicitis. Dig Surg 2017;34:103-7.

72. Roberts KE, Starker LF, Duffy AJ, Bell RL, Bokhari J. Stump appendicitis: a surgeon's dilemma. JSLS 2011;15:373-8.

73. Taban S, Dema A, Lazar D, Sporea I, Lazar E, Cornianu M. An unusual "tumor" of the cecum: the inverted appendiceal stump. Rom J Morphol Embryol 2006;47:193-6.

74. Ciani S, Chuaqui B. Histological features of resolving acute, non-complicated phlegmonous appendicitis. Pathol Res Pract 2000;196:89-93.

75. Yilmaz M, Akbulut S, Kutluturk K, et al. Unusual histopathological findings in appendectomy specimens from patients with suspected acute appendicitis. World J Gastroenterol 2013;19:4015-22.

76. Mazziotti MV, Marley EF, Winthrop AL, Fitzgerald PG, Walton M, Langer JC. Histopathologic analysis of interval appendectomy specimens: support for the role of interval appendectomy. J Pediatr Surg 1997;32:806-9.

77. Misdraji J. Mucinous epithelial neoplasms of the appendix and pseudomyxoma peritonei. Mod Pathol 2015;28(Suppl 1):S67-79.

78. Pal K. Granulomatous appendicitis in children: a single institutional experience. Afr J Paediatr Surg 2014;11:26-31.

79. Clarke H, Pollett W, Chittal S, Ra M. Sarcoidosis with involvement of the appendix. Arch Intern Med 1983;143:1603-4.

80. Ripolles T, Martinez MJ, Morote V, Errando J. Appendiceal involvement in Crohn's disease: gray-scale sonography and color Doppler flow features. AJR Am J Roentgenol 2006;186:1071-8.

81. Han H, Kim H, Rehman A, Jang SM, Paik SS. Appendiceal Crohn's disease clinically presenting as acute appendicitis. World J Clin Cases 2014;2:888-92.

82. Bronner MP. Granulomatous appendicitis and the appendix in idiopathic inflammatory bowel disease. Semin Diagn Pathol 2004;21:98-107.

83. Yantiss RK, Sapp HL, Farraye FA, et al. Histologic predictors of pouchitis in patients with chronic ulcerative colitis. Am J Surg Pathol 2004;28:999-1006.

84. Goldblum JR, Appelman HD. Appendiceal involvement in ulcerative colitis. Mod Pathol 1992;5:607-10.

85. Kooij IA, Sahami S, Meijer SL, Buskens CJ, Te Velde AA. The immunology of the vermiform appendix: a review of the literature. Clin Exp Immunol 2016;186:1-9.

86. Myrelid P, Landerholm K, Nordenvall C, Pinkney TD, Andersson RE. Appendectomy and the risk of colectomy in ulcerative colitis: a national cohort study. Am J Gastroenterol 2017;112:1311-9.

87. Kroft SH, Stryker SJ, Rao MS. Appendiceal involvement as a skip lesion in ulcerative colitis. Mod Pathol 1994;7:912-4.

88. Groisman GM, George J, Harpaz N. Ulcerative appendicitis in universal and nonuniversal ulcerative colitis. Mod Pathol 1994;7:322-5.

89. Davison AM, Dixon MF. The appendix as a 'skip lesion' in ulcerative colitis. Histopathology 1990;16:93-5.

90. van Spreeuwel JP, Lindeman J, Bax R, Elbers HJ, Sybrandy R, Meijer CJ. Campylobacter-associated appendicitis: prevalence and clinicopathologic features. Pathol Annu 1987;22(Pt 1):55-65.

91. Campbell LK, Havens JM, Scott MA, Lamps LW. Molecular detection of Campylobacter jejuni in archival cases of acute appendicitis. Mod Pathol 2006;19:1042-6.

92. Lamps LW, Madhusudhan KT, Greenson JK, et al. The role of Yersinia enterocolitica and Yersinia pseudotuberculosis in granulomatous appendicitis: a histologic and molecular study. Am J Surg Pathol 2001;25:508-15.

93. Lamps LW, Havens JM, Gilbrech LJ, Dube PH, Scott MA. Molecular biogrouping of pathogenic Yersinia enterocolitica: development of a diagnostic PCR assay with histologic correlation. Am J Clin Pathol 2006;125:658-64.

94. Lamps LW, Madhusudhan KT, Havens JM, et al. Pathogenic Yersinia DNA is detected in bowel and mesenteric lymph nodes from patients with Crohn's disease. Am J Surg Pathol 2003;27:220-7.

95. Chis B, Dudric V, Fodor D. Tuberculous appendicitis. A case report. Med Ultrason 2017;19:333-5.

96. Singh MK, Arunabh, Kapoor VK. Tuberculosis of the appendix—a report of 17 cases and a suggested aetiopathological classification. Postgrad Med J 1987;63:855-7.

97. Lamps LW. Appendicitis and infections of the appendix. Semin Diagn Pathol 2004;21:86-97.

98. Garner JP, Macdonald M, Kumar PK. Abdominal actinomycosis. Int J Surg 2007;5:441-8.

99. Lee SY, Kwon HJ, Cho JH, et al. Actinomycosis of the appendix mimicking appendiceal tumor: a case report. World J Gastroenterol 2010;16:395-7.

100. Jarry J, Shekher M, Imperato M, Michel P. Appendicitis: when there is more than meets the eye. Clin Res Hepatol Gastroenterol 2011;35:765-7.

101. Hickey K, McKenna P, O'Connell PR, Gillan JE. Actinomycosis presenting as appendicitis in pregnancy. Br J Obstet Gynaecol 1993;100:595-6.

102. Gomez-Torres GA, Ortega-Garcia OS, Gutierrez-Lopez EG, et al. A rare case of subacute appendicitis, actinomycosis as the final pathology reports: a case report and literature review. Int J Surg Case Rep 2017;36:46-9.

103. Guarner J, de Leon-Bojorge B, Lopez-Corella E, et al. Intestinal intussusception associated with adenovirus infection in Mexican children. Am J Clin Pathol 2003;120:845-50.

104. Richardsen I, Schob DS, Ulmer TF, et al. Etiology of appendicitis in children: the role of bacterial and viral pathogens. J Invest Surg 2016;29:74-9.

105. Canterino JE, McCormack M, Gurung A, Passarelli J, Landry ML, Golden M. Cytomegalovirus appendicitis in an immunocompetent host. J Clin Virol 2016;78:9-11.

106. Dieterich DT, Kim MH, McMeeding A, Rotterdam H. Cytomegalovirus appendicitis in a patient with acquired immune deficiency syndrome. Am J Gastroenterol 1991;86:904-6.

107. Kothari A, Caradine KD, Rico Crescencio JC, et al. Cytomegalovirus appendicitis after hematopoietic stem cell transplantation. Transpl Infect Dis 2017;19.

108. Neumayer LA, Makar R, Ampel NM, Zukoski CF. Cytomegalovirus appendicitis in a patient with human immunodeficiency virus infection. Case report and review of the literature. Arch Surg 1993;128:467-8.

109. Faldetta KF, Kattakuzhy S, Wang HW, Sereti I, Sheikh V. Cytomegalovirus immune reconstitution inflammatory syndrome manifesting as acute appendicitis in an HIV-infected patient. BMC Infect Dis 2014;14:313.

110. Lopez-Navidad A, Domingo P, Cadafalch J, Farrerons J, Allende L, Bordes R. Acute appendicitis complicating infectious mononucleosis: case report and review. Rev Infect Dis 1990;12:297-302.

111. Paik SY, Oh JT, Choi YJ, Kwon KW, Yang WI. Measles-related appendicitis. Arch Pathol Lab Med 2002;126:82-4.

112. Pancharoen C, Ruttanamongkol P, Suwangool P, Likitnukul S, Thisyakorn U. Measles-associated appendicitis: two case reports and literature review. Scand J Infect Dis 2001;33:632-3.

113. Stadlmann S, Lenggenhager DM, Alves VA, et al. Histopathologic characteristics of the transitional stage of measles-associated appendicitis: case report and review of the literature. Hum Pathol 2011;42:285-90.

114. Lamps LW, Molina CP, West AB, Haggitt RC, Scott MA. The pathologic spectrum of gastrointestinal and hepatic histoplasmosis. Am J Clin Pathol 2000;113:64-72.

115. ter Borg F, Kuijper EJ, van der Lelie H. Fatal mucormycosis presenting as an appendiceal mass with metastatic spread to the liver during chemotherapy-induced granulocytopenia. Scand J Infect Dis 1990;22:499-501.

116. Larbcharoensub N, Boonsakan P, Kanoksil W, et al. Fungal appendicitis: a case series and review of the literature. Southeast Asian J Trop Med Public Health 2013;44:681-9.

117. Altun E, Avci V, Azatcam M. Parasitic infestation in appendicitis. A retrospective analysis of 660 patients and brief literature review. Saudi Med J 2017;38:314-8.

118. Arca MJ, Gates RL, Groner JI, Hammond S, Caniano DA. Clinical manifestations of appendiceal pinworms in children: an institutional experience and a review of the literature. Pediatr Surg Int 2004;20:372-5.

119. Wiebe BM. Appendicitis and Enterobius vermicularis. Scand J Gastroenterol 1991;26:336-8.

120. Cook GC. Enterobius vermicularis infection. Gut 1994;35:1159-62.

121. Botes SN, Ibirogba SB, McCallum AD, Kahn D. Schistosoma prevalence in appendicitis. World J Surg 2015;39:1080-3.

122. Nash TE, Cheever AW, Ottesen EA, Cook JA. Schistosome infections in humans: perspectives and recent findings. NIH conference. Ann Intern Med 1982;97:740-54.

123. Gryseels B, Polman K, Clerinx J, Kestens L. Human schistosomiasis. Lancet 2006;368:1106-18.

124. Onuigbo WI. Appendiceal schistosomiasis. Method of classifying oviposition and inflammation. Dis Colon Rectum 1985;28:397-8.

125. Satti MB, Tamimi DM, Al Sohaibani MO, Al Quorain A. Appendicular schistosomiasis: a cause of clinical acute appendicitis? J Clin Pathol 1987;40:424-8.

126. Nutman TB. Human infection with Strongyloides stercoralis and other related Strongyloides species. Parasitology 2017;144:263-73.

127. Komenaka IK, Wu GC, Lazar EL, Cohen JA. Strongyloides appendicitis: unusual etiology in two siblings with chronic abdominal pain. J Pediatr Surg 2003;38:E8-10.

128. Aroukatos P, Verras D, Vandoros GP, Repanti M. Myxoglobulosis of the appendix: a case associated with ruptured diverticulum. Case Rep Med 2010;2010.

129. Williams R. Neuroma of the appendix. In: Williams RA, Myers P, eds. Pathology of the appendix and its durgical treatment. London: Chapman and Hall Medical Press; 1994:126-36.

130. Di Sebastiano P, Fink T, di Mola FF, et al. Neuroimmune appendicitis. Lancet 1999;354:461-6.

131. Nemeth L, Reen DJ, O'Briain DS, McDermott M, Puri P. Evidence of an inflammatory pathologic condition in "normal" appendices following emergency appendectomy. Arch Pathol Lab Med 2001;125:759-64.

132. Franke C, Gerharz CD, Bohner H, et al. Neurogenic appendicopathy: a clinical disease entity? Int J Colorectal Dis 2002;17:185-91.

133. Chaudhary P, Nabi I, Arora MP. Periappendicitis: our 13 year experience. Int J Surg 2014;12:1010-3.

134. Prystowsky JB, Stryker SJ, Ujiki GT, Poticha SM. Gastrointestinal endometriosis. Incidence and indications for resection. Arch Surg 1988;123:855-8.

135. Ortiz-Hidalgo C, Cortes-Aguilar D, Ortiz de la Pena J. Endometriosis of the vermiform appendix (EVA) is an uncommon lesion with a frequency < 1% of all cases of pelvic endometriosis. Recent case. World J Surg 1999;23:427.

136. Yantiss RK, Clement PB, Young RH. Endometriosis of the intestinal tract: a study of 44 cases of a disease that may cause diverse challenges in clinical and pathologic evaluation. Am J Surg Pathol 2001;25:445-54.

137. Sriram PV, Seitz U, Soehendra N, Schroeder S. Endoscopic appendectomy in a case of appendicular intussusception due to endometriosis, mimicking a cecal polyp. Am J Gastroenterol 2000;95:1594-6.

138. Nycum LR, Moss H, Adams JQ, Macri CI. Asymptomatic intussusception of the appendix due to endometriosis. South Med J 1999;92:524-5.

139. Misdraji J, Lauwers GY, Irving JA, Batts KP, Young RH. Appendiceal or cecal endometriosis with intestinal metaplasia: a potential mimic of appendiceal mucinous neoplasms. Am J Surg Pathol 2014;38:698-705.

140. Kim J, Russell P, Arendse M, Lim C, Kedziora A. Endometriosis in appendix and adjacent caecum with intestinal gland differentiation. Pathology 2013;45:513-6.

141. Cajigas A, Axiotis CA. Endosalpingiosis of the vermiform appendix. Int J Gynecol Pathol 1990;9:291-5.

142. McCluggage WG, Clements WD. Endosalpingiosis of the colon and appendix. Histopathology 2001;39:645-6.

143. Corben AD, Nehhozina T, Garg K, Vallejo CE, Brogi E. Endosalpingiosis in axillary lymph nodes: a possible pitfall in the staging of patients with breast carcinoma. Am J Surg Pathol 2010;34:1211-6.

144. Chai D, Wijesuriya R. Deciduosis of the appendix: diagnostic dilemma continues despite MRI evidence. Ann R Coll Surg Engl 2016;98:e200-2.

145. Suster S, Moran CA. Deciduosis of the appendix. Am J Gastroenterol 1990;85:841-5.

146. Bellizzi AM, Rock J, Marsh WL, Frankel WL. Serrated lesions of the appendix: a morphologic and immunohistochemical appraisal. Am J Clin Pathol 2010;133:623-32.

147. Yantiss RK, Panczykowski A, Misdraji J, et al. A comprehensive study of nondysplastic and dysplastic serrated polyps of the vermiform appendix. Am J Surg Pathol 2007;31:1742-53.

148. Choi CI, Kim DH, Jeon TY, Kim DH, Shin NR, Park DY. Solitary Peutz-Jeghers-type appendiceal hamartomatous polyp growing into the terminal ileum. World J Gastroenterol 2014;20:4822-6.

149. Kaneko M, Nozawa H, Kitayama J, et al. A case of hereditary hemorrhagic telangiectasia (Osler-Weber-Rendu disease) with multiple polyps arising in the cecum and appendix. Acta Gastroenterol Belg 2011;74:352-4.

8 DISEASES OF THE ANUS

CONGENITAL AND ACQUIRED STRUCTURAL ANOMALIES

Anorectal Malformations

Definition. *Persistent cloaca* occurs when the rectum, vagina, and urinary tract form a single channel. *Atresia* is the lack of continuity between the large intestine and anus in combination with an absent anal opening on the skin surface. A *fistula* is an aberrant communication between the distal rectum and the urogenital tract, scrotum, or vagina.

Clinical Features. Anorectal malformations occur in approximately 1/5,000 births, and show an equal predilection for boys and girls. Risk has been linked to maternal obesity and heavy smoking, although familial clustering in some cases suggests a heritable component (1,2). Most malformations are accompanied by an imperforate anus, which is generally evident upon physical examination. Patients who are not treated immediately after birth develop intestinal obstruction after feedings followed by progressive abdominal distention and vomiting of fecal material. Contrast-enhanced pelvic imaging and ultrasound facilitate delineation of the anatomy and identify fistulous tracts between the gastrointestinal tract and other organs (3).

Anorectal malformations are often accompanied by other congenital anomalies, including the VACTERL (vertebral anomalies, anal atresia, cardiovascular anomalies, tracheoesophageal fistula, esophageal atresia, renal and/or radial anomalies, limb defects) syndrome, trisomies 18 and 21, caudal regression syndrome, and *HLXB9* mutations. Anorectal malformations are classified in three groups: persistent cloaca, low lesions, and high lesions depending on the presence of fistulae and associated abnormalities of the urogenital tract.

Pathogenesis. The urorectal septum divides the cloaca into ventral urogenital and dorsal hindgut cavities by the 10th week of gestation. The cloacal membrane covers the end of the dorsal hindgut until the end of the 7th gestational week, when it ruptures to create continuity between the endoderm of the hindgut and the ectoderm of the proctodeum. Squamous epithelium extends caudally from the proctodeum, ultimately transitioning to the glandular epithelium of the lower gastrointestinal tract. Thus, the upper anus is derived from the endoderm and the distal anus develops from the ectoderm. Developmental abnormalities reflect deviations from this sequence of events and defective formation of the urorectal septum.

Gross and Microscopic Findings. The rectum, lower urinary tract, and vagina are fused to form a single lumen in individuals with persistent cloaca. Patients with low lesions have an imperforate anus with stenosis in close proximity to a blind-ended rectal pouch (fig. 8-1A,B). High lesions occur in the pelvis and usually feature a fistula between the rectum and bladder, urethra, or vagina, in addition to imperforate anus (fig. 8-1C,D). Resected anorectal malformations contain all the elements of the rectal wall at their proximal end, and show variable amounts of fibrosis and inflammation distally. The mucosa may be ulcerated or inflamed; mural fibrosis causes disruption of the muscularis propria (4).

Treatment and Prognosis. Surgical correction of anal atresia with creation of a hole in the anal skin overlying the sphincter is the only treatment option. Atresias accompanied by fistulae to other organs are managed with temporary colostomy followed by the creation of an anal orifice. Unfortunately, many patients continue to have continence issues or constipation (5).

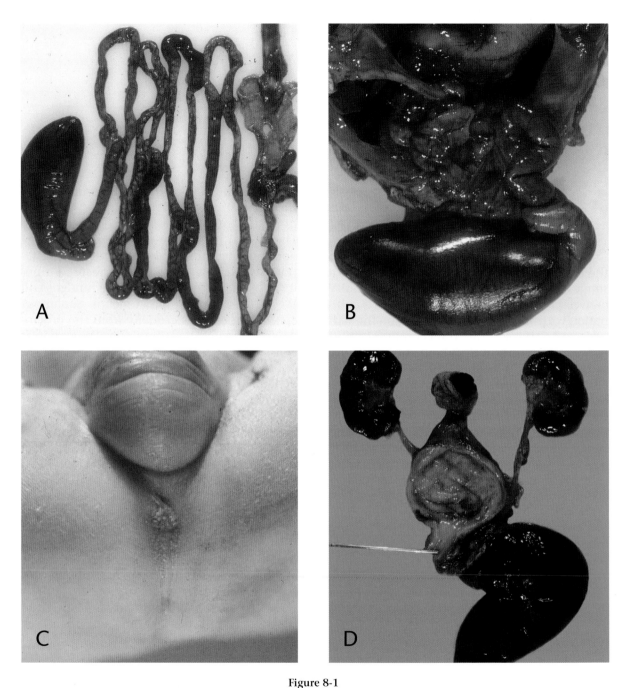

Figure 8-1

ANORECTAL MALFORMATIONS

A stillborn infant with multiple congenital anomalies also had rectal atresia (A); the rectum ends in a dilated blind pouch (B). An imperforate anus features a pucker, but no opening, in the skin overlying the anal sphincter (C). This abnormality is associated with a rectovaginal fistula (D). (Courtesy of Dr. D. Beneck, New York, NY.)

Tailgut Cyst

Definition. *Tailgut cyst* is a post-natal remnant of the hindgut located in the presacral space. Synonyms include *retrorectal cystic hamartoma, cyst of postanal intestine, enterogenous cyst, myoepithelial hamartoma of rectum,* and *retrorectal cyst.*

Clinical Features. Tailgut cysts are rare congenital malformations with an estimated incidence of 1/40,000 (6–8). There is a strong female predominance, with a female to male ratio of 5 to 1 (6). Most tailgut cysts are asymptomatic; those that come to clinical attention are usually detected in adults between 30 and 60 years of age. Symptoms include rectal bleeding, discomfort while sitting, difficulty in urination or defecation, and sciatica due to compression of adjacent structures (6,7). Occasional cysts prolapse through the anus. They also become infected, in which case they simulate the clinical features of perirectal abscesses.

Digital rectal exam may reveal a non-tender, extrinsic mass compressing the rectum, although it often fails to detect small lesions with low fluid tension (6). Low abdominal and pelvic imaging are critical to establishing a diagnosis (8).

Pathogenesis. The hindgut extends into an embryonic tail during the 4th week of gestation. This tailgut segment is located caudal to the site of the future anus. It normally disappears by the 8th week of gestation. Incomplete regression presumably gives rise to tailgut cysts (6,7).

Gross Findings. Tailgut cysts range from 2 to 12 cm in diameter. The cystic cavity is well circumscribed and may be unilocular or multiloculated. Cysts are usually surrounded by a dense fibrous rind adherent to adjacent soft tissue and skeletal muscle (2). Most contain clear yellow or green, slightly viscous fluid, although some are filled with thick brown, pasty material. The cyst lining may be erythematous or denuded (fig. 8-2).

Microscopic Findings. The cyst wall is mostly fibrous. It contains circumferentially arranged aggregates of smooth muscle cells of the muscularis propria, but they are often disrupted by fibrosis and attenuated in many areas (fig. 8-3A). The epithelium consists of multiple cell types, including stratified squamous, cuboidal, transitional, and columnar cells (fig. 8-3B,C). Columnar cells may be ciliated or mucinous; the latter have a gastric or goblet cell phenotype. Cysts can be denuded with abundant inflammation, fibrosis, and cholesterol clefts (fig. 8-3D).

Differential Diagnosis. Other cystic lesions that are unrelated to the gastrointestinal tract occur in the presacral space; these entities should be considered in the differential diagnosis of tailgut cysts. Epidermoid cysts tend to be unilocular and

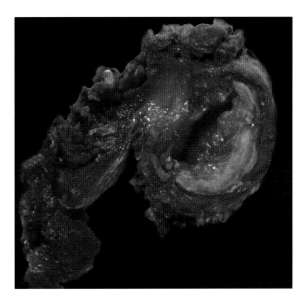

Figure 8-2

TAILGUT CYST

The cystic cavity has an erythematous lining and is surrounded by a dense fibrotic wall that blends imperceptibly with surrounding soft tissues.

are lined by stratified squamous epithelium; they lack skin appendages and smooth muscle cells (9). Dermoid cysts resemble epidermoid cysts but contain dermal appendages. Rectal duplication cysts are unilocular lesions with a well-developed muscularis propria and colonic-type epithelium. Distinction between tailgut cysts and teratomas rests on the detection of all three germ layers in the latter (10).

Treatment and Prognosis. Uncomplicated tailgut cysts are cured by excision. Rarely, well-differentiated endocrine tumors (i.e., carcinoid tumors) and intestinal-type adenocarcinomas develop in these lesions and, thus, complete excision is recommended whenever tailgut cysts are detected (7).

Ectopic Tissues

Definition. *Ectopic tissue* is histologically normal tissue in an abnormal location. The term derives from the Greek, meaning "other place." Synonyms include *heterotopia* and *choristoma*.

Clinical Features. Several types of heterotopia have been described in the anal and perianal region, all of which are uncommon. Clinical manifestations are similar regardless of histologic subtype. Most patients are asymptomatic. Those

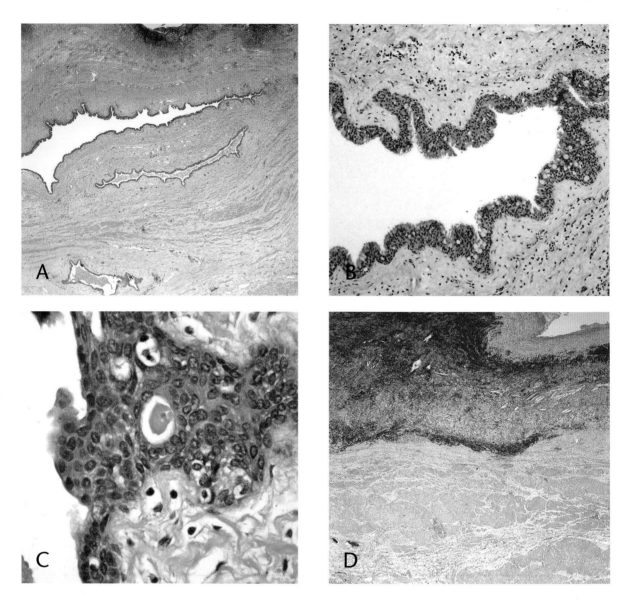

Figure 8-3

TAILGUT CYST

The cyst lining is surrounded by abundant fibrous tissue and attenuated bundles of smooth muscle cells (A). It contains a mixed population of transitional and intestinal-type epithelium with scattered goblet cells (B). Squamoid cells are present in association with short columnar epithelium (C). Inflamed cysts contain hemorrhagic contents with abundant inflammation and cholesterol clefts (D).

who come to clinical attention usually have gastric heterotopias that cause pain, itching, and bleeding related to local irritation (11–13). Anal polyps may also be detected by the patient or identified at the time of clinical examination.

Gross Findings. Ectopic tissues typically produce small sessile polyps that simulate fibroepithelial polyps. Irritated ectopic rests and those composed of acid-producing gastric mucosa can ulcerate (11,13,14).

Microscopic Findings. Anogenital mammary-like glands have been considered to represent ectopic elements, but they are detected frequently enough that some authors consider them to represent a normal finding in the anogenital region (15). They contain lobules of variably

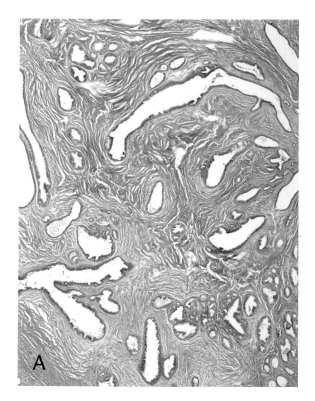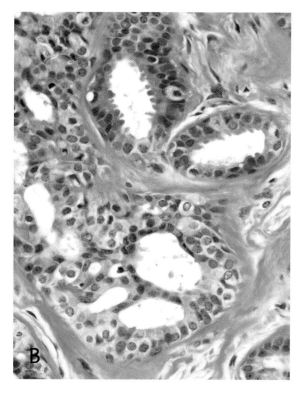

Figure 8-4

MAMMARY-TYPE GLANDS

Irregularly distributed, slightly ectatic ducts are associated with sclerotic stroma (A). Glands are arranged in lobules and contain a dual population of luminal cuboidal to columnar cells and myoepithelial cells (B).

dilated glands lined by cuboidal or columnar cells accompanied by myoepithelial cells (fig. 8-4). Apocrine metaplasia is frequently present and the surrounding stroma may be hyalinized.

Gastric and prostatic tissues are also detected in the anal mucosa. Gastric heterotopias are typically composed of clustered oxyntic glands surfaced by foveolar-type epithelium (fig. 8-5) (12,16). Prostatic glands are arranged in rounded aggregates and contain a dual population of luminal secretory cells and basaloid cells (14).

Treatment and Prognosis. Symptomatic heterotopic tissue is generally excised. Complete resection is associated with a resolution of symptoms and excellent prognosis.

Hemorrhoids

Definition. *Hemorrhoids* are enlarged, downwardly displaced anal cushions containing vascular plexuses.

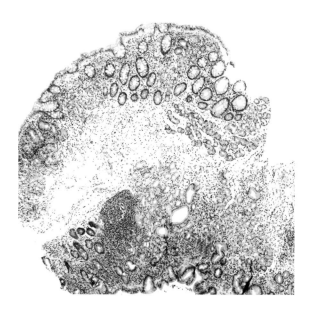

Figure 8-5

ECTOPIC GASTRIC MUCOSA IN ANORECTUM

Tightly packed aggregates of gastric glands are present in association with colonic glands.

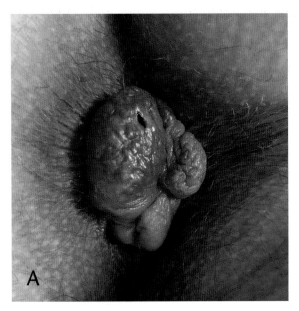
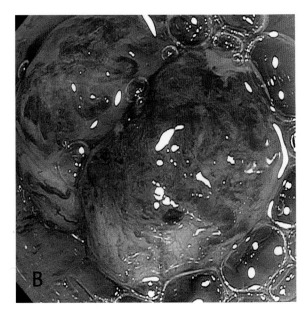

Figure 8-6

HEMORRHOIDS

A large external hemorrhoid presents as a polypoid, skin-covered lesion at the anal canal. The areas of blue discoloration represent the engorged veins (A). Internal hemorrhoids are bulging, erythematous polyps in the upper anus (B). (Courtesy of Dr. K. Garrett, New York, NY.)

Clinical Features. Hemorrhoids affect at least 5 percent of the general population, although the precise prevalence is unknown. Many patients are asymptomatic or treat themselves without seeking medical attention, and others attribute unrelated anorectal symptoms to hemorrhoids (17–19). Hemorrhoids occur with equal frequency in men and women. They most commonly affect patients 45 to 65 years of age and are rare before age 20 (17).

Typical symptoms include hematochezia, itching, and prolapse with straining (18). Bleeding is typically associated with defecation. Pain rarely occurs in patients with uncomplicated hemorrhoids; it usually signals thrombosis of an external hemorrhoid (17).

Pathogenesis. The mechanisms by which hemorrhoids develop remain poorly understood. The most popular theory is that age-related deterioration of connective tissues within the anal cushions facilitates their downward displacement; increased intravascular pressure leads to venous dilatation. Any condition that promotes increased pressure within the vascular plexus can contribute to hemorrhoid formation (19). Although constipation, hard stools, and low-fiber diet have been implicated in their pathogenesis, recent data do not support the notion that these factors play an important role in hemorrhoid development (17,18,20). Pregnancy is a risk factor for hemorrhoids, but the condition usually resolves or improves after delivery (17).

Gross Findings. External hemorrhoids are derived from the external/inferior hemorrhoidal plexus below the dentate line and are covered by skin or squamous mucosa. They appear as polypoid, skin-covered lesions with a blue tint, reflecting engorged veins (fig. 8-6, left) (16). Internal hemorrhoids are derived from the superior hemorrhoidal plexus above the dentate line; they are surfaced by rectal or transitional mucosa and contain protruding, dilated vessels (fig. 8-6, right).

Microscopic Findings. Dilated, engorged veins expand the submucosa (fig. 8-7). Thrombi that display various degrees of organization are often present, especially in external lesions (fig. 8-8). The vessel walls may be thick or thin. Inflammatory changes, surface ulceration, and features of mucosal prolapse are frequent findings (fig. 8-9). Occasional hemorrhoid excision specimens display

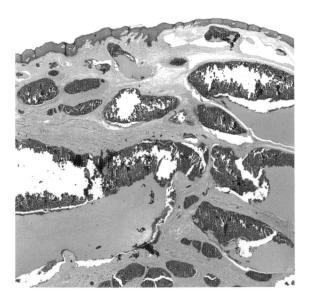

Figure 8-7

HEMORRHOIDS

Multiple dilated thin-walled veins expand the submucosa.

evidence of infection, squamous neoplasia, or melanocytic neoplasms (21–24).

Differential Diagnosis. Anal melanoma can simulate the clinical appearance of a thrombosed hemorrhoid because it typically presents as a dark brown anal polyp in middle-aged or older patients (23). Mucosal prolapse polyps may be mistaken for hemorrhoids for similar reasons, but they lack the dilated vessels and fibromuscular stroma of a hemorrhoid. Skin tags lack dilated vessels and fibromuscular stroma as well.

Treatment and Prognosis. Some patients are effectively treated with dietary modification and topical analgesics or anti-inflammatory drugs. Sclerotherapy, rubber band ligation, cryotherapy, radiofrequency ablation, and infrared coagulation represent non-surgical options. Surgical management is indicated when other interventions fail or lead to local complications (17–20).

Fissures

Definition. *Fissures* are linear tears or disruptions of the mucosa.

Clinical Features. Patients complain of blood-streaked stools and pain with defecation. Parents with young children who have fissures often report that their children cry with defecation. These lesions may be associated with hypertrophic anal papillae.

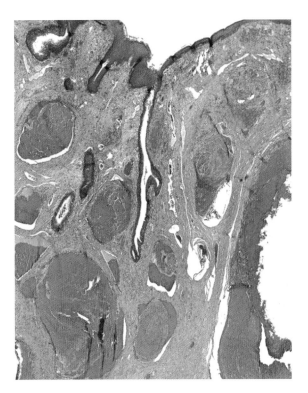

Figure 8-8

HEMORRHOIDS

An external hemorrhoid contains multiple thrombi, some with recanalization.

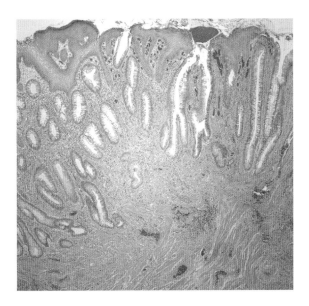

Figure 8-9

HEMORRHOIDS

A large internal hemorrhoid shows features of mucosal prolapse. Bundles of smooth muscle cells emanate from the muscularis mucosae into the lamina propria.

449

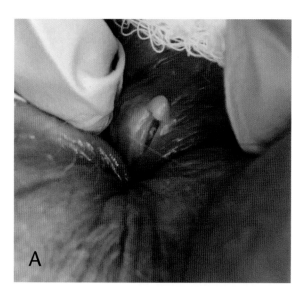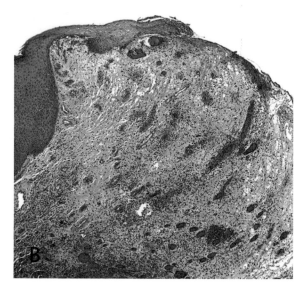

Figure 8-10

ANAL FISSURE

A linear tear in the mucosa is present in the posterior midline. The lesion has a clean base and erythematous edges (A). The histologic features are nonspecific; ulcerated, reactive squamous epithelium overlies inflammation and granulation tissue (B). (A: courtesy of Dr. K. Garrett, New York, NY.)

Pathogenesis. Many conditions contribute to the formation of anal fissures, including constipation and trauma from passing hard stools, chronic diarrhea, childbirth or other perineal injury, and stress-related clenching of sphincters (25,26). Patients with fissures have increased resting anal pressure compared with controls, which may contribute to diminished mucosal perfusion (26).

Gross Findings. Fissures are mucosal disruptions in the distal anal canal overlying the internal sphincter muscle (fig. 8-10A). Most are located in the posterior midline where the anal sphincter bifurcates to encircle the rectum; only 10 to 15 percent occur in the anterior midline. Lesions that do not develop in the midline may be multifocal or reflect an underlying condition, as described below.

Microscopic Findings. The histologic features of anal fissures are non-specific. Acute and chronic inflammation are accompanied by ulcers, granulation tissue, fibrosis, and reactive epithelial changes (fig. 8-10B). Persistent lesions are associated with dense fibrosis, hyperplasia, hyperkeratosis, and parakeratosis of the adjacent squamous epithelium.

Differential Diagnosis. Non-healing, painless fissures should be evaluated for underlying pathology, such as Crohn disease, neoplasia, or infection, especially when they are multifocal or occur away from the midline (26). Non-necrotic granulomas and lymphoid aggregates suggest Crohn disease (25,26).

Treatment and Prognosis. Nonsurgical treatment options include stool softeners, topical analgesics, botulinum injections, and drugs directed at decreasing sphincter tone (26). Persistent symptoms may be surgically managed with sphincterotomy, although this option is typically avoided in children due to risk of injury to the sphincters, and may also result in incontinence in adult patients. Inadequately treated anal fissures pursue a chronic course of intermittent exacerbation over many years.

Fistulae

Definition. *Fistulae* (*fistula-in-ano*) are inflammatory tracts that communicate between the lumen of the anal canal and skin, perianal soft tissues, or musculature.

Clinical Features. Most anal fistulae result from trauma or infection (27). They also develop in patients with radiation treatment, neoplasia, and Crohn disease (28–30). The main presenting symptom is intermittent or continuous discharge, which may be bloody, watery, or

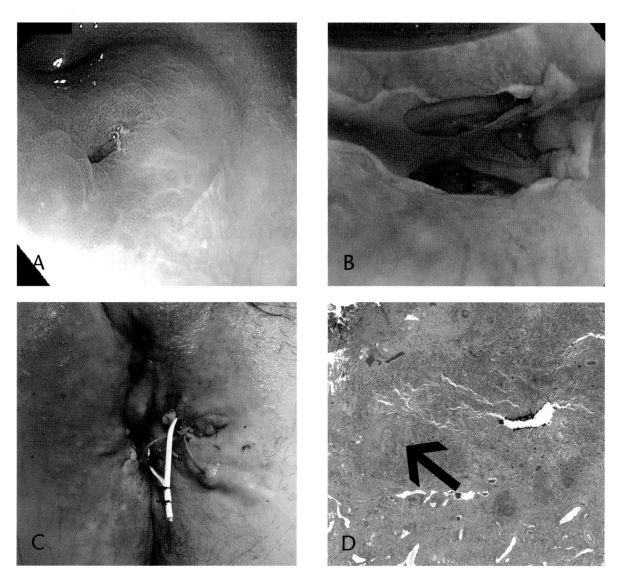

Figure 8-11

ANAL FISTULAE

The opening of an anal fistula is surrounded by mildly edematous and erythematous mucosa (A). Multiple internal openings are surrounded by purulent material in a patient with Crohn disease (B). A patient with Crohn disease has multiple fistulae around the anus. Setons facilitate drainage and healing (C). A fistulous tract is lined by granulation tissue and squamous epithelium (arrow); it is surrounded by marked acute and chronic inflammation (D). (C: courtesy of Dr. K. Garrett, New York, NY.)

purulent. Fistulae are often painful and can be complicated by superimposed infection (31).

Gross Findings. The external opening of the fistula often extrudes pus and is surrounded by raised erythematous skin. The internal opening is usually surrounded by edematous or erythematous mucosa that may be accompanied by purulent exudates (fig. 8-11A,B). Both the internal and external openings become increasingly fibrotic

over time, and the entire fistulous tract may be so scarred that it forms a palpable cord. Fistulous tracts can be simple or display extremely complex anatomy, with multiple communications between the anus and skin (fig. 8-11C). Crohn disease-related fistulae are often complex and painless, with irregular edges and little induration.

Microscopic Findings. Fistulous tracts are lined by granulation tissue with variable

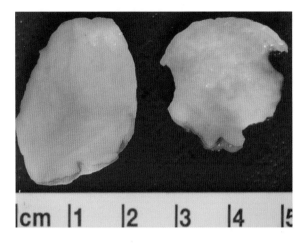

Figure 8-12

FIBROEPITHELIAL POLYP

The cut surface is fibrous, homogeneous, and covered by squamous epithelium.

amounts of acute and chronic inflammation (fig. 8-11D). The epithelium at both openings is often hyperplastic, with mild reactive cellular changes; epithelium may grow into either end of the fistulous tract and completely surface the fistula. A foreign body giant cell reaction to luminal material is often present in association with organizing abscesses and fibrosis. This type of poorly formed granulomatous inflammation is a non-specific finding and should not be confused with the non-necrotic granulomas occasionally present in Crohn disease-related fistulae.

Treatment and Prognosis. Small fistulae often heal with a combination of supportive care and antibiotic therapy, and those related to Crohn disease resolve following treatment with tumor necrosis factor-alpha (TNF-α) inhibitors. However, many patients with complicated or large fistulae require surgery. Operative approaches optimize healing of the fistula and recurrence prevention with preservation of continence (27,31,32). Patients with fistulizing Crohn disease have a small but definite risk for developing either squamous cell carcinoma or adenocarcinoma in the fistula tract (33).

POLYPS OF THE ANUS

Fibroepithelial Polyp

Definition. *Fibroepithelial polyp* is a benign polypoid lesion composed of fibrovascular tissue and squamous epithelium. Synonyms include *hypertrophic anal papilla* and *anal tag.*

Clinical Features. Anal fibroepithelial polyps are similar to their cutaneous counterparts. Many patients are asymptomatic, although some lesions grow large enough to cause a mass sensation or prolapse (34). Itching is a common complaint and bleeding occurs occasionally.

Pathogenesis. Anal papillae enlarge as a result of inflammation, edema, or fibrosis. Intermittently increased luminal pressure promotes their elongation within the anal canal, and may cause them to prolapse outside the anus. Fibroepithelial polyps are associated with chronic anal ulcers and fissures (34).

Gross Findings. Fibroepithelial polyps of the anal canal are located at the dentate line. Most measure 0.5 to 1.5 cm, although some are up to 4 cm (35). The cut surface is firm, homogeneous, and tan-white (fig. 8-12).

Microscopic Findings. These benign lesions are covered by squamous epithelium that displays mild hyperplasia, with parakeratosis or hyperkeratosis (35). The stroma is paucicellular, with a loose and fibrillary appearance in most cases; older lesions contain dense hyalinized collagen (fig. 8-13A) (35,36). Scattered spindled or stellate stromal cells with large, often multiple, nuclei are usually present (fig. 8-13B). These atypical cells are CD34 positive and likely represent activated fibroblasts (37).

Differential Diagnosis. Fibroepithelial polyps simulate the clinical features of hemorrhoids, but they lack the dilated vessels, hemorrhage, and thrombosis typical of the latter. Their pink-white color and location on the distal side of the dentate line should facilitate distinction from adenomatous polyps (34).

Treatment and Prognosis. Symptomatic fibroepithelial polyps are excised and generally do not recur. Associated fissures and ulcers are managed as previously described.

Inflammatory Cloacogenic Polyp

Definition. *Inflammatory cloacogenic polyp*, also termed *mucosal prolapse polyp*, results from anal mucosal prolapse.

Clinical Features. Inflammatory cloacogenic polyps are the most distal form of mucosal prolapse polyp (38–40). Most patients present with minor anorectal bleeding, passage of mucus, or tenesmus,

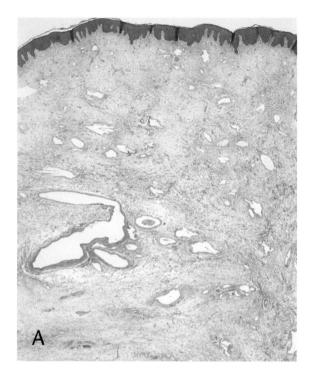
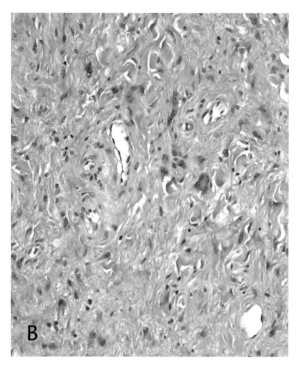

Figure 8-13

FIBROEPITHELIAL POLYP

The polyp contains paucicellular fibrous stroma and prominent thin-walled vessels (A). Scattered stellate and multinucleated stromal cells are present in dense collagenous stroma (B).

and often complain of straining to defecate (41). Lesions occur in both adults and children.

Pathogenesis. Mucosal prolapse is associated with impaired relaxation of the pelvic musculature (41). Increased resting tone and intermittent straining lead to repetitive bouts of ischemic mucosal injury. Prolapse-type polyps also occur in patients with chronic idiopathic inflammatory bowel disease, diverticular disease, and adjacent to hemorrhoids.

Gross Findings. Inflammatory cloacogenic polyps are soft and friable at the surface, but contain a thick muscular base. They usually occur on the anterior wall of the anorectum and span 1 to 2 cm (fig. 8-14). Larger polyps range up to 5 cm (40). Polyps may be single or multiple, and are often associated with ulcers or mucosal erythema.

Microscopic Findings. Inflammatory cloacogenic polyps contain a combination of glandular colorectal-type mucosa, anal stratified squamous epithelium, and transitional epithelium, reflecting their location at the junction between

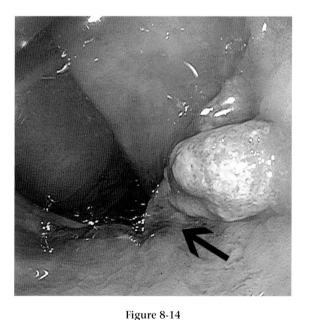

Figure 8-14

INFLAMMATORY CLOACOGENIC (PROLAPSE) POLYP

A large fibrotic prolapse polyp is present at the proximal edge of the squamous mucosa (arrow). Unlike hemorrhoids, there are no visible engorged vessels.

453

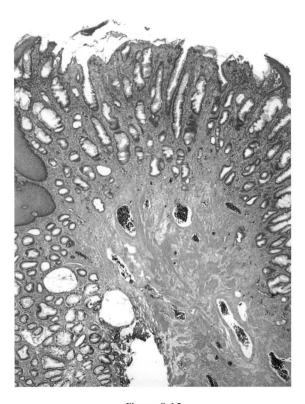

Figure 8-15

INFLAMMATORY CLOACOGENIC (PROLAPSE) POLYP

The polyp contains intestinal epithelium and squamous epithelium with central erosion.

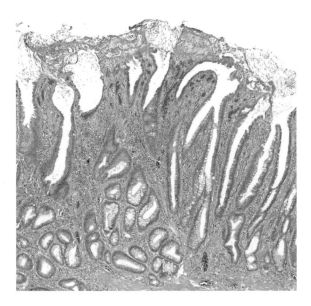

Figure 8-16

INFLAMMATORY CLOACOGENIC (PROLAPSE) POLYP

This polyp shows villiform glandular mucosa with adherent mucoid membranes overlying superficial erosions. Engorged capillaries in the lamina propria and perpendicular extension of the muscularis mucosae in the mucosa are seen.

squamous and colonic epithelium (fig. 8-15). Similar to other prolapse polyps, the muscularis mucosae is thick and disorganized, with aggregates of smooth muscle cells extending into the lamina propria in a perpendicular fashion. Additional features include stromal hyalinization with prominent capillaries; elongated, hyperplastic, and irregular crypts that occasionally extend into the submucosa; and surface erosions (39,40). The surface epithelium often has a striking villiform appearance with erosions and pseudomembranes at the surface (fig. 8-16) (39).

Differential Diagnosis. Mucosal prolapse polyps in the anus are often mistaken for hemorrhoids (39,40). Those that occur in children can be confused with hamartomatous polyps. Clues to the diagnosis include the presence of ischemic-type mucosal changes, crypt serration, fibromuscularization of the lamina propria, and confinement of polyps to the distal colorectum. The villiform appearance can mimic a villous adenoma, especially when accompanied by

regenerative cytologic atypia in crypt epithelium (41). Nevertheless, prolapse changes can complicate low rectal adenomas and, thus, lack of maturation and cytologic abnormalities at the polyp surface should not be dismissed simply because the muscularis mucosae is prominent or shows splaying in the lamina propria (42).

Treatment and Prognosis. Polypectomy is typically performed to establish the diagnosis and control bleeding symptoms. Recurrence is common (40,41).

Condyloma Acuminatum

Definition. *Condyloma acuminatum* is a human papillomavirus (HPV)-associated wart or polyp. Synonyms include *anogenital wart, low-grade squamous intraepithelial lesion,* and *anal intraepithelial neoplasia 1.*

Clinical Features. Condyloma acuminatum is derived from the Greek "kondyloma," meaning "knuckle" or "knob" and Latin "acuminatum," meaning "pointed" or "tapered." It is the most common and well-recognized HPV-associated lesion (43). The incidence of condyloma acuminatum is rising, particularly among homosexual men who practice anal receptive intercourse or are human immunodeficiency virus (HIV) positive (44,45). The disease, however, still shows a slight female predominance, reflecting the increased risk for anal involvement among patients with HPV-related disease of the vagina and cervix (46).

Patients typically present with anal bleeding or discharge, pain, and itching. Screening programs for high-risk populations use high-resolution anoscopy in combination with anal Pap smear (47). As in the cervix, acetic acid can be applied to highlight the lesions (48).

The terminology for HPV-associated anal lesions is confusing and non-standardized because many diagnostic terms used in cervical and cutaneous pathology have been inconsistently applied to the anal mucosae. The College of American Pathologists (CAP) and the American Society for Colposcopy and Cervical Pathology (ASCCP) recommend uniform terminology for anogenital squamous lesions (49,50). Participants in the Lower Anogenital Squamous Terminology (LAST) project classify anal squamous dysplasia with a two-tiered system: low-grade (LSIL) and high-grade intraepithelial (HSIL) dysplasia, although anal intraepithelial neoplasia (AIN) and perianal intraepithelial neoplasia (PAIN) persist in the LAST nomenclature (49). The former is reserved for squamous lesions within the anal canal and the latter refers to lesions of the perianal skin that are located within 5 cm of the anal verge. Current criteria equate koilocytic atypia of condylomata acuminata and mild dysplasia (i.e., AIN1) to LSIL, whereas HSIL encompasses both moderate and severe dysplasia (i.e., AIN2 and AIN3). Anal squamous lesions that are classified as LSIL and HSIL can be further described using the PAIN or AIN grades to facilitate clinical communication (e.g., HSIL [AIN3]).

Pathogenesis. Most condylomata acuminata are associated with HPV genotypes 6 and 11, which have a lower risk of progression to malignancy than high-risk genotypes. Lesions with high-grade dysplasia are usually associated with HPV genotypes 16 and 18 (51,52). It is important to recognize, however, that some low-grade lesions can harbor high-risk HPV genotypes, and low-risk genotypes are detected in occasional high-grade lesions (46). Some patients, especially those with HIV infection, may be infected by multiple HPV genotypes (51). Immunosuppressed patients with multifocal disease appear to be at the highest risk of progression.

Gross Findings. Condylomata can be single or multiple, and typically appear as fleshy, pink-white papillary or "cauliflower-like" masses (fig. 8-17A). They often occur in clusters, and may cover large areas of skin or mucosa. Squamous lesions in the anal canal are white, pigmented, or erythematous papules and plaques; they are often multicentric (fig. 8-17B) (48).

Microscopic Findings. Condylomata have a cauliflower-like polypoid appearance that reflects a proliferation of mature-appearing squamous epithelium supported by lamina propria (fig. 8-18A). The surface epithelium is expanded, with irregular peaks topped by layers of compact parakeratosis (fig. 8-18B). Supporting lamina propria contains multiple, slightly dilated vessels (fig. 8-18C). Viral infection usually induces koilocytic change in mature keratinocytes, although this feature can be inconspicuous in some cases. Koilocytes display wrinkled nuclear contours, lending a "raisinoid" appearance, as well as sharply demarcated perinuclear clearing of cytoplasm, which produces a halo (fig. 8-18D). Binucleation is a common feature and scattered dyskeratotic keratinocytes are common features. Morphologic changes of HPV infection can occur within the context of a condyloma or flat mucosa.

Low-grade neoplasia (i.e., LSIL, AIN1) is characterized by slightly disorganized and enlarged keratinocytes restricted to the basal third of the epithelium. High-grade neoplasia (i.e., HSIL, AIN2, and AIN3) displays more severe nuclear abnormalities in keratinocytes occupying at least two thirds of the mucosal thickness (fig. 8-19A,B) (49,50). Dysplastic cells show nuclear membrane irregularities, hyperchromasia, enlargement, and pleomorphism. Atypical parakeratosis and mitotic figures in the upper third of the mucosa are frequently present.

Both LSIL and HSIL show increased Ki-67 immunolabeling, with nuclear positivity in the upper two thirds of the epithelium (fig. 8-19C). High-risk HPV genotypes also upregulate p16 (a tumor suppressor gene product that is a surrogate marker of HPV infection), which drives cellular proliferation. As a result, HSIL typically shows

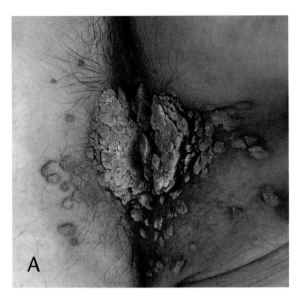
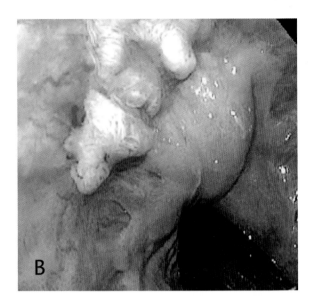

Figure 8-17

CONDYLOMA ACUMINATUM

Multiple raised white-gray, fleshy papillary and cauliflower-like lesions are at the anal orifice and on the perianal skin (A). A white, papillary mass is present at the anorectal junction (B). (A: courtesy of Dr. K. Garrett, New York, NY.)

diffuse, block-like nuclear and cytoplasmic p16 staining, whereas LSIL and non-neoplastic conditions are negative for this marker or show patchy staining (fig. 8-19D) (53–55).

Differential Diagnosis. Condyloma lata of syphilis, fibroepithelial polyps, nevi, and molluscum contagiosum share similar clinical features with those of condyloma acuminatum and, thus, biopsy should be performed to establish a diagnosis in all suspected cases (43,48). Several reactive and neoplastic conditions mimic the histologic features of condylomata acuminata and squamous intraepithelial neoplasia. Glycogenated squamous cells can simulate koilocytes, although they generally lack a sharp perinuclear halo and contain small nuclei with evenly dispersed chromatin. Inflamed squamous mucosa and skin often display reactive nuclear atypia and increased mitotic activity; a diagnosis of low-grade dysplasia in the setting of an ulcer or abundant active inflammation should be carefully made.

The anal transition zone contains multilayered transitional epithelium that can feature enlarged, crowded nuclei. These changes resemble those of HSIL, particularly when superimposed reactive changes are present. Immunohisto-

chemical stains directed against Ki-67 and p16 are helpful in these situations.

Treatment and Prognosis. Condylomata acuminata without high-grade neoplasia can be managed with a number of topical agents that can be administered by the patient, including podophyllotoxin, Imiquimod, and sinecatechins. These agents obliterate the lesions but do not eliminate HPV and, thus, recurrence is common, ranging from 6 to 69 percent depending on the agent used (56–58). Trichloroacetic acid is a potent topical agent that must be administered by a health care provider; it is highly effective at eliminating lesions, but more than 30 percent of patients develop recurrent disease (56,57). Other nonsurgical options include cryotherapy, electrocautery, laser ablation, and radiofrequency ablation. These treatments offer minimal morbidity but recurrence rates range from 25 to 90 percent depending on HIV status. Surgical curettage and excision are also associated with significant recurrence rates (56). Patients with anal LSIL progress to HSIL at a rate of 12 to 24 percent over 1 to 3 years, and the risk is higher among HIV-positive patients (58). Early data suggest that the HPV vaccine effectively prevents anogenital warts (57).

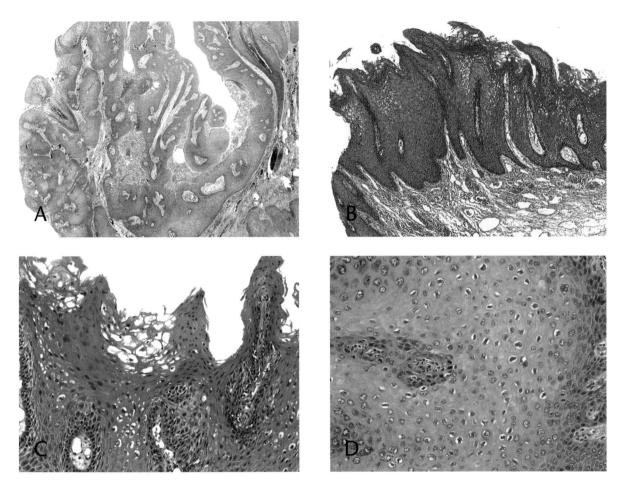

Figure 8-18

CONDYLOMA ACUMINATUM

An excised condyloma shows markedly thickened squamous epithelium with abundant parakeratosis and hyperkeratosis, typical of condyloma acuminatum (A). The surface epithelium displays undulating peaks of epithelium surfaced by parakeratosis (B). Thick, compact layers of parakeratosis and prominent thin-walled vessels in the superficial lamina propria are characteristic (C). Koilocytes are characterized by wrinkled or "raisinoid" nuclear contours, sharply demarcated perinuclear halos, and binucleation (D).

INFLAMMATORY DISEASES OF THE ANUS

Herpes Simplex Virus

Definition. Herpes simplex infection is caused by herpes simplex virus (HSV)1 or HSV2.

Clinical Features. HSV is a member of the Herpesviridae family, which includes varicella zoster virus, cytomegalovirus, Epstein-Barr virus, and human herpesviruses types 6 and 8. Most anorectal isolates are type HSV2, but HSV1 can cause identical disease (59). Genital HSV remains one of the most common infections in HIV-positive persons. It is also common in immunocompromised patients who are at risk

for dissemination and life-threatening illness. Immunocompetent patients may develop infection, although it is generally self-limited. Transmission occurs through anal intercourse or oral and anal contact; risk is increased in patients with multiple partners who engage in high-risk sexual behavior (59).

Presenting symptoms include severe anorectal pain, tenesmus, constipation, mucopurulent discharge, hematochezia, and fever; occasional patients are asymptomatic. Concomitant neurologic symptoms, such as difficulty in urination, impotence, and paresthesias of the buttocks and upper thigh, are common, as are

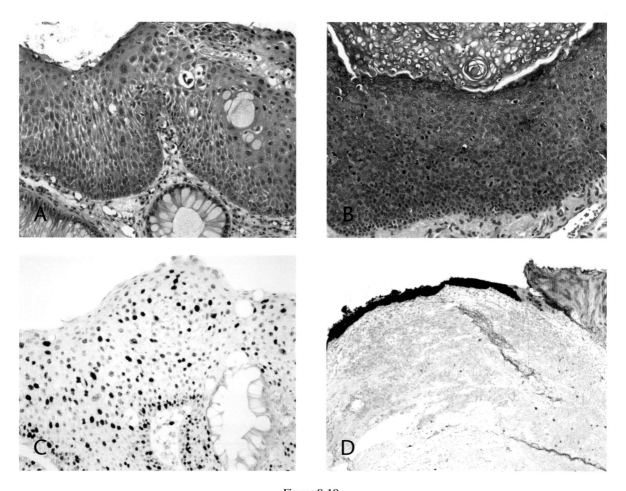

Figure 8-19

ANAL SQUAMOUS INTRAEPITHELIAL LESIONS

This condyloma with low-grade dysplasia (LSIL) contains slightly disorganized keratinocytes with enlarged nuclei near the basement membrane (A). Another lesion with high-grade dysplasia (HSIL) displays full-thickness dysmaturation with numerous mitotic figures (B). Immunolabeling with Ki-67 is present at all levels in the mucosa of a low-grade lesion (C). A p16 immunostain demonstrates intense, full-thickness "block" positivity in the high-grade lesion on the left and weak patchy staining in the low-grade focus on the right (D).

inguinal lymphadenopathy and fever (59,60). Serologic studies can facilitate a diagnosis when antibody titers are very high or rising, but are of limited clinical use because latent infections can persist for years. More recent type-specific (HSV1 and HSV2) antibodies can aid distinction between reactivated and newly acquired HSV infection in some circumstances (61).

Pathogenesis. Herpes simplex viruses reside in dorsal ganglia after primary infection. They travel along sensory neurons to replicate in target tissues when reactivated (62). The virus is shed in secretions from infected individuals and transmitted via contact with mucous membranes.

Gross Findings. Primary infection of the perianal skin and anal canal can extend proximally into the rectum. Herpetic vesicles, pustules, or ulcers are often present on the external surface (fig. 8-20). Chronic lesions can produce indurated, ulcerated masses that simulate neoplasia. Mucosal ulceration and friability may occur in some cases. Colitis proximal to the anorectum is extremely rare and limited to patients with underlying malignancy, immunodeficiency, or immunosuppression.

Microscopic Findings. The histologic features of HSV1 and HSV2 infection are essentially identical. Infection causes severe, inflammatory

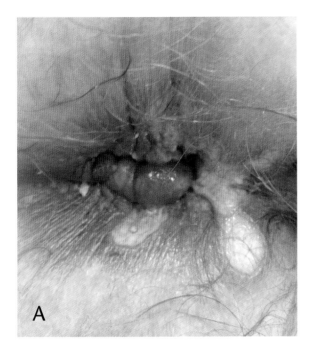 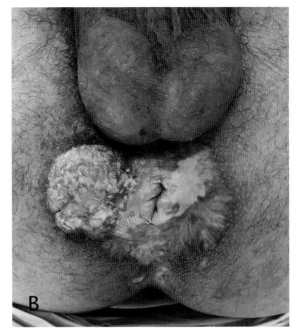

Figure 8-20

ANAL HERPES SIMPLEX VIRUS (HSV) INFECTION

A large anal ulcer is accompanied by peripheral vesicles. Multiple confluent, shallow ulcers are surfaced by a fibrinous exudate (A). An older lesion appears as a large ulcer with sharp borders and an indurated base (B). (Courtesy of Dr. K. Garrett, New York, NY.)

injury to the anorectal mucosa. Ulcers are accompanied by an exuberant neutrophil-rich infiltrate as well as an exudate containing sloughed squamous cells, cellular debris, and macrophages (fig. 8-21A) (60). The best place to search for viral inclusions is within the squamous epithelium at the edges of ulcers and in sloughed cells within the exudates. Two types of nuclear inclusions may be found: homogeneous "ground-glass" (i.e., Cowdry B) inclusions and less frequent acidophilic (i.e., Cowdry A) inclusions with a surrounding clear halo and marginated chromatin (fig. 8-21B). Infected cells can contain a single or multiple nuclei with inclusions. They have irregular nuclear contours and display nuclear molding.

Immunohistochemical stains for HSV1 and HSV2 are commercially available (fig. 8-22). Rectal swabs can be used for viral culture as well as serologic detection of antigen (61,62). Polymerase chain reaction (PCR) is increasingly used to establish a diagnosis.

Differential Diagnosis. The differential diagnosis includes cytomegalovirus (CMV), adenovirus, and varicella zoster virus (VZV), which also

rarely infects the gastrointestinal tract (63). The "owl's eye" inclusions of CMV are morphologically distinct from the "ground-glass" inclusions of HSV and are located in endothelial cells, stromal cells, and macrophages, rather than squamous epithelial cells (fig. 8-23). Varicella zoster virus (VZV) produces histologic lesions identical to those of HSV, but patients are often systemically ill with a rash, and VZV rarely causes lesions confined to the anogenital region (64). Molluscum contagiosum can affect the anogenital area and is recognized as a sexually transmitted infection. It produces one or more pearly white papules rather than an ulcer. The papules consist of inverted, hyperplastic squamous mucosa containing aggregates of infected cells that harbor characteristic molluscum bodies (fig. 8-24) (65). Immunohistochemical stains against viruses can be helpful in difficult cases.

Treatment and Prognosis. Anal HSV, similar to genital infection, is treated with acyclovir.

Syphilis

Definition. *Syphilis* is caused by the bacteria *Treponema pallidum.*

459

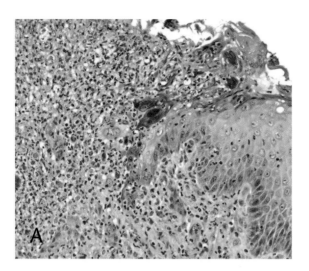 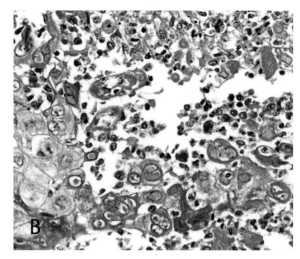

Figure 8-21

ANAL HERPES SIMPLEX VIRUS INFECTION

Typical lesions show superficial erosions, with an inflammatory infiltrate that contains neutrophils and macrophages. "Ground-glass" viral inclusions are easily seen within epithelial cells at the edge of the ulcer (A). Detached squamous cells contain "ground-glass inclusions" with marginated chromatin (B).

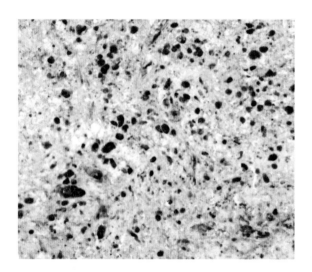 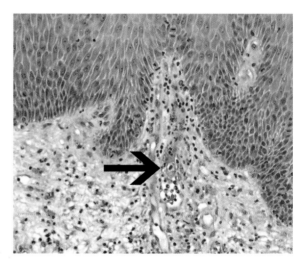

Figure 8-22

ANAL HERPES SIMPLEX VIRUS INFECTION

Immunohistochemistry demonstrates numerous HSV-infected cells in the inflammatory infiltrate.

Figure 8-23

ANAL CYTOMEGALOVIRUS (CMV) INFECTION

A large "owl's eye" CMV inclusion (arrow) is present within an endothelial cell at the edge of an anal ulcer in a patient receiving chemotherapy for leukemia.

Clinical Features. Gastrointestinal infection with *Treponema pallidum*, the causative agent of syphilis, commonly involves the anorectum. Infection can produce either proctitis of the distal rectum or anal lesions. Primary anal syphilis usually produces a chancre, whereas secondary syphilis presents with persistent chancre, rash, lymphadenopathy, fever, or condyloma lata (66).

The incidence of syphilis is increasing, especially in men who practice anal receptive intercourse. Homosexual males, particularly those who also have HIV infection, are at particularly high risk of infection. Many authorities believe that anorectal syphilis is underdiagnosed due to its variable clinical findings and low index of clinical

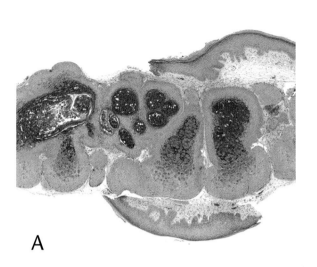
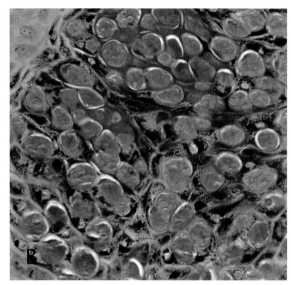

Figure 8-24

ANAL MOLLUSCUM CONTAGIOSUM

A characteristic papule is composed of inverted lobules of squamous epithelium with central collections of infected cells containing molluscum bodies (A). Multiple large eosinophilic inclusions are present in association with hypergranulosis (B).

suspicion. Infection can be spread through both unprotected anal sex and oral sex (67).

Condyloma lata are moist, wart-like lesions of the perianal skin and squamous mucosa (68).

The diagnosis often requires serologic studies because the organism cannot be easily cultured. Non-treponemal serologic tests, such as VDRL and RPR, measure levels of antibodies to substances (e.g., cardiolipin) that are produced in response to tissue damage (69). They can be used as screening tests for potential infection, as well for assessing disease activity. Treponemal serologic tests measure treponeme-specific antibodies. Although treponemal tests were historically used to confirm a nontreponemal positive result, many laboratories now use treponemal tests for screening purposes because they are automated, more specific, and subject to a lesser degree of variability with respect to interpretation.

Pathogenesis. *T. pallidum* is an obligate human pathogen that is transmitted sexually or from an infected mother to the fetus (70). Syphilis was recognized as a sexually transmitted disease as early as the sixteenth century, long before the bacteria was identified in 1905 (71). Clinical manifestations result from the host immune response to bacterial replication and subsequent tissue damage.

Primary syphilis features chancres on areas of sexual contact, often with concomitant adenopathy, that resolve without treatment. The secondary phase occurs 6 to 8 weeks later and features fever, rash, and other systemic manifestations. As the secondary phase subsides, patients enter a latent phase that can last several years. Although they are asymptomatic, patients with latent disease may still be infectious. Many untreated patients ultimately develop tertiary syphilis, which can cause severe cardiac, neurological, and visceral injury and destructive bony lesions (70).

Gross Findings. Patients with primary anorectal syphilis develop chancres and/or mild proctitis. The latter are indurated, annular lesions spanning up to 2 cm in diameter; they may be solitary or multiple and are variably tender (66,72,73). Signs of secondary syphilis typically present 6 to 8 weeks later, and include masses, mucocutaneous rash, and condyloma lata. These lesions are raised, moist, smooth warts that are often associated with itching, a foul odor, and inguinal adenopathy. Simultaneous features of both primary and secondary

461

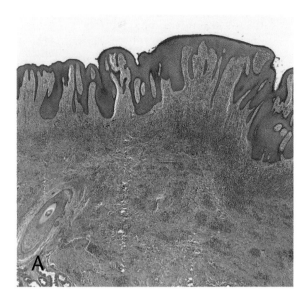
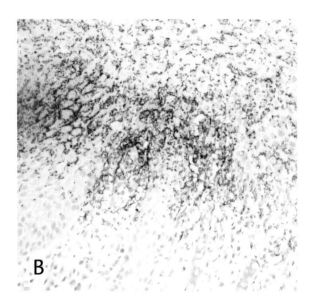

Figure 8-25

ANAL SYPHILIS

Condyloma lata feature hyperplastic squamous epithelium with a dense plasmacytic infiltrate at the base; perivascular inflammation extends into the deep dermis (A). Immunohistochemistry directed against treponemes demonstrates innumerable organisms within the squamous epithelium (B).

infection occasionally coexist. The mass lesions of secondary syphilis may mimic malignancy; surgical removal without a prior biopsy should be avoided (73).

Microscopic Findings. Condyloma lata feature hyperplastic squamous epithelium with a band-like plasma cell-rich infiltrate at the base of the lesion that extends along vessels and nerves into the deeper soft tissues (fig. 8-25A). Ulcers and neutrophilic inflammation are often present in the superficial epithelium (74).

Immunohistochemical stains directed against *T. pallidum* are commercially available and are much more sensitive than silver impregnation stains, such as Warthin-Starry, Steiner, and Dieterle (fig. 8-25B). Darkfield examination of anorectal discharge may show organisms, although they must be distinguished from spirochetes that comprise the normal gut flora as well as intestinal spirochetosis (75).

Differential Diagnosis. Chancres simulate the clinical features of anal fissures, fistulas, and traumatic lesions. The clinicopathologic features of syphilitic proctitis can mimic those of many other sexually transmitted proctocolitides (76). Condyloma lata simulates the gross appearance of condylomata acuminatum and squamous cell

carcinoma (73,74,76). However, both condyloma acuminata and squamous cell carcinomas tend to be more dry, papillary, and keratinized than condyloma lata (76). Condyloma lata also lack parakeratosis, koilocytosis, and cytologic features of dysplasia. They also display marked plasma cell-rich inflammation that is generally lacking in HPV-related disease and carcinomas. Immunohistochemistry, HPV testing, and serologic testing for syphilis can facilitate distinction between syphilitic lesions and condylomata acuminata in difficult cases.

Treatment and Prognosis. Syphilis is usually treated with penicillin injections followed by disease monitoring with nontreponemal serologic tests. Recurrent infections are common, particularly among men who practice anal receptive intercourse. The risk of recurrence is markedly increased in HIV-positive patients (77).

Lymphogranuloma Venereum

Definition. *Lymphogranuloma venereum* (LGV) is a sexually transmitted infection caused by *Chlamydia trachomatis*.

Clinical Features. *Chlamydia trachomatis* serotypes L1, L2, and L3 are responsible for LGV. The incidence of LGV has increased remarkably in industrialized countries during the past 15 years, particularly among men who practice anal receptive intercourse. Infection is often associated with HIV positivity and concomitant sexually transmitted infections (77,78). The anorectum is the most commonly affected gastrointestinal site.

Patients usually present with an ulcer at the inoculation site followed by lymphadenopathy, fever, bleeding, and anal pain, although not all findings are present in all patients (77). Patients with LGV proctitis present with mucoid or bloody discharge, anal pain, fever, tenesmus, and constipation (see also chapter 4).

Pathogenesis. Infection by *C. trachomatis* stimulates both the humoral and cell-mediated arms of the immune system, leading to T-cell activation and antibody formation. Chronic inflammation and tissue injury causes fibrosis and scarring if untreated. The organism may remain in epithelial cells for some time, causing persistent and recurrent infection. Infection is likely serotype specific, and patients infected by one serovar are vulnerable to infection with different serovars (79).

Gross Findings. Infected patients usually have visible ulcers accompanied by mucosal granularity, erythema, and friability (72,80). Inguinal lymphadenopathy is a common feature.

Microscopic Findings. The typical inflammatory pattern is that of a dense lymphohistiocytic infiltrate with prominent plasma cells. Some cases display neuromatous hyperplasia, deep lymphoid aggregates, extensive submucosal fibrosis, and occasional granulomas (81). Active neutrophilic inflammation, crypt architectural distortion, and Paneth cell metaplasia may be present in colonic samples, but are not conspicuous.

There is no histochemical method for detecting the organism and, thus, ancillary tests are required to establish a diagnosis. Serologic testing from a rectal swab or lymph node aspirate is the gold standard for diagnosis. This method detects the organism and also aids in distinguishing LGV *C. trachomatis* infection from infection by other serovars that are treated differently (77).

Differential Diagnosis. Histologic features of LGV are indistinguishable from those of syphilitic proctitis; distinction relies on immunohistochemistry for spirochetes and results of serologic tests. The disease also causes inflammatory changes that are easily confused with those of

chronic idiopathic inflammatory bowel disease (83). In contrast to Crohn disease and ulcerative colitis, however, cases of LGV typically display only mild to moderate acute inflammation and well-developed changes of mucosal remodeling, such as basal plasmacytosis, architectural distortion, and Paneth cell metaplasia, are less prominent than are typically seen in untreated chronic idiopathic inflammatory bowel disease.

Treatment and Prognosis. Treatment consists of antibiotic therapy with doxycycline or erythromycin. Sexual partners of infected persons should also be treated, even if they are asymptomatic (69). Longstanding cases may lead to abscess formation, strictures, and fistulae, further simulating features of idiopathic inflammatory bowel disease (78).

Granuloma Inguinale

Definition. *Granuloma inguinale* is caused by the gram-negative pleomorphic bacteria *Klebsiella* (formerly *Calymmatobacterium*) *granulomatis*. *Donovanosis* is a synonym.

Clinical Features. Granuloma inguinale is a progressive, indolent infection occurring widely throughout tropical and subtropical regions of the world, particularly Papua New Guinea, the Aboriginal community in Australia, and parts of South Africa, India, and Brazil (82,83). It typically affects the cutaneous and subcutaneous tissues of the genitals, perineum, and anus. Hematogenous spread to bone, joints, and visceral organs also occurs. Lymphadenopathy is uncommon.

Most infections are sexually transmitted, although other routes of infection include vaginal birth and fecal contamination. The typical presentation is a papule that develops into a painless ulcer that bleeds readily; ulcers are associated with extensive tissue necrosis and scarring (84). Infection with HIV tends to promote extensive tissue destruction and requires prolonged antibiotic therapy (85).

Pathogenesis. Study of *K. granulomatis* has been limited by the fact that the organism is very difficult to culture. The precise mechanism by which it infects cells and produces tissue damage remains unknown (86).

Gross Findings. Ulcers are indurated and erythematous, and bleed easily (84). Some have irregular, heaped-up edges, whereas others are

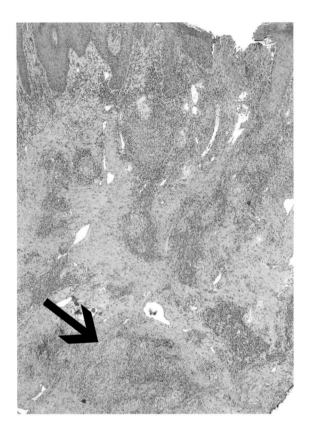

Figure 8-26

PERIANAL CROHN DISEASE

An ulcer is associated with dense lymphoplasmacytic infiltrates, lymphoid aggregates, and fibrosis. Scattered non-necrotic epithelioid granulomas are present (arrow).

necrotic. Extensive fibrosis and scarring are characteristic.

Microscopic Findings. The histologic features of granuloma inguinale are non-specific. Tissue samples contain a macrophage-rich inflammatory infiltrate with variable numbers of neutrophils and mononuclear cells (86). Macrophages contain Donovan bodies, or intracytoplasmic inclusion bodies, which represent encapsulated intracellular bacteria. Older lesions may consist predominantly of granulation tissue.

Slides can be prepared from swabbed lesions and stained with Giemsa, Wright, or Warthin-Starry stains to reveal the Donovan bodies (84). Culture is extremely difficult; PCR exists but is not widely available.

Differential Diagnosis. The differential diagnosis includes other ulcerative infections, including syphilis, HSV, and LGV. Distinction between these entities often relies on immunohistochemical demonstration of pathogens, cultures, and serologic studies.

Treatment and Prognosis. Treatment consists of antibiotic therapy with azithromycin, co-trimoxazole, or doxycycline until complete healing is achieved (84). Relapse may occur within 6 to 18 months despite apparent healing. Sclerotic lesions cause anal stenosis; extensive scarring of the inguinal region may result in lymphedema (87).

Crohn Disease

Definition. *Crohn disease* is an idiopathic immune-mediated disorder of the gastrointestinal tract and anus, often accompanied by other systemic manifestations.

Clinical Features. Patients develop a wide variety of anal manifestations, ranging from skin tags to severe fistulizing disease. Reported rates of anal involvement by Crohn disease range from 10 to 80 percent; variable reported rates reflect differences in definitional criteria for peri-anal disease, duration of follow-up, and composition of the patient population (88). Inflammatory anal disease is generally considered a marker of more severe luminal injury.

Gross Findings. The anal manifestations of Crohn disease are variable and include strictures, fissures, fistulae, ulcers, abscesses, and skin tags. Patients with disease of the lower gastrointestinal tract are more likely to have perianal manifestations than those with disease confined to the upper gastrointestinal tract (96).

Microscopic Findings. Histologic findings include non-necrotic epithelioid granulomas accompanied by chronic inflammation, lymphoid aggregates, fibrosis, and multinucleated giant cells (fig. 8-26) (90,91). Erosions, ulcers, and intense neutrophilic inflammation are commonly present in patients with active disease.

Differential Diagnosis. The differential diagnosis of Crohn disease is broad and includes entities such as hidradenitis suppurativa, sarcoidosis, and granulomatous infections (fig. 8-27). However, most patients with Crohn disease have inflammation of the gastrointestinal tract as well. The diagnosis may be particularly challenging if the patient does not have a known history of Crohn disease.

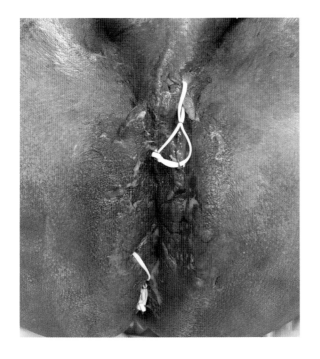

Figure 8-27

HIDRADENITIS SUPPURITIVA

Hidradenitis suppuritiva causes cutaneous disease that simulates anal Crohn disease. Multiple fistulous tracts are surrounded by induration. (Courtesy of Dr. K. Garrett, New York, NY.)

Treatment and Prognosis. Most patients with fistulizing Crohn disease are treated with TNF-α inhibitors. Patients have a slightly increased risk anal carcinoma, especially when they have longstanding or severe perianal disease with fistulae (92,93).

REFERENCES

1. Teerlink CC, Bernhisel R, Cannon-Albright LA, et al. A genealogical assessment of familial clustering of anorectal malformations. J Hum Genet 2018;63:1029-34.
2. Svenningsson A, Gunnarsdottir A, Wester T. Maternal risk factors and perinatal characteristics of anorectal malformations. J Pediatr Surg 2018;53:2183-8.
3. Hosokawa T, Yamada Y, Hsokawa M, et al. Ultrasound imaging of the anorectal malformation during the neonatal period: a comprehensive review. Jpn J Radiol 2018;36:581-91.
4. Xiao H, Huang R, Cui DX, Xiao P, Diao M, Li L. Histopathologic and immunohistochemical findings in congenital anorectal malformations. Medicine (Baltimore) 2018;97:e11675.
5. Tainaka T, Uchida H, Tanaka Y, et al. Long-term outcomes and complications after laparoscopic-assisted anorectoplasty vs. Posterior sagittal anorectoplasty for high- and intermediate-type anorectal malformation. Pediatr Surg Int 2018;34:1111-5.
6. Haydar M, Griepentrog K. Tailgut cyst: a case report and literature review. Int J Surg Case Rep 2015;10:166-8.
7. Prasad AR, Amin MB, Randolph TL, Lee CS, Ma CK. Retrorectal cystic hamartoma: report of 5 cases with malignancy arising in 2. Arch Pathol Lab Med 2000;124:725-9.
8. Shetty AS, Loch R, Yoo N, Mellnick V, Fowler K, Narra V. Imaging of tailgut cysts. Abdom Imaging 2015;40:2783-95.
9. Azatcam M, Altun E, Avci V. Histopathological diagnostic dilemma in retrorectal developmental cysts: report of a case and review of the literature. Turk Patoloji Derg 2018;34:175-8.
10. Bullard Dunn K. Retrorectal tumors. Surg Clin North Am 2010;90:163-71.

11. Cheng DW, Sekhon HK, Toutounjian R, Abbas MA. Heterotopic gastric mucosa of the anus associated with anal ulcer. Tech Coloproctol 2012;16:167-8.

12. Mannan A, Vieth M, Khararjian A, et al. The outlet patch: gastric heterotopia of the colorectum and anus. Histopathology 2018;73:220-9.

13. Steele SR, Mullenix PS, Martin MJ, et al. Heterotopic gastric mucosa of the anus: a case report and review of the literature. Am Surg 2004;70:715-9.

14. Tekin K, Sungurtekin U, Aytekin FO, et al. Ectopic prostatic tissue of the anal canal presenting with rectal bleeding: report of a case. Dis Colon Rectum 2002;45:979-80.

15. Kazakov DV, Spagnolo DV, Stewart CJ, et al. Fibroadenoma and phyllodes tumors of anogenital mammary-like glands: a series of 13 neoplasms in 12 cases, including mammary-type juvenile fibroadenoma, fibroadenoma with lactation changes, and neurofibromatosis-associated pseudoangiomatous stromal hyperplasia with multinucleated giant cells. Am J Surg Pathol 2010;34:95-103.

16. Iacopini F, Gotoda T, Elisei W, et al. Heterotopic gastric mucosa in the anus and rectum: first case report of endoscopic submucosal dissection and systematic review. Gastroenterol Rep (Oxf) 2016;4:196-205.

17. Lohsiriwat V. Hemorrhoids: from basic pathophysiology to clinical management. World J Gastroenterol 2012;18:2009-17.

18. Madoff RD, Fleshman JW, Clinical Practice Committee, American Gastroenterological Association. American gastroenterological association technical review on the diagnosis and treatment of hemorrhoids. Gastroenterology 2004;126:1463-73.

19. Sneider EB, Maykel JA. Diagnosis and management of symptomatic hemorrhoids. Surg Clin North Am 2010;90:17-32.

20. Ganz RA. The evaluation and treatment of hemorrhoids: a guide for the gastroenterologist. Clin Gastroenterol Hepatol 2013;11:593-603.

21. Daniel F, Trak-Smayra V, Ziade N. A prolapsing pile revealing anal squamous cell carcinoma. Am J Gastroenterol 2016;111:454.

22. Lemarchand N, Tanne F, Aubert M, et al. Is routine pathologic evaluation of hemorrhoidectomy specimens necessary? Gastroenterol Clin Biol 2004;28:659-61.

23. Meguerditchian AN, Meterissian SH, Dunn KB. Anorectal melanoma: diagnosis and treatment. Dis Colon Rectum 2011;54:638-44.

24. Val-Bernal JF, Mayorga M, Val D. Incidental melanocytic nevi in hemorrhoidectomy specimens. Am J Dermatopathol 2016;38:278-82.

25. Jamshidi R. Anorectal complaints: hemorrhoids, fissures, abscesses, fistulae. Clin Colon Rectal Surg 2018;31:117-20.

26. Madoff RD, Fleshman JW. AGA technical review on the diagnosis and care of patients with anal fissure. Gastroenterology 2003;124:235-45.

27. Simpson JA, Banerjea A, Scholefield, JH. Management of anal fistula. BMJ 2012;345:e6705.

28. Gopal DV. Diseases of the rectum and anus: a clinical approach to common disorders. Clin Cornerstone 2002;4:34-48.

29. Marks CG, Ritchie JK. Anal fistulas at St Mark's Hospital. Br J Surg 1977;64:84-91.

30. Shwaartz C, Munger JA, Deliz JR, et al. Fistula-associated anorectal cancer in the setting of crohn's disease. Dis Colon Rectum 2016;59:1168-73.

31. Panes J, Rimola J. Perianal fistulizing Crohn's disease: pathogenesis, diagnosis and therapy. Nat Rev Gastroenterol Hepatol 2017;14:652-64.

32. Tabry H, Farrands PA. Update on anal fistulae: surgical perspectives for the gastroenterologist. Can J Gastroenterol 2011;25:675-80.

33. Wisniewski A, Flejou JF, Siproudhis L, Abramowitz L, Svrcek M, Beaugerie L. Anal neoplasia in inflammatory bowel disease: classification proposal, epidemiology, carcinogenesis, and risk management perspectives. J Crohns Colitis 2017;11:1011-8.

34. Gupta PJ. Hypertrophied anal papillae and fibrous anal polyps, should they be removed during anal fissure surgery? World J Gastroenterol 2004;10:2412-4.

35. Beer TW, Carr NJ. Fibroepithelial polyps of the anus with epithelial vacuolation. Am J Surg Pathol 1999;23:488-89.

36. Groisman GM, Polak-Charcon S. Fibroepithelial polyps of the anus: a histologic, immunohistochemical, and ultrastructural study, including comparison with the normal anal subepithelial layer. Am J Surg Pathol 1998;22:70-6.

37. Sakai Y, Matsukuma S. CD34+ stromal cells and hyalinized vascular changes in the anal fibroepithelial polyps. Histopathology 2002;41:230-5.

38. Abid S, Khawaja A, Bhimani SA, Ahmad Z, Hamid S, Jafri W. The clinical, endoscopic and histological spectrum of the solitary rectal ulcer syndrome: a single-center experience of 116 cases. BMC Gastroenterol 2012;12:72.

39. Chetty R, Bhathal PS, Slavin JL. Prolapse-induced inflammatory polyps of the colorectum and anal transitional zone. Histopathology 1993;23:63-7.

40. Saul SH. Inflammatory cloacogenic polyp: relationship to solitary rectal ulcer syndrome/mucosal prolapse and other bowel disorders. Hum Pathol 1987;18:1120-5.

41. Poon KK, Mills S, Booth IW, Murphy MS. Inflammatory cloacogenic polyp: an unrecognized cause of hematochezia and tenesmus in childhood. J Pediatr 1997;130:327-9.

42. Parfitt JR, Shepherd NA. Polypoid mucosal prolapse complicating low rectal adenomas: beware the inflammatory cloacogenic polyp! Histopathology 2008;53:91-6.

43. Echenique I, Phillips BR. Anal warts and anal intradermal neoplasia. Clin Colon Rectal Surg 2011;24:31-8.

44. Daling JR, Madeleine MM, Johnson LG, et al. Human papillomavirus, smoking, and sexual practices in the etiology of anal cancer. Cancer 2004;101:270-80.

45. Nelson RA, Levine AM, Bernstein L, Smith DD, Lai LL. Changing patterns of anal canal carcinoma in the United States. J Clin Oncol 2013;31:1569-75.

46. Stier EA, Sebring MC, Mendez AE, Ba FS, Trimble DD, Chiao EY. Prevalence of anal human papillomavirus infection and anal HPV-related disorders in women: a systematic review. Am J Obstet Gynecol 2015;213:278-309.

47. Smyczek P, Singh AE, Romanowski B. Anal intraepithelial neoplasia: review and recommendations for screening and management. Int J STD AIDS 2013;24:843-51.

48. Handsfield HH. Clinical presentation and natural course of anogenital warts. Am J Med 1997;102:16-20.

49. Darragh TM, Colgan TJ, Cox JT, et al. The lower anogenital squamous terminology standardization project for HPV-associated lesions: background and consensus recommendations from the College of American Pathologists and the American Society for Colposcopy and Cervical Pathology. Arch Pathol Lab Med 2012;136:1266-97.

50. Maniar KP, Nayar R. HPV-related squamous neoplasia of the lower anogenital tract: an update and review of recent guidelines. Adv Anat Pathol 2014;21:341-58.

51. Tamalet C, Obry-Roguet V, Ressiot E, Bregigeon S, Del Grande J, Poizot-Martin I. Distribution of human papillomavirus genotypes, assessment of HPV 16 and 18 viral load and anal related lesions in HIV positive patients: a cross-sectional analysis. J Med Virol 2014;86:419-25.

52. Wong AK, Chan RC, Aggarwal N, Singh MK, Nichols WS, Bose S. Human papillomavirus genotypes in anal intraepithelial neoplasia and anal carcinoma as detected in tissue biopsies. Mod Pathol 2010;23:144-50.

53. Bean SM, Eltoum I, Horton DK, Whitlow L, Chhieng DC. Immunohistochemical expression of p16 and Ki-67 correlates with degree of anal intraepithelial neoplasia. Am J Surg Pathol 2007;31:555-61.

54. Pirog EC, Quint KD, Yantiss RK. P16/CDKN2A and Ki-67 enhance the detection of anal intraepithelial neoplasia and condyloma and correlate with human papillomavirus detection by polymerase chain reaction. Am J Surg Pathol 2010;34:1449-55.

55. Samama B, Lipsker D, Boehm N. P16 expression in relation to human papillomavirus in anogenital lesions. Hum Pathol 2006;37:513-9.

56. Lacey CJ, Woodhall SC, Wikstrom A, Ross J. 2012 European guideline for the management of anogenital warts. J Eur Acad Dermatol Venereol 2013;27:e263-70.

57. Leszczyszyn J, Lebski I, Lysenko L, Hirnle L, Gerber H. Anal warts (condylomata acuminata)—current issues and treatment modalities. Adv Clin Exp Med 2014;23:307-11.

58. Roberts JR, Siekas LL, Kaz AM. Anal intraepithelial neoplasia: a review of diagnosis and management. World J Gastrointest Oncol 2017;9:50-61.

59. Rompalo AM. Diagnosis and treatment of sexually acquired proctitis and proctocolitis: an update. Clin Infect Dis 1999;28(Suppl 1):S84-90.

60. Goodell SE, Quinn TC, Mkrtichian E, Schuffler MD, Holmes KK, Corey L. Herpes simplex virus proctitis in homosexual men. Clinical, sigmoidoscopic, and histopathological features. N Engl J Med 1983;308:868-71.

61. LeGoff J, Pere H, Belec L. Diagnosis of genital herpes simplex virus infection in the clinical laboratory. Virol J 2014;11:83.

62. Steiner I, Kennedy PG, Pachner AR. The neurotropic herpes viruses: herpes simplex and varicella-zoster. Lancet Neurol 2007;6:1015-28.

63. You DM, Johnson MD. Cytomegalovirus infection and the gastrointestinal tract. Curr Gastroenterol Rep 2012;14:334-42.

64. Winter ST. Anorectal ulcer in chicker pox. Br Med J 1955;1:1070-1.

65. Chen X, Anstey AV, Bugert JJ. Molluscum contagiosum virus infection. Lancet Infect Dis 2013;13:877-88.

66. Mindel A, Tovey SJ, Timmins DJ, Williams P. Primary and secondary syphilis, 20 years' experience. 2. Clinical features. Genitourin Med 1989;65:1-3.

67. Marcus U, Bremer V, Hamouda O, et al. Understanding recent increases in the incidence of sexually transmitted infections in men having sex with men: changes in risk behavior from risk avoidance to risk reduction. Sex Transm Dis 2006;33:11-7.

68. Hamlyn E, Taylor C. Sexually transmitted proctitis. Postgrad Med J 2006;82:733-6.

69. Morshed MG, Singh AE. Recent trends in the serologic diagnosis of syphilis. Clin Vaccine Immunol 2015;22:137-47.

70. Peeling RW, Mabey D, Kamb ML, Chen XS, Radolf JD, Benzaken AS. Syphilis. Nat Rev Dis Primers 2017;3:17073.

71. Tampa M, Sarbu I, Matei C, Benea V, Georgescu SR. Brief history of syphilis. J Med Life 2014;7:4-10.

72. Arnold CA, Limketkai BN, Illei PB, Montgomery E, Voltaggio L. Syphilitic and lymphogranuloma venereum (LGV) proctocolitis: clues to a frequently missed diagnosis. Am J Surg Pathol 2013;37:38-46.

73. Gopal P, Shah RB. Primary anal canal syphilis in men: the clinicopathologic spectrum of an easily overlooked diagnosis. Arch Pathol Lab Med 2015;139:1156-60.

74. Tayal S, Shaban F, Dasgupta K, Tabaqchali MA. A case of syphilitic anal condylomata lata mimicking malignancy. Int J Surg Case Rep 2015;17:69-71.

75. Esteve M, Salas A, Fernandez-Banares F, et al. Intestinal spirochetosis and chronic watery diarrhea: clinical and histological response to treatment and long-term follow up. J Gastroenterol Hepatol 2006;21:1326-33.

76. Bruins FG, van Deudekom FJ, de Vries HJ. Syphilitic condylomata lata mimicking anogenital warts. BMJ 2015;350:h1259.

77. Hoentjen F, Rubin DT. Infectious proctitis: when to suspect it is not inflammatory bowel disease. Dig Dis Sci 2012;57:269-73.

78. de Vrieze NH, van Rooijen M, Schim van der Loeff MF, de Vries HJ. Anorectal and inguinal lymphogranuloma venereum among men who have sex with men in amsterdam, the netherlands: trends over time, symptomatology and concurrent infections. Sex Transm Infect 2013;89:548-52.

79. Land JA, Evers JL. Chlamydia infection and subfertility. Best Pract Res Clin Obstet Gynaecol 2002;16:901-12.

80. Stoner BP, Cohen SE. Lymphogranuloma venereum 2015: clinical presentation, diagnosis, and treatment. Clin Infect Dis 2015;61(Suppl 8):S865-73.

81. de la Monte SM, Hutchins GM. Follicular proctocolitis and neuromatous hyperplasia with lymphogranuloma venereum. Hum Pathol 1985;16:1025-32.

82. O'Farrell N, Moi, H, Board, IWESgE. European guideline for the management of donovanosis, 2010. Int J STD AIDS 2010;21:609-10.

83. Soni S, Srirajaskanthan R, Lucas SB, Alexander S, Wong T, White JA. Lymphogranuloma venereum proctitis masquerading as inflammatory bowel disease in 12 homosexual men. Aliment Pharmacol Ther 2010;32:59-65.

84. O'Farrell N. Donovanosis. Sex Transm Infect 2002;78:452-7.

85. Basta-Juzbasic A, Ceovic R. Chancroid, lymphogranuloma venereum, granuloma inguinale, genital herpes simplex infection, and molluscum contagiosum. Clin Dermatol 2014;32:290-8.

86. Kharsany AB, Hoosen AA, Naicker T, Kiepiela P, Sturm AW. Ultrastructure of calymmatobacterium granulomatis: comparison of culture with tissue biopsy specimens. J Med Microbiol 1998;47:1069-73.

87. Velho PE, Souza EM, Belda Junior W. Donovanosis. Braz J Infect Dis 2008;12:521-5.

88. Eglinton TW, Barclay ML, Gearry RB, Frizelle FA. The spectrum of perianal Crohn's disease in a population-based cohort. Dis Colon Rectum 2012;55:773-7.

89. Kanaan Z, Ahmad S, Bilchuk N, Vahrenhold C, Pan J, Galandiuk S. Perianal Crohn's disease: Predictive factors and genotype-phenotype correlations. Dig Surg 2012;29:107-14.

90. Taylor BA, Williams GT, Hughes LE, Rhodes J. The histology of anal skin tags in Crohn's disease: an aid to confirmation of the diagnosis. Int J Colorectal Dis 1989;4:197-9.

91. Hernandez Z, Almeida P, Borrego L, Hernandez J. Infiltrated perianal plaques. Perianal crohn's disease. Int J Dermatol 2013;52:23-4.

92. Frisch M, Johansen C. Anal carcinoma in inflammatory bowel disease. Br J Cancer 2000;83:89-90.

93. Sjodahl RI, Myrelid P, Soderholm JD. Anal and rectal cancer in Crohn's disease. Colorectal Dis 2003;5:490-5.

Index*

*In a series of numbers, those in boldface indicate the main discussion of the entity.